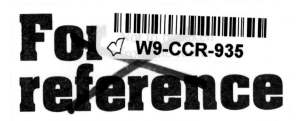

ENCYCLOPEDIA OF
DISABILITY

ENCYCLOPEDIA OF DISABILITY

A History in Primary Source Documents

VOLUME EDITORS

SHARON L. SNYDER

University of Illinois at Chicago

DAVID T. MITCHELL

University of Illinois at Chicago

ILLUSTRATIONS EDITOR

SHARON L. SNYDER

GENERAL EDITOR
GARY L. ALBRECHT
University of Illinois at Chicago

VOLUME V

A SAGE Reference Publication

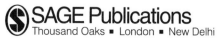

SAGE Publications
Thousand Oaks ▪ London ▪ New Delhi

Tim Lowly. *Beacon: Bless the Bastard.* 1991. 48" by 60." Tempera on panel. Reprinted by generous permission of the artist.

For information:

 Sage Publications, Inc.
2455 Teller Road
Thousand Oaks, California 91320
E-mail: order@sagepub.com

Sage Publications Ltd.
1 Oliver's Yard
55 City Road
London EC1Y 1SP
United Kingdom

Sage Publications India Pvt. Ltd.
B-42, Panchsheel Enclave
Post Box 4109
New Delhi 110 017 India

Printed in the United States of America

Library of Congress Cataloging-in-Publication Data

Encyclopedia of disability / general editor, Gary L. Albrecht.
     p. cm.
Includes bibliographical references and index.
ISBN 0–7619–2565–1 (cloth)
   1. People with disabilities—Encyclopedias. 2. Sociology of disability—Encyclopedias.
3. Disability studies—Encyclopedias. I. Albrecht, Gary L.
HV1568.E528 2006
362.4′03—dc22   2005018301

This book is printed on acid-free paper.

05   06   07   10 9   8   7   6   5   4   3   2   1

Publisher:	Rolf A. Janke
Developmental Editor:	Sara Tauber
Project Editor:	Diana E. Axelsen
Copy Editor:	Kate Peterson, Judy Selhorst, Gillian Dickens, Rachel Hile Bassett
Typesetter:	C&M Digitals (P) Ltd.
Proofreader:	Colleen Brennan
Indexer:	Mary Mortensen
Cover Designer:	Michelle Lee Kenny

CONTENTS

Part One: Origins of Disability

The Ancient World

The Ancient World: Sumeria/Mesopotamia

The Ancient World: South Asia

The Bible

Hebrew Bible: The Old Testament

Apocrypha

New Testament: Christian Scriptures

Middle Ages

Part Two: Modernity and Normalization

1500–1800

1800–1945

Part Three: Culture and Resistance

1946–present

LIST OF ILLUSTRATIONS

Part One: Origins of Disability

The Ancient World

The Bible

The Middle Ages

Part Two: Modernity and Normalization

1500–1800

1800–1945

Part Three: Culture and Resistance

(1946-present)

LIST OF ENTRIES

Reader's Guide

The Reader's Guide is provided to help readers locate entries and primary sources by topical category. It classifies the A–Z entries (Volumes I–IV) and primary source documents (Volume V) into twenty-five categories: Accessibility, Arts, Biographies, Children and Infants, Deafness and Deaf Culture, Disability Studies, Economics and Employment, Education, Ethical Issues, Experience of Disability, Health and Medicine, Health Care, History of Disability, Information Technology, Language of Disability, Law and Social Policy, Models, Organizations, Politics, Rehabilitation, Rehabilitative Engineering and Assistive Technology, Religion, Science, Sports, and Therapies. Some entries and documents may appear in more than one category.

Page numbers for primary source documents and illustrations can be found in the Table of Contents and List of Illustrations for Volume V, which appear in the front matter of each volume, and in the index.

ACCESSIBILITY

Accessibility
Accessibility Codes and Standards
Accessible Internet
Air Carrier Access
Computer Software Accessibility
Public Transportation
Sexual Access
Visitability
Worksite Modification

ARTS

Aesthetics
Art Therapy
Autobiography
Cartooning
Dance
Disability Arts
Documentary Film
Drama and Performance
Film
Kyōgen Comedy
Literature, Folly

Moscow Theater of Mime and Gesture
Music
Music and Blindness
National Theatre of the Deaf (United States)
Nonti Natakam (Tamil Cripple Drama)
Novel, The
Poetry
Representations of Disability, History of
Sign Poetry
Television

Readings in Volume V

Addison, Joseph, from *The Spectator*
Anderson, Sherwood, from *Winesburg, Ohio*
Barbauld, Anna Laeticia, from "An Inquiry into Those Types of Distress That Excite Agreeable Sensations"
Bradstreet, Anne, "The Author to Her Book"
Brontë, Charlotte, from *Jane Eyre*
Brooks, Gwendolyn, from *A Street in Bronzeville*
Byron, Lord, from *The Deformed Transformed*
Clay, Sally, "People Who"
Coleridge, Samuel Taylor, from "Dejection: An Ode"
Conrad, Joseph, from *The Secret Agent*
Crane, Stephen, from *The Monster*

BIOGRAPHIES

Readings in Volume V

CHILDREN AND INFANTS

Children with Disabilities, Rights of
Feral Children
Infant Stimulation Programs
Infanticide
Maternal Imagination
Parental Advocacy
Parental Narratives
Pediatric Rehabilitation
Poster Child
Prematurity

Readings in Volume V

Dickens, Charles, from *A Christmas Carol*
Dodd, William, from *A Narrative of William Dodd: Factory Cripple*
Goddard, Henry Herbert, "The Improvability of Feeble-Minded Children"
Kelley, Florence, "Injurious Employments"
Korean Child Welfare Committee, from *Handicapped Children's Survey Report*
Kuroyanagi, Tetsuko, *Totto-chan: The Little Girl at the Window*
Meltzer, Ewald, *Survey to German Parents of 162 Disabled Children*
Nation, Carry A., from *The Use and Need of the Life of Carry A. Nation*
Smart, Isabelle Thompson, from *Studies in the Relation of Physical Inability and Mental Deficiency to the Body Social*
Spyri, Johanna, *Heidi*
Story of Enkidu (Wolf Child)

DEAFNESS AND DEAF CULTURE

Audism
Deaf, History of the
Deaf Culture
Deaf People at the Ottoman Court
Deaf People in African Histories
Deafblindedness
Deafness, Milan Congress of 1880 on
Deafness, on Martha's Vineyard
Hearing Impairment
Moscow Theater of Mime and Gesture
National Theatre of the Deaf (United States)
Oralism
Sign Language
Sign Language Interpretation
Sign Poetry

Readings in Volume V

Al-Jahiz, *The Book of Animals, IV*
Baudier, Michel, on the Ottoman Empire
Bobovi's Description of the Ottoman Court
Bon, Ottaviano, Description of the Ottoman Court
Busbecq on the Murder of Mustapha
Dallam, Thomas, *Account of an Organ Carryed to the Grand Seignor*
Deaf and Deaf-Mute Servants in the Sultan's Court
Flournoy, John J., to William Turner, "A Mighty Change"
"Position of the Students, Faculty and Staff of Gallaudet University"
Rycaut, Sir Paul, from *The History of the Present State of the Ottoman Empire*
Sandys, George, from *A Relation of a Journey . . .*

DISABILITY STUDIES

Alienation
Anthropology
Attitudes
Body, Theories of
Canadian Centre on Disability Studies
Cultural Context of Disability
Disability Studies
Disability Studies: Australia
Disability Surveys
Epidemiology
Explanatory Legitimacy Theory
Feminism
Humanities
Pedagogy and Curriculum Design
Queer/Disability Studies
Research
Sociology
Translating Theory and Research into Practice

Readings in Volume V

The Hunter College Disability Studies Project, "Definition of Disability Studies"

ECONOMICS AND EMPLOYMENT

Advertising
Affirmative Businesses
Begging

Substitute Decision Making
Values

Readings in Volume V

Not Dead Yet
Nussbaum, Susan, *Parade*
Talbot, Margaret, "The Executioner's I.Q. Test"

EXPERIENCE OF DISABILITY

Ableism
Accidents
Activities of Daily Living (ADLs)
Aging
Aging, International
Capacity Building
Chronically Sick and Disabled Persons Act of 1970
   (United Kingdom)
Communication
Community Living and Group Homes
Consumer Control
Consumer Satisfaction
Decision Making
Deformity
Developing World
Disability Culture
Disability in Contemporary Africa
Disability Management
Disability Pride
Disabled Veterans
Empowerment and Emancipation
Experience
Family
Family, International
Gender
Gender, International
Geography and Disability
Hand and Arm Manipulation
Home Support
Identity
Inclusion and Exclusion
Independent Living
Inspiration
Institutionalization and Segregation
Invalid Women
IQ
Isolation
Journalism

Latino Health
Leadership
Oppression
Parenting
Participation
Passing
Peer Support
Personal Assistance and Direct Payment
Personal Care Attendants
Public Stripping
Quality of Life
Race and Ethnicity
Racism
Rape
Recreation
Representations of Disability, Social
Self-Sufficiency
Sex Industry, International
Sexuality
Siblings of People with Disabilities
Sick Role
Social Networks
Social Support
Stigma
Stigma, International
Stress
Suicide
Supported Services
Telethons
Tokenism
Transgression
Travel
Universalism
Violence
Visibility and Invisibility
Xenodisability

Experience in Specific Countries

Disability in Contemporary Australia
Disability in Contemporary China
Disability in Contemporary India
Experience of Disability: Brazil
Experience of Disability: China
Experience of Disability: Colombia
Experience of Disability: Costa Rica
Experience of Disability: India
Experience of Disability: Ireland
Experience of Disability: Japan
Experience of Disability: New Zealand

HEALTH AND MEDICINE

Conditions, Mental

Readings in Volume V

Conditions, Physical

Readings in Volume V

HEALTH CARE

HISTORY OF DISABILITY

INFORMATION TECHNOLOGY

LANGUAGE OF DISABILITY

REHABILITATIVE ENGINEERING AND ASSISTIVE TECHNOLOGY

RELIGION

The Son of David
Taoist Scripture: Chuang-Tzu
Tobit's Blindness
The Uruk Incantation
Westminster Larger Catechism
The Zend-Avesta

SCIENCE

Biological Determinism
Evolutionary Theory
Genetics
Molecular, Cellular, and Tissue Engineering
Mutation Theory

Readings in Volume V

Darwin, Charles, from *The Descent of Man*
Spencer, Herbert, *Social Statics or Order*

SPORTS

Classification in Paralympic Sport
Doping in Paralympic Sport
Paralympics
Sports and Disability
Sydney Paralympics

THERAPIES

Antipsychiatry Movement
Art Therapy
Aversive Therapies
Behavior Therapy
Clever Hans
Complementary and Alternative Medicine
Discredited Therapies

Early Childhood Intervention
Exercise and Physical Activity
Gene Therapy
Group Therapy
Mindfulness Meditation
Neuropsychiatry
Neuropsychology
Orthopedics
Physical Activity
Physical Therapy
Psychiatry
Psychology
Rehabilitation Psychology
Sex Therapy
Social Work

Readings in Volume V

Chamberlin, Judi, from "Confessions of a
    Noncompliant Patient"
Chamberlin, Judi, from *On Our Own: Patient-
    Controlled Alternatives to the Mental Health
    System*
Dendron News
Fernald, Walter, from *The History of the Treatment
    of the Feeble-Minded*
Foucault, Michel, from *The Birth of the Clinic*
Goffman, Erving, from *Asylums: Essays on the
    Social Situation of Mental Patients and Other
    Inmates*
Laing, R. D., from *The Politics of Experience*
"N-P": The Case of Neuropsychiatric Disability
Séguin, Edouard Onesimus, *Idiocy: And Its
    Treatment by the Physiological Method*
Szasz, Thomas, from *The Myth of Mental Illness*
Zinman, Sally, Howie T. Harp, and Su Budd, from
    *Reaching Across: Mental Health Clients Helping
    Each Other*

ILLUSTRATIONS: A NOTE TO THE READER

The illustrations in Volume V offer the reader examples of how disability has been viewed in a variety of cultures across thousands of years, from ancient Egypt and medieval Europe to nineteenth-century America and twenty-first-century Japan. The visual elements in Volume V are not intended to illustrate specific documents. Instead, they invite the reader to explore the history of disability through images of the myriad ways in which disability has been viewed by artists and politicians, religious leaders and movie directors, and contemporary disability rights activists from Mumbai to Chicago.

This visual history of disability complements both the documentary history presented through primary sources in Volume V and the many entries in Volumes I through IV that deal with the history of disability throughout the world. We encourage you to use these images to enlarge your understanding of how men and women over the centuries have experienced and conceptualized the complex phenomenon of disability and its meaning for individuals and cultures.

TOWARD A HISTORY OF DISABILITY IN PRIMARY SOURCES

Throughout history, disability has provided opportunities for the display of bodily aberration. This exhibitionistic tendency often seeks to cater to prurient human interests about embodied differences while also referencing physical and cognitive variations as a metaphor for human calamity. Whether this demand to conceptualize disability involves the revision of physical space, communication modes, the provision of care, or bodily compensation, the need to interpret difference among human communities remains relatively consistent. It is the one possible "universal" claim that the materials included in this volume demonstrate. The uniqueness of bodies and minds causes us to encounter the degree to which the made-world proves exclusionary. For instance, the ancient Greek temple at Delphi once had a series of ramped slopes visitors traversed to arrive at the oracle. Only later did the Romans insert marble stairs, which effectively cut off access to the hallowed site for many. Likewise, some two millennia later, the disabled physicist Stephen Hawking's visit to India prompted the government to construct a variety of ramps and other accommodations so that he could visit various historic sites. This instant access (however flawed, in that bathrooms remained inaccessible, and usable transportation continued to be nonexistent) had previously been resisted for years, despite Indian disabled peoples' active protests and requests. Our external and attitudinal environments require alteration, because they are so often organized around invented obstacles. Our environments are created to meet inflexible standards—they presume a set of common bodily capacities, and those who don't conform find themselves left out.

While this point may seem obvious, it has a rather serious set of consequences for disabled people. As populations experience their bodies as "mis-fit" for routine participation, they not only find themselves excluded but also experience constant scrutiny regarding their insufficiencies. Human communities have found it much easier to contemplate the inadequacies of bodies rather than the inadequacies of human-made spaces. Thus, disability arrives at our own moment as one of the most thought-about differences in history. This history proves both rich and disturbing. As one traces out the history of disabled peoples, a seemingly inevitable encounter with ways of conceptualizing differences of all kinds comes to the forefront. Whether we read prophecies of ancient Sumer distilled from the analysis of disabled fetuses; the origin stories of Shinto, Native American, and African communities, which often turn on warnings about the devaluation of disabled bodies; the miraculous cure missions of religious and secular prophets' scientifically backed efforts to rid nations of their disabled populations; the establishment of utopian communities both with and without disabled bodies; spaces of cultural segregation transformed into creative communities of alternative embodiment; or the ironic reversals of disability rights movements holding up mirrors to expose various degrading cultural contexts, disability perseveres as a site of difference that we cannot live without. One might say that disabled peoples' bodies, therefore, provide the impetus to contemplate the inadequacies of places, peoples, and beliefs. The common practice of exhibiting disabled people as fools, oddities, marvels, and misfits brings these tensions forth. However, this exhibitionistic tendency among many cultures becomes a matter of grave concern for those designated as "deviant" or "deficient."

This volume compiles transhistorical and transcultural materials pertinent to a consideration of disabled people's lives. We intend it as a starting point for the analysis of disability as a difference of great social import. Despite the enormity of the task, even an encyclopedic undertaking of this scale can be offered in only the most cursory way. Consequently, we do not claim to provide an exhaustive collection of disability history to any extent. However, the materials gathered here seek to shore up two insufficiencies in our current disability knowledge base: (a) the state of the field of disability history has only recently generated significant scholarly attention; and (b) this first effort at compiling primary source materials on disability unveils that the history of human differences has been relegated to the dustbin of human concerns. Often like the bodies that they describe, discussions of disabled people (under any name) have been erased from historical records. Without an adequate interpretive lens with which to approach the historical situation of disability, individual and collective experiences remain only vaguely comprehended. Not only do the materials gathered herein represent fragments of fragments of our current disability knowledge base (in fact, we have assembled the bulk of material in Volume V as brief excerpts from longer works), these materials demonstrate the degree to which our thinking about the history of embodied differences has only begun.

There are few recognized traditions of discussion about disability by disabled people, for instance—although this volume identifies disabled perspectives operating in every cultural and historical moment. Nor does this volume's overrepresentation of U.S. and European sources provide a reliable glimpse into those cultural locations beyond the "West." We have tried to draw from an international archive of materials, but ultimately, even these materials provide little more than glimpses of Western thinkers contemplating disability in cultures markedly alien to their own sensibilities. Thus, the "non-Western" sources here prove interesting largely to the extent that they help capture a portrait of displaced Westerners contemplating disability as a metaphor for their own feelings of displacement. The culturally alienated spend a significant amount of time imposing their own understanding of bodily estrangement upon those who may or may not experience their lives in this manner. While entries can be found from distinctive cultural traditions such as Africa, the Middle East, Korea, and Australia, they show disability as a continuing topic of concern for English-speaking subjects. Additionally, they also underscore how many observers actively look for disability in other cultures

as a barometer of insufficient "modernity" when contrasted with the viewer's home culture.

In this volume, we use the term *disability* to serve as a retrospective label across periods that did not use the designation to group or describe those classified as exceptionally variant. Consequently, the identification of disability history is a self-consciously undertaken task, one that proves thoroughly retrospective and, therefore, imposed to a degree from our own historical moment. For our purposes, disability provides a nodal point from which to gather experiences that share little in common beyond a stigmatized existence based on perceived biologically based differences. Readers will find the language of other historical moments referencing bodies as monstrous, crippled, lame, mute, deaf and dumb, lunatic, and so on. But the volume endeavors to bring these referencing strategies together to construct a shared history, a history of those identified as exceptionally different because of real or perceived incapacities of some major life function. As in the Americans with Disabilities Act (1990), we emphasize "perceived" differences, because the language of human embodiment occurs fully within the domain of representation.

One common point that we'd like this work to demonstrate, then, is the contingent status of "deviance." Given that differences worthy of special social recognition change radically from era to era (in fact, one could potentially use these shifts to reliably mark historical periods themselves), disability cannot be said to *exist*. Differences worthy of note in any period come fully mediated by language and the particularity of cultural investments. The clarity behind identifications of human variance proves consistently unstable, and what passes for a devalued difference in one period often loses import in another. Like bodies, language tends to break down in its goal of describing difference in a reliable, universal, and transhistorical manner. This lack of a definitional heart to disability defines bodies that *differ* from each other as much as they are believed to depart from the norms. As norms shift, so do expressions of embodiment qualifying as exceptional.

Portrayals of disability often situate subjects as those to be viewed, consumed, gazed upon, and gawked at by others secure in their positions of normalcy. The contemplation of disability—the meaning-making acts spawned by human differences—situates observers with the power to evaluate one variation as acceptable and another as pathological. In doing so, the definers solidify their own membership among the norms as an effect of designating others as deficient. Encounters with variation arrive replete with evaluative notions of deficiency. To some extent, we have lost even the medieval ability to marvel at the range of variations that exist or to experience awe at the adaptive capacities of all human beings in general. When we delve into histories of disability, it is difficult not to be struck by the degree to which disabled lives have been explained by others. The voices of disabled people—particularly in nonartistic media—are largely absent in the various proclamations of medicine, policy, law, philosophy, and so forth. As an effort to compensate for this rhetorical insufficiency, we have constructed this volume as a dialectic between artistic and other explanatory forms. Not that the arts themselves do not falter in this arena, but they represent a historical conversation that sometimes yields significant disabled subjectivities.

Whereas artists and literary authors may occupy their own marginalized societal roles, their portrayal of disabled people can often be mined for unexpected insights. For instance, in Raphael's last painting, *The Transfiguration* (1517–1520), the "lunatic boy" in the lower right corner is presented as an object of spectacle. Those who gaze, gesture, and point would mark his extreme difference from their own bodies. His awkwardly twisting body, perhaps rigid from hypertonia, becomes an opportunity to solidify the assembled audience's sense of self-possession. Further, those of us examining the painting participate in a parallel viewing situation; our own autonomy may be confirmed as participants in the witnessing of the "lunatic boy" as Other. His spastic body separates him from the flowing anonymity of the bodies of the gazers. Yet, perhaps ironically, Raphael makes their replicated physical uniformity blend each into the other while the lunatic body remains unintegrated. With this portrayal, Raphael provides a window onto a significant swath of disability history. The disabled individual is infantilized and patronized in her or his portrayal; the different body is first *set off* from the majority and then *set out* as visual fodder for consumption. The excessiveness of this objectifying process becomes so noticeable that the reader of this volume may find him- or herself struck by the sheer repetition of the situation—whether it occurs in the town square, on the freak show stage, in televisual disease-of-the-week dramas, or in the privacy of the medical office.

Yet, the patronization of disabled subjects forms only one base upon which the triangular foundation of disability rests. If we return to the Raphael painting momentarily, we may also realize the reluctance—even

terror—of those seeking an intervention on the lunatic boy's behalf. If we imagine the figure frozen by the painter in the midst of a seizure that the gathered crowd cannot adequately restrain, then the scene transforms from one of passivity into an odd power exercised. While the application of a treatment—in this case the disciples' contemplation of miraculous cure once Christ has left them alone—seeks to domesticate and manage the contorting body before them, the effort becomes an operation on the theater of the lunatic boy's presumed grotesquerie. His difference must be mastered to alleviate his "suffering" perhaps, but the real struggle resides in the gathered crowd's discomfort. The lunatic boy's loss of control—bound up in the representation of seizure, spasticity, and temporary immobilization—seems orchestrated from elsewhere, perhaps through some more metaphysical line of communication. *The Transfiguration* leaves those in the lower half of the painting encumbered by the material scene of disability, while the boy alone gestures toward the transfiguration taking place in the top half of the painting. His difference provides a vantage point that others fail to realize—without him, the scene above would go unremarked.

An ironic reversal has occurred, and disability, treated as misfortune by those around the boy, proves unexpectedly revelatory. Situating disability at this important nexus—as an object of scrutiny, as the power of the stigmatized, and as alternative vision—shows us that human variation elicits strong (and sometimes opposing) sensations. Some viewers stare, while others look away with expressions of repulsion or, at best, consternation. But the visceral nature of responses to the disabled body becomes a vantage point from which we may view the world anew. As the religious and medical communities become fixated on the material "problem" before them, efforts to tame, manage, or contain the power of difference are countered by the alternative economy of disability-based desire. When they have sought to give voice to their experiences, disabled people often position their own interests quite differently. Rather than the restitution of their bodies to some less conspicuous existence, disabled people seek redress of a wider social network of obstacles, as if the body were not an isolated entity but rather an active participant in a socially mediated process. This adjusted analytical focus from individual insufficiency to socially created deviance informs the social model of disability. Rather than faulty bodies, the social model seeks to recognize faulty systems of human devising.

The entries in this volume provide myriad examples of ways to view disability, but its ultimate objective remains committed to influencing perceptions. The collection seeks to expose the process of seeing human differences as received belief rather than naturalized divisions. Just as the British philosopher John Berger (1973), in his aptly entitled book *Ways of Seeing,* explains that the figure of Vanity (usually portrayed as a nude woman holding a mirror in narcissistic rapture) represents an expression of the artist's desire rather than her own, our effort here follows a similar strategy. Rather than simply accepting historical depiction, we want to offer these works as the product of interests devised largely outside of disabled peoples' perspectives. Repeated images of short-statured people as maniacal dwarfs, blind people as metaphysical seers, individuals with epilepsy as demonically possessed, and limping figures as archetypal villains receive their power through generational reiteration. These visions are detrimental not merely because they undermine the ability of disabled people to fully participate in activities of culture making, but also because they bestow a deterministic fate. Disability often leads one to be scorned on behalf of a socially bestowed fate as beggar, idol, and pariah.

One result of this approach to disability is that disability-based social marginalization becomes misrecognized as the product of individual incapacities. In his painting *The Cripples* (1568), the Flemish painter Brueghel bitterly scribbled on the back of the portrait: "Cripples go and be prosperous!"—as if a reduction to panhandling on the streets provides a secretly lucrative occupation based on the sympathies of unsuspecting passersby. The foxtails pinned to the beggars' clothes evidence the work of those who would approach disabled bodies to glean "luck" or to fend off their own potential vulnerabilities. In treating disabled people as the objects of social ritual, the community is denied even the basic right of self-reflection. Such has been the case for other devalued communities, such as women and people of color. It is rare that one witnesses a disabled subject staring back at the viewer in full possession of his or her humanity. Moments where disabled people return the gaze rather than function as the pure object of others' scrutiny can be found in works such as Velasquez's *Las Meninas,* where the royal dwarf stares out knowingly from the scene. But parallel depictions are few and far between.

At the same time, and in spite of this treatment, disabled people have used their rejected bodies as sites of cultural transformation. The history of artistic expression presented in this volume may also be viewed as surprisingly synonymous with the expressive creativity of people with disabilities. Discussions of the works of disabled artists have often avoided the question of the impact of their bodies on their work, as in the cases of Claude Monet—visual impairment; Henri Toulouse-Lautrec—short-statured; Paul Klee—scleroderma; Edvard Munch—schizophrenia; Francisco Goya—deafness; Vincent van Gogh—mental illness; Auguste Renoir—arthritis; and Frida Kahlo—spina bifida. However, we would like to present the work of individuals such as these as an opportunity to imagine how the unique visions of their work draw directly from their experiences of disability. Many have portrayed their experiences directly, as in Goya's renditions of deafness or Kahlo's depictions of her scarred body, back brace, physicians, and lengthy confinements to her bed. Likewise, van Gogh painted his own medical attendants and his cell at the Arles institution. Because disabled people have found themselves restricted to rather narrow locations, their work explores that space as if it were a universe unto itself.

In addition to the impoverishment of the visual arts, one would find literature equally depreciated by the absence of disabled peoples' poems and stories. For instance, we would lose the work of key literary figures such as Homer—blind; John Milton—blind; Samuel Johnson—Tourette's syndrome; Alexander Pope—scoliosis; Lord Byron—Little's disease; John Keats—tuberculosis; Emily Dickinson—visual impairment; Walt Whitman—mobility impairment; Stephen Crane—tuberculosis; Virginia Woolf—depression; James Joyce—visual impairment; Jorge Luis Borges—blind; Flannery O'Connor—lupus; and others. In truth, if one were to subtract disability experience from the traditions identified here, we would immediately lose much innovation in the history of all arts. All of these individuals sought to transform cultural attitudes about human differences by exploring disability experience as distinctive in its own right.

The conflicts identified and even generated by such representations are certainly formidable. Each image arrives saturated with the workings of power as certain bodies become targets for pathological ascriptions. As Foucault argues, "History is at war with the body." This volume pays homage to the wages of this war on bodies deemed disabled by virtue of capacity, aesthetic, race, gender, and class. We recognize such portrayals as static patterns of narrative investment.

Our intention is to open up these representations for scrutiny as a step toward cultivating a need for further nuance. If language determines interpretive options to a significant extent, then exposing the limits of meaning gestures toward a more complex register of narrative possibilities. Likewise, many of these excerpts expose the extent to which disability has served as a productive arena of contemplation. Those who have explored disability experiences as a meaningful aspect of human embodiment (rather than outside of or somehow apart from other experiences) demonstrate that we fail if we continue to view bodies as passively imprinted by environments. Rather, bodies serve as active mediators of our interactions between ourselves, others, and the environments we inhabit.

Finally, while bodies can function as a source of division between individuals and communities, feelings of estrangement produced by these encounters are hardly inevitable. Instead, they largely come from a historical lack of intimacy with bodily, sensory, and cognitive differences. As disabled people found themselves incarcerated, segregated, isolated, and ostracized (sometimes voluntarily but usually imposed by others), their social invisibility further alienated them from those who moved more freely in the world. Their absence increased a distance from others and made their pending reintegration even less likely.

Without the participation of disabled people, environments continue to be imagined for the use of a narrow range of capacities; without the participation of disabled people, we all grow desensitized to our own bodies; without the participation of disabled people, our own vulnerability seems more threatening; without the participation of disabled people, we allow ourselves to imagine human existence as independent rather than interdependent; without the participation of disabled people, we ultimately deny variation in the name of a destructive and mythical homogeneity. In other words, rather than existing on the fringes of embodied experience, disability is central to our ability to envision ourselves in meaningful ways.

As psychiatric institutions in Nazi Germany systematically exterminated "lives unworthy of life," the net of in-valid bodies expanded. Those who participated in the exterminations participated in hedonistic rituals such as parties on the occasion of the 10,000th killing, staff orgies, and brutal devaluations of each other. The devaluation of disabled lives is ultimately tantamount to a disregard for all lives.

Yet, in spite of the devastation wrought by the advent of institutionalization, disabled people participated in developed social networks of their own. Asylums, institutions, clinics, hospitals, and segregated schools all became sites of community development where disabled people created a refuge for the value of variation. These cordoned-off sites sometimes became havens as well as alienating locations. They served as source for the cultivation of shared politics and critique—the two values that most define shared human endeavor. Many of us are unfamiliar with these alternative social groupings, and thus the materials here help to better acquaint readers with the specificity of an "outside" community now made newly available for contemplation. One might use this volume as a means for exploring the ways in which even derided embodiment gives birth to an alternative economy of difference. All of these facets of disability experience have remained relatively unthought. The materials presented here seek to dispel this defining lack of familiarity to whatever extent possible.

Note

1. Philip Sandblom, author of *Creativity and Disease* (1997), has researched birth records kept by Kahlo's doctor that diagnose her with spina bifida.

Reference

Berger, John. 1973. *Ways of Seeing.* New York: Viking Press.
Sandblom, Philip. 1997. *Creativity and Disease: How Illness Affects Literature, Art, and Music.* London: Marion Boyers.

ACKNOWLEDGMENTS

In many ways, all books are collective efforts. They come about, as Virginia Woolf wrote, as the distillation of generations of thinking in common. This is absolutely the case in the work of creating an encyclopedia. One contributor referred to the collection project throughout its design as the Cyclops. He thus invoked the monstrosity behind the mission making us all Dr. Frankensteins when many had felt themselves instead an ally of the monster. But he also invoked the mundane monster-making that an odyssey must find in concealed places—"look, here be monsters."

Such an intellectual, cultural, geographical, and historical undertaking inevitably resonates with an eighteenth-century effort to catalogue all species and name every item. Nothing could be further from the case with the volume before you. In this case, given no financial incentive and little potential scholarly credit, those who extended their efforts in the name of this project did so out of a deep commitment to the cultivation of disability history. Volume 5, in particular, developed as an extended international effort with scholars contributing sources from five continents. Without the input, wisdom, community, and scrupulous scholarly contributions of our editorial team, we could not have completed this project.

Consequently, the editors, both formal and informal, for this primary source volume merit full credit for the range of sources and outreach efforts of the materials represented herein. We all recognized that the task before us was not really feasible given the state of interest and early point in the advent of global transmission technologies so we sought to confine our tracking efforts to themes and strands of available resources. A serious caveat, then: This volume represents collective efforts but is by no means exhaustive or even representative. Instead, it reflects the range

that we could pull together in a limited amount of time and with minimal financial resources as well as the serious barriers of restricting this volume to English text sources alone. In spite of these factors, the participants acknowledged here went to great lengths to make the volume as international as possible.

A significant contribution to the ancient history section of this volume has been collected and introduced by Martha Rose. She worked from beginning to end on this project and assured that materials from Greece, Rome, and other early civilizations gave the volume serious historical sweep. Likewise, Kerry Wood organized and introduced important materials from the Old and New Testament on disability. Penny Richards provided materials from women's literature and history, education, and disability parenting literature, as well as various insertions into nineteenth- and early twentieth-century sources for the United States. Kumur B. Selim, who worked to improve the non-Western range of the volume despite its representational barriers, contributed materials from many locations and across all time periods. Without this contribution, the volume would be further impoverished as to what it might tell us about disability in non-western contexts. To an endlessly giving colleague Tobin Siebers, we offer our appreciation for work in European and American sources of the Romantic period. David Gerber provided expert guidance on the inclusion of materials pertinent to disabled veterans in the United States. Disability historian Sandy Suffian added some of her own previously untapped sources with respect to institutional history in Africa, Israel, and elsewhere. In Germany, we were fortunate to have the leadership provided by Anne Waldschmidt to ensure that the history of German disabled people and institutions were adequately addressed. Anne orchestrated her own editorial team to assure the volume of historical scope and cross disability sources from German literature and history. Similarly, Helen Meekosha did the same for sources on disability history in Australia. She gathered up scholars, activists, and community participants from many sectors and professions, all of whom made important additions to an oft neglected geographical locale rich in disability history. Further, we want to acknowledge Yerker Andersson, who assembled his own impressive group of scholars in the field of Deaf Studies and Deaf History. This volume only scratches the surface of the international undertakings that are underway in deaf history. Whatever merits this volume may have go to the credit of these individuals who worked and contributed of their time, materials, and expertise on behalf of their shared commitment to the need for developing a comparative disability history. Finally, we acknowledge the work of Eunjung Kim, who researched important sources from the history of disability in Korea to include in this compilation. The significant contributions of all our editors make this volume a monument in collective scholarly output. They have our sincere thanks for their generosity, candor, and expertise.

As we neared completion of the final section on globalization, British disability film historian Paul Darke provided as with a timely set of stills from the history of disability in cinema. He also provided access to his voluminous disability stamp collection from around the world. For these two important contributions alone, we owe Paul a great debt. We received several important disability sources in Japan from our friend Patrick Drazen, whose knowledge of Japanese popular culture never ceases to amaze us. In a parallel effort, we offer our deep appreciation to Yangling Li, who researched some key Chinese sources for the twentieth century. Japanese disability advocate Nagase Osamu and Indian disability scholar and activist Meenu Bhambhani contributed visual and textual sources from their country's respective disability civil rights movements. Serbian disability scholar and activist Vladimir Cuk generously provided materials to include the activities of the Serbian disabled students' movement. Disability activists, scholars, and archivists in Canada, Australia, and Britain also pitched in to have their movements represented. Many thanks to Tomato Lichy, Mitzi Waltz, Karen Soldatic, Graeme Bacque, Geoffrey Reaume, Penny Bould, and Lilith Finkler—and particularly Tony Baldwinson,

who also provided visual materials from the history of blind individuals in Britain and the Soviet Union. We are greatly heartened by these global commitments and also by those who believe they matter enough to record the real life experiences of disabled constituencies everywhere with care and insight.

Sara Vogt, a researcher who also pursues scholarship in comparative studies of U.S. and German disability policy, skillfully translated German language source materials. Ingrid Hoffman at the University of Minnesota also undertook crucial German translation work along with Liz Winters from her outpost in St. Louis. Without the expertise of anti-psychiatry researcher Pamela Wheelock, this volume would find itself largely bereft of materials documenting the U.S. anti-psychiatry movement from the 1950s onward. The combined efforts of these scholars proved the sole reason why the volume was able to include these primary source texts. Such donated participation has proven essential in helping us demonstrate the international scope of political struggles around disability and other marginalized peoples.

Of course, no volume such as this can come to fruition without a committed and knowledgeable administrative staff. Most importantly we want to recognize Michelle Jarman, who, in addition to providing key sources herself, also led an early research, collection, and proofreading effort in which many Ph.D. students in disability studies at the University of Illinois participated. Michelle's scrupulous skills in review and research are greatly appreciated. Those who assisted locally in bringing the volume to realization include Michael Gill, Eunjung Kim, Sharon Lamp, Yanling Li, Sarah Rose, Mark Sherry, Shilpaa Anand, Heather Stone, Terri Thrower, Sara Vogt, Carlos Drazen, and Pamela Wheelock. Each contributed of their time, expertise, scholarly imagination, and good will. Their collaborative work together on the Sage encyclopedia project has resulted in the generative formation for a new graduate student organization, the Disability History and Culture Collective at the University of Illinois in Chicago.

Another critical impetus for the planning of this volume came in a faculty and teacher summer institute in disability studies sponsored by the first National Endowment for the Humanities. The scholars who contributed their time, expertise, and readings for this institute formed the initial skeleton of the current volume. Those who participated in the Including Disability in K-12 project include Linda Ware, Douglas Baynton,

Helen Deutsch, Jim Ferris, Martha Rose, David Gerber, Martha Stoddard Holmes, Carrie Sandahl, Tobin Siebers, Rosemarie Garland-Thomson, and Brenda Brueggemann. Their fine work—individually and collectively—has continued to prod and inspire our own. This volume is very much the fruit of their labors as well.

Additionally, longtime colleagues and newer research associates who participated as members of the American and Canadian faculty research group at the Einstein Forum for the 2004 summer institute on T-4 and the legacies of eugenics deserve recognition here as well. All showed remarkable potential for collective scholarship in action on the crossings among German, U.S., and Canadian disability history. The Germany summer institute participants include Adrienne Asch, Brenda Brueggemann, Sally Chivers, Sumi Colligan, Gerald O'Brien, Ingrid Hoffman, Nicole Markotic, Sandy O'Neill, Walton Schalick, Rosemarie Garland Thomson, Kanta Kochar-Lindgren, Debjani Mukherjee, Sara Vogt, Pamela Wheelock, and Emma Mitchell. Our month-long stint with this group gave us all a career's worth of future research topics as well as a camaraderie rarely experienced among academics engaged in a shared intellectual enterprise.

Of course, for us, no project would be complete without the input, investment, and counseling provided by artist Riva Lehrer. Her vision and creative insight give our own musings a sense of grander insight, cultural necessity, and aesthetic belonging.

Lehrer's ability to recognize connections across seemingly unlike things has cultivated our understanding of history as belonging to the different as well as the differentiated. Additionally, our acquaintance with Brian Zimmerman has re-fueled our commitments to reading as an occupation of significance. Their presence in this volume is significant even if largely absent on the surface of things (but, then again, this is how they contribute some of their greatest work).

In a larger sense, the entire encyclopedia project would not have occurred without the leadership of Gary Albrecht and the other participants in Sage's interdisciplinary "Noah's Ark." Jerome Bickenbach and Walton Schalick deserve particular recognition as disability scholars of integrity who worked alongside of us to pull off this massive endeavor. Our admiration of the scholarship, leadership capacities, and integrity of these individuals remains high. Our especial appreciation go to Tamar Heller, Joe Flaherty, Eduardo Encinas, and Dudley Childress, who participated in the long march of meetings that ultimately culminated in this five-volume work.

And, finally, to the "Buffy the Vampire Slayer" fan club who didn't need to imagine another world in order to understand the importance of this one. As Buffy once said, "You know what they say–those of us who failed history . . . doomed to repeat it in summer school." Let's hope we all have summers off from this time forward as a result of good historical karma.

ABOUT THE ENCYCLOPEDIA COVERS: VISUALIZING VARIATION

Sharon L. Snyder

The five covers for the *Encyclopedia of Disability* represent a selection of artistic impressions across a range of cultures, time periods, and multiple disabilities. They also render some of the unique orbits for the complex relationships that disability experiences provoke. Each is purposely nontragic and discourages pathos or too easy sentiment. Instead, the covers emphasize the creative and self-inventive side of disability experience. All make disability a window onto diverse landscapes for the body different.

Taken collectively, they may even suggest an odd refuge in disability—the degree to which incapacities can be viewed as protecting us, and motivating creative agency, even as they may render us most vulnerable. Perhaps someone such as Frida Kahlo, who lived so intensely in her body, could identify the lure of incapacity to this extent. She wrote in her diaries:

> We take refuge in, we take flight into irrationality, magic, abnormality, in fear of the extraordinary beauty of truth of matter and dialectics, of whatever is healthy and strong—we like being sick to protect ourselves. Someone—something—always protects us from the truth—Our own ignorance and fear. (*The Diary* 1995:248–249)

Thought about in such a way, disability no longer means a condition, an incapacity, or lack that belongs to a body, but rather a product of the interactions between self, society, body, and the variety of interactions (from political economies to personal commitments) that they engender. Disabled bodies, then, are artifacts—found or experienced while saturated with the meaning of our own investments, concerns, hopes, and insignificance in the world.

That the relations precipitated by human differences so often become detrimental to people with disabilities, turning even families or institutions devoted to their care into warehouses or danger zones, does not lessen their significance. Analysis of disability from a social perspective reveals the extent to which cultures prove creative at inventing endless varieties of human diminishment. In response, one finds counter-creativity demanded of disabled people. Their own livelihood, and sometimes their very lives, can rely on an ability to subvert supernatural views held about their conditions, contest medical fascination with their corporeality as "specimens," or spend years finding the means to escape confinement from back wards, closets, and institutions. The art depicted on the covers of this five-volume set, then, present us with this multisided nature of disability experience. Each portrays individuals both marked as undeniably different and actively transforming of the social terms of their reception.

The bronze sculpture of the Nigerian King Oba (cover of Volume IV) speaks directly to this idea of disability as urgently necessary renegotiation of the terms by which the nondisabled may see us. The king stands between the dual supports of his personal assistants with his mudfish legs on full display to the viewer. Rather than a story of personal diminishment by paralysis, the king explains his condition, contrariwise, as a deepening of his power. Mudfish represented a revered species in Nigerian culture at the time of this event. A king who awakens to discover himself immobile—particularly when the appearance of physical or cognitive disability in a ruler results, by law, in exile or execution from his subjects—can avert certain catastrophe only by such inventive quick thinking. Instead of concealing his paralysis, the king parades his body transformation before more lethal rumors can begin to circulate.

The Oba's explanation for his sudden mobility impairment draws directly upon insider understanding: Difference of form does not equate with absence of kingly capacity. Legs bow out and gradually modify into the heads and forelegs of the mudfish as the product of a powerful formulation of the meaning of body changes. The king tells his subjects that he can now pass between earthly and spiritual realms just as the mudfish navigate land and sea as half-reptile and half-fish. Circling the human figures, a series of four amphibian heads stare out as totemic sentries. The artist admires the flexibility of such an in-between space occupied by the Oba in his claimed role as a mediator now between human assistants and animal protectors.

Both Oba and artist participate in the recognition that variation exists across species and hence offers to us a rich array of explanations for the value of bodily configurations that might otherwise be cast out as undesirable. The sculpture posits continuity to natures, creatures, cohabitants, in a portrayal of paralysis: mudfish legs, human assistants with partially truncated torsos, pineapples, elephant trunk, snake, and swamp tangle. All life forms mesh in a symbiotic system of mutual belonging despite intense differences of capacity. Diversity teems across the bronze figure's vertical and horizontal axes. A celebration of varying capacities from human to animal culminates in the exhibition of Oba's bowing legs in order that variations across bodies in nature can provide context for a human body with paralyzed legs without a lessening of value.

The nineteenth-century Japanese triptych *Hua T'o Treating an Instance of Necrosis on the Arm of the Warrior Guan Yu* (cover of Volume III, 1853) by the famous printmaker Utagawa Kuniyoshi, depicts a historical event from fourteenth-century China. To the far left of the work we witness a surgeon, dwarfed in the presence of the massive body of Guan Yu, plying his trade in spite of the recreational distractions taking place around him. The physician, Hua T'o, meaning "miracle working doctor" (or "divine physician" based on the Japanese word *shenyi*), concentrates on a lesion eating away at the general's right arm. His localized treatment effort contrasts with the social frivolity portrayed in the rest of the painting. Medicine pursues its healing art as the world continues on indifferent to the work of bodily salvage. In this reading, we could situate ourselves as admirers of precise medical application as the "patient" stubbornly pursues other desires with a reckless lack of concern: Medicine

works against time and gross inattention to attend to human vulnerability. We are situated as admirers of medical technique; the physician's perseverance is sustained in spite of activities that might prove distracting to the treatment effort.

Likewise, a viewer of the painting may also contemplate the work as a commentary on war. Bodies are wantonly exposed to violence and disability, disease, and death. Human wreckage is exposed as the primary product of militarized clashes between individuals, tribes, and nations. The painting depicts Guan Yu calmly receiving treatment following a battle wound caused by a poison arrow. The warrior ignores the cleaning of the wound down to the bone as an example of the power of the first administration of anesthetic. He has adopted an attitude that places his body as fully secondary to more immediate concerns, whether the task at hand is a battle or gamesmanship. In the unfinished disability play *The Deformed Transformed* (1822), the renowned Romantic poet Lord Byron, argued that masculine able-bodiedness seemed to require that men put their healthy bodies at risk of violation, as if they could not feel their lives as "real" enough without exposing themselves to the potential of disability. The thrill of physical threats pursued and then evaded. The painting of Hua T'o suggests a similar reading in that the development of necrosis suggests a near-gangrenous wound progressing to the point of a serious medical condition. A poor result might yield the loss of a limb or disuse of his arm because the general has refused to attend to the initial laceration in a timely manner. This patient inattention to the poisoning produces an even graver medical predicament. From this vantage point, a viewer might choose to indict the warrior's indifference to his own health concerns or grow further weary of war's destruction.

Alternatively, one may also glimpse a cultivated demeanor in Guan Yu's laissez-faire attitude toward medical attention. We might draw an interesting parallel to the experience of medicalization by disabled persons—particularly in the case of individuals who have spent significant time "under the knife." While medicine demands the full attention of the patient to participate in its own healing mission, those exposed to continuous medical care often refuse this singular attention paid to their bodies. Undergoing medical care requires a multitasking mission, or the rest of one's life comes to a full stop. In this view, we might think of medicine as the disruptive event against which the rest of one's life must be experienced. A certain capacity develops among disabled people to handle their other "business" as the medical industry rages around them. In fact, there's a form of patient *cool* where one refuses to allow a medical event to eclipse the myriad other demands on one's life—such an attitude can be found on display in the Kuniyoshi print as the game of Go continues in the face of surgery. In fact, the medical activity is reduced to a mere third of the triptych while the game occupies the remainder of the artist's interest. The social interaction requires as much seriousness as the presence of necrosis itself.

Likewise, Tim Lowly's *Beacon (Bless the Bastard)* (cover of Volume V, 1991) emphasizes independent coexistence among bodies occupying shared space. Rocks, river, grass, and other earthly elements populate the scene with an adult care provider and a disabled child positioned a few feet away. The two female figures, out of doors and beyond the traditional confines of domesticity, do not show shame or efforts to hide from the world's discomfort with disability. The caregiver looks off in the distance responding to some unknown force with a stem wielded over her shoulder in the gesture of a blessing. Behind and below the caregiver, a child (the artist's daughter Temma) lies on a bright blue pallet that cushions her from the ground—the same ground on which her mother's bare feet are firmly planted. The disabled girl's body, illuminated in the landscape and sprawled beneath the sky, wears a one-piece playsuit with socks and shoes, carefully swaddled despite the apparent warmth of the day. The relationship between the two figures, emphasized by the colors in the child's garment and repeated in the mother's striped dress, openly proclaims their identification. This is Temma's consciously placed residence in the world; she might be lying there contemplating a future yet to be articulated by the adults around her. The daughter's figure, aimed like a magnetic compass arrow toward the bridge in the upper left canvas, serves as a beacon to the artist, and, in this landscape, literally could be cast in a red outfit as if a signal translated from one location to another. The way a painter selects and places a subject onto a canvas in a highly self-conscious act parallels how Temma's caregiver has consciously situated her in this setting. In other works, Temma lies near a muddy puddle, a pond, on a day bed, across a desert floor, near a wooded river stream; her figure a geographic nomad yet without apparent mobility. These portraits capture Temma's vantage point as contemplative of universes unrevealed in ordinary landscapes—and strangely altered by the insertion of a disabled body. The historical absence of disabled

people in routine places makes every appearance potentially transgress audience expectations. Conversely, every insertion undermines the belief that there are some places disabled persons should not go.

Just below the bridge, a small group clusters around a makeshift stone altar and, in a rather ritualistic manner, evokes a history of atonement practices. These ritualistic acts often occur in response to a mystery disability seems to evoke. Why me? Or what did I do to deserve this fate? Or what does this difference mean for the community? Are we culpable in some way? Piled stones reference all the hard things humans negotiate, arrange, and work with, just as the allegorical landscape offers hugely divergent elements, from spongy riverbed to wooden platform, to inhabit. Each formation seems to be selected for its yielding principles. Fjords— irregular land and water masses—remind us of the non-standard geometries of embodiment and mirror the daughter's figure akimbo on land. Bodies of water and of land encroach on and define each other—clearly etched by nonregimented and unpredictable shorelines. The work on the makeshift altar occurs while the determined "blessing" of the mother above also redoubles as a fending off of outside forces and even our gaze, as viewers prying into a private scene. As if we must first fathom the precision of the mother's expression and gesture in the foreground before gaining access to the proceedings beyond her, she stands as a cautious gatekeeper before the rest of the painting.

The subtitle, *Bless the Bastard,* refers not to the child but to the concept of flinging back insults with a shield of mercy. The artist explains the idea as a matter of how one might bless those who curse one with additional punch. The mother's determined motions, her turning outward and her gesture toward the past, and her daughter's resident outside location, present them as participants in a fully parallel existence. The story of disability unveils that even the most ordinary outing requires a variety of self-conscious placements and protective gestures.

Finally, a white building perched near the skyline in the upper-right-hand corner recalls, as well, the Olson house on the upper horizon of Andrew Wyeth's famous painting *Christina's World*. As in the Lowly work, the house in Wyeth's painting also makes a young disabled woman's predicament into an allegory. The disabled figure in each work lies in the foreground staring off into the distance—relatively immobile or alternatively mobile in body but imaginatively engaged in future prospects unknown to, and unimagined by, viewers. In *Beacon,* the far-off residence appears like a temple amid a landscape that is filled with objects that catch a viewer's eye. Each item serves as a potential enhancement or barrier to navigation across it. Certainly, both disability paintings place a demand on the viewer to acknowledge these scenes as complete worlds. In them an ordinary morning scene, the forthrightly mundane world, is lent a hue of studied complexity toward a disability's self-conscious placement therein. *Beacon* offers Temma's figure as a guidepost rather than repulsion. The disability-wise gestures of the figures themselves are understood to occur in the face of a modern hyperrational clarity that would dispense with disability experience as some all-too-obvious tragedy. The paintings provide a lesson in how to live in the world with severe disability. Both ask us to reexamine this premise by requiring that we look closely enough to discern the disability coordinates of lives that might at first glance appear wasted.

Whereas Lowly and Wyeth represent intimate works about disability by nondisabled artists, Frida Kahlo's work supplies an example of artistic traditions spawned by disabled artists themselves (cover of Volume I). Responses to the disability context of Kahlo's work and life have ranged from incredulity to simple disability disavowal: "Frida Kahlo—she's a national treasure. How could she be a disabled woman?" Contrariwise, the complex disability perspectives that inform her subject matter and the terms of her artistic exploration can become so central that disability interests may overwhelm all else in her work. Certainly, few artists since the Middle Ages made the topic of personal suffering such a wellspring for creative figuration. For disability critics, one must note the inventiveness that informs Kahlo's access to artistic practices, from painting on canvasses suspended over her bed to laptop easels to the elaborate journal she kept detailing her pain, confinement, and multiple surgeries (including the amputation of her right leg in 1955). Such investments in the ability of art to provide her with immense joy "in spite of my long illness" led her to have her four-poster bed dismantled and reconstructed in the national museum of Mexico City. The unusual accommodation occurred on an evening prior to the one exhibition during her lifetime in her home country for the purpose of being able to view the exhibit herself in comfort.

Kahlo's life, whether conceived as utterly conditioned by disability or as having disability merely incidental to it, has served as the topic of children's books and films. Controversies rage over the terms and origins of her multiple impairments. Some have identified her disability as resulting from a bus accident when she was 16 years old in 1926; others with the effects of polio contracted at the age of 6; and still others, such as Philip Sandblom author of *Creativity and Disease* (1997), propose that she was born with the congenital condition of spina bifida, which she spent her life concealing. We may be discussing some combination of all of these events in one body as well. These discussions are as interesting for the fears and concerns interpreters express about the meanings of congenital (as opposed to acquired) disabilities for stories of artistic achievement. Acquired disability makes one a hapless victim of circumstances while congenital disability signifies a status as metaphysical pawn.

Nevertheless, the latter attribution of spina bifida as an initial source of her disabilities becomes most provocative given her preoccupation with the spinal column in her work. Her paintings commonly depict Mexico as an ionic column with wings. In addition, she also uses duality or twinning such as in her work, *The Two Fridas* (1939), where we see her heart beating and a circulatory system that feeds the nearby identical body image with which she clasps hands. The work depicted here, painted in 1946 amid a flurry of surgeries and hospital stays, *Arbol de la Esperanza Mantente Firme* (*Tree of Hope—Stand Firm!*), associates an ironic meaning to the figure holding a back brace in one half and wounds along the supine figure's spine in the other. The sense of strength that Kahlo must have felt in herself—particularly through her political commitments to Communist revolution—resound as both a plea (make me strong in the face of pain) and a command to others (stand firm in your political convictions). These words, *"arbol de la esperanza mantente firme,"* which one of her biographers, Hayden Herrera, identified as the lyrics to a song she knew, would also appear a year later in a diary entry celebrating the 30th anniversary of the Bolshevik revolution. For Kahlo, debilitating physical anguish could be offset to some degree with a merger of disability and political images in that both coexist without eclipsing the other: The most disabled also embody the fiercest commitments for social justice. The two often become a self-referencing system in the body of her works.

Compositionally, the contrasted backgrounds of night and day suggest a confluence of binary associations between light and dark, health and illness, passive hospital patient and active revolutionary. Yet the painting throws such easy oppositions into question in that all coexist, and enlightenment may come from either source. The more medical image appears in the day where one might expect to find her more "public"—that is, less vulnerable—self. Thus, the work is an emblem of Kahlo's artistic *oeuvre* in that these versions of the self do not simply balance the subject but rather serve as wellsprings for creative vision in their own right. The pink brace grasped securely in the hands of the formally dressed figure who waves a small flag contrasts with the night and small moon on the right side of the canvas. The body of the fully draped figure situated at a perfect right angle to the reposed figure on the wheeled operating table function as two supports along the canvas's vertical and horizontal planes. The figure on the left displays open seeping wounds across a back that is exposed between pulled-apart sheets as if to unveil her body in a surgical cut-away.

Likewise, spinal lesions echo across both halves of the painting. They duplicate cracks and ridges that split dry earth across which the stretcher seems precariously perched. This yawning crevasse is exactly the same size as the wheeled bed. A surreal glittery ball stands for the sun, and her flowery headdress hovers suspended in this cosmic stratosphere. The velvet dress suggests a more formal version of the Aztec clothing that she wore throughout her adult life. It's also a chosen legacy rescued from a colonized past. Hence the more surreal aspect of this painting: The body left behind, ruptured, and lying across night and day is juxtaposed to the upright, dressed red figure who gazes at the viewer while holding the brace in full display. It also appears that the seated figure wears a similar corset-like apparatus beneath the dress because the bulbous endings appear around her chest and match the same design of the brace in her hands. In a *Time* magazine article of April 27, 1953, Kahlo insisted that "I never painted dreams. I painted my own reality" (p. 90). The painting may most of all render homage to her prosthetic back brace and her investments in it. Today, one can find the same pink back brace with personal decorations in a visit to her home, now a national museum. In either case, both portraits echo with Kahlo's disability markers that worked to flaunt, as opposed to mask them, from the viewer.

Kahlo's work has been often attributed to the influence of northern Dutch painters such as Pieter Brueghel the Elder, and particularly, Hieronymus Bosch (Jeroen Van Aken: 1450–1516). While Brueghel painted mimetic images of everyday northern peasant life, Bosch's impact on Kahlo is often identified through his portrayals of bizarre imaginings such as the events captured in his work *Extraction of the Stone of Madness (The Cure of Folly)* (ca. 1475) (cover of Volume II). Whereas Kahlo followed Vincent van Gogh in portraying her physicians in respectful portraits as a sign of appreciation, Bosch participates in a less reverent approach. In this painting, Bosch satirizes the medieval medical practice of removing stones from the head as a treatment for madness, traumatic brain injury, and insanity. In addition, the other two onlookers—a friar and a nun—represent alternative religious domains where madness was commonly addressed with alms and prayer. Thus, Bosch assembles the surgery's audience carefully in his effort to draw the three figures into the net of this parody—as if every charlatan, barber, and pious practitioner of his day comes together in this unholy gathering to witness someone else's suffering. Their own moral stature in the community depends on catering to those residing among the "less fortunate."

The subject of the surgery—a patient drawn in the guise of various "fools" of the day—undergoes a risky intervention. Hopes for release from such conditions as insanity resulted in a willingness to expose oneself to disastrous—and often life-threatening—efforts to alleviate symptoms. Similar practices for the treatment of mental illness were widespread in Bosch's day. Evidence also suggests that in spite of critiques such as this one, the practice continued into the Renaissance where similar procedures are documented as late as the sixteenth century. Like Kahlo, Bosch rarely ventured far from home, and his works include details of familiar scenes within a tightly circumscribed area. Yet, as in this work, Bosch's paintings place the rituals of life in question by unveiling the violence that often resides just beneath the surface. Consequently, *Extraction of the Stone of Madness* suggests that "deviant" behavior may be found on both sides of the treatment divide.

Bosch's painting, inspired by various folk tales and critiques of the physicians' guilds of his time, appears fairytale-like in its allegorical assemblage of medical and religious personnel. In each figure, the primary treatment tools come on display—from the barber's scalpel to the friar's chalice-like vessel to the nun who balances a book on her head. The physician applies his effort directly to the body, the male priest talks and gestures toward the patient during the ordeal as if performing an exorcism of demons, and the nun looks on in contemplation as if patiently awaiting inspiration from the text above. Each intervention strategy seems poised to encourage equal levels of suspicion. Rather than a stone, the surgery results in the extraction of a flower from the man's head. This is a curious object in that the flower appears much more at home in the naturalistic setting while the human practitioners seem out of place. The town situated off in the distance further emphasizes their displacement. As one commentator puts it:

> Moreover, this work of art bears the inscription 'Master, take away the stone, my name is Lubbert Das.' It is worth pointing out that Lubbert Das was a comical character that originates in the Dutch literature of that time. The stone is represented as a flower (tulip) on the head of the patient near the surgeon's knife, because of the similarity between the words tulip (*tulp*) and madness in Dutch. (Babiloni et al. 2003:1)

This direct parallel between organic life and insanity may suggest Bosch's effort to equate both objects with the forces of nature that ultimately evade human control.

While madness may be commonly represented as severe distraction from the applications of daily living, only the patient's gaze breaks the painting's plane as he looks out uncertainly toward the artist capturing the event and/or the hapless viewer consuming the event. His look of personal concern contrasts with the concentrated efforts of the others as they attend directly to the site of conflict—namely, his brain as resident location for the "disorder"—and thus the "patient's" objectification turns out to be at least threefold on behalf of the barber, artist, and viewer. We participate as consumers of the discomforting scene. Bosch captures the worst kind of medical theater, one that not only subjects one to painful procedures of dubious merit but also is witnessed by others to further deepen the stigma.

The painting also comments on a long-standing belief in medicine that the body functions as symptomatic surface for otherwise ephemeral "cognitive" phenomena (i.e., madness in this case). Without a tangible bodily location, medicine would prove at a loss as to how to proceed in its material correctives. The concept of a "stone" of madness then takes an abstract matter of behavior perceived as deviant and objectifies it in physical terms. Thus, various bodily zones get targeted as the seat/source of intangible phenomena. In the eugenics period (1840–1940), "idiocy" was theorized as a lack of control of the will, and "docile" bodies

were targeted through physical exercises, concentration rituals (e.g., standing in one place for minutes at a time), and hygienic grooming practices—a presentable body represents a compliant citizen. In each instance, exerting force on the physical body provided a route through which to impose control over minds.

In sum, these artistic works demonstrate that disability is both a product of specific local contexts *and* shared, even global, disability perspectives. Africa, Japan, the United States, Mexico, and the Netherlands all contribute to a multinational mosaic of disability representation; in doing so, disability transcends geography, culture, and history in its situation as a metaphorical and pragmatic device of social meaning making. The question "What do we do with our disabled people?" resonates in most cultures and across historical moments. In the midst of its invocation as perpetual crisis, disability can expose ruses to the control and mastery of human variation, give expression to individual assertions of difference and group identity, portray indifference or excruciating investment in the denial of deviance, resignify incapacity into unexpected ability, or provide opportunities of interdependency among human vulnerabilities in search of mutual support. On each cover of Volumes I through V, disability serves as the medium through which artists—and, consequently, the viewers of their art—may ponder cultural responses to the persistence of human heterogeneity. Difference prompts myriad social schemes of suppression in futile efforts to contain variation within a narrower range of expression. Artists of disability are not in any way immune to the homogenizing projects of cultures, but their work gives us perspective on how we might improve the future by contemplating the limitations of tolerance in our past.

Further Readings

Babiloni, F., C. Babiloni, F. Carducci, F. Cincotti, and P. M. Rossini. 2003. "'The Stone of Madness' and the Search for the Cortical Sources of Brain Diseases with Non-Invasive EEG Techniques." *Clinical Neurophysiology* 114: 1775–1780.

The Diary of Frida Kahlo: An Intimate Self-Portrait. 1995. New York: Harry M. Abrams.

Herrera, Hayden. 2002. *Frida Kahlo: The Paintings.* New York: Perennial.

Sandblom, Philip. 1996. *Creativity and Disease: How Illness Affects Literature, Art and Music,* 12th ed. New York: Marion Boyers.

ABOUT THE GENERAL EDITOR

Gary L. Albrecht is Professor of Public Health and of Disability and Human Development at the University of Illinois at Chicago. His current work focuses on the quality of life of disabled people based on National Institutes of Health (NIH)–funded studies of disabled women experiencing the menopausal transition and a study of disability risk in the United Kingdom, France, and the United States. Complementary work on the experience of disability in the inner city has been funded by the National Institute on Disability and Rehabilitation Research (NIDRR). He is past Chair of the Medical Sociology Section of the American Sociological Association, a member of the Executive Committee of the Disability Forum of the American Public Health Association, an early member of the Society for Disability Studies, and an elected member of the Society for Research in Rehabilitation (UK). He has received the Award for the Promotion of Human Welfare and the Eliot Freidson Award for the book *The Disability Business: Rehabilitation in America.* He also has received a Switzer Distinguished Research Fellowship, Schmidt Fellowship, New York State Supreme Court Fellowship, Kellogg Fellowship,

National Library of Medicine Fellowship, World Health Organization Fellowship, the Lee Founders Award from the Society for the Study of Social Problems, the Licht Award from the American Congress of Rehabilitation Medicine, and the University of Illinois at Chicago Award for Excellence in Teaching.

He has been elected Fellow of the American Association for the Advancement of Science (AAAS) and is a frequent Visiting Fellow at the University of Oxford and Scholar in Residence at the Maison des Sciences de l'Homme, Paris. He has led scientific delegations in rehabilitation medicine to the Soviet Union and the People's Republic of China and served on study sections, grant review panels, and strategic planning committees on disability in Australia, Canada, the European Community, France, Ireland, Poland, Sweden, South Africa, the United States, and the World Health Organization, Geneva. His most recent books are *The Handbook of Social Studies in Health and Medicine* (Sage, 2000, edited with Ray Fitzpatrick and Susan Scrimshaw) and the *Handbook of Disability Studies* (Sage, 2001, edited with Katherine D. Seelman and Michael Bury).

About the Editors of Volume V

David T. Mitchell is Associate Professor of Disability Studies at the University of Illinois at Chicago. From 2000 to 2004, he served as Director of the first Ph.D. program in disability studies. He has also served as president of the Society for Disability Studies and as Chair and founding member of the Modern Language Association's Committee on Disability Issues. He has served on the Board of Directors for Chicago's Independent Living Center, Progress Center, and as an editor on numerous editorial boards including that of the journal *Disability & Society*. He earned his Ph.D. from the Program in American Culture at the University of Michigan, Ann Arbor.

Most recently, Dr. Mitchell has been concerned with the inclusion and advancement of students with disabilities in higher education. Disability studies takes as its charge the goal of making classrooms and the university more accessible. Similarly, fields of inquiry need to become more answerable for their embedded assumptions about disability. Part of this work involves querying the role that disabled persons play as objects for different kinds of knowledge acquisition about them. Consequently, he directed the first National Endowment for the Humanities Summer Institute in Disability Studies for Educators. In addition, he has traveled and lectured extensively on these and other disability studies topics, in the United States, Canada, Germany, Ireland, Russia, Britain, and Costa Rica. In 2004, he codirected a seminar project team that researched euthanasia murder files and original documentation from psychiatric institutions in National Socialist Germany. This commission remains committed to making the history of disability genocide more known, studied about, and understood.

He is coauthor of *Cultural Locations: Discourses of Disability* (2005), coeditor of *Eugenics in America: A History in Primary Sources* (2005), coauthor of *Narrative Prosthesis: Disability and the Dependencies of Discourse* (2000), coeditor of *The Body in Physical Difference: Discourses of Disability* (1998), coeditor of a special issue of *Disability Studies Quarterly* on disability studies in the humanities, and coeditor of a special issue on disability issues in writing by the American author Herman Melville for the journal *Leviathan*.

Sharon L. Snyder is Assistant Professor in the Department of Disability and Human Development at the University of Illinois at Chicago. She is a founding member of the Modern Language Association's Committee on Disability Issues and of the Disability Studies Discussion Group. As a faculty member in the first Ph.D. program in disability studies in the United States, she has developed graduate courses including disability in film, the history of eugenics, representational history, globalization and political economies, and curriculum development for disability studies. In 2004, she directed the Legacies of Eugenics, a DAAD (German Academic Exchange Service) seminar for U.S. and Canadian faculty at the Einstein Forum, Potsdam, Germany. She has codirected a National Endowment for the Humanities Summer Institute and served as a faculty lecturer at the University of Costa Rica.

Dr. Snyder is coauthor of *Cultural Locations of Disability* (2005), coeditor of *Eugenics in America* (2005), coeditor of *Disability Studies: Enabling the Humanities* (2003), coauthor of *Narrative Prosthesis: Disability and the Dependencies of Discourse* (2000), and coeditor of the first collection of essays on disability studies in the humanities, *The Body and Physical Difference: Discourses of Disability* (1997). As the series editor for Corporealities: Discourses of Disability, she has been instrumental in encouraging scholarly work in the new analytical field of disability studies. Her essays on disability theory, disability culture, and representational history have been published widely and translated for many international professional journals.

The founder of the independent production company Brace Yourselves Productions, she is also a documentary filmmaker whose work includes *Self-Preservation: the Art of Riva Lehrer, Disability Takes on the Arts, A World without Bodies*, and *Vital Signs: Crip Culture Talks Back*. Awards for her films include the Festival Grand Prize at Rehabilitation International's Film Festival, Achievement and Merit Awards at Superfest, and Best of the Festival at Moscow's Breaking Down Barriers.

Origins of Disability

◉ The Ancient World ◉ The Bible ◉ The Middle Ages

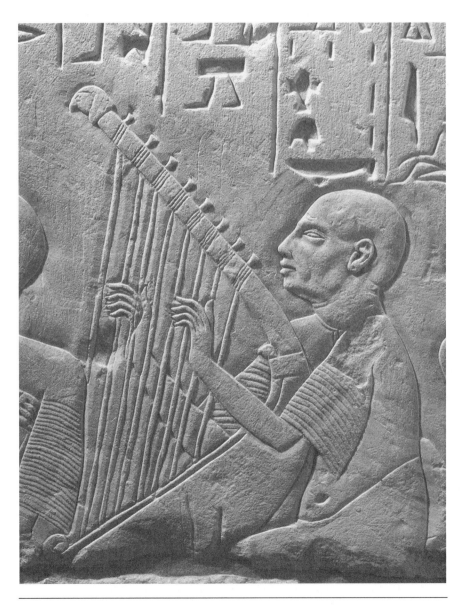

Blind harpist, Nineteenth Dynasty. One of the oldest traditions involves the participation of blind and visually impaired individuals in the profession of music. This detail of a relief was created during the Nineteenth Dynasty, New Kingdom (ca. 1250 bce).

Source: Rijksmuseum van Oudheden, Leiden, The Netherlands. Photo credit: Erich Lessing/Art Resource, New York.

The Ancient World: Sumeria/Mesopotamia

▣ Proverbs from Ki-en-gir (Sumer) (2000 BCE)*

As an early agricultural empire, the Mesopotamian valley hosted the cultivation of a complex system of management that oversaw the investment, production, and distribution of crops throughout the region. Written on clay tablets, the proverbs excerpted below are primarily secular beliefs that seek to sort out the consequences of various virtues and vices associated with human differences. Most proverbs also demonstrate uneven power relationships between disabled and nondisabled participants.

In the city of the lame, the halt are couriers.

How [. . .] the halt stand up?

After a lion had caught a "bush-pig," he roared, "Until now your flesh has not filled my mouth, but your squeals have made me deaf!"

Being strong does not compare to having intelligence.

A fool who was "overwhelmed" at his behind stuck his hand into his behind.

A man whose knees are paralyzed. Nintu has not conceived him, as they say.

A lame man spoke as follows to his mother: "At a place where a man sleeps on a couch let it not please his bones!" His mother spoke as follows: "As if (?) you were afraid of anything, when (?) have we seen you running?"

A lame man saw some runners. "The people who disappeared, where did they go?" he asked.

A lame man came running out from [. . .] and spoke as follows: "As long as I was lame, I could not have done it!"

The poor man caused all kinds of trouble for the wealthy man [. . .] a lasting skin disease.

The lame (?) took a reed basket. For (?) his words a man beats him.

His mother was lame, and his arms are paralyzed.

Source: Alster, Bendt, ed. and trans. 1997. *Proverbs of Ancient Sumeria: The World's Earliest Proverb Collections*. New York: CDL Press.

*A word followed by "(?)" indicates uncertainty on the part of the translator. Lacunae in the text are indicated by [. . .].

▣ The Babylonian Theodicy (ca. 2000 BCE)

This text was created in the form of a dialogue between two actors—one who plays the role of a skeptic (or longtime sufferer) and one who functions as a believer. In this excerpt, the speaker argues that his lot has been so unfair that even cripples and fools enjoy higher social standing.

Your reasoning is a cool breeze, a breath of fresh air for mankind,

Most particular friend, your advice is excellent,

Let me put but one matter before you;

Those who seek not after a god can go the road of favor,

Those who pray to a goddess have grown poor and destitute,

Indeed, in my youth I tried to find out the will of my god,

3

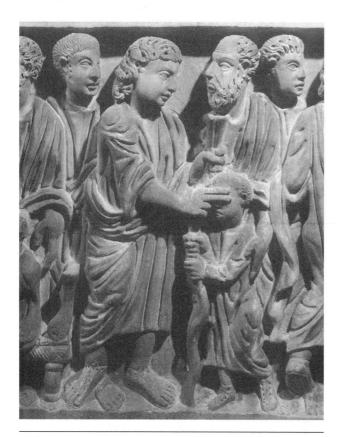

Mythological "scarface" genie from Baktriana, in eastern Iran. Late third to early second century BCE. The "scarface" genie has a body covered with snake scales. It wears a skirt, and its long facial scar symbolizes a destructive ritual.

Source: Louvre, Paris. Erich Lessing/Art Resource, New York.

With prayer and supplication I besought my goddess.
I bore a yoke of profitless servitude,
My god decreed for me poverty instead of wealth
A cripple rises above me, a fool is ahead [of] me,
Rogues are in the ascendant, I am demoted.

Among the friend's standard pious replies, we find:

Adept scholar, master of erudition,
You blaspheme in the anguish of your thoughts,
Divine purpose is as remote as innermost heaven,
It is too difficult to understand, people cannot understand it.

Source: Pritchard, James B., ed. 1958. Pp. 160–168 in *The Ancient Near East: Volume II. A New Anthology of Texts and Pictures.* Princeton, NJ: Princeton University Press.

▣ Hammurabi's Code of Laws
(ca. 1780 BCE)

Following a genealogy of the royal lineage of Hammurabi, a list of some 282 laws make up the Babylonian kingdom's judicial code. Among these laws are the familiar prescriptions of bodily injuries as atonement for various crimes (e.g., an eye for an eye, a tooth for a tooth).

Code of Laws

Battery

195. If a son strike his father, they shall cut off his fingers.

196. If a man destroy the eye of another man, they shall destroy his eye.

197. If one break a man's bone, they shall break his bone.

198. If one destroy the eye of a freeman or break the bone of a freeman, he shall pay one mina of silver.

199. If one destroy the eye of a man's slave or break a bone of a man's slave he shall pay one-half his price.

200. If a man knock out a tooth of a man of his own rank, they shall knock out his tooth.

201. If one knock out the tooth of a freeman, he shall pay one-third mina of silver.

202. If a man strike the person of a man (*i.e.,* commit an assault) who is his superior, he shall receive sixty strokes with an ox-tail whip in public.

203. If a man strike another man of his own rank, he shall pay one mina of silver.

209. If a man strike a man's daughter and bring about a miscarriage, he shall pay ten shekels of silver for her miscarriage.

210. If that woman die, they shall put his daughter to death.

211. If, through a stroke, he bring about a miscarriage to the daughter of a freeman, he shall pay five shekels of silver.

212. If that woman die, he shall pay one-half mina of silver.

Physicians

215. If a physician operate on a man for a severe wound (or make a severe wound upon a man) with a bronze lancet and save the man's life; or if he open an

abscess (in the eye) of a man with a bronze lancet and save that man's eye, he shall receive ten shekels of silver (as his fee).

216. If he be a freeman, he shall receive five shekels.

217. If it be a man's slave, the owner of the slave shall give two shekels of silver to the physician.

218. If a physician operate on a man for a severe wound with a bronze lancet and cause the man's death; or open an abscess (in the eye) of a man with a bronze lancet and destroy the man's eye, they shall cut off his fingers.

221. If a physician set a broken bone for a man or cure his diseased bowels, the patient shall give five shekels of silver to the physician.

Source: Harper, Robert Francis, trans. 1904. *The Code of Hammurabi, King of Babylon, About 2250 B.C.*, 2nd ed. Chicago: University of Chicago Press.

◉ The Laws of Eshunna
(ca. 1770 BCE)*

Dadusha of Eshunna was one of the first to document laws in the Babylonian language. The document consists of 60 paragraphs. It begins with the establishment of tariffs and then discusses ships and grain, family and slaves, physical wounds, animals, and the construction of houses. In this excerpt from the section on physical wounds, injuries to various body parts are assigned a hierarchical sum in terms of their value to the injured.

42: If a man bites the nose of a(nother) man and severs it, he shall pay 1 mina of silver. (For) an eye (he shall pay) 1 mina of silver; (for) a tooth 1/2 mina; (for) an ear 1/2 mina; (for) a slap in the face 10 shekels of silver.

43: If a man severs a(nother) man's finger, he shall pay two-thirds of a mina of silver.

44: If a man throws a(nother) man to the floor in an *altercation* and breaks his *hand,* he shall pay 1/2 mina of silver.

45: If he breaks his foot, he shall pay 1/2 mina of silver.

46: If a man assaults a(nother) man and breaks his [. . .], he shall pay two-thirds of a mina of silver.

47: If a man *hits* a(nother) man *accidentally,* he shall pay 10 shekels of sliver.

Source: Schley, Donald G., trans. 1985. "Law." Chapter 10 in *The Ancient Orient: An Introduction to the Study of the Ancient Near East,* Wolfram Von Soden, ed. Grand Rapids, MI: William B. Eerdmans.

*Lacunae in the text are indicated by [. . .].

◉ Ludlul Bêl Nimeqi (Sumerian Wisdom Text: Man and His God) (ca. 1700 BCE)*

Zugagib, one of the early kings of Sumer, is said to have ruled for 840 years. His story in this excerpt provides striking images of suffering and the attendant amelioration that healing can offer. Many scholars believe this document to be an early source for the biblical tale of Job.

53. [He who made woman] and created man
Marduk, has ordained (?) that he be encompassed with sickness (?) [. . .]

54. And [. . .] in whatever [. . .]
He said: "How long will he be in such great affliction and distress?
What is it that he saw in his vision of the night?"
"In the dream Ur-Bau appeared
A mighty hero wearing his crown

55. A conjurer, too, clad in strength,
Marduk indeed sent me;
Unto Shubshi-meshri-Nergal he brought abundance;
In his pure hands he brought abundance. . . ."

58. . . . He approached (?) and the spell which he had pronounced (?) . . .

59. He sent a storm wind to the horizon;
To the breast of the earth it bore a blast
Into the depth of his ocean the disembodied spirit vanished (?);
Unnumbered spirits he sent back to the under-world.
The [. . .] of the hag-demons he sent straight to the mountain.

60. The sea-flood he spread with ice;

The roots of the disease he tore out like a plant.

The horrible slumber that settled on my rest

Like smoke filled the sky [. . .]

With the woe he had brought, unrepulsed and bitter, he filled the earth like a storm.

61. The unrelieved headache which had overwhelmed the heavens

He took away and sent down on me the evening dew.

My eyelids, which he had veiled with the veil of night

He blew upon with a rushing wind and made clear their sight.

My ears, which were stopped, were deaf as a deaf man's

62. He removed their deafness and restored their hearing.

My nose, whose nostril had been stopped from my mother's womb—

He eased its deformity so that I could breathe.

My lips, which were closed he had taken their strength—

He removed their trembling and loosed their bond.

63. My mouth which was closed so that I could not be understood—

He cleansed it like a dish, he healed its disease.

My eyes, which had been attacked so that they rolled together—

He loosed their bond and their balls were set right.

The tongue, which had stiffened so that it could not be raised

64. He relieved its thickness, so its words could be understood.

The gullet which was compressed, stopped as with a plug—

He healed its contraction, it worked like a flute.

My spittle which was stopped so that it was not secreted—

He removed its fetter, he opened its lock.

Source: Pritchard, James B., ed. 1958. Pp. 148–160 in *The Ancient Near East: Volume II. A New Anthology of Texts and Pictures.* Princeton, NJ: Princeton University Press.

*A word followed by "(?)" indicates uncertainty on the part of the translator. Lacunae in the text are indicated by [. . .].

▣ *The Omen Series Summa Izbu*
(ca. 1300 BCE)*

These tablets, compiled in the Mesopotamian region over a period of 2000 years, recorded predictions of good or bad events (including events of national significance) thought to be signaled by the birth of a human or animal with a physical deformity. According to Leichty, "Late in the Middle Babylonian period," the records were systematized in order "to cover all the possible [occurrences] of abnormal births" (p. 24). Some examples not included in the excerpt include the following: "If a woman of the palace gives birth to a deaf child—the possessions of the king will be lost" (p. 70), and "If a woman of the palace gives birth, and (the child) has six fingers on its left hand, the prince will plunder the land of his enemy" (p. 71).

If a woman is pregnant, and her foetus cries—the land will experience mis-fortune.

If a woman gives birth to a male idiot—troubles; scattering of the house of the man.

If a woman gives birth to a female idiot—the house of the man will [. . .]

If a woman gives birth to a male dwarf—troubles; the house of the man will be scattered.

If a woman gives birth to a female dwarf—correspondingly.

If a woman gives birth to a boy cripple—the house of the man will suffer.

If a woman gives birth to a girl cripple—the house of the man will be scattered; ditto (i.e., will suffer).

If a woman gives birth to a male form—good news will arrive in the land.

If a woman gives birth to a female form—that house will get ahead; he (i.e., the father) will have good luck.

If a woman gives birth to a blind child—the land will be disturbed; the house of the man will not prosper.

If a woman gives birth to [. . .]—that city will experience destruction outside (?).

If a woman gives birth to a cripple (lit. a contorted one)—the land will be disturbed; the house of the man will be scattered.

If a woman gives birth to a deaf child—that house will prosper outside (of its city).

If a woman gives birth to a giant, either male or female—a sinful man impregnated that woman in the street.

If a woman gives birth to a child with two faces—the reign of a despotic king will be changed.

If a woman gives birth to an albino (?)—that house will not prosper.

If a woman gives birth to half of a human form—that house will be scattered.

If a woman gives birth, and (the child) is half a cubit tall, he is bearded, he can talk, he can walk, and he has teeth; his is called "tigrilu"—reign of Nergal; a fierce attack; there will be a mighty person in the land; pestilence; one street will be hostile to the other; one house will plunder the other.

If a woman gives birth to two boys—there will be hard times in the land; the land will experience unhappiness; there will be bad times for the house of their father.

If a woman gives birth to two boys, and they have one abdomen (between them)—

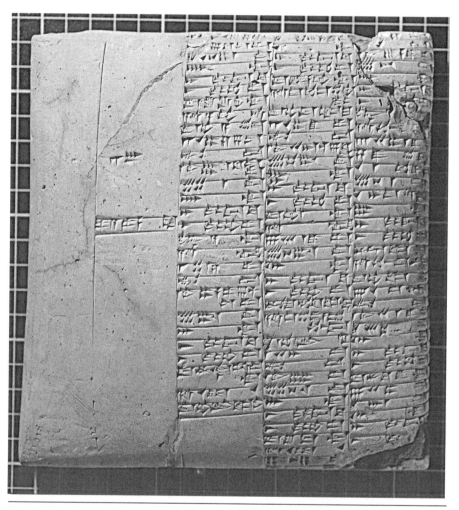

Ancient Sumerian cuneiform tablet (1300 BCE) describing a science of foretelling future events from the features of disabled fetuses and irregularly shaped animal livers.

Source: British Museum, London. Photo credit: Sharon Snyder.

(there will be) dissension (between) man and wife; the house [. . .].

If a woman gives birth to two (children), and they are joined like the "Bull(god), son of Samas"—the king will conquer his enemies.

If a woman gives birth to two (children), and they are connected at their spine, but their faces are opposite (each other)—the land's gods will leave it; (there will be) dissension (between) the king and his sons.

If a woman gives birth to two (children), and they have neither nose nor feet—the land of the king will become waste.

If a woman gives birth to twins for a second time—that land will disappear; the house of the man will be scattered.

If a woman gives birth to twins, and they are joined at their rib(s)—two will rule the land which one ruled.

If a woman gives birth to twins, and they are joined at their rib(s), and the right one has no right hand—an enemy will defeat me in battle, and diminish the land, (and) make it weak; he will defeat my army.

If a woman gives birth to twins, and ditto (i.e. they are joined at their ribs), and the left one has no left hand—you will defeat the enemy in battle, and correspondingly.

Source: Leichty, Erle, ed. and trans. 1970. *The Omen Series Summa Izbu*. Locust Valley, NY: Augustin.

*A word followed by "(?)" indicates uncertainty on the part of the translator. Lacunae in the text are indicated by [. . .].

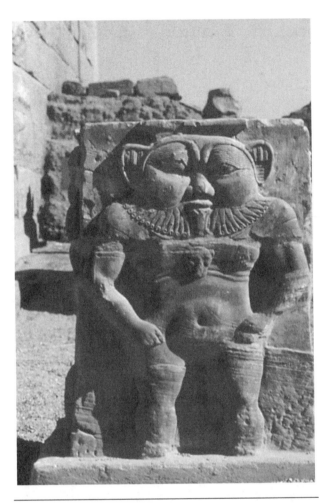

The god Besh, usually shown as a dwarf, is a domestic god, protector of women in childbirth, and is also associated with music and dance.

Source: Temple of Hathor, Dendera, Egypt. Photo credit: Erich Lessing/Art Resource, New York.

◉ Nabonidus and His God (539 BCE)

The excerpt below records a fragment of the words of the prayer said by King Nabonidus of Babylonia after being cured of the ulcer that had afflicted him for seven years. Two facts about Nabonidus can be corroborated by referring to other texts: Nabonidus was believed to have a mental illness, and he insulted the Babylonian clergy by being monotheistic. The text below may have been modified to fit the prohibitions on priestly purity identified in Leviticus.

Words of the prayer, said by Nabonidus, king of Babylonia, the great king, when afflicted with an ulcer on command of the most high God in Temâ:

I, Nabonidus, was afflicted with an evil ulcer for seven years, and far from men I was driven, until I prayed to the most high God. And an exorcist pardoned my sins. He was a Jew from among the children of the exile of Judah, and said: "Recount this in writing to glorify and exalt the name of the most high God." Then I wrote this: "When I was afflicted for seven years by the most high God with an evil ulcer during my stay at Temâ, I prayed to the gods of silver and gold, bronze and iron, wood, stone and lime, because I thought and considered them gods [. . .]

Source: Pritchard, James B., ed. 1958. Pp. 108–112 in *The Ancient Near East: Volume II. A New Anthology of Texts and Pictures.* Princeton, NJ: Princeton University Press.

◉ The Zend-Avesta
(6th c. BCE ?)

The Avesta, the earliest sacred text of Zoroastrianism, dates possibly from the sixth century BCE, and its meanings are not entirely transparent to modern interpreters. One section, the Vendidad (more correctly transcribed as Videvdat), gives an early sketch of an imagined "new world," utopia, or paradise, from which disability, disease, and behavioral weaknesses are excluded, perhaps by selective breeding or eugenics (Vendidad, Fargard II, 27–37, pp. 17–19 in this translation). The disabilities and unpleasant behavior seem to be attributed to the activity of Angra Mainyu, the power of darkness in the Avestan cosmology. Some interpreters understand the list of "disabilities" as referring to moral depravity rather than to physical impairment.

Fargard II

21 (42). The Maker, Ahura Mazda, of high renown in the Airyana Vaêgô, by the good river Dâitya, called together a meeting of the celestial gods.

The fair Yima, the good shepherd, of high renown in the Airyana Vaêgô, by the good river Dâitya, called together a meeting of the excellent mortals.

To that meeting came Ahura Mazda, of high renown in the Airyana Vaêgô, by the good river Dâitya; he came together with the celestial gods.

To that meeting came, the fair Yima, the good shepherd, of high renown in the Airyana Vaêgô, by the good river Dâitya; he came together with the excellent mortals.

22 (46). And Ahura Mazda spake unto Yima, saying: 'O fair Yima, son of Vîvanghat! Upon the material world the fatal winters are going to fall, that shall bring the fierce, foul frost; upon the material world the fatal winters are going to fall, that shall make snow-flakes fall thick, even an aredvî deep on the highest tops of mountains.

23 (52). And all the three sorts of beasts shall perish, those that live in the wilderness, and those that live on the tops of the mountains, and those that live in the bosom of the dale, under the shelter of stables.

24 (57). Before that winter, those fields would bear plenty of grass for cattle: now with floods that stream, with snows that melt, it will seem a happy land in the world, the land wherein footprints even of sheep may still be seen.

25 (61). Therefore make thee a Vara, long as a riding-ground on every side of the square, and thither bring the seeds of sheep and oxen, of men, of dogs, of birds, and of red blazing fires.

Therefore make thee a Vara, long as a riding-ground on every side of the square, to be an abode for men; a Vara, long as a riding-ground on every side of the square, to be a fold for flocks.

26 (65). There thou shalt make waters flow in a bed a hâthra long; there thou shalt settle birds, by the ever-green banks that bear never-failing food. There thou shalt establish dwelling places, consisting of a house with a balcony, a courtyard, and a gallery.

27 (70). Thither thou shalt bring the seeds of men and women, of the greatest, best, and finest kinds on this earth; thither thou shalt bring the seeds of every kind of cattle, of the greatest, best, and finest kinds on this earth.

28 (74). Thither thou shalt bring the seeds of every kind of tree, of the greatest, best, and finest kinds on this earth; thither thou shalt bring the seeds of every kind of fruit, the fullest of food and sweetest of odour. All those seeds shalt thou bring, two of every kind, to be kept inexhaustible there, so long as those men shall stay in the Vara.

29 (80). There shall be no humpbacked, none bulged forward there; no impotent, no lunatic; no poverty, no lying; no meanness, no jealousy; no decayed tooth, no leprous to be confined, nor any of the brands wherewith Angra Mainyu stamps the bodies of mortals.

30 (87). In the largest part of the place thou shalt make nine streets, six in the middle part, three in the smallest. To the streets of the largest part thou shalt

bring a thousand seeds of men and women; to the streets of the middle part, six hundred; to the streets of the smallest part, three hundred. That Vara thou shalt seal up with the golden ring, and thou shalt make a door, and a window self-shining within.

31 (93). Then Yima said within himself: 'How shall I manage to make that Vara which Ahura Mazda has commanded me to make?'

And Ahura Mazda said unto Yima: 'O fair Yima, son of Vîvanghat! Crush the earth with a stamp of thy heel, and then knead it with thy hands, as the potter does when kneading the potter's clay.'

32. And Yima did as Ahura Mazda wished; he crushed the earth with a stamp of his heel, he kneaded it with his hands, as the potter does when kneading the potter's clay. [Paragraph 32 is found in an alternate version of the text.]

33 (97). And Yima made a Vara, long as a riding-ground on every side of the square. There he brought the seeds of sheep and oxen, of men, of dogs, of birds, and of red blazing fires. He made Vara, long as a riding-ground on every side of the square, to be an abode for men; a Vara, long as a riding-ground on every side of the square, to be a fold for flocks.

34 (101). There he made waters flow in a bed a hâthra long; there he settled birds, by the evergreen banks that bear never-failing food. There he established dwelling places, consisting of a house with a balcony, a courtyard, and a gallery.

35 (106). There he brought the seeds of men and women, of the greatest, best, and finest kinds on this earth; there he brought the seeds of every kind of cattle, of the greatest, best, and finest kinds on this earth.

36 (110). There he brought the seeds of every kind of tree, of the greatest, best, and finest kinds on this earth; there he brought the seeds of every kind of fruit, the fullest of food and sweetest of odour. All those seeds he brought, two of every kind, to be kept inexhaustible there, so long as those men shall stay in the Vara.

37 (116). And there were no humpbacked, none bulged forward there; no impotent, no lunatic; no poverty, no lying; no meanness, no jealousy; no decayed tooth, no leprous to be confined, nor any of the brands wherewith Angra Mainyu stamps the bodies of mortals.

38 (123). In the largest part of the place he made nine streets, six in the middle part, three in the smallest. To the streets of the largest part he brought a thousand seeds of men and women; to the streets of the

middle part, six hundred; to the streets of the smallest part, three hundred. That Vara he sealed up with the golden ring, and he made a door, and a window self-shining within.

39 (129). O Maker of the material world, thou Holy One! What (lights are there to give light) in the Vara which Yima made? [The material in parentheses is found in an alternate version of the text.]

40 (131). Ahura Mazda answered: 'There are uncreated lights and created lights. There the stars, the moon, and the sun are only once (a year) seen to rise and set, and a year seems only as a day.

41 (33). 'Every fortieth year, to every couple two are born, a male and a female. And thus it is for every sort of cattle. And the men in the Vara which Yima made live the happiest life.'

42 (137). O Maker of the material world, thou Holy One! Who is he who brought the law of Mazda into the Vara which Yima made?

Ahura Mazda answered: 'It was the bird Karshipta, O holy Zarathustra!'

43 (140). O Maker of the material world, thou Holy One! Who is the lord and ruler there?

Ahura Mazda answered: 'Urvata*d*-nara, O Zarathustra! and thyself, Zarathustra.'

Source: Darmesteter, James, trans. 1880. *Sacred Books of the East: Vol. 4. The Zend-Avesta: Part I. The Vendidad.* Oxford, UK: Oxford University Press.

▣ The Uruk Incantation
(ca. 3rd c. BCE)

The Uruk incantation is an example of spoken chants offered by incantation priests in temple. It may have been written around 1600 BCE by Sin-leqe-unnini, the master scribe of the Gilgamesh epic during the Kassite period in Mesopotamia. The following excerpt invokes miraculous cures for various disabilities.

I have taken a (magic) bond from the wooden roof, in silence, from the threshold of the gate. I have put it underneath my tongue. I have entered a house full of words, a tongue-tied table, a mixing bowl (full) of poison. When they saw me, the house full of words fell silent, the tongue-tied table was upset, the mixing bowl (full) of poison was poured out.

I have been successful, and I am successful . . . before adults and children, women and men, . . . and

those assembled and sitting at the gate, before so-and-so, from *everything.*

Remove, drive out pains! Defective one, be wh(ole)! Lame one, run! Find companions, excessive one! *Finally,* (you all) rise!

Speak, dumb one! Rise, silent one!

Who is angry, who is enraged, who is clothed in the garment of anger, (has) fire in his mouth, (has) *mixtures (of spittle)* underneath his tongue? So-and-so, the son of so-and-so, is angry and enraged, is clothed in the garment of anger, (has) fire in his mo[uth], (has) *mixtures (of spittle)* underneath his tongue, I am wise . . .

I have taken a (magic) knot from [*the threshold?*], soundless(ly), from the room [(*below) the roof*]. I have entered into the presence of so-and-so . . . I have made him take off the garment of anger. I have clothed him in the garment of . . . I have taken the fire from his mouth, the *mixtures (of spittle)* from underneath [*his tongue*]. My good things from his mouth [*come forth*], my evil things from *his posterior* [. . .], before adults and children, women and men, [. . . and those assembled] and sitting at the gate, and before s[o-and-so . . .].

[*Remove, drive out pains!*] Defective one, [be whole]! Lame one, run! Find companions, excessive one! *Finally,* (you all) rise!

Speak dumb one! Rise, silent one!

Source: Pritchard, James B., ed. 1958. Pp. 220–221 in *The Ancient Near East: Volume II. A New Anthology of Texts and Pictures.* Princeton, NJ: Princeton University Press.

▣ Story of Enkidu (Wolf Child)
(2nd c. BCE)

The Epic of Gilgamesh, possibly from the second millennium BCE, appears to include an early description of a "feral child and young man" named Enkidu. He is primitive and hairy, was raised on wild asses' milk, eats grass with gazelles and drinks at cattle's water holes, and is unfamiliar with ordinary human food and drink. After his seduction and education by a temple prostitute, Enkidu joins Gilgamesh in his quest. He experiences an episode of paralysis but recovers and helps his friend in battle. Many conflicting interpretations of this part of the epic have been proposed.

So the Goddess of Creation took and formed in her mind
This image, and there it was conceived—in her mind, and it was made of material
That composes the Great God,
He of the Firmament.
She then plunged her hands down into water and pinched off a little clay.
She let it drop in the wilderness
Thus the noble Enkidu was made. For this was he the very strength of Ninurta, the God of War, was his form, rough bodied, long hair,
His hair waved like corn filaments—Yes, like the hair of that goddess
Who is the corn, she, Nisaba. Matted hair was all over his body, like the skins of the cattle.
Yes, like the body of that god.
Who is the cattle, he, Samugan.
This Enkidu was innocent of mankind.
He knew not the cultivated land.
Enkidu was in the hills
With the gazelles—
They jostled each other
With all the herds
He too loved the water-hole.
But one day by a water hole
A trapper met him
Yes, face to face,
Because the herds of wild game
Had strayed into his territory.
On three days face to face—
Each day the trapper was terrified,
Frozen stiff with fear.
With his game he went home,
Unable to speak, numb with fright.
The trapper's face altered, new—
A long journey does that to one,
Gives a new visage upon returning—
The trapper, his heart all awe, told his father:
'Father, what a man! No other like him! He comes from the hills, strongest alive!
A star in heaven his strength,
Of the star essence of An, the Sky Father
Over the hills with the beasts
Eating grass
Ranges across all your land,
Goes to the wells.
I fear him, stay far away.
He fills in my pits
Tears up my game traps

Helps the beasts escape;
Now all the game slips away—
Through my fingers.'
His father opened his mouth,
Told the son, the trapper:
'My son, in Uruk lives Gilgamesh.
None can withstand him,
None has surpassed him,
As a star in heaven his strength
Of the star-essence of An, the Sky Father.
Go to Uruk, find Gilgamesh
Praise the wild man's strength ask for a temple hierodule from the Temple of Love,
Such a child of pleasure;
Bring her and let her power of woman
Subdue this wild man.
When he goes to the wells,
He will embrace the priestess
And the wild beasts will reject him.'
To Uruk the trapper went
And said to Gilgamesh:
'Like no other, wild,
Roaming in the pastures,
A star in heaven his strength
Of the star-essence of An, the Sky Father.
I am afraid, stay far away; he helps the beasts escape
Fills in my pits
Tears up my game traps.'
Gilgamesh said:
'Trapper, return,
Take a priestess, child of pleasure—
When he goes to the wells
He will embrace the priestess
And the wild beasts will reject him.'
Then returned with the hierodule
And three days to the drinking hole,
There sat down
Hierodule facing the trapper,
Waiting for the game.
First day, nothing.
Second day, nothing.
Third day, yes.
The herds came to drink, and Enkidu—
Glad for the water were the small wild beasts,
And Enkidu was glad for the water—
He of the gazelles and wild grass,
Born in the hills.
The priestess saw this man
Wild from the hills.
'There, woman,' the trapper,

'Bare your breasts now;
This is he,
Have no shame, delay not,
Welcome his love,
Let him see you naked,
Let him possess your body.
As he approaches, take off your clothes,
Lie with him, teach him,
The savage, your art of woman,
For as he loves you, then
The wild beasts, his companions,
They will reject him.'
She had no shame for this,
Made herself naked
Welcomed his eagerness
Incited him to love,
Taught the woman's art.
Six days, seven nights,
That time lying together,
Enkidu had forgotten his home
Had forgotten the hills
After that time he was satisfied.
Then he went back to the wild beasts—
But the gazelles saw him and ran,
The wild beasts saw him and ran.
Enkidu would follow, but weak,
His strength gone through woman;
Wisdom was in him,
Thoughts in his head— a man's.
So he returned to the priestess.
At her feet he listened intently
'You have wisdom, Enkidu.
Now you are as a god.
Why the beasts? Why the hills?
Come to Uruk of the strong walls
To Inanna's Temple of Love,
And to the Eanna,
Where the Sky God An can be found.
Gilgamesh is there, strong,
Raging like a wild bull, over all
Is his strength.'
Favourably as he speaks, he hears her words.
He comes to know his own heart
And his desire to find a friend.
He tells her, the priestess:
'Take me, girl, to the sacred pure
Dwelling of Love and Sky God's house
Where lives Gilgamesh of perfect strength,
He who rages like a bull over all,
And I will summon him forth and challenge him

And I will shout in Uruk:
"I am the mightiest!
Yes, I can change the order of what is!
Anyone born on the steppe is mighty and has strength"'
'Then let us go that he may see your face
And I will show you Gilgamesh, for I know well where he is.
Come Enkidu, to Uruk of ramparts,
Where all are dressed for festival,
Where each day is a festival,
Where there are boys,
Where there are girls,
Deliciously ripe and perfumed,
Who drive the great ones from their fretted couches
To you, Enkidu, of joy in life
I will show Gilgamesh of joy in life
See him, see his face
Radiant is his manhood, of full-bodied vigour
His body ripe with beauty in every part.
So exceeding you in strength,
Needing no sleep by day or by night.
Restrain your folly, Enkidu.
Gilgamesh—Shamash the Sun is proud,
Also An, the God of Firmament,
Also valiant Enlil, his son,
And Enki, his son also—
All have given wisdom.
Before you come from the open plains
Gilgamesh will have dreamed of it.'
And so Gilgamesh rose from his bed
And to his mother, in revealing dreams, said:
'Mother, I saw in a dream last night
That there were stars in heaven
And a star descended upon me like unto
The essence of An, the Sky God.
I tried to lift it up, but it was too heavy for me,
I tried to move it, but it would not be moved.
The land of Uruk was around it,
The land was placed round about it.
All the people were pressing towards it.
All the nobles also came round it,
And all my friends kissed its feet.
I was drawn towards it as to a woman
And I laid it at your feet
And you said it was my equal.'
She, the Wise, the Custodian of Knowledge,
Says to her lord—
She, Ninsun, Custodian of Knowledge,
Says to Gilgamesh:

'Your equal was a star of heaven
Which descended upon you like unto
The essence of An who is the God of the Firmament
You tried to lift it but it would not be moved
And I called it your equal, comparing it to you.
You were drawn to it as to a woman.
The meaning of this
Is of a strong friend who saves his companion
He is the strongest of the land; he has strength.
As a star in heaven his strength,
The strength of An of the Firmament and his host.
So that you are drawn to him overwhelmingly.
And this means he will never forsake you.
Such is your dream.'
Gilgamesh says again to his mother:
'Mother, another dream
In Uruk of the ramparts lay an axe—All were gathered around it,
Uruk-land was standing round about it.
The people pressed towards it;
I laid it at your feet.
I was drawn to it as to a woman.

For you called it my equal.'
She, the Wise Custodian of Knowledge, says to her son—
'The axe is a man
You were drawn to it as to a woman
For I called it your equal
And it was to rival you.
This means a strong friend standing by his friend
He is the strongest of the land; he has strength.
The essence of An of the Firmament, is his,
So strong is he.'
Gilgamesh then spoke to his mother
'Now according to the word of God Enlil
Let a counsellor and friend come to me
That I may acquire a companion
And to him I shall be friend and counsellor also.'
And as Gilgamesh revealed his dream
The girl was speaking to Enkidu
As they sat together.

Source: Temple, Robert, trans. 1991. *The Epic of Gilgamesh*. London: Rider.

The Ancient World: South Asia

▣ *Caraka Samhita*
(400–200 BCE)

This ancient text, which helped establish the philosophical foundations of Indian medicine, describes the ideal characteristics of a physician. According to the Caraka, health and disease are not necessarily predetermined, and life may be prolonged by human efforts.

3.8.8: He should be peaceful, noble in disposition, incapable of any mean act, with straight eyes, face and nose, with slim body, having a clean and red tongue, without distortion of teeth or lips, with clear voice (i.e. with voice neither indistinct nor nasal), preserving, without egotism, intelligent, endowed with powers of reasoning and good memory, with broad mind, inclined to medical study either because of being born in the family of physicians or by natural aptitude, with eagerness to have the knowledge of truth, with no deformity of body and no defect of sense-organs, by nature modest and gentle, contemplating on the true nature of things, without anger and without addiction, endowed with good conduct, cleanliness, good habits, love, skill and courtesy, desirous of the welfare of all living beings, devoid of greed and laziness and having full loyalty and attachment to the teacher.

4.2.31–38: The mind is indeed bound by passion and ignorance and, in the absence of knowledge, all disorders are brought about by them. This mind along with its disorders and the force of past actions are the causes of transmigration of the self from life to life as well as for righteous and unrighteous conduct.

Source: Sharma, P. V., trans. 1981. Pp. ix–xxxii in *Caraka Samhita.* Varanasi, India: Chaukhamba Orientalia.

▣ Jataka Tales: "The Tricky Wolf and the Rats" (3rd c. BCE)

The Buddhist Jatakas consist of some 538 lively stories of events during the incarnations of the Buddha, compiled perhaps in the third century BCE. They were handy teaching tools, ranging from short to very long, each embodying one or more moral lessons. Itinerant monks spread them across South and East Asia over centuries, and many different language versions exist. Several Jatakas are specifically on disability themes, and disabled people appear casually in many others. Some portray unexpected features, such as a warrior dwarf, a cripple who is an ace stone-thrower, and a blind sea pilot who sees more with his hands than other men do with two eyes.

Once upon a time a Big Rat lived in the forest, and many hundreds of other Rats called him their Chief.

A Tricky Wolf saw this troop of Rats, and began to plan how he could catch them. He wanted to eat them, but how was he to get them? At last he thought of a plan. He went to a corner near the home of the Rats and waited until he saw one of them coming. Then he stood up on his hind legs.

The Chief of the Rats said to the Wolf, "Wolf, why do you stand on your hind legs?"

"Because I am lame," said the Tricky Wolf. "It hurts me to stand on my front legs."

"And why do you keep your mouth open?" asked the Rat.

"I keep my mouth open so that I may drink in all the air I can," said the Wolf. "I live on air; it is my only food day after day. I can not run or walk, so I stay here. I try not to complain." When the Rats went away the Wolf lay down.

The Chief of the Rats was sorry for the Wolf, and he went each night and morning with all the other Rats to talk with the Wolf, who seemed so poor, and who did not complain.

Each time as the Rats were leaving, the Wolf caught and ate the last one. Then he wiped his lips, and looked as if nothing had happened.

Each night there were fewer Rats at bedtime. Then they asked the Chief of the Rats what the trouble was. He could not be sure, but he thought the Wolf was to blame.

So the next day the Chief said to the other Rats, "You go first this time and I will go last."

They did so, and as the Chief of the Rats went by, the Wolf made a spring at him. But the Wolf was not quick enough, and the Chief of the Rats got away.

"So this is the food you eat. Your legs are not so lame as they were. You have played your last trick, Wolf," said the Chief of the Rats, springing at the Wolf's throat. He bit the Wolf, so that he died.

And ever after the Rats lived happily in peace and quiet.

Source: Babbitt, Ellen C., trans. 1922. "The Tricky Wolf and the Rats." Pp. 11–14 in *More Jataka Tales*. New York: Appleton-Century.

▣ *The Mahabharata*
(3rd c. BCE)

The blind King Dhritarashtra appears throughout the Mahabharata—not really in the battle books, but he is there in the background having the awful scenes verbally described to him, which is how we also get to hear about it all. Some mention is included of "idiots," "stupidity," "fools," "undeveloped mind," and so forth, yet it is clear that the use of such terms ranges from descriptions of people with what is now called mental handicap or intellectual disability (identifiable through references to a lack of spiritual discernment) to mere personal abuse.

Adi Parva

[Editor's note: The following provides paraphrases of relevant sections of the *Mahabharata*, with explanatory notes in brackets where necessary and occasional quotations for especially important points.]

[Several reasons were offered to explain Dhritarashtra's blindness, as follows.]

I Dhritarashtra refers to his blindness as being among the reasons why he could not prevent the dispute between his sons and nephews.

LXVII Dhritarashtra was blind through his mother's fault and the wrath of the Rishi.

CVI [Note that in this section, for *blind,* J. A. B. van Buitenen's translation (1973, 1975) has "with the eyesight of wisdom."] To perpetuate the Bharata line the Rishi Dwaipayana (Vyasa) is called upon to impregnate the widows of his half-brother Vichitravirya. The first of these princesses, afraid of the rishi's grim appearance, closes her eyes in fear and keeps them shut. The son (Dhritarashtra) is thereby doomed to be born blind. The second widow keeps her eyes open, but she is pale with fear. Her son, Pandu (i.e., "the pale") is therefore pale. The first widow is later asked to try for a second son, but she sends her Sudra maid instead. From her, Vidura is born.

[Debates ensue about blindness as an appropriate reason to exclude Dhritarashtra from becoming king.]

CIX Pandu becomes king, Dhritarashtra being disqualified by his blindness, Vidura by having a Sudra mother.

CX King Suvala, with some qualms, gives his daughter Gandhari to wed the blind Dhritarashtra. Gandhari takes to wearing a blindfold, through respect for her future husband.

CXXXVI Dhritarashtra regrets that, because he is blind, he cannot see the weapons skills display given by his sons on the completion of their education. As it proceeds, Vidura describes the feats to Dhritarashtra, Kunti and Gandhari.

CXLIII Discussion of whether it was right that Dhritarashtra, being blind, took over the kingdom after Pandu's death.

CXLVII Blind men given as an example of ignorance.

Sabha Parva

[Editor's note: Early medical attitudes toward human variation and further discrimination experienced by Dhritarashtra.]

V Instruction from the Rishi Narada to King Yudhishthira includes the questions:

Seekest thou to cure bodily diseases by medicines and fasts, and mental illness with the advice of the aged? I hope that the physicians engaged in looking after thy health are well conversant with the eight kinds of treatment and are all attached and devoted to thee.

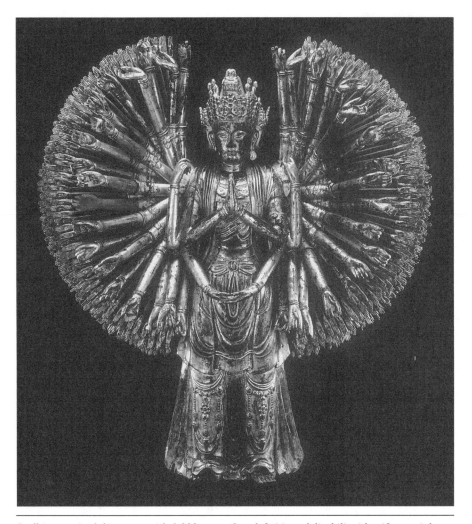

Bodhisattva Avalokitesvara with 1,000 arms. One definition of disability identifies social perceptions of human forms based on too much or too little body. The supernatural powers of gods are often identified in this manner, but it is unclear what impact this presentation mode had on the experiences of disabled people of the time. Frontal view. Chinese wood sculpture, 160 120 50 cm.

Source: Musée des Arts Asiatiques-Guimet, Paris. Photo by Thierry Ollivier. Photo credit: Réunion des Musées Nationaux/Art Resource, New York.

V "Cherishest thou like a father, the blind, the dumb, the lame, the deformed, the friendless, and ascetics that have no homes?"

X The husband of Uma, three-eyed Mahadeva, is described as being surrounded by hundreds and thousands of spirits, "some of dwarfish stature, some of fierce visage, some hunch-backed," and so on.

XVII Vrihadratha, king of Magadha, marries twin wives but has no son. He obtains a blessed mango, which his wives divide and eat. They conceive, and each bears half a baby, which their two midwives wrap and throw out at the back door. A rakshasa woman, Jara, collects and unites the pieces, which

then become a living child, Jarasandha.

XXIII Before unarmed combat between Jarasandha and Bhima, a priest brings "various excellent medicines for restoring lost consciousness and alleviating pain."

XXX Among various conquests by Sahadeva is "a wild tribe by the name of the Kerakas who were men with one leg."

XLII Sisupala is born with three eyes and four hands. His parents, the king of Chedi and his wife, consider abandoning the child, but a voice forbids them. Many visitors come to see the monster. Later the child's spare arms fall off and the third eye disappears when he is placed on the lap of Damodara.

L Among the visitors failing to gain admission to the court of King Yudhishthira are some tribes with three eyes, some with eyes on their foreheads, and many with only one leg.

LI Yajnaseni (Draupadi) daily attends to the needs of everybody, "including even the deformed and the dwarfs," before taking food herself.

LV The "weak-minded" Dhritarashtra, "deprived of reason by Fate," gives in to the plan to seize the wealth of Pandu's sons by gambling.

LXIII Vidura, knowing that his rebukes to Dhritarashtra and Duryodhana are unwelcome, tells the king that "if thou wishest to hear words that are agreeable to thee, in respect of all acts good or bad, ask thou women and idiots and cripples or persons of that description."

LXXII Dhritarashtra, trying to placate Pandu's sons after their defeat in the first gambling match, appeals to them with the fact that he is "old and blind."

LXXX Sanjaya remarks to Dhritarashtra, about Duryodhana, that "The gods first deprive that man of his reason unto whom they send defeat and disgrace."

Vana Parva

II Saunaka counsels Yudhishthira for depression:

Sensible physicians first seek to allay the mental sufferings of their patients by agreeable converse and the offer of desirable objects. And as a hot iron bar thrust into a jar makes the water therein hot, even so doth mental grief bring on bodily agony. And as water quenches fire, so doth true knowledge allay mental disquietude. And the mind attaining ease, the body findeth ease also.

XLIX Dhritarashtra complains that "seeing me void of eye-sight, and incapable of exerting myself actively, my wretched son, O charioteer, believeth me to be a fool, and listeneth not to my words."

LXX King Nala, after abandoning his wife Damayanti, goes to Ayodhya and becomes charioteer to king Rituparna. He adopts the name Vahuka, his appearance becomes "unsightly," and he has short arms as a result of an encounter with a snake (LXVI). [Others say he became a dwarf or was "deformed."]

CVII People were harassed by the "dull-headed sons of Sagara." One of them, Asamanjas, "used to seize by the throat the feeble children of the townsmen, and threw them while screaming into the river."

CXIX Valarama censures Dhritarashtra's behavior, saying that "He doth not now see with his mind's eye how he hath become so sightless, and on account of what act he hath grown blind among the kings of this entire earth."

CXXXII–CXXXIV Account of Ashtavakra (i.e., "crooked in eight parts of the body"). The learned Kahoda's wife becomes pregnant. The fetus, already well-versed in the Vedas, criticizes mistakes in his father's reading, causing Kahoda to curse his child to be crooked in eight parts. The sage is then defeated in debate by Vandin and forfeits his life at the court of king Janaka. Later, Ashtavakra goes to Janaka but is turned away by a warder. Ashtavakra asserts his right of way, as a Brahmin, over "the blind, the deaf, the women, carriers of burdens, and the king respectively." He gains admittance and defeats Vandin in debate. Kahoda reappears and says, "Weak persons may have sons endued with strength; dunces may have intelligent sons; and the illiterate may have sons possessed of learning." Later, Ashtavakra enters the river Samanga, and his limbs are straightened.

CXXXVI–CXXXVII Yavakri, attempting to flee into his father's Agnihotra room, is prevented and seized by "a blind Sudra warder."

CXLIX Among advice on statecraft, from Hanuman to Bhima: In secret affairs, women, sots, boys, covetous or mean-minded persons, and "he that betrayeth signs of insanity" should not be consulted. Dunces "should in all affairs be excluded."

CLXLIX Advice on religious practice from Markandeya to King Yudhishthira: "If they that are to be employed in *Sraddhas* happen to be dumb, blind, or deaf, care should be taken to employ them along with Brahmanas conversant with the Vedas."

CCVI Markandeya connects the decay of virtue to kingly sins:

And when all this taketh place the subjects of the kingdom begin to decay. And it is then, O Brahmana, that ill-looking monsters, and dwarfs, and hunchbacked and large-headed wights, and men that are blind or deaf or those that have paralysed eyes or are destitute of the power of procreation, begin to take their birth. It is from the sinfulness of kings that their subjects suffer numerous mischiefs.

CCVIII

The diseases from which man suffer, are undoubtedly the result of their own *karma*. They then behave like small deer at the hands of hunters, and they are racked with mental troubles. And, O Brahmana, as hunters intercept the flight of their game, the progress of those diseases is checked by able and skilful physicians with their collections of drugs.

CCXXIX Various spirits are described that oppress children. Some causes of madness are given, such as seeing gods in a dream.

The man who loses his reason on account of his mind being demoralised with vices, runs mad in no time, and his illness must be remedied according to methods prescribed in the *Sastras*. Men also run mad from perplexity, from fear, as also on beholding hideous sights. The remedy lies in quieting their minds. There are three classes of spirits, some are frolicsome, some are gluttonous, and some sensual. Until men attain the age of three score and ten, these evil influences continue to torment them, and then fever becomes the only evil spirit that afflicts sentient beings.

CCLXLII–CCLXLVI Savitri marries the son of blind, exiled King Dyumatsena. When Yama comes to take her husband, Savitri pleads strongly with him, obtaining a return of the eyesight and kingdom of Dyumatsena and eventually winning back her husband's life. When Dyumatsena's usurper has been killed, his subjects demand that Dyumatsena return, saying "Whether possessed of sight or not, even he shall be our king!"

Udyoga Parva

XXX Yudhishthira, sending greetings via Sanjaya, includes the entire court of Dhritarashtra, including "the many hump-back and lame ones" among the servants, and inquires after the welfare of those who are

> defective in limb, those that are imbecile, the dwarfs to whom Dhritarashtra gives food and raiment from motives of humanity, those that are blind, and all those that are aged, as also to the many that have the use only of their hands being destitute of legs.

XXXIII Vidura, imparting wisdom proverbs to Dhritarashtra: "Of the five senses beholding to man, if one springeth a leak, then from that single hole runneth out all his intelligence, even like water running out from a perforated leathern vessel."

XXXIV Vidura to Dhritarashtra:

> He to whom the gods ordain defeat, hath his senses taken away, and it is for this that he stoopeth to ignoble deeds. When the intellect becometh dim and destruction is nigh, wrong, looking like right, firmly sticketh to the heart.

LXIV Honey from the northern mountain, Gandhamadana, which would cause a sightless man to obtain sight.

LXIX Men deprived of sense by avarice and desire, are "like blind men [falling into pits] when led by the blind."

LXXI Dhritarashtra says that he envies sighted people who may see the beauty of Vasudeva.

XCII Vidura notes that "no wise man would spend his breath for nothing, like a singer before the deaf"; he notes also that the sons of Kuru have been "blinded by prosperity and pride."

CXXX Duryodhana and friends plot to seize Krishna when he acts as the Pandavas' ambassador to Dhritarashtra. Satyaki describes them as "like idiots and children desiring to seize a blazing fire by means of their garments."

CXLVII Bhishma to Duryodhana: "Thy father was born blind, and in consequence of this congenital defect of a sense, he could not become king."

CXLIX Dhritarashtra informs Duryodhana that even his own great-grandfather Devapi, the eldest of three princes, could not inherit the kingdom because he had a skin disease. "The gods do not approve a king that is defective of a limb." [Any distinction between absent limb and skin disease is not made clear.]

Drona Parva

LI Brahma instructs Death to "kill all creatures including idiots and seers at my command."

CXLII "It is evident that with the decrepitude of the body one's intellect also becomes decrepit" [spoken as an insult].

CLXXXII One of the celestial weapons was snatched "like a fruit from the hand of a cripple, with a withered arm, by a strong person."

CCII The companions of Mahadeva (or Rudra) are

> celestial beings of diverse forms, some of whom are dwarfs, some have matted locks, some with bald heads, some with short necks, some with large stomachs, some with huge bodies, some possessed of great strength and some of long ears. All of them, O Partha, have deformed faces and mouths and legs and strange attires.

Karna Parva

IV Refers to Dhritarashtra as one "who had knowledge only for his eye"—with footnote "A respectful epithet for a blind man."

Sauptika Parva

VI

> One should not cast weapons upon kine, Brahmanas, kings, women, friends, one's own mother, one's own preceptor, a weak man, an idiot, a blind man, a sleeping man, a terrified man, one just risen from sleep, an intoxicated person, a lunatic and one that is heedless.

Stree Parva

XII When the Pandavas go to meet Dhritarashtra, Krishna presents the blind king with an iron statue, in place of Bhima. The king seizes this and crushes it in his embrace, suffering much bruising and vomiting blood as a result. He believes he has killed Bhima, and after the passion has passed, they tell him that he has destroyed an iron statue.

Santi Parva (i)

IX Yudhishthira decides to give up earthly glory. "Without conversing with anybody, I shall assume the outward form of a blind and deaf idiot, while living in contentment."

XIV Draupadi complains that Yudhishthira has gone mad:

That person who through dullness of intellect acts in this way never succeeds in winning prosperity. The man that treads along the path of madness should be subjected to medical treatment by the aid of incense and collyrium, of drugs applied through the nose, and of other medicines.

XVI "Without doubt, mental diseases spring from physical ones. Similarly physical diseases spring from mental ones." "Goodness, passion and darkness [*sattvas, rajas, tamas*] are the three attributes of the mind. The existence of these three in harmony is the sign of [mental] health."

XXIII Story of a person who ate fruit to which he was not entitled and suffered amputation of both hands. On bathing in a sacred stream, his hands are restored.

XXV "If the Time does not come, the infant does not acquire power of speech."

XXV "They that are highly stupid and they that are masters of their souls enjoy happiness here. They however, that occupy an intermediate place suffer misery."

XXVI "That men give unto the undeserving and refrain from giving unto the deserving is due to inability to discriminate between the deserving and the undeserving. For this reason the practice of even the virtue of charity is difficult."

XXXVII A virtuous man would not make a gift [probably refers to a formal gift, not to alms] to various listed people, including to

one that is insane, or unto a thief, or unto a slanderer, or unto an idiot, or unto one that is pale of hue, or unto one that is defective of a limb, or unto a dwarf, or unto a wicked person

XLIII "The puissant king, with great compassion, extended his favours to the destitute and the blind and the helpless by giving them food, clothes and shelter."

LXIX When the king's city is under threat, "all beggars, eunuchs, lunatics, and mimes" should be driven out of town.

LXXXIII

There should be no dwarfs, no hump-backed persons, no one of an emaciated constitution, no one who is lame or blind, no one who is an idiot, no woman, and no eunuch, at the spot where the king holds his consultations. Nothing should move there before or behind, above or below, or in transverse directions.

XC

When the king does not restrain vice, a confusion of castes follows, and sinful *Rakshasas,* and persons of neutral sex, and children destitute of limbs or possessed of thick tongues, and idiots, begin to take birth in even respectable families.

CLVII Might makes right, and therefore it is prudent to overlook wrongs done by a stronger person "even as one should overlook (from compassion) the acts of a child, an idiot, or one that is blind or deaf."

CLX The only problem with self-control is that "a person who has self-control is regarded by men as weak and imbecile."

CLXIII "Compassion proceeds from a sight of the helpless and miserable persons with whom the world abounds. That sentiment disappears when one understands the strength of virtue." [Compassion, like any sort of passion, is a weakness to be overcome. If a righteous person acts in a kindly way toward a disabled person, it should be out of the realization of duty, rather than because of the passing sentiment.]

Anusasana Parva (i)

XVII Reference to "the sciences of palmistry and phrenology and other branches of knowledge treating of the physical frame as the indicator of mental peculiarities."

XXIII

All Brahmanas that have been outcasted (on account of the commission of heinous sins), as also Brahmanas that are idiots and out of mind, do not deserve to be invited to Sraddhas in which offerings are made to either the deities or the *Pitris.* That Brahmana who is afflicted with leucoderma, or he that is destitute of virility, or he that has got leprosy, or he that has got phthisis or he that is labouring under epilepsy (with delusions of the sensorium), or he that is blind, should not, O king, be invited.

XXIV "Thou shouldst know that man to be guilty of Brahmanicide who robs the blind, the lame, and idiots of their all."

XXVI

Those who, although possessed of the physical ability, do not seek to have a sight of the auspicious Ganga of sacred current, are, without doubt, to be likened to persons afflicted with congenital blindness or those that are [deaf] or those that are destitute of the power of locomotion through palsy or lameness

XXVI "Verily, Ganga . . . is competent to bestow the fruition of all their wishes upon them that are blind, them that are idiots, and them that are destitute of all things."

Anusasana Parva (ii)

XXXVIII On the weaknesses of women:

Even those women that are loved by their husbands and treated with great respect, are seen to bestow their favours upon men that are hump-backed, that are blind, that are idiots, or that are dwarfs. Women may be seen to like the companionship of even those men that are destitute of the power of locomotion or those men that are endued with great ugliness of features.

XL Sakra, capable of assuming any form, "sometimes appears as an idiot destitute of all intelligence."

LXI "The king should protect the wealth of those that are old, of those that are minors, of those that are blind, and of those that are otherwise disqualified."

LXXXV An unwise parrot is informed that a speech defect will be inflicted on it. "Like that of a child or an old man, thy speech shall be sweet and indistinct and wonderful."

XC At Sraddhas, unworthy Brahmanas should not be invited. "A Brahmana that is blind stains sixty individual[s] of the line; one that is destitute of virile power a hundred; while one that is afflicted with white leprosy stains as many as he looks upon, O king."

XCIX "One that steals a light becomes blind. Such a man has to grope through darkness (in the next world) and becomes destitute of resplendence."

CIV

One should not taunt a person that is defective of a limb or that has a limb in excess, or one that is destitute of learning, or one that is miserable, or one that is ugly or poor, or one that is destitute of strength.

CIV Advice on the choice of a wife and the importance of avoiding

a woman that is deficient of any limb . . . as also one that has any malformation; as also one that has been born in the race to which one's mother belongs. . . . or one that is afflicted with leprosy, or born in a family in which there has been epilepsy.

CXXVI Vishnu points out that the sight of a Brahmana of dwarfish stature is lucky, because he took such a disguise when defeating Vali.

CXLV Refers to those who do, and those who do not, make charitable gifts to blind, distressed, or mendicant people.

CXLV Why are some men born blind? Their eyes had earlier coveted their neighbor's wife.

CXLVI Even a woman can accumulate merit, if she feeds distressed, blind, or destitute Brahmanas.

Aswamedha Parva

VII A Brahmana, "raving like a lunatic," stated, "I am afflicted with a cerebral disorder, and, I always act according to the random caprices of my own mind."

XXXVI Very sinful men sink down to take birth in the brute creation, becoming

immobile entities, or animals, or beasts of burden; or carnivorous creatures, or snakes, or worms, insects, and birds; or creatures, of the oviparous order, or quadrupeds of diverse species, or lunatics, or deaf or dumb human beings, or men that are afflicted by dreadful maladies and regarded as unclean.

Others slowly make progress upward. "Coming to sinful births and becoming Chandalas or human beings that are deaf or that lisp indistinctly, they attain to higher and higher castes."

LIX Krishna returns home, amid great celebrations: "Gifts were being ceaselessly made to those that were distressed, or blind, or helpless."

XC At the end of Yudhishthira's horse sacrifice, where "all the poor, the blind, and the helpless ones had been gratified," a mongoose arrives and announces that the horse sacrifice was worth less than the small quantity of barley given away by a certain Brahmana engaged in ascetic practices.

Asramavasika Parva

V "Apes and birds and other animals that can imitate human beings should all be excluded from the council chamber, as also idiots and lame and palsied individuals."

XV Sighted Kunti walks ahead, with eye-bandaged Gandhari's hand on her shoulder; blind Dhritarashtra follows, with his hand on Gandhari's shoulder.

XXXV Vyasa has arranged for the living to meet with the dead. He then grants sight to Dhritarashtra so that he can actually see his sons for the first time, even after they have died.

Source: Ganguli, Kisari Mohan, trans. 1883–1896. *The Mahabharata of Krishna-Dwaipayana Vyasa.* Available at http://www.sacred-texts.com/hin/maha/

The Ancient World: East Asia

◉ Analects of Confucius
(ca. 500 BCE)

These sayings of the famous Chinese philosopher Confucius were compiled and expanded after his death. In these comments, we find Confucius's notion of virtue defined by his idea of positive character traits to which one should aspire. The analects include a variety of behaviors prescribed for encounters with disabled people.

6.8: Leprosy

Po Niu was sick and Confucius came to see him. He held his hand through the window and said, "He is dying! How awful it is that this kind of man should be sick like this! How awful it is that this kind of man should be sick like this!"

9:9: Blindness

If the master saw someone in mourning, or in full ceremonial dress, or a blind person, even if they were young, he would collect himself. If he had to pass by them, he would do it quickly.

10:16: Blindness

In bed he avoids lying in the posture of a corpse. When at home he does not use ritual attitudes. When appearing before anyone in mourning, however well he knows him, he must put on altered expression, and when appearing before anyone in sacrificial garb, or a blind man, even informally, he must be sure to adopt the appropriate attitude. On meeting anyone in deep mourning he must bow across the bar of his chariot; he also bows to people carrying and he should rise to his feet. Upon hearing a sudden clap of thunder or a violent gust of wind, he must change countenance.

15.41: Blindness

The music master, Mien, having called upon him, when they came to the steps, the Master said, "Here are the steps." When they came to the mat for the guest to sit upon, he said, "Here is the mat." When all were seated, the Master informed him, saying, "So and so is here; so and so is here."

The music master, Mien, having gone out, Tsze-chang asked, saying, "Is it the rule to tell those things to the music master?"

The Master said, "Yes. This is certainly the rule for those who lead the blind."

16:6: Blindness

Confucius said: "There are three common mistakes made by those who are of rank:

(1) To speak when there is nothing to be said; this is imprudence.

(2) To be silent when there is something to be said; this is deception.

(3) To speak without paying attention to the expression on the person's face; this is called blindness."

18:5: Madness

Chieh Yü, the madman of Ch'u, came past Master K'ung, singing as he went:
Oh phoenix, phoenix
How dwindled is your power!
As to the past, reproof is idle,
But the future may yet be remedied.
Desist, desist!

Great in these days is the peril of those who fill office.

Master K'ung got down, desiring to speak with him; but the madman hastened his step and got away, so that Master K'ung did not succeed in speaking to him.

Source: Legge, James, trans. 1861. *The Chinese Classics: Analects of Confucius.* Oxford, UK: Clarendon Press.

◙ Taoist Scripture: Chuang-Tzu
(ca. 3rd c. BCE)

These writings, dating from the fourth to second centuries BCE, include disabled people in the Seven Inner Chapters (that portion of the work considered most likely to have been written by Chuang-Tzu himself), and some of the disabled people described are depicted as being advanced on the Way. Chuang-tzu (Zhuangzi) may have been the first to imagine a social dimension to disability, suggesting that a powerful spirit may, as a result of the defects in the society in which it is born, inhabit a deformed human shape. This writing includes many disabled characters and illustrates the Taoist belief that nature should remain as it is rather than be fixed or altered by human intervention.

There was a hunchback named Su. His jaws touched his navel. His shoulders were higher than his head. His neck bone stuck out toward the sky. His viscera were turned upside down. His buttocks were where his ribs should have been. By tailoring, or washing, he was easily able to earn his living. By sifting rice he could make enough to support a family of ten. When orders came down for a conscription, the hunchback walked about unconcerned among the crowd. And similarly, in government conscription for public works, his deformity saved him from being called. On the other hand, when it came to government donations of grain for the disabled, the hunchback received as much as three chung and of firewood, ten faggots. And if physical deformity was thus enough to preserve his body until the end of his days, how much more should moral and mental deformity avail!

Deformities, or Evidence of a Full Character

In the state of Lu there was a man, named Wang T'ai, who had had one of his legs cut off. His disciples were as numerous as those of Confucius. Ch'ang Chi asked Confucius, saying, "This Wang T'ai has been mutilated, yet he has as many followers in the Lu State as you. He neither stands up to preach nor sits down to give discourse; yet those who go to him empty, depart full. Is he the kind of person who can teach without words and influence people's minds without material means? What manner of man is this?"

"He is a sage," replied Confucius, "I wanted to go to him, but am merely behind the others. Even I will go and make him my teacher,—why not those who are lesser than I? And I will lead, not only the State of Lu, but the whole world to follow him."

"The man has been mutilated," said Ch'ang Chi, "and yet people call him 'Master.' He must be very different from the ordinary men. If so, how does he train his mind?"

"Life and Death are indeed changes of great moment," answered Confucius, "but they cannot affect his mind. Heaven and earth may collapse, but his mind will remain. Being indeed without flaw, it will not share the fate of all things. It can control the transformation of things, while preserving its source intact."

"How so?" asked Ch'ang Chi. "From the point of view of differentiation of things," replied Confucius, "we distinguish between the liver and the gall, between the Ch'u State and the Yueh State. From the point of view of their sameness, all things are One. He who regards things in this light does not even trouble about what reaches him through the senses of hearing and sight, but lets his mind wander in the moral harmony of things. He beholds the unity in things, and does not notice the loss of particular objects. And thus the loss of his leg is to him as would be the loss of so much dirt."

"But he cultivates only himself," said Ch'ang Chi. "He uses his knowledge to perfect his mind, and develops his mind into the Absolute Mind. But how is it that people flock around him?"

"A man," replied Confucius, "does not seek to see himself in running water, but in still water. For only what is itself still can instill stillness into others. The grace of earth has reached only the pines and cedars; winter and summer alike, they are green. The grace of God has reached to Yao and to Shun, who alone attained rectitude. Happily he was able to rectify himself and thus become the means through which all were rectified. For the possession of one's original (nature) is evidenced in true courage.

"A man will, single-handed, brave a whole army. And if such a result can be achieved by one in search of fame through self control, how much greater courage can be shown by one who extends his sway over heaven and earth and gives shelter to all things, who, lodging temporarily within the confines of a body with contempt for the superficialities of sight and sound, brings his knowledge to level all knowledge and whose mind never dies! Besides, he (Wang T'ai) is only awaiting his appointed hour to go up to Heaven. Men indeed flock to him of their own accord. How can he take seriously the affairs of this world?"

Shent'u Chia had only one leg. He studied under Pohun Wujen ("Muddle-Head No-Such-Person") together with Tsech'an of the Cheng State. The latter said to him, "When I leave first, do you remain behind. When you leave first, I will remain behind." Next day, when they were again together sitting on the same mat in the lecture-room, Tsech'an said, "When I leave first, do you remain behind. Or if you leave first, I will remain behind. I am now about to go. Will you remain or not? I notice you show no respect to a high personage. Perhaps you think yourself my equal?"

"In the house of the Master," replied Shent'u Chia, "there is already a high personage (the Master). Perhaps you think that you are the high personage and therefore should take precedence over the rest. Now I have heard that if a mirror is perfectly bright, dust will not collect on it, and that if it does, the mirror is no longer bright. He who associates for long with the wise should be without fault. Now you have been seeking the greater things at the feet of our Master, yet you can utter words like these. Don't you think you are making a mistake?"

"You are already mutilated like this," retorted Tsech'an, "yet you are still seeking to compete in virtue with Yao. To look at you, I should say you had enough to do to reflect on your past misdeeds!"

"Those who cover up their sins," said Shent'u Chia, "so as not to lose their legs, are many in number. Those who forget to cover up their misdemeanors and so lose their legs (through punishment) are few. But only the virtuous man can recognize the inevitable and remain unmoved. People who walked in front of the bull's-eye when Hou Yi (the famous archer) was shooting, would be hit. Some who were not hit were just lucky. There are many people with sound legs who laugh at me for not having them. This used to

make me angry. But since I came to study under our Master, I have stopped worrying about it. Perhaps our Master has so far succeeded in washing (purifying) me with his goodness. At any rate, I have been with him nineteen years without being aware of my deformity. Now you and I are roaming in the realm of the spiritual, and you are judging me in the realm of the physical. Are you not committing a mistake?" At this Tsech'an began to fidget and his countenance changed, and he bade Shent'u Chia to speak no more.

There was a man of the Lu State who had been mutilated, by the name of Shushan No-toes. He came walking on his heels to see Confucius; but Confucius said, "You were careless, and so brought this misfortune upon yourself. What is the use of coming to me now?" "It was because I was inexperienced and careless with my body that I hurt my feet," replied No-toes. "Now I have come with something more precious than feet, and it is that which I am seeking to preserve. There is no man, but Heaven shelters him; and there is no man, but the Earth supports him. I thought that you, Master, would be like Heaven and Earth. I little expected to hear these words from you."

"Pardon my stupidity," said Confucius. "Why not come in? I shall discuss with you what I have learned." But No-toes left. When No-toes had left, Confucius said to his disciples, "Take a good lesson. No-toes is one-legged, yet he is seeking to learn in order to make atonement for his previous misdeeds. How much more should those who have no misdeeds for which to atone?"

No-toes went off to see Lao Tan (Laotse) and said, "Is Confucius a Perfect One or is he not quite? How is it that he is so anxious to learn from you? He is seeking to earn a reputation by his abstruse and strange learning, which is regarded by the Perfect One as mere fetters."

"Why do you not make him regard life and death, and possibility and impossibility as alternations of one and the same principle," answered Lao Tan, "and so release him from these fetters?"

"It is God who has thus punished him," replied No-toes. "How could he be released?"

Duke Ai of the Lu State said to Confucius, "In the Wei State there is an ugly person, named Ait'ai (Ugly) T'o. The men who have lived with him cannot stop thinking about him. Women who have seen him, would say to their parents, 'Rather than be another man's wife, I would be this man's concubine.' There are scores of such women. He never tries to lead others, but only follows them. He wields no power of a ruler by which he may protect men's lives. He has no hoarded wealth by which to gratify their bellies, and is besides frightfully loathsome. He follows but does not lead, and his name is not known outside his own State. Yet men and women alike all seek his company. So there must be some thing in him that is different from other people. I sent for him, and saw that he was indeed frightfully ugly. Yet we had not been many months together before I began to see there was something in this man. A year had not passed before I began to trust him. As my State wanted a Prime Minister, I offered him the post. He looked sullenly before he replied and appeared as if he would much rather have declined. Perhaps he did not think me good enough for him! At any rate, I gave the post to him; but in a very short time he left me and went away. I grieved for him as for a lost friend, as though there were none left with whom I could enjoy having my kingdom. What manner of man is this?"

"When I was on a mission to the Ch'u State," replied Confucius, "I saw a litter of young pigs sucking their dead mother. After a while they looked at her, and then all left the body and went off. For their mother did not look at them any more, nor did she seem any more to have been of their kind. What they loved was their mother; not the body which contained her, but that which made the body what it was. When a man is killed in battle, his coffin is not covered with a square canopy. A man whose leg has been cut off does not value a present of shoes. In each case, the original purpose of such things is gone. The concubines of the Son of Heaven do not cut their nails or pierce their ears. Those (servants) who are married have to live outside (the palace) and cannot be employed again. Such is the importance attached to preserving the body whole. How much more valued is one who has preserved his virtue whole? Now Ugly T'o has said nothing and is already trusted. He has achieved nothing and is sought after, and is offered the government of a country with the only fear that he might decline. Indeed he must be the one whose talents are perfect and whose virtue is without outward form!"

"What do you mean by his talents being perfect?" asked the Duke. "Life and Death," replied Confucius, "possession and loss, success and failure, poverty and wealth, virtue and vice, good and evil report, hunger and thirst, heat and cold—these are

changes of things in the natural course of events. Day and night they follow upon one another, and no man can say where they spring from. Therefore they must not be allowed to disturb the natural harmony, nor enter into the soul's domain. One should live so that one is at ease and in harmony with the world, without loss of happiness, and by day and by night, share the (peace of) spring with the created things. Thus continuously one creates the seasons in one's own breast. Such a person may be said to have perfect talents."

"And what is virtue without outward form?"

"When standing still," said Confucius, "the water is in the most perfect state of repose. Let that be your model. It remains quietly within, and is not agitated without. It is from the cultivation of such harmony that virtue results. And if virtue takes no outward form, man will not be able to keep aloof from it."

Some days afterwards Duke Ai told Mintse saying, "When first I took over the reins of government, I thought that in guiding the people and caring for their lives, I had done all my duty as a ruler. But now that I have heard the words of a perfect man, I fear that I have not achieved it, but am foolishly squandering my bodily energy and bringing ruin to my country. Confucius and I are not prince and minister, but friends in spirit."

Hunchback-Deformed-No-Lips spoke with Duke Ling of Wei and the Duke took a fancy to him. Big-Jar-Goiter spoke with Duke Huan of Ch'i, and the Duke took a fancy to him. As for the well-formed men, he thought their necks were too scraggy. Thus it is that when virtue excels, the outward form is forgotten. But mankind forgets not that which is to be forgotten, forgetting that which is not to be forgotten. This is forgetfulness indeed!

And thus the Sage sets his spirit free, while knowledge is regarded as extraneous growths—agreements are for cementing relationships, goods are only for social dealings, and the handicrafts are only for serving commerce. For the Sage does not contrive, and therefore has no use for knowledge; he does not cut up the world, and therefore requires no cementing of relationships; he has no loss, and therefore has no need to acquire; he sells nothing, and therefore has no use for commerce. These four qualifications are bestowed upon him by God, that is to say, he is fed by God. And he who is thus fed by God has little need to be fed by man.

He wears the human form without human passions. Because he wears the human form he associates with men. Because he has not human passions the questions of right and wrong do not touch him. Infinitesimal indeed is that which belongs to the human; infinitely great is that which is completed in God.

Hueitse said to Chuangtse, "Do men indeed originally have no passions?"

"Certainly," replied Chuangtse.

"But if a man has no passions," argued Hueitse, "what is it that makes him a man?"

"Tao," replied Chuangtse, "gives him his expressions, and God gives him his form. How should he not be a man?"

"If then he is a man," said Hueitse, "how can he be without passions?"

"Right and wrong (approval and disapproval)," answered Chuangtse, "are what I mean by passions. By a man without passions I mean one who does not permit likes and dislikes to disturb his internal economy, but rather falls in line with nature and does not try to improve upon (the materials of) living."

"But how is a man to live this bodily life," asked Hueitse. "He does not try to improve upon (the materials of) his living?"

"Tao gives him his expression," said Chuangtse, "and God gives him his form. He should not permit likes and dislikes to disturb his internal economy. But now you are devoting your intelligence to externals, and wearing out your vital spirit. Lean against a tree and sing; or sit against a table and sleep! God has made you a shapely sight, yet your only thought is the hard and white."

Joined Toes

Joined toes and extra fingers seem to come from nature, yet, functionally speaking they are superfluous. Goiters and tumors seem to come from the body, yet in their nature, they are superfluous. And (similarly), to have many extraneous doctrines of charity and duty and regard them in practice as parts of a man's natural sentiments is not the true way of Tao. For just as joined toes are but useless lumps of flesh, and extra fingers but useless growths, so are the many artificial developments of the natural sentiments of men and the extravagances of charitable and dutiful conduct but so many superfluous uses of intelligence.

People with superfluous keenness of vision put into confusion the five colors, lose themselves in the forms and designs, and in the distinctions of greens and yellows for sacrificial robes. Is this not so?

Of such was Li Chu (the clear-sighted). People with superfluous keenness of hearing put into confusion the five notes, exaggerate the tonic differences of the six pitch-pipes, and the various timbres of metal, stone, silk, and bamboo of the Huang-chung, and the Ta-lu. Is this not so? Of such was Shih K'uang (the music master). People who abnormally develop charity exalt virtue and suppress nature in order to gain a reputation, make the world noisy with their discussions and cause it to follow impractical doctrines. Is this not so? Of such were Tseng and Shih.

People who commit excess in arguments, like piling up bricks and making knots, analyzing and inquiring into the distinctions of hard and white, identities and differences, wear themselves out over mere vain, useless terms. Is this not so? Of such were Yang and Mo.

All these are superfluous and devious growths of knowledge and are not the correct guide for the world. He who would be the ultimate guide never loses sight of the inner nature of life. Therefore with him, the united is not like joined toes, the separated is not like extra fingers, what is long is not considered as excess, and what is short is not regarded as wanting. For duck's legs, though short, cannot be lengthened without dismay to the duck, and a crane's legs, though long, cannot be shortened without misery to the crane. That which is long in nature must not be cut off, and that which is short in nature must not be lengthened. Thus will all sorrow be avoided. I suppose charity and duty are surely not included in human nature. You see how many worries and dismays the charitable man has! Besides, divide your joined toes and you will howl: bite off your extra finger and you will scream. In the one case, there is too much, and in the other too little; but the worries and dismays are the same. Now the charitable men of the present age go about with a look of concern sorrowing over the ills of the age, while the non-charitable let loose the desire of their nature in their greed after position and wealth. Therefore I suppose charity and duty are not included in human nature. Yet from the time of the Three Dynasties downwards what a commotion has been raised about them! Moreover, those who rely upon the arc, the line, compasses, and the square to make correct forms injure the natural constitution of things. Those who use cords to bind and glue to piece together interfere with the natural character of things. Those who seek to satisfy the mind of man by hampering it with ceremonies and music and affecting charity and devotion have lost their original nature. There is an original nature in things. Things in their original nature are curved without the help of arcs, straight without lines, round without compasses, and rectangular without squares; they are joined together without glue and hold together without cords. In this manner all things live and grow from an inner urge and none can tell how they come to do so. They all have a place in the scheme of things and none can tell how they come to have their proper place. From time immemorial this has always been so, and it may not be tampered with. Why then should the doctrines of charity and duty continue to remain like so much glue or cords, in the domain of Tao and virtue, to give rise to confusion and doubt among mankind? Now the lesser doubts change man's purpose, and the greater doubts change man's nature. How do we know this? Ever since the time when Shun made a bid for charity and duty and threw the world into confusion, men have run about and exhausted themselves in the pursuit thereof. Is it not then charity and duty which have changed the nature of man?

Therefore I have tried to show that from the time of the Three Dynasties onwards, there is not one who has not changed his nature through certain external things. If a common man, he will die for gain. If a scholar, he will die for fame. If a ruler of a township, he will die for his ancestral honors. If a Sage, he will die for the world. The pursuits and ambitions of these men differ, but the injury to their nature resulting in the sacrifice of their lives is the same. Tsang and Ku were shepherds, and both lost their sheep. On inquiry it appeared that Tsang had been engaged in reading with a shepherd's stick under his arm, while Ku had gone to take part in some trials of strength. Their pursuits were different, but the result in each case was the loss of the sheep. Po Yi died for fame at the foot of Mount Shouyang.

Robber Cheh died for gain on the Mount Tungling. They died for different reasons, but the injury to their lives and nature was in each case the same. Why then must we applaud the former and blame the latter? All men die for something, and yet if a man dies for charity and duty the world calls him a gentleman; but if he dies for gain, the world calls him a low fellow. The dying being the same, one is nevertheless called a gentleman and the other called a low character. But in point of injury to their lives and nature, Robber Cheh was just another Po Yi. Of what use then is the distinction of 'gentleman' and 'low fellow' between them? Besides, were a man to apply himself to charity and duty until he were the equal of Tseng or Shih, I would not call it good. Or to savors, until he were the equal of Shu Erh (famous cook), I would not call it good. Or to sound, until he were the equal of Shih K'uang, I would not call it good. Or to colors, until he were the equal of Li Chu, I would not call it good. What I call good is not what is meant by charity and duty, but taking good care of virtue. And what I call good is not the so-called charity and duty, but following the nature of life. What I call good at hearing is not hearing others but hearing oneself. What I call good at vision is not seeing others but seeing oneself. For a man who sees not himself but others, or takes possession not of himself but of others, possessing only what others possess and possessing not his own self, does what pleases others instead of pleasing his own nature. Now one who pleases others, instead of pleasing one's own nature, whether he be Robber Cheh or Po Yi, is just another one gone astray. Conscious of my own deficiencies in regard to Tao, I do not venture to practise the principles of charity and duty on the one hand, nor to lead the life of extravagance on the other.

On Tolerance

Of old, the Yellow Emperor first interfered with the natural goodness of the heart of man, by means of charity and duty. In consequence, Yao and Shun wore the hair off their legs and the flesh off their arms in endeavoring to feed their people's bodies. They tortured the people's internal economy in order to conform to charity and duty. They exhausted the people's energies to live in accordance with the laws and statutes. Even then they did not succeed. Thereupon, Yao (had to) confine Huantou on Mount Ts'ung, exile the chiefs of the Three Miaos and their people into the Three Weis, and banish the Minister of Works to Yutu, which shows he had not succeeded. When it came to the times of the Three Kings, the empire was in a state of foment. Among the bad men were Chieh and Cheh; among the good were Tseng and Shih. By and by, the Confucianists and the Motseanists arose; and then came confusion between joy and anger, fraud between the simple and the cunning, recrimination between the virtuous and the evil-minded, slander between the honest and the liars, and the world order collapsed.

Then the great virtue lost its unity, men's lives were frustrated. When there was a general rush for knowledge, the people's desires ever went beyond their possessions. The next thing was then to invent axes and saws, to kill by laws and statutes, to disfigure by chisels and awls. The empire seethed with discontent, the blame for which rests upon those who would interfere with the natural goodness of the heart of man.

In consequence, virtuous men sought refuge in mountain caves, while rulers of great states sat trembling in their ancestral halls. Then, when dead men lay about pillowed on each other's corpses, when cangued prisoners jostled each other in crowds and condemned criminals were seen everywhere, then the Confucianists and the Motseanists bustled about and rolled up their sleeves in the midst of gyves and fetters! Alas, they know not shame, nor what it is to blush!

Until I can say that the wisdom of Sages is not a fastener of cangues, and that charity of heart and duty to one's neighbor are not bolts for gyves, how should I know that Tseng and Shih were not the singing arrows (forerunners) of (the gangsters) Chieh and Cheh? Therefore it is said, "Abandon wisdom and discard knowledge, and the empire will be at peace."

The Yellow Emperor sat on the throne for nineteen years, and his laws obtained all over the empire. Hearing that Kuangch'engtse was living on Mount K'ungt'ung, he went there to see him, and said, "I am told that you are in possession of perfect Tao. May I ask what is the essence of this perfect Tao? I desire to obtain the essence of the universe to secure good harvests and feed my people. I should like also to control the yin and yang principles to fulfill the life of all living things."

"What you are asking about," replied Kuangch'engtse, "is merely the dregs of things. What you wish to control are the disintegrated factors thereof. Ever since the empire was governed by you, the clouds have rained before thickening, the foliage of trees has fallen before turning yellow, and the brightness of the sun and moon has increasingly paled. You have the shallowness of mind of a glib talker. How then are you fit to speak of perfect Tao?"

The Yellow Emperor withdrew. He resigned the Throne. He built himself a solitary hut, and sat upon white straw. For three months he remained in seclusion, and then went again to see Kuangch'engtse.

The latter was lying with his head towards the south. The Yellow Emperor approached from below upon his knees. Kowtowing twice upon the ground, he said, "I am told that you are in possession of perfect Tao. May I ask how to order one's life so that one may have long life?"

Kuangch'engtse jumped up with a start. "A good question indeed!" cried he. "Come, and I will speak to you of perfect Tao. The essence of perfect Tao is profoundly mysterious; its extent is lost in obscurity.

"See nothing; hear nothing; guard your spirit in quietude and your body will go right of its own accord.

"Be quiet, be pure; toil not your body, perturb not your vital essence, and you will live forever.

"For if the eye sees nothing, and the ear hears nothing, and the mind thinks nothing, your spirit will stay in your body, and the body will thereby live for ever.

"Cherish that which is within you, and shut off that which is without for much knowledge is a curse.

"Then I will take you to that abode of Great Light to reach the Plateau of Absolute Yang. I will lead you through the Door of the Dark Unknown to the Plateau of the Absolute Yin."

Source: Legge, James, trans. 1890. *The Complete Chuang Tzu*. Oxford, UK: Clarendon Press.

◉ *The Kojiki* (712 CE)

In the following legend from The Kojiki, a historical compilation that includes many ancient Japanese legends, unusual births are explained by looking to the sexual relationship of the parents. Specifically, this selection describes the offspring of Izanagi and Izanami, whose children included the Japanese islands as well as various disabled children whom they did not acknowledge as their own. By consulting the gods, they learn that their children's deformities arose from the fact that the wife initiated the sexual contact that led to their procreation.

Part I. The Birth of the Deities

Courtship of the Deities: The Male-Who-Invites and the Female-Who-Invites

Having descended from Heaven on to this island, they saw to the erection of a heavenly august pillar, they saw to the erection of a hall of eight fathoms. Then Izanagi, the Male-Who-Invites, said to Izanami, the Female-Who-Invites, "We should create children"; and he said, "Let us go around the heavenly august pillar, and when we meet on the other side let us be united. Do you go around from the left, and I will go from the right." When they met, Her Augustness, the Female-Who-Invites, spake first, exclaiming, "Ah, what a fair and lovable youth!" Then His Augustness said, "Ah what a fair and lovable maiden!" But afterward he said, " It was not well that the woman should speak first!" The child which was born to them was Hiruko (the leech-child), which when three years old was still unable to stand upright. So they placed the leech-child in a boat of reeds and let it float away. Next they gave birth to the island of Aha. This likewise is not reckoned among their children.

Hereupon the two deities took counsel, saying: "The children to whom we have now given birth are not good. It will be best to announce this in the august place of the Heavenly deities." They ascended forthwith to Heaven and inquired of Their Augustnesses the Heavenly deities. Then the Heavenly deities commanded and found out by grand divination, and ordered them, saying: "they were not good because the woman spoke first. Descend back again and amend your words." So thereupon descending back, they again went round the heavenly august pillar. Thereupon his Augustness the Male-Who-Invites spoke first: "Ah! what a fair and lovely maiden!" Afterward his younger sister Her Augustness the Female-Who-Invites spoke: "Ah! what a fair and lovely youth!" Next they gave birth to the Island of Futa-na in Iyo. This island has one body and four faces, and each face has a name. So the Land of Iyo is called Lovely-Princess; the Land of Sanuki is called Princess-Good-Boiled-Rice; the Land of Aha is called the Princess-of-Great-Food, the Land of Tosa is called Brave-Good-Youth. Next they gave birth to the islands

of Mitsu-go near Oki, another name for which islands is Heavenly-Great-Heart-Youth. This island likewise has one body and four faces, and each face has a name. So the Land of Tsukushi is called White-Sun-Youth; the Land of Toyo is called Luxuriant-Sun-Youth; the Land of Hi is called Brave-Sun-Confronting-Luxuriant-Wondrous-Lord-Youth; the Land of Kumaso is called Brave-Sun-Youth. Next they gave birth to the Island of Iki, another name for which is Heaven's One-Pillar. Next they gave birth to the Island of Tsu, another name for which is Heavenly-Hand-Net-Good-Princess. Next they gave birth to the Island of Sado. Next they gave birth to Great-Yamato-the-Luxuriant-Island-of-the-Dragon-fly, another name for which is Heavenly-August-Sky-Luxuriant-Dragon-fly-Lord-Youth. The name of "Land-of-the-Eight-Great-Islands" therefore originated in these eight islands having been born first. After that, when they had returned, they gave birth to the Island of Koo-zhima in Kibi, another name for which island is Brave-Sun-Direction-Youth. Next they gave birth to the Island of Adzuki, another name for which is Oho-Nu-De-Hime. Next they gave birth to the Island of Oho-shima, another name for which is Oho-Tamaru-Wake. Next they gave birth to the Island of Hime, another name for which is Heaven's-One-Root. Next they gave birth to the Island of Chika, another name for which is Heavenly-Great-Male. Next they gave birth to the islands of Futa-go, another name for which is Heaven's Two-Houses. (Six islands in all from the Island of Ko in Kibi to the Island of Heaven's-Two-Houses.)

Source: Chamberlain, Basil Hall, trans. 1883. *The Kojiki*. Tokyo: Asiatic Society of Japan.

The Ancient World: Africa

▣ *The Satire of the Trades*
(2025–1700 BCE)

A Middle Kingdom work preserved in later Ancient Egyptian literature. The stories document the difficulties and sufferings of workers in various trades.

The beginning of the teaching which the man of Tjel named Dua-Khety made for his son named Pepy, while he sailed southwards to the Residence to place him in the school of writings among the children of the magistrates, the most eminent men of the Residence.

So he spoke to him: Since I have seen those who have been beaten, it is to writings that you must set your mind. Observe the man who has been carried off to a work force. Behold, there is nothing that surpasses writings! They are a boat upon the water. Read then at the end of the Book of Kemyet this statement in it saying: As for a scribe in any office in the Residence, he will not suffer want in it.

When he fulfills the bidding of another, he does not come forth satisfied. I do not see an office to be compared with it, to which this maxim could relate. I shall make you love books more than your mother, and I shall place their excellence before you. It is greater than any office. There is nothing like it on earth. When he began to become sturdy but was still a child, he was greeted (respectfully). When he was sent to carry out a task, before he returned he was dressed in adult garments.

I do not see a stoneworker on an important errand or in a place to which he has been sent, but I have seen a coppersmith at his work at the door of his furnace. His fingers were like the claws of the crocodile, and he stank more than fish excrement.

Every carpenter who bears the adze is wearier than a fieldhand. His field is his wood, his hoe is the axe. There is no end to his work, and he must labor excessively in his activity. At nighttime he still must light his lamp.

The jeweler pierces stone in stringing beads in all kinds of hard stone. When he has completed the inlaying of the eye-amulets, his strength vanishes and he is tired out. He sits until the arrival of the sun, his knees and his back bent at (the place called) Aku-Re. ["his back bent": Tables were used only rarely in ancient Egypt. Most craftsmen worked crouching with their workpieces on the ground.]

The barber shaves until the end of the evening. But he must be up early, crying out, his bowl upon his arm. He takes himself from street to street to seek out someone to shave. He wears out his arms to fill his belly, like bees who eat (only) according to their work. ["The barber shaves": Considering the tools they had, shaving must have been pretty exhausting for the barber and quite an ordeal for his client. Copper and bronze tools are not known for their razor-sharp edges.]

The reed-cutter goes downstream to the Delta to fetch himself arrows. He must work excessively in his activity. When the gnats sting him and the sand fleas bite him as well, then he is judged.

The potter is covered with earth, although his lifetime is still among the living. He burrows in the field more than swine to bake his cooking vessels. His clothes being stiff with mud, his head cloth consists only of rags, so that the air which comes forth from his burning furnace enters his nose. He operates a pestle with his feet with which he himself is pounded, penetrating the courtyard of every house and driving earth into every open place.

I shall also describe to you the bricklayer. His kidneys are painful. When he must be outside in the wind, he lays bricks without a garment. His belt is a cord for his back, a string for his buttocks. His strength has vanished through fatigue and stiffness, kneading all his excrement. He eats bread with his fingers, although he washes himself but once a day. ["His kidneys are painful": much of the work was done bending over while lifting quite heavy loads.]

It is miserable for the carpenter when he planes the roof-beam. It is the roof of a chamber 10 by 6 cubits. A month goes by in laying the beams and spreading the matting. All the work is accomplished. But as for the food which is to be given to his household (while he is away), there is no one who provides for his children.

The vintner carries his shoulder-yoke. Each of his shoulders is burdened with age. A swelling is on his neck, and it festers. He spends the morning in watering leeks and the evening with corianders, after he has spent the midday in the palm grove. So it happens that he sinks down (at last) and dies through his deliveries, more than one of any other profession.

The fieldhand cries out more than the guinea fowl. His voice is louder than the raven's. His fingers have become ulcerous with an excess of stench. When

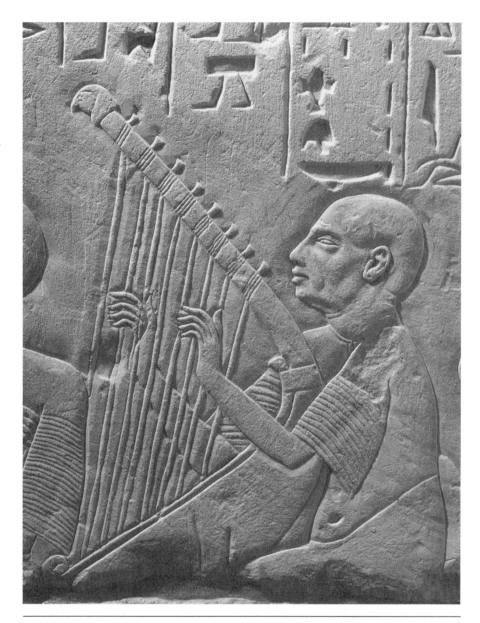

Blind harpist. One of the oldest traditions involves the participation of blind and visually impaired individuals in the profession of music. This detail of a relief was created during the Nineteenth Dynasty, New Kingdom (ca. 1250 BCE).

Source: Rijksmuseum van Oudheden, Leiden, The Netherlands. Photo credit: Erich Lessing/Art Resource, New York.

he is taken away to be enrolled in Delta labour, he is in tatters. He suffers when he proceeds to the island, and sickness is his payment. The forced labour then is tripled. If he comes back from the marshes there, he reaches his house worn out, for the forced labor has ruined him.

The weaver inside the weaving house is more wretched than a woman. His knees are drawn up against his belly. He cannot breathe the air. If he

wastes a single day without weaving, he is beaten with 50 whip lashes. He has to give food to the doorkeeper to allow him to come out to the daylight.

The arrow maker, completely wretched, goes into the desert. Greater than his own pay is what he has to spend for his she-ass for its work afterwards. Great is also what he has to give to the fieldhand to set him on the right road to the flint source. When he reaches his house in the evening, the journey has ruined him.

The courier goes abroad after handing over his property to his children, being fearful of the lions and the Asiatics. He only knows himself when he is back in Egypt. But his household by then is only a tent. There is no happy homecoming.

The furnace-tender, his fingers are foul, the smell thereof is as corpses. His eyes are inflamed because of the heaviness of smoke. He cannot get rid of his dirt, although he spends the day at the reed pond. Clothes are an abomination to him. [In a country where wood was rare and any combustible matter might serve as fuel, the use of clean-burning charcoal was probably not widespread.]

The sandal maker is utterly wretched carrying his tubs of oil. His stores are provided with carcasses, and what he bites is hides.

The washerman launders at the riverbank in the vicinity of the crocodile. I shall go away, father, from the flowing water, said his son and his daughter, to a more satisfactory profession, one more distinguished than any other profession. His food is mixed with filth, and there is no part of him which is clean. He cleans the clothes of a woman in menstruation. He weeps when he spends all day with a beating stick and a stone there. One says to him, dirty laundry, come to me, the brim overflows.

The fowler is utterly weak while searching out for the denizens of the sky. If the flock passes by above him, then he says: would that I might have nets. But God will not let this come to pass for him, for He is opposed to his activity.

I mention for you also the fisherman. He is more miserable than one of any other profession, one who is at his work in a river infested with crocodiles. When the totalling of his account is made for him, then he will lament. One did not tell him that a crocodile was standing there, and fear has now blinded him. When he comes to the flowing water, so he falls as through the might of God.

See, there is no office free from supervisors, except the scribe's. He is the supervisor!

But if you understand writings, then it will be better for you than the professions which I have set before you. Behold the official and the dependent pertaining to him. The tenant farmer of a man cannot say to him: Do not keep watching me. What I have done in journeying southward to the Residence is what I have done through love of you. A day at school is advantageous to you. Seek out its work early, while the workmen I have caused you to know hurry on and cause the recalcitrant to hasten.

I will also tell you another matter to teach you what you should know at the station of your debating. Do not come close to where there is a dispute. If a man reproves you, and you do not know how to oppose his anger, make your reply cautiously in the presence of listeners.

If you walk to the rear of officials, approach from a distance behind the last. If you enter while the master of the house is at home, and his hands are extended to another in front of you, sit with your hand to your mouth. Do not ask for anything in his presence. But do as he says to you. Beware of approaching the table. ["But do as he says to you": i.e., but react to him when addressed.]

Be serious, and great as to your worth. Do not speak secret matters. For he who hides his innermost thoughts is one who makes a shield for himself. Do not utter thoughtless words when you sit down with an angry man. ["Be serious, and great as to your worth": i.e., be serious with anyone greater in dignity when you sit down with an angry man, but take your seat with the reliable.]

When you come forth from school after midday recess has been announced to you, go into the court-yard and discuss the last part of your lesson book.

When an official sends you as a messenger, then say what he said. Neither take away nor add to it. He who abandons a chest of books, his name will not endure. He who is wise in all his ways, nothing will be hidden from him, and he will not be rebuffed from any station of his.

Do not say anything false about your mother. This is an abomination to the officials. The offspring who does useful things, his condition is equal to the one of yesterday. Do not indulge with an undisciplined man, for it is bad after it is heard about you. When you have eaten three loaves of bread and swallowed two jugs of beer, and the body has not yet had enough, fight against it. But if another is satiated, do not stand, take care not to approach the table.

See, you send out a large number. You hear the words of the officials. Then you may assume the characteristics of the children of men, and you may walk in their footsteps. One values a scribe for his understanding, for understanding transforms an eager person. You are to stand when words of welcome are offered. Your feet shall not hurry when you walk. Do not approach a trusted man, but associate with one more distinguished than you. But let your friend be a man of your generation.

See, I have placed you on the path of God. The fate of a man is on his shoulders on the day he is born. He comes to the judgement hall and the court of magistrates which the people have made. See, there is no scribe lacking sustenance, (or) the provisions of the royal house. It is Meskhenet who is turned toward the scribe who presents himself before the court of magistrates. Honour your father and mother who have placed you on the path of the living. Mark this, which I have placed before your eyes, and the children of your children.

I have placed you on the path of God: Abundance is on the path of the god the court of magistrates which the people have made: that court of officials is the one allotting people to him.

It has come to an end in peace.

Source: Ermann, A., trans; Dollinger, André, ed. and annotated. 2004. "The Satire of the Trades, or, The Instructions of Dua-Khety." Available at http://nefertiti.iwebland.com/texts/instructions_of_kheti.htm

▣ "Fire from Heaven!" A Story of the Wagogo

Africa contributes many Origin tales to the world's heritage as well as many stories in which people travel in search of fire. Some Origin accounts address disability and may embody a code of inclusive practice with disabled people. An intriguing story from the Wagogo people of Tanzania involves all these elements, plus some sharp psychology, a deity running a competition game show, and an ending that appeals to women everywhere.

Long ago there was no fire on earth; so a man went up into the sky to look for fire. When he got to the first heaven he met a number of individuals who were only half men (i.e. having only one side) whereupon he commenced to laugh, and they asked him whether he was laughing at their deformity, and he replied in the affirmative, saying that there were no such people in his country. He then ascended higher until he reached the second heaven, where he saw men walking on their heads. They, too, asked him whether he was laughing at them; and he replied in the affirmative. Not yet having found fire, he ascended still higher, until he got to the third heaven, when he saw men going on their knees; and they also asked him if he was laughing at their deformity, and he replied as he did before, in the affirmative. In reply to his enquiries about fire they told him that he had almost arrived at his destination; and they told him to go straight on until he came to God's house, where he would find God himself standing outside, as that was the place where he was always to be found. He pursued his course as directed, and was not long before he reached the abode of *Mulungu* (God), which was situated in the fourth heaven. Everywhere the sight was ravishing. The man approached near and saluted *Mulungu*. The salutation being over *Mulungu* asked him what brought him there. He replied saying he had come in search of fire, as in his country there was no fire. *Mulungu* showed him a room in which to sleep and told him that on the morrow he would find fire. Next morning *Mulungu* came and called him and showed him a room in which the most beautiful vessels were placed, all of which had covers; but besides the very beautiful vessels there were two other very inferior vessels placed by themselves. He chose a very beautiful pot and went outside, where he met *Mulungu*, who told him to remove the cover. Having done so he found ashes and charcoal in the pot. Whereupon he asked, 'Lord, have you no fire?' *Mulungu* replied saying, 'How was it that on the journey here you laughed at my children? Is there nothing lacking in your country, and if so what has brought you here?' Thereupon he ordered him to return to his home.

A second and a third man went who had the same experience. At last a woman went; and when she got to the first heaven, the one-sided people came to greet her, and she sang and they danced; and when she was tired of singing, the strange beings showed her the way without her asking any questions. When she got to the second and third heavens she also sang and the inhabitants danced; and when they asked her whether people in her country had deformities, she said many were afflicted in that way, and she went on to tell them that some walked on their ears, others on their toes, and others again were blind. When she had rested she resumed her journey, and ere long she arrived at the house of *Mulungu*. He (*Mulungu*) asked her her business, and when she had told her errand he showed her a room in which to sleep the night. The next morning he called her and showed her the lovely vessels which he had previously shown to the three men and told her to choose one; but she shrank from doing so, fearing to touch such lovely vessels. Glancing, however, in the direction of the two inferior pots she summoned up courage to take one of them. Having chosen a pot she went outside and saw *Mulungu,* who told her to uncover the pot; and when she had done so, lo! there was the long-looked-for fire inside! Mulungu praised her for the way in which she behaved toward his children on her way thither; and he presented her with an ox in recognition of her kindness. Here she remained two days feasting on the meat, and on the third day *Mulungu* told her she might go and take the fire with her, which would be sufficient for all the world. It was a day of great rejoicing when the woman returned to the earth. Multitudes came to hear the news and to procure fire from the pot. The men with one accord applauded the woman, and declared that the women have more sense than the men.

Source: Cole, H. 1902. "Notes on the Wagogo of German East Africa." *Journal of the Anthropological Institute of Great Britain and Ireland* 32:305–338.

The Ancient World: Pre-Columbian Americas

▣ The Legend of the Pyramid of the Dwarf (569–1000 CE)

John Stephens transcribed this story in 1840 from the local inhabitants of Uxmal (the site in present-day Mexico of an ancient Mayan city) in 1840. Note that this transcription is only one of many versions of this story, suggesting its importance in the imagination of the community.

There was an old woman who lived in a hut that was located on the exact spot where the finished pyramid now stands. This old woman was a witch who one day went into mourning that she had no children. One day, she took an egg and wrapped it in cloth and placed it in a corner of her small hut. Every day she went to look at the egg until one day it hatched and a small creature, closely resembling a baby, came from the enchanted egg.

The old woman was delighted and called the baby her son. She provided it with a nurse and took good care of it so that within a year it was walking and talking like a man. It stopped growing after a year and the old woman was very proud of her son and told him that one day he would be a great Lord or King.

One day, she told her son to go the House of the Governor and challenge the King to a trial of strength. The dwarf didn't want to go at first but the old woman insisted and so to see the King he went. The guards let him in and he threw down his challenge to the King. The King smiled, and told the dwarf to lift a stone that weighed three *arrobas* (75 pounds). At this the dwarf cried and ran back to his mother. The witch was wise, and told her son to tell the King that if the King would lift the stone first, then he would lift it also. The dwarf returned and told the King what his mother told him

to say. The king lifted the stone and the dwarf did the same. The King was impressed, and a little nervous, and tested the dwarf for the rest of the day with other feats of strength. Each time the King performed an act, the dwarf was able to match it.

The King became enraged that he was being matched by a dwarf, and told the dwarf that in one night he must build a house higher than any other in the city or he would be killed. The dwarf again returned crying to his mother who told him to not lose hope, and that he should go straight to bed. The next morning the city awoke to see the Pyramid of the Dwarf in its finished state, larger than any other building in the city.

The King saw this building from his palace and was again enraged and summoned the dwarf. The King told the dwarf he had one final test of strength. The dwarf had to collect two bundles of *Cogoil* wood, a very strong and heavy wood, and the king would break the wood over the head of the dwarf, and after that the dwarf could have his turn to break the wood over the King's head.

The dwarf again ran to his mother for help. She told him not to worry and placed an enchanted tortillia on his head as a crown. The trial was performed in front of all the great men of the city. The King broke the whole of his bundle over the dwarfs head one at a time without hurting or bothering the dwarf in the least. The King then tried to bow out of his challenge, but in front of all the [city's] great men he knew he had no choice but to go ahead and let the dwarf have his turn.

The second stick of the bundle broke the Kings skull into pieces and he fell dead at the foot of the dwarf who[m] everyone acknowledged as the new King.

The dwarf returned to tell his mother what had transpired, but found that she had died. But she died happy to know that her son had indeed become King.

Legend has it that in the town of Mani, seventeen leagues distant, there is a deep well that opens into a cave that leads all the way to Merida. In this cave, on the bank of a stream under the shade of a large tree, sits an old woman . . . with a serpent by her side. She begs occasionally or sells water. Not for money, but for a *criatura* or baby to feed to her serpent.

This old woman is the mother of the dwarf.

Source: Stephens, John, trans. 1840. *Pyramid of the Dwarf.* Available at http://ancientsites.com/aw/Post/259572

▣ Ee-ee-toy's Song: When He Made the World Serpents

At this point in the story three key Pima Gods, Ee-ee-toy, Toehahvs, and Juhwerta Mahkai, decide to have a contest to make the best first people to occupy the land. However, unbeknownst to the others, Mahkai has already invented a people to begin civilization, and he seeks to protect their privilege by making imperfect dolls.

I know what to do;
I am going to move the water
Both ways.

But the water was still running in the valleys, and Ee-ee-toy took a hair from his head and made it into a snake—*Vuck-vahmuhtl.* And with this snake he pushed the waters south, but the head of the snake was left lying to the west and his tail to the east.

But there was more water, and Ee-ee-toy took another hair from his head and made another snake, and with this snake pushed the rest of the water north. And the head of this snake was left to the east and his tail to the west. So the head of each snake was left lying with the tail of the other.

And the snake that has his tail to the east, in the morning will shake up his tail to start the morning wind to wake the people and tell them to think of their dreams.

And the snake that has his tail to the west, in the evening will shake up his tail to start the cool wind to tell the people it is time to go in and make the fires and be comfortable.

And they said: "We will make dolls, but we will not let each other see them until they are finished."

And Ee-ee-toy sat facing the west, and Toehahvs facing the south, and Juhwerta Mahkai facing the east.

And the earth was still damp and they took clay and began to make dolls. And Ee-ee-toy made the best. But Juhwerta Mahkai did not make good ones, because he remembered some of his people had escaped the flood thru a hole in the earth, and he intended to visit them and he did not want to make anything better than they were to take the place of them. And Toehahvs made the poorest of all.

Then Ee-ee-toy asked them if they were ready, and they all said yes, and then they turned about and showed each other the dolls they had made.

And Ee-ee-toy asked Juhwerta Mahkai why he had made such queer dolls.

"This one," he said, "is not right, for you have made him without any sittingdown parts, and how can he get rid of the waste of what he eats?"

But Juhwerta Mahkai said: "He will not need to eat, he can just smell the smell of what is cooked."

Then Ee-ee-toy asked again: "why did you make this doll with only one leg—how can he run?" But Juhwerta Mahkai replied: "He will not need to run; he can just hop around."

Then Ee-ee-toy asked Toehahvs why he had made a doll with webs between his fingers and toes—"How can he point directions?" But Toehahvs said he had made these dolls so for good purpose, for if anybody gave them small seeds they would not slip between their fingers, and they could use the webs for dippers to drink with.

And Ee-ee-toy held up his dolls and said: "These are the best of all, and I want you to make more like them." And he took Toehahv's dolls and threw them into the water and they became ducks and beavers. And he took Juhwerta Mahkai's dolls and threw them away and they all broke to pieces and were nothing.

And Juhwerta Mahkai was angry at this and began to sink into the ground; and took his stick and hooked it into the sky and pulled the sky down while he was sinking. But Ee-ee-toy spread his hand over his dolls, and held up the sky, and seeing that Juhwerta Mahkai was sinking into the earth he sprang and tried to hold him and cried, "Man, what are you doing! Are you going to leave me and my people here alone?"

But Juhwerta Mahkai slipped through his hands, leaving in them only the waste and excretion of his skin. And that is how there is sickness and death among us.

Source: Lloyd, J. William, trans. 1911. *Aw-aw-tam Indian Nights: The Myths and Legends of the Pimas.* Available at http://www .sacred-texts.com/nam/sw/ain/ain07.htm

▣ Ciqneqs Myth

Using the fieldwork of J. P. Harrington as a basis, Thomas Blackburn compiled oral narratives of the Chumash Indians from coastal California. Ciqneqs myths are similar to European tales about cognitively disabled individuals, such as "simple Simon."

Once there was a village with only a few families living in it, and in two of these families there was a man and woman who married one another when they came of age. After their marriage, they began to have children, and their first twelve children were all boys. The last, however, was a girl. The children all grew up, and one day it was discovered that the girl was pregnant. . . . [section about a makeshift paternity test omitted here]

When the child was born the brothers called the ?alaxlaps to come and name him. (The ?alaxlaps was a kind of priest. He could tell whether or not a person would be fortunate in his transactions, and also by the planet of a person what would be his or her fate. He was an anatomist, physiognomist, and astrologer.) The ?alaxlaps asked who the child's father was. One brother said to ask the child's mother. Then the mother said her baby was a sowing of the clouds. When the ?alaxlaps heard this, he said to her: "Ah, girl, you were born to be happy. For it is your lot to give birth to this child of the clouds. Name him Ciqneqs."

When the child, Ciqneqs, grew old enough to go on errands, there was an old woman in the village who was his grandmother's sister. This old lady was very much inclined to be a sorceress. Ciqneqs knew about this. One day one of his uncles asked the boy to take his old woman over to his camp on the beach where he was clamming. She was quite old and was blind. Ciqneqs led the old lady to the camp, which was close to a precipice. Noticing this, the boy left the old woman at the camp and looked over the cliff. He saw there was a cave at the foot of the cliff that would be covered by water at high tide, but which was now dry, and that there were many large rocks scattered around the entrance.

He went back to the old woman and said: 'Let's go a little further.' He gave her her cane and led her down the edge of the cliff into the cave. He told her: 'While you're here, I'm going over to the house and I'll return.' Then he left quietly. Once outside the cave, he began to pile up stones until the entrance was completely blocked. Sometime later, the uncle noticed that it was high tide and thought to ask Ciqneqs how the old

woman was. 'No animal will harm her,' said Ciqneqs. 'Is she away from the reach of the tide?' asked the uncle. 'Yes,' said the boy. Later, another old woman, missing her neighbor, told the uncle: 'You had better go and see what Ciqneqs has done with his grandmother's sister.' The uncle went, and not finding the old lady anywhere returned and said: 'She is not there.' Then the other old lady said to Ciqneqs: 'What did you do with her?' The boy answered: 'I put her in a cave.' 'Why did you put her in there?' 'She fooled the world too much by means of her black magic.' Then the old woman exclaimed: 'You really are a child of the clouds, and only the clouds can punish you. But we must be patient with you, because if the clouds punish you by means of a deluge of water, the punishment will fall on us also.'

Editors' Note: There are other Ciqneqs stories, but this one has most of the usual elements: taking orders literally, giving weird or cryptic answers to all inquiries, and going unpunished because he's a "child of the clouds." He frustrates the Yowoyow, the devil, in another story, with his strange conversational style, until the devil gives up and goes away disgusted. He sings a creepy song to scare away his fellow villagers, ending with the line, "I am son of the dead, and therefore I am hungry." He kills a little brother in his care by misconstruing the directions his parents left him. He tries to bed his sister after misunderstanding his grandmother's instructions to marry. "Siqneqs did many other stupid things, but his parents always sent him on errands anyway," explains one storyteller. "And even today, when parents scold their children they're apt to say, 'That's just like Siqneqs!'"

Source: Blackburn, Thomas C. 1975. *December's Child: A Book of Chumash Oral Narratives.* Berkeley: University of California Press.

▣ Qöyáwaima (Oraíbi)

An ethnographical account of the legends, myths, and stories of the Hopi. A number of the stories address disability as a key, providing moments of revelation that are revered in the tribal histories.

42. The Blind Man and the Lame Man

A long time ago there was an earthquake at Oraíbi. It was a very nice day; people had eaten their breakfast

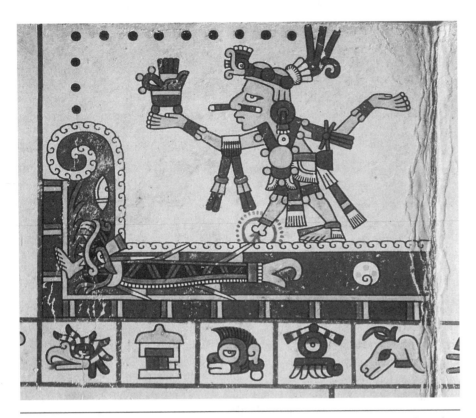

Tezcatlipoca tempting the Earth Monster. A panel from the Codex Fejervary-Mayer shows how Tezcatlipoca tempted the Earth Monster to the surface of the great waters by using his foot as bait. In swallowing his foot, she loses her lower jaw. As a result of this disability she was unable to sink, and thus the earth was created from her body. Mayan manuscript, Mixtec style, with date glyphs. Beaten deer skin and limewash.

Source: Liverpool Museum, Liverpool, Great Britain. Photo credit: Werner Forman/Art Resource, New York.

as usual, and were happy. Then towards noon the earth and the houses began to move and to tremble, and very soon there was a great noise like thunder, but nothing could be seen and the people did not know where it came from. They ran to their houses and everywhere to see what was the matter. Sometime in the afternoon the earth trembled very much, and a large piece of ground sank down at Skeleton gulch (Másvövee), so called because at one time a great many slain people were thrown there. This is situated about half a mile northeast of Oraíbi; the piece that sank down reached nearly to the village of Oraíbi. There was also a very large crack right on the public square or plaza of the village.

By this time the people got frightened very much, and all left the village, running toward the north. In the village there lived in one of the houses a blind man, and in another house a cripple who could not walk. When these noticed that some serious disturbance was taking place, they got very much

frightened, and the blind man called over to the cripple asking for information. The latter answered that the earth had been trembling and the village had been in motion, and that all the people had left the village. The cripple then asked the blind man to come over to his house. The blind man asked the cripple to come over to his house, but after a while the cripple prevailed, and the blind man, taking a stick and feeling his way before himself, tried to reach the house of the cripple, the latter directing him which way to go. When he had arrived at the house the cripple said: "Let us also flee. You carry me on your back, and I shall show you the way." This they did, the cripple turning the head of the blind man in the direction in which he wanted him to turn and to go. Thus they left the village, also in a northerly direction, following the others.

A short distance north of the village a large elk met them, coming from the north. "O my! what is that?" the cripple said, on the back of the blind man. "What is it?" the latter asked. "Something very large. It is nearly black, and yet it is not quite black." The blind man, who had been a great hunter in his youth, when he still had his eyesight, at once suspected what it might be, and asked for details, and soon concluded that it must be an elk. Before leaving the village the blind man had suggested that they take a bow and arrows along so that, in case they needed some food, they could kill some game. When they had come opposite the elk the cripple suggested that the blind man shoot the elk, as his own hands were also somewhat crippled, and he was unable to handle a bow. He put an arrow on the bow, and the blind man got the bow ready, the cripple doing the aiming for him. The elk was now standing west of them, and at the proper time the cripple told the blind man to shoot. He shot and killed the elk.

They were now very anxious to roast some of the meat, but had nothing to skin the animal or cut the meat with; so they went there and with one of their arrows they dug out the eyes of the elk. The blind man then, being directed by the lame man, gathered some sticks of wood and they built a fire, starting the fire by rubbing wood and fire sticks together. They placed the two eyes on the fire and waited. When the eyes got very hot they burst with a great report. "Hihiyá!" the men exclaimed, and both jumped up, the lame man finding that he could walk, and the blind man finding his eyes opened. "Ishutí," the blind man said. "What is it (hintí)?" "My eyes are open." "Yes, and I can walk," the other man replied. By this time it had become evening. "Now let us remain awake all night," the man who had been blind said, "because if we go to sleep my eyes might stick together again." "Yes, if I lie down I might find that I cannot walk again in the morning," the other one replied. So the first one handed the other a small twig of ö'cvi (Ephedra), saying to him, "If you see that I go to sleep, you prick my eyes so that I

awake." The other one handed the blind man, as we shall call him for brevity's sake, also some prickly weed, saying, "If you see me sit down you prick my body so that I remain standing." Thus they remained awake all night watching each other.

Early in the morning they concluded that they would follow the tracks of the inhabitants of the village who had fled. They finally found them in a timber quite a distance to the north. "What has happened to you?" they said. "Why, you were blind and lame, and now you can see and walk." "Yes," they said, "something has happened to us: and now let us go back again to the village. There is nothing the matter there any more." So the people all returned to the village, these two taking the lead, and that is the reason why Oraíbi is again inhabited. If these two had not brought the people back they would never have returned.

Source: Voth, H. R., trans. 1905. *The Traditions of the Hopi* (Field Columbian Museum Publication 96, Anthropological Series Vol. 8). Chicago: Field Columbian Museum.

The Ancient World: Norse Culture

▣ "The Death of Balder"
(ca. 1250 CE)

The name of Balder (or Baldr) means "the glorious," but he was also identified as the "god of tears." He was the son of Odin and Frigg and described as one of the wisest gods in Norse mythology. The excerpt below occurs on the heels of Balder's foreboding dream about his own death. As a protective measure, his mother, Frigg, asks all things not to hurt him, but she doesn't ask the mistletoe, because it seems young and harmless. Later, disguised as an old woman, the trickster Loki makes a dart out of mistletoe and tricks the blind god Hod into throwing it at Balder, precipitating his death. Thus, the story becomes a tale of Loki's treachery toward other gods' singular weaknesses.

A servant hurried up and offered Loki wine. Loki drained the cup at one draught and then sauntered across the spacious hall, behind the semi-circle of the gods and their followers. He sidled up to Hod and poked him in the ribs.

'That can only be Loki,' said Hod.

'None other,' said a voice in his ear.

'Well?' said Hod.

'Why don't you join in? Why aren't you throwing darts at your brother?'

'Because I can't see where he is,' said Hod.

Loki sucked his cheeks.

'Another thing,' said Hod. 'I have no weapon.'

'This is not as it should be,' said Loki with measured indignation. 'They do wrong to ignore you—and your brother.'

Hod's expression did not alter. He had long since learned to accept his fate. 'Nothing comes,' he said, 'of ranking resentment.'

Hod's words were drowned in a roar of laughter.

'What is that?' he asked.

'Only more of the same,' said Loki. 'A dart well aimed. But now it's your turn, Hod. You should pay your respects like everybody else.'

'I have no weapon,' Hod repeated.

'Take this twig then,' said Loki, and he put the sharpened mistletoe between Hod's hands. 'I'll show you where he's standing. I'll stand behind you and guide your hand.'

Loki's eyes were on fire now. His whole body was on fire. His face was ravaged by wolfish evil and hunger.

Hod grasped the mistletoe and lifted his right arm. Guided by Loki, he aimed the dart at his brother Balder.

The mistletoe flew through the hall and it struck Balder. It pierced him and passed right through him. The god fell on his face. He was dead.

There was no sound in Gladsheim, no sound, only the roaring of silence. The gods could not speak. They looked at the fairest and most wise of them all, shining and lifeless, they could not even move from where they stood to lift him.

The gods stared at each other and then they turned to stare at Hod and Loki. They had no doubt. They were all of one mind about who had caused Balder's death and yet none of them were able to take vengeance.

The ground of Gladsheim was hallowed and no one was ready to shed blood in the sanctuary.

Hod could not see the fearsome gaze of that gathering. Loki could not withstand it. He loped towards the doors of Gladsheim and slunk away into the darkness.

Source: Mabie, Hamilton Wright, trans. 1901. *Norse Stories Retold from the Eddas.* New York: Dodd, Mead and Company. Available at http://www.mainlesson.com/display.php?author=mabie&book=norse&story=balder

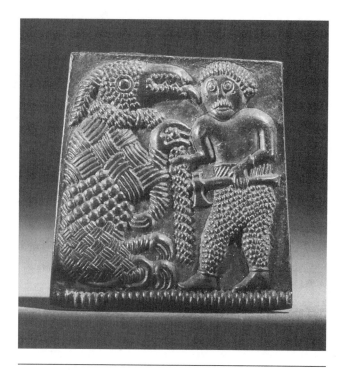

Tyr, the original sky god of the Germanic tribes, with a chained wolf, Fenrir, whom Tyr fettered at the cost of his own hand. Although the other Norse gods laugh at his willingness to sacrifice a bodily appendage, the story emphasizes the heroism of suffering on behalf of the community. Sixth century, bronze. Matrix used in the manufacture of helmet plaques.

Source: Torslunda Parish, Oland, Sweden. Statens Historiska Museet, Stockholm, Sweden. Photo credit: Werner Forman/Art Resource, New York.

◉ "The Binding of the Wolf" (ca. 1250 CE)

The wolf, Fenrir (Fenrer in this version), is the oldest child of the trickster god Loki (Loke in this version) and the giantess Angrboda. Of all the gods, only Tyr is brave enough to feed Fenrir as he roams the fields of Asgard. As the gods grow increasingly leery of the wolf's size and power they decide to try and bind him with a variety of strong materials. Finally, the dark dwarves of Svartalfheim create a silky rope that can hold the wolf. However, in the process of binding the wolf, Tyr loses his hand and forearm. As a result, Tyr's shortened arm becomes a symbol of personal sacrifice for the good of others.

Loke looked like a god and had many of the wonderful gifts which the gods possessed, but at heart he was one of those giants who were always trying to cross Bifrost, the shining rainbow-bridge, at the heavenly end of which Heimdal kept guard day and night, with eyes so keen that in the darkness as easily as in the light he could see a hundred miles distant, and with ears so sharp that he could hear the noiseless blossoming of the grass in the deepest valley, and the growing of the wool upon the backs of sheep browsing along the hill-tops. Loke had the mind of the gods, who were always working to bring order and beauty into the world, but he had the heart of the giants, who were striving to undo the good and cover the earth with howling storms and icy desolation. After he had been in Asgard for a time he wanted to get back to Jotunheim, where his true home was. There he married a terrible giantess, and three children were born to him, more repulsive than their mother, Hel, the Midgard-serpent, and the Fenris-wolf. These monsters grew to be very strong and horrible to look upon before the gods thought of destroying them; but one day, as Odin looked over the worlds from his throne, a shadow fell upon his face, for he saw how powerful the children of Loke were becoming, and he knew they would work endless mischief and misery for gods and men; so he sent some of the gods to bring the monsters to Asgard. It was a strange sight when Loke's children were brought into heaven, Hel's terrible face turning into stone every one who looked, unless he were a god; the Midgard-serpent coiling its immense length into great circles over which the glittering eyes wandered restlessly; and the Fenris-wolf growling with a deep, cruel voice. Odin looked sternly at Loke, the evil god who had brought such savage beings among men, and then with a dark brow he cast Hel down into the dusky kingdoms of the dead, and hurled the snake into the deep sea, where he grew until he coiled around the whole earth; but Fenrer, the wolf, was permitted to grow up in Asgard. He was so fierce that only Tyr, the sword-god, could feed him. He roamed about Asgard, his huge body daily growing stronger, and his hungry eyes flashing more and more fiercely.

After a time another shadow fell upon Odin's face, for Fenrer was fast becoming the most terrible enemy of the gods, and the oracles who could look into the future, said that at the last great battle he would destroy Odin himself. So Odin called all the gods together, and as they came into the great hall the wolf crouched at the door, with a look that made even their strong hearts shudder.

"Our most dangerous enemy is growing stronger every day under our roof and by our hands," said

Odin, "and we shall cease to be gods if we are so blind as to nourish our own destroyer."

"Kill him!" muttered some one.

"No," said Odin; "although he is to devour me, no blood shall stain the sacred seats of the gods."

"Chain him!" said Thor.

That was a good plan, they all agreed, but how was it to be done?

"Leave that to me," answered Thor, full of courage, for he had done many wonderful things, and there was nothing of which he was afraid.

That night the fires in the great smithy blazed and roared so fiercely that the heavens far around were lighted with the glow, and in the dusky light the strong forms of the gods moved to and fro as they worked on the chain with which they meant to bind the Fenris-wolf. All night Thor's mighty strokes rang on the hard iron, and when the morning came the chain was done, and they called it Leding. Then the gods called Fenrer, spread out the chain, and asked him to show his wonderful strength by breaking it.

The wolf knew better than the gods how strong he had grown, and that the breaking of Leding would be a very small matter for him; so he permitted them to bind the great links around his shaggy body and about his feet, and to rivet the ends so fast that it seemed as if nothing on earth could ever break them apart again. When it was all done, and Thor's eyes were beginning to smile at his success, the wolf got quietly upon his feet, stretched himself as easily as if a web of silk were cast over him, snapped the massive chain in a dozen places, and walked off, leaving the gods to gather up the broken links.

"He has grown terribly strong," said Odin, looking at the great pieces of iron.

"Yes," answered sturdy Thor, "stronger than I thought; but I will forge another chain, which even he cannot break."

Again the red glow shone in the sky over Asgard, the fires flashed and blazed, and the great hammers rang far into the night, and the next day the mighty chain Drome, twice as strong as Leding, was finished.

"Come, Fenrer," said Thor, "you already famous for your strength; if you can break this chain no [one] will ever be able to deny your strength, and you will win great honour among gods and men."

The wolf growled as he looked at the great chain, for he knew that the gods feared him and wanted to make him harmless. He knew also that he could break the chain which they had forged with so much toil to bind

him with, and so he let them fasten him as before. When all was done, the gods began to smile again, for they had made the strongest chain that ever was or could be made, and now surely the wolf was forever harmless.

But Fenrer knew better than they. He rose slowly, with the massive links bound closely about him, shook himself fiercely, stretched himself, and then with a mighty effort dashed himself on the ground; the earth shook, the chain burst, and its links flew through the air and buried themselves in the ground, so tremendous was the effort with which the wolf freed himself. A fierce joy gleamed in his eyes as he walked away with deep growls, leaving the gods to console themselves as best they might, for there were no more chains to be made.

Long and anxiously they talked together, but no one could think of anything which could hold Fenrer until Odin called to Skirner, Frey's swiftest messenger: "Go to Svartalfheim as fast as the flash of Thor's hammer, and the dwarfs shall make us an enchanted chain which even he cannot break."

Skirner was off almost before Odin had done speaking. Travelling over land and sea he soon came to the dark entrance of the under-world where the dwarfs lived, and in a very short time he was in the dusky home of the wonderful little workers in iron. They were rushing about with black faces and dirty hair when Skirner called them together and said, "You must make for the gods an enchanted chain so slight that Fenrer will be willing to be bound by it, and so strong that when he has allowed himself to be tied he cannot break loose again."

The dwarves whispered together for a few moments, and then scattered in every direction; for they were going to make the most wonderful chain that was ever put together, and there were many things to be looked after before it could be done. Skirner sat in the darkness until the busy little workers had finished the band, and then he carried it quickly to Asgard, where all the gods were waiting anxiously for his coming and Fenrer was stealthily stealing from place to place through the city. Skirner spread the string out for the gods to look at, and they could hardly believe it was strong enough. It was very long, but so small and soft that it seemed no more than silken twine; it was made out of such things as the sound of a cat's footsteps, the roots of the mountains, the breath of a fish, and the sinews of a bear, and nothing could break it.

The gods were so happy in the hope of being relieved of their enemy that they could not thank

Skirner enough. They all went to a rocky island in a lake called Amsvartner, taking the wolf with them. Thor showed the silken twine to Fenrer. "You have broken Leding and Drome," he said, "and now you will break this also, although it is somewhat stronger than one would think, to look at it."

Then he handed the magic cord from one god to another and each tried to break it, but no one succeeded.

"We cannot do it," they all said after it had been handed around the circle, "but Fenrer can."

The wolf looked at it suspiciously.

"It is such a slender thread," he answered, "that I shall get no credit if I break it, and if it is made with magic, slight as it looks I shall never get loose from it again."

The gods looked at one another and smiled.

"Oh, you will easily break so slim a band as that," they replied, "since you have already broken the heaviest chains in the world; and if you cannot break it we will loosen you again."

"If you bind me so fast that I am not able to get myself free, I shall get little help from you," said the wolf truthfully enough. "I am very unwilling to have this twine bound about me; but that you may not be able to call me cowardly, I will do it if some one of you will lay his hand in my mouth as a pledge that there is no deceit about this thing."

The gods looked at each other when they heard these words. Fenrer had spoken the truth, there was no denying that. He must be chained now, however, or they would all be destroyed; but who would lose a hand to save the rest? Thor's hands were needed to swing the hammer against the giants, and everybody could think of some very good reason why his hand should not be lost. There was an awful pause, and then Tyr, the god of honour and courage, who had never stood still when he ought to go forward, stretched out his right hand and laid it in the wolf's hungry mouth.

Then the gods bound the slender cord tightly around Fenrer, fold on fold, winding its whole length about him and tying the ends tightly together. It was so slight that it seemed as if it must break in fifty places as soon as the wolf began to stretch himself. So perhaps thought Fenrer himself; but the harder he strove to break loose, the closer the cord drew about him. He sprang from side to side, he threw himself on the ground, he stretched his mighty limbs with all his strength, but the twine only cut the deeper. Then a mighty rage filled the wolf because he had suffered himself to be deceived, his eyes flamed with fury, and the foam ran out of his mouth. The gods were so delighted when they found the wolf really fast at last that they began to laugh, all except brave Tyr, who lost his right hand.

They took the wonderful silken chain and drew it through the middle of a rock and sunk the rock so deep in the earth that nothing but an earthquake could stir it. Fenrer, wild with pain and rage, rushed from side to side so violently that the earth rocked beneath him, and opening his tremendous jaws sprang upon the gods; whereupon they thrust a sword into his cruel jaws so that the hilt stood on his lower jaw and the point pierced the roof of the mouth.

So the Fenris-wolf was bound and made fast to the rocky island, his jaws spread far apart, foaming and growling until the last great day.

Source: Mabie, Hamilton Wright, trans. 1901. *Norse Stories Retold from the Eddas.* New York: Dodd, Mead and Company. Available at http://www.mainlesson.com/display.php?author= mabie&book=norse&story=wolf

The Ancient World: Greece

▣ Tiresias

Tiresias sits at the origin of a long tradition of blind prophets who, though they have lost their literal vision, compensate by seeing accurately into the future. This excerpt provides a well-known nineteenth-century commentary on his ancestry and his powers of foresight.

Early in the contest Eteocles consulted the soothsayer Tiresias as to the issue. Tiresias in his youth had by chance seen Minerva bathing. The goddess in her wrath deprived him of his sight, but afterwards relenting gave him in compensation the knowledge of future events. When consulted by Eteocles, he declared that victory should fall to Thebes if Menoeceus, the son of Creon, gave himself a voluntary victim. The heroic youth, learning the response, threw away his life in the first encounter.

Source: Bulfinch, Thomas. 1855. *Bulfinch's Mythology: The Age of Fables or Stories of Gods and Heroes.* Available at http://etext.library .adelaide.edu.au/b/bulfinch/thomas/b93fab/chap23.html

▣ Homer, the *Iliad* (ca. 750 BCE)

The Homeric writings contain several references to disabled people and provide hints about the meaning of disability. In both passages, the appearance of the person is noted; in Thersites' case, his appearance is noted disparagingly; in the case of Hephaestus, it is merely described. Note, though, that both Thersites and Hephaestus are playing important community roles. Regardless of physical appearance, Thersites is a soldier; Hephaestus is a craftsman.

From Book 2

The rest now took their seats and kept to their own several places, but Thersites still went on wagging his unbridled tongue—a man of many words, and those unseemly; a monger of sedition, a railer against all who were in authority, who cared not what he said, so that he might set the Achaeans in a laugh. He was the ugliest man of all those that came before Troy—bandy-legged, lame of one foot, with his two shoulders rounded and hunched over his chest. His head ran up to a point, but there was little hair on the top of it. Achilles and Ulysses hated him worst of all, for it was with them that he was most wont to wrangle; now, however, with a shrill squeaky voice he began heaping his abuse on Agamemnon. The Achaeans were angry and disgusted, yet none the less he kept on brawling and bawling at the son of Atreus.

"Agamemnon," he cried, "what ails you now, and what more do you want? Your tents are filled with bronze and with fair women, for whenever we take a town we give you the pick of them. Would you have yet more gold, which some Trojan is to give you as a ransom for his son, when I or another Achaean has taken him prisoner? Or is it some young girl to hide and lie with? It is not well that you, the ruler of the Achaeans, should bring them into such misery. Weakling cowards, women rather than men, let us sail home, and leave this fellow here at Troy to stew in his own meeds of honour, and discover whether we were of any service to him or no. Achilles is a much better man than he is, and see how he has treated him—robbing him of his prize and keeping it himself. Achilles takes it meekly and shows no fight; if he did, son of Atreus, you would never again insult him."

Thus railed Thersites, but Ulysses at once went up to him and rebuked him sternly. "Check your glib tongue, Thersites," said be, "and babble not a word further. Chide not with princes when you have none to back you. There is no viler creature come before Troy with the sons of Atreus. Drop this chatter about kings, and neither revile them nor keep harping about going home. We do not yet know how things are going to be, nor whether the Achaeans are to return with good success or evil. How dare you gibe at Agamemnon because the Danaans have awarded him so many prizes? I tell you, therefore—and it shall surely be—that if I again catch you talking such nonsense, I will either forfeit my own head and be no more called father of Telemachus, or I will take you, strip you stark naked, and whip you out of the assembly till you go blubbering back to the ships."

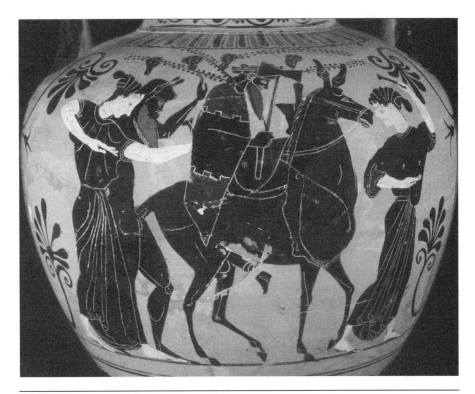

Hephaestus, god of fire, bronzework, and craftsmen, is returned to Olympus by his nondisabled brother, Dionysus. The story explains the contest of Zeus's decision to exclude Hephaestus from the domain of the gods. The image uses the common visual identifier of an inverted foot to characterize his mobility impairment. Black-figured Attic amphora, end of sixth century BCE. Terra cotta, height 40 cm, diameter 27.3 cm.

Source: Kunsthistorisches Museum, Vienna, Austria. Photo credit: Erich Lessing/Art Resource, New York.

On this he beat him with his staff about the back and shoulders till he dropped and fell a-weeping. The golden sceptre raised a bloody weal on his back, so he sat down frightened and in pain, looking foolish as he wiped the tears from his eyes. The people were sorry for him, yet they laughed heartily, and one would turn to his neighbour saying, "Ulysses has done many a good thing ere now in fight and council, but he never did the Argives a better turn than when he stopped this fellow's mouth from prating further. He will give the kings no more of his insolence."

From Book 14

Thereon laughter-loving Venus said, "I cannot and must not refuse you, for you sleep in the arms of Jove who is our king."

As she spoke she loosed from her bosom the curiously embroidered girdle into which all her charms had been wrought—love, desire, and that sweet flattery which steals the judgement even of the most prudent. She gave the girdle to Juno and said, "Take this girdle wherein all my charms reside and lay it in your bosom. If you will wear it I promise you that your errand, be it what it may, will not be bootless."

When she heard this Juno smiled, and still smiling she laid the girdle in her bosom.

Venus now went back into the house of Jove, while Juno darted down from the summits of Olympus. She passed over Pieria and fair Emathia, and went on and on till she came to the snowy ranges of the Thracian horsemen, over whose topmost crests she sped without ever setting foot to ground. When she came to Athos she went on over the waves of the sea till she reached Lemnos, the city of noble Thoas. There she met Sleep, own brother to Death, and caught him by the hand, saying, "Sleep, you who lord it alike over mortals and immortals, if you ever did me a service in times past, do one for me now, and I shall be grateful to you ever after. Close Jove's keen eyes for me in slumber while I hold him clasped in my embrace, and I will give you a beautiful golden seat, that can never fall to pieces; my clubfooted son Vulcan shall make it for you, and he shall give it a footstool for you to rest your fair feet upon when you are at table."

From Book 18

And Juno answered, "Dread son of Saturn, why should you say this thing? May not a man though he be only mortal and knows less than we do, do what he can for another person? And shall not I—foremost of all goddesses both by descent and as wife to you who reign in heaven—devise evil for the Trojans if I am angry with them?"

Thus did they converse. Meanwhile Thetis came to the house of Vulcan, imperishable, star-bespangled, fairest of the abodes in heaven, a house of bronze wrought by the lame god's own hands. She found him busy with his bellows, sweating and hard at work, for he was making twenty tripods that were to stand by the wall of his house, and he set wheels of gold under them all that they might go of their own selves to the assemblies of the gods, and come back again—marvels indeed to see. They were finished all but the ears of cunning workmanship which yet remained to be fixed to them: these he was now fixing, and he was hammering at the rivets. While he was thus at work silver-footed Thetis came to the house. Charis, of graceful head-dress, wife to the far-famed lame god, came towards her as soon as she saw her, and took her hand in her own, saying, "Why have you come to our house, Thetis, honoured and ever welcome—for you do not visit us often? Come inside and let me set refreshment before you."

The goddess led the way as she spoke, and bade Thetis sit on a richly decorated seat inlaid with silver; there was a footstool also under her feet. Then she called Vulcan and said, "Vulcan, come here, Thetis wants you"; and the far-famed lame god answered, "Then it is indeed an august and honoured goddess who has come here; she it was that took care of me when I was suffering from the heavy fall which I had through my cruel mother's anger—for she would have got rid of me because I was lame. It would have gone hardly with me had not Eurynome, daughter of the ever-encircling waters of Oceanus, and Thetis, taken me to their bosom. Nine years did I stay with them, and many beautiful works in bronze, brooches, spiral

armlets, cups, and chains, did I make for them in their cave, with the roaring waters of Oceanus foaming as they rushed ever past it; and no one knew, neither of gods nor men, save only Thetis and Eurynome who took care of me. If, then, Thetis has come to my house I must make her due requital for having saved me; entertain her, therefore, with all hospitality, while I put by my bellows and all my tools."

On this the mighty monster hobbled off from his anvil, his thin legs plying lustily under him. He set the bellows away from the fire, and gathered his tools into a silver chest. Then he took a sponge and washed his face and hands, his shaggy chest and brawny neck; he donned his shirt, grasped his strong staff, and limped towards the door. There were golden handmaids also who worked for him, and were like real young women, with sense and reason, voice also and strength, and all the learning of the immortals; these busied themselves as the king bade them, while he drew near to Thetis, seated her upon a goodly seat, and took her hand in his own, saying, "Why have you come to our house, Thetis honoured and ever welcome—for you do not visit us often? Say what you want, and I will do it for you at once if I can, and if it can be done at all."

Thetis wept and answered, "Vulcan, is there another goddess in Olympus whom the son of Saturn has been pleased to try with so much affliction as he has me? Me alone of the marine goddesses did he make subject to a mortal husband, Peleus son of Aeacus, and sorely against my will did I submit to the embraces of one who was but mortal, and who now stays at home worn out with age. Neither is this all. Heaven vouchsafed me a son, hero among heroes, and he shot up as a sapling. I tended him as a plant in a goodly garden and sent him with his ships to Ilius to fight the Trojans, but never shall I welcome him back to the house of Peleus. So long as he lives to look upon the light of the sun, he is in heaviness, and though I go to him I cannot help him; King Agamemnon has made him give up the maiden whom the sons of the Achaeans had awarded him, and he wastes with sorrow for her sake. Then the Trojans hemmed the Achaeans in at their ships' sterns and would not let them come forth; the elders, therefore, of the Argives besought Achilles and offered him great treasure, whereon he refused to bring deliverance to them himself, but put his own armour on Patroclus and sent him into the fight with much people after him. All day long they fought by the Scaean gates and would have taken the city there and then, had not Apollo vouchsafed glory to Hector and slain the valiant son of Menoetius after he had done the Trojans much evil. Therefore I am suppliant at your knees if haply you may be pleased to provide my son, whose end is near at hand, with helmet and shield, with goodly greaves fitted with ancle-clasps, and with a breastplate, for he lost his own when his true comrade fell at the hands of the Trojans, and he now lies stretched on earth in the bitterness of his soul."

And Vulcan answered, "Take heart, and be no more disquieted about this matter; would that I could hide him from death's sight when his hour is come, so surely as I can find him armour that shall amaze the eyes of all who behold it."

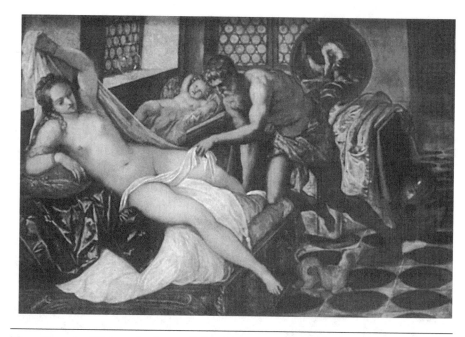

Mars, Venus, and Vulcan, *by Jacopo Robusti Tintoretto (1518–1594). Illustration of the well-known myth of Vulcan's (the Roman name for the disabled god Hephaistos) discovery of the goddess of beauty's infidelity to him with the god of war, Mars. Unlike the Athenians, who erected a major temple to the crook-footed god, the Romans tended to lavish more attention on his debasement.*

Source: Art Resource, New York.

Source: Butler, Samuel, trans. 1898. *The Iliad by Homer.* Available at http://www.iclasses.org/assets/literature/iliad.cfm

◉ Homer on Hephaistos
(ca. 750 BCE)

In this excerpt from the Odyssey, *Hephaistos, the crook-footed Greek god, sets a trap to catch Venus and Mars in the midst of an affair. Hephaistos pleads to Jove for help because he has been cuckolded because of his lameness.*

Now Venus was just come in from a visit to her father Jove, and was about sitting down when Mars came inside the house, and said as he took her hand in his own, "Let us go to the couch of Vulcan: he is not at home, but is gone off to Lemnos among the Sintians, whose speech is barbarous."

She was nothing loth, so they went to the couch to take their rest, whereon they were caught in the toils which cunning Vulcan had spread for them, and could neither get up nor stir hand or foot, but found too late that they were in a trap. Then Vulcan came up to them, for he had turned back before reaching Lemnos, when his scout the sun told him what was going on. He was in a furious passion, and stood in the vestibule making a dreadful noise as he shouted to all the gods.

"Father Jove," he cried, "and all you other blessed gods who live for ever, come here and see the ridiculous and disgraceful sight that I will show you. Jove's daughter Venus is always dishonouring me because I am lame. She is in love with Mars, who is handsome and clean built, whereas I am a cripple—but my parents are to blame for that, not I; they ought never to have begotten me. Come and see the pair together asleep on my bed. It makes me furious to look at them. They are very fond of one another, but I do not think they will lie there longer than they can help, nor do I think that they will sleep much; there, however, they shall stay till her father has repaid me the sum I gave him for his baggage of a daughter, who is fair but not honest."

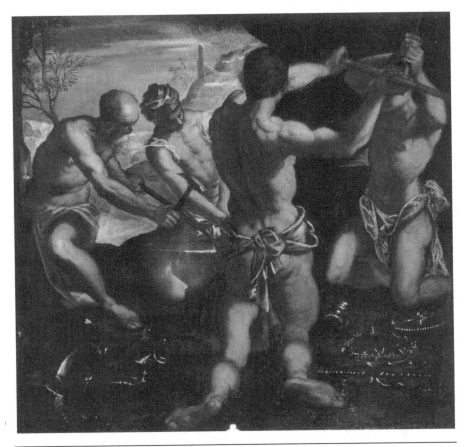

The Forge of Vulcan (1576), by Jacopo Robusti Tintoretto (1518–1594). A late Italian Renaissance painting of the disabled god Vulcan's supervision of the forge, emphasizing his stature as an innovator of technology for bodies. The painting portrays Vulcan's legs as massive and muscular to foreground his ability. Images known as Classical tend to drop out any identification of disability.

Source: Art Resource, New York.

On this the gods gathered to the house of Vulcan. Earth-encircling Neptune came, and Mercury the bringer of luck, and King Apollo, but the goddesses stayed at home all of them for shame. Then the givers of all good things stood in the doorway, and the blessed gods roared with inextinguishable laughter, as they saw how cunning Vulcan had been, whereon one would turn towards his neighbour saying:

"Ill deeds do not prosper, and the weak confound the strong. See how limping Vulcan, lame as he is, has caught Mars who is the fleetest god in heaven; and now Mars will be cast in heavy damages."

Thus did they converse, but King Apollo said to Mercury, "Messenger Mercury, giver of good things, you would not care how strong the chains were, would you, if you could sleep with Venus?"

"King Apollo," answered Mercury, "I only wish I might get the chance, though there were three times as

many chains—and you might look on, all of you, gods and goddesses, but would sleep with her if I could."

The immortal gods burst out laughing as they heard him, but Neptune took it all seriously, and kept on imploring Vulcan to set Mars free again. "Let him go," he cried, "and I will undertake, as you require, that he shall pay you all the damages that are held reasonable among the immortal gods."

"Do not," replied Vulcan, "ask me to do this; a bad man's bond is bad security; what remedy could I enforce against you if Mars should go away and leave his debts behind him along with his chains?"

"Vulcan," said Neptune, "if Mars goes away without paying his damages, I will pay you myself." So Vulcan answered, "In this case I cannot and must not refuse you."

Thereon he loosed the bonds that bound them, and as soon as they were free they scampered off, Mars to Thrace and laughter-loving Venus to Cyprus and to Paphos, where is her grove and her altar fragrant with burnt offerings. Here the Graces bathed her, and anointed her with oil of ambrosia such as the immortal gods make use of, and they clothed her in raiment of the most enchanting beauty.

Thus sang the bard, and both Ulysses and the seafaring Phaeacians were charmed as they heard him.

Source: Butler, Samuel, trans. 1900. *The Odyssey*. Republished 2004. eBooks@Adelaide. Available at http://etext.library.adelaide.edu.au/h/homer/h8o/index.html

◨ **Plato,** *Republic* (380–370 BCE)

Plato, the fifth-/fourth-century philosopher and mentor to Aristotle, devises a highly regulated utopian state in

his Republic, *a philosophical analysis of justice. Sometimes taken as evidence of actual Greek practice, this model community—a utopia, after all—does not resemble familiar Greek patterns. In other passages (not excerpted here), in contrast to the actual classical Greek world, some women have roles of leadership (451 c–457 c); the family is abolished (457 c–461 e); and the city's inhabitants do not disagree with each other (462 a–466 d). In the* Laws, *written many years after his* Republic, *Plato again comments on the perfect community, suggesting that one might be exempt from marrying someone "suffering from defects of mind or body." Plato's musings confirm the established practice in ancient Greece: one married whom one was contracted to marry, regardless of aesthetic or mental characteristics. The following excerpt is in the form of a dialogue between different individuals.*

These, he said, and none other; for what can be more ridiculous than for them to utter the names of family ties with the lips only and not to act in the spirit of them?

Then in our city the language of harmony and concord will be more often heard than in any other. As I was describing before, when anyone is well or ill, the universal word will be "with me it is well" or "it is ill."

Most true.

And agreeably to this mode of thinking and speaking, were we not saying that they will have their pleasures and pains in common?

Yes, and so they will.

And they will have a common interest in the same thing which they will alike call "my own," and having this common interest they will have a common feeling of pleasure and pain?

Yes, far more so than in other States.

And the reason of this, over and above the general constitution of the State, will be that the guardians will have a community of women and children?

That will be the chief reason.

And this unity of feeling we admitted to be the greatest good, as was implied in our comparison of a well-ordered State to the relation of the body and the members, when affected by pleasure or pain?

That we acknowledged, and very rightly.

Then the community of wives and children among our citizens is clearly the source of the greatest good to the State?

Certainly.

And this agrees with the other principle which we were affirming—that the guardians were not to have houses or lands or any other property; their pay was to be their food, which they were to receive from the other citizens, and they were to have no private expenses; for we intended them to preserve their true character of guardians.

Right, he replied.

Both the community of property and the community of families, as I am saying, tend to make them more truly guardians; they will not tear the city in pieces by differing about "mine" and "not mine"; each man dragging any acquisition which he has made into a separate house of his own, where he has a separate wife and children and private pleasures and pains; but all will be affected as far as may be by the same pleasures and pains because they are all of one opinion about what is near and dear to them, and therefore they all tend toward a common end.

Certainly, he replied.

And as they have nothing but their persons which they can call their own, suits and complaints will have no existence among them; they will be delivered from all those quarrels of which money or children or relations are the occasion.

Of course they will.

Neither will trials for assault or insult ever be likely to occur among them. For that equals should defend themselves against equals we shall maintain to be honorable and right; we shall make the protection of the person a matter of necessity.

That is good, he said.

Yes; and there is a further good in the law; viz., that if a man has a quarrel with another he will satisfy his resentment then and there, and not proceed to more dangerous lengths.

Certainly.

To the elder shall be assigned the duty of ruling and chastising the younger.

Clearly.

Nor can there be a doubt that the younger will not strike or do any other violence to an elder, unless the magistrates command him; nor will he slight him in any way. For there are two guardians, shame and fear, mighty to prevent him: shame, which makes men refrain from laying hands on those who are to them in the relation of parents; fear, that the injured one will be succored by the others who are his brothers, sons, fathers.

That is true, he replied.

Then in every way the laws will help the citizens to keep the peace with one another?

Yes, there will be no want of peace.

And as the guardians will never quarrel among themselves there will be no danger of the rest of the city being divided either against them or against one another.

None whatever.

I hardly like even to mention the little meannesses of which they will be rid, for they are beneath notice: such, for example, as the flattery of the rich by the poor, and all the pains and pangs which men experience in bringing up a family, and in finding money to buy necessaries for their household, borrowing and then repudiating, getting how they can, and giving the money into the hands of women and slaves to keep—the many evils of so many kinds which people suffer in this way are mean enough and obvious enough, and not worth speaking of.

Yes, he said, a man has no need of eyes in order to perceive that.

Source: Spens, H., trans. 1906. *The Republic*. London: Dent.

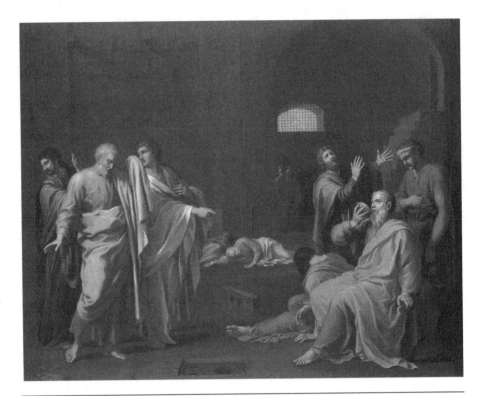

The Death of Socrates *(1650), by Charles Alphonse Dufresnoy (1611–1668). Recreation of Socrates' death sentence. Socrates was required to drink a draft of hemlock by an Athenian jury who found him guilty of corrupting the city's youth and interfering with religious practices. The German philosopher Nietzsche comments that Socrates was the "ugliest man in Greece" because of his facial deformity and that his philosophy championed the beauty of intellect as a redress for his society's emphasis on surface appearance. Oil on canvas, 122 × 155 cm.*

Source: Galleria Palatina, Palazzo Pitti, Florence, Italy. Photo credit: Alinari/Art Resource, New York.

▣ Aristotle, *Politics* (ca. 350 BCE)

In his Politics, *the fourth-century BCE philosopher Aristotle proposes the ideal society. He suggests that the intelligence of men is constitutionally determined, and that men should take roles according to their constitution. In this excerpt, Aristotle goes on to suggest that in the ideal state, "no deformed child shall be reared."*

From Book VII:

Since the legislator should begin by considering how the frames of the children whom he is rearing may be as good as possible, his first care will be about marriage—at what age should his citizens marry, and who are fit to marry? In legislating on this subject he ought to consider the persons and the length of their life, that their procreative life may terminate at the same period, and that they may not differ in their bodily powers, as will be the case if the man is still able to beget children while the woman is unable to bear them, or the woman able to bear while the man is unable to beget, for from these causes arise quarrels and differences between married persons. Secondly, he must consider the time at which the children will succeed to their parents; there ought not to be too great an interval of age, for then the parents will be too old to derive any pleasure from their affection, or to be of any use to them. Nor ought they to be too nearly of an age; to youthful marriages there are many objections—the children will be wanting in respect to the parents, who will seem to be their contemporaries, and disputes will arise in the management of the household. Thirdly, and this is the point from which we digressed, the legislator must mold to his will the frames of newly-born children. Almost all these objects may be secured by attention to one point. Since the time of generation is commonly limited within the age of seventy years in the case of a man, and of fifty in the case of a woman, the commencement of the union should conform to these periods. The union of male and female when too young is bad for the procreation of children; in all other animals the offspring of the young are small and in-developed, and with a tendency to produce female children, and therefore also in man, as is proved by the fact that in those cities in which men and women are accustomed to marry young, the people are small and weak; in childbirth also younger women suffer more, and more of them die; some persons say that this was the meaning of the response once given to the Troezenians— the oracle really meant that many died because they married too young; it had nothing to do with the ingathering of the harvest. It also conduces to temperance not to marry too soon; for women who marry early are apt to be wanton; and in men too the bodily frame is stunted if they marry while the seed is growing (for there is a time when the growth of the seed, also, ceases, or continues to but a slight extent). Women should marry when they are about eighteen years of age, and men at seven and thirty; then they are in the prime of life, and the decline in the powers of both will coincide. Further, the children, if their birth takes place soon, as may reasonably be expected, will succeed in the beginning of their prime, when the fathers are already in the decline of life, and have nearly reached their term of three-score years and ten.

Thus much of the age proper for marriage: the season of the year should also be considered; according to our present custom, people generally limit marriage to the season of winter, and they are right. The precepts of physicians and natural philosophers about generation should also be studied by the parents themselves; the physicians give good advice about the favorable conditions of the body, and the natural philosophers about the winds; of which they prefer the north to the south.

What constitution in the parent is most advantageous to the offspring is a subject which we will consider more carefully when we speak of the education of children, and we will only make a few general remarks at present. The constitution of an athlete is not suited to the life of a citizen, or to health, or to the procreation of children, any more than the valetudinarian or exhausted constitution, but one which is in a mean between them. A man's constitution should be inured to labor, but not to labor which is excessive or of one sort only, such as is practiced by athletes; he should be capable of all the actions of a freeman. These remarks apply equally to both parents.

Women who are with child should be careful of themselves; they should take exercise and have a nourishing diet. The first of these prescriptions the legislator will easily carry into effect by requiring that they shall take a walk daily to some temple, where they can worship the gods who preside over birth. Their minds, however, unlike their bodies, they ought to keep quiet, for the offspring derive their natures from their mothers as plants do from the earth.

As to the exposure and rearing of children, let there be a law that no deformed child shall live, but that on the ground of an excess in the number of children, if the established customs of the state forbid this (for in our state population has a limit), no child is to be exposed, but when couples have children in excess, let abortion be procured before sense and life have begun; what may or may not be lawfully done in these cases depends on the question of life and sensation.

And now, having determined at what ages men and women are to begin their union, let us also determine how long they shall continue to beget and bear offspring for the state; men who are too old, like men who are too young, produce children who are defective in body and mind; the children of very old men are weakly. The limit then, should be the age which is the prime of their intelligence, and this in most persons, according to the notion of some poets who measure life by periods of seven years, is about fifty; at four or five years or later, they should cease from having families; and from that time forward only cohabit with one another for the sake of health; or for some similar reason.

As to adultery, let it be held disgraceful, in general, for any man or woman to be found in any way unfaithful when they are married, and called husband and wife. If during the time of bearing children anything of the sort occur, let the guilty person be punished with a loss of privileges in proportion to the offense.

Source: Jowett, Benjamin, trans. 1900. *The Politics of Aristotle.* New York: Colonial Press.

▣ Lysias 24, "On the Refusal of a Pension" (ca. 404 BCE)

Lysias 24 was probably meant for presentation—whether or not it actually was presented—before the Athenian Boule, the council that ran the affairs of state on behalf of the entire citizen body. The speech probably dates to the closing years of the fifth century BCE. The defendant had been classed among the unable and had been receiving a state pension. Now, the pension was in danger of being rescinded. The defendant was obviously disabled in the modern sense of the term, yet he could not merely display his disabled body before the Boule as proof that he deserved to keep the pension. Rather, he had to point to conditions such as his aged mother, whom he had to support. This document points to the ancient lack of codification and assumptions about people with what we call disabilities.

I can almost find it in me to be grateful to my accuser, gentlemen of the Council, for having involved me in these proceedings. For previously I had no excuse for rendering an account of my life; but now, owing to this man, I have got one. So I will try to show you in my speech that this man is lying, and that my own life until this day has been deserving of praise rather than envy; for it is merely from envy, in my opinion, that he has involved me in this ordeal.

But I ask you, if a man envies those whom other people pity, from what villainy do you think such a person would refrain? Is it possible that he hopes to get money by slandering me? And if he makes me out an enemy on whom he seeks to be avenged, he lies; for his villainy has always kept me from having any dealings with him either as a friend or as an enemy.

So now, gentlemen, it is clear that he envies me because, although I have to bear this sore misfortune, I am a better citizen than he is. For indeed I consider, gentlemen, that one ought to remedy the afflictions of the body with the activities of the spirit; for if I am to keep my thoughts and the general tenor of my life on the lever of my misfortune, how shall I be distinguished from this man?

Well, in regard to those matters, let these few words of mine suffice; I will now speak as briefly as I can on the points with which I am here concerned. My accuser says that I have no right to receive my civil pension, because I am able-bodied and not classed as disabled, and because I am skilled in a trade which would enable me to live without this grant.

In proof of my bodily strength, he instances that I mount on horseback; of the affluence arising from my trade, that I am able to associate with people who have means to spend. Now, as to the affluence for my trade and the nature of my livelihood in general, I think you are all acquainted with these: I will, however, make some brief remarks of my own.

My father left me nothing, and I have only ceased supporting my mother on her decease two years ago; while as yet I have no children to take care of me. I possess a trade that can give me but slight assistance: I already find difficulty in carrying it on myself, and as yet I am unable to procure someone to relieve me of the work. I have no other income besides this dole, and if you deprive me of it I might be in danger of finding myself in the most grievous plight.

Do not, therefore, gentlemen, when you can save me justly, ruin me unjustly; what you granted me when I was younger and stronger, do not take from me when I am growing older and weaker; not, with your previous reputation for showing the utmost compassion even towards those who are in no trouble, be moved now by this man to deal harshly with those who are objects of pity even to their enemies; nor, by having the heart to wrong me, cause everyone else in my situation to despond. And indeed, how extraordinary the case would be, gentlemen! When my misfortune was but simple, I am found to have been receiving this pension; but now, when old age, diseases, and the ills that attend on them are added to my trouble, I am to be deprived of it!

The depth of my poverty, I believe, can be revealed more clearly by my accuser than by anyone else on earth. For if I were charged with the duty of producing tragic drama, and should challenge him to an exchange of property, he would prefer being the producer ten times over to making the exchange once. Surely it is monstrous that he should now accuse me of having such great affluence that I can consort on equal terms with the wealthiest people, while, in the event of such a thing as I have suggested, he should make that choice. Why, what could be more villainous?

As to my horsemanship, which he has dared to mention to you, feeling neither awe of fortune nor shame before you, there is not much to tell. For I, gentlemen, am of the opinion that all who suffer from some affliction make it their single aim and constant study to manage the condition that has befallen them with the least amount of discomfort. I am such an one, and in the misfortune that has stricken me I have devised this facility for myself on the longer journeys that I find necessary.

But the strongest proof, gentlemen, of the fact that I mount horses because of my misfortune, and not from insolence, as this man alleges, is this: if I were a man of means, I should ride on a saddled mule, and would not mount other men's horses. But in fact, as I am unable to acquire anything of the sort, I am compelled, now and again, to use other men's horses.

Well, I ask you, gentlemen, is it not extraordinary that, if he saw me riding on a saddled mule, he would hold his peace, for what could he say?—and then, because I mount borrowed horses, he should try to persuade you that I am able-bodied; and that my using two sticks, while others use one, should not be argued by him against me as a sign of being able-bodied, but my mounting horses would be advanced by him as a proof to you that I am able-bodied? For I use both aids for the same reason.

So utterly has he surpassed the whole human race in impudence that he tries with his single voice to persuade any of you on this point, gentlemen, what hinders me from drawing a lot for election as one of the nine archons, and you from depriving me of my obol as having sound health, and voting it unanimously to this man as being a cripple? For surely, after you have deprived a man of the grant as being able-bodied, the law officers are not going to debar this same person, as being disabled, from drawing a lot!

Nay, indeed you are not of the same opinion as he is, nor is he either, and rightly so. For he has come here to dispute over my misfortune as if over an heiress, and he tries to persuade you that I am not the sort of man that you all see me to be; but you—as is incumbent on men of good sense—have rather to believe your own eyes than this person's words. . . .

For insolence is not likely to be shown by poor men laboring in the utmost indigence, but by those who possess far more than the necessaries of life; nor by men disabled in body, but by those who are still young and have a youthful turn of mind.

For the wealthy purchase with their money escape from the risks that they run, whereas the poor are compelled to moderation by the pressure of their want. The young are held to merit indulgence from their elders; but if their elders are guilty of offence, both ages unite in reproaching them.

The strong are at liberty to insult whomsoever they will with impunity, but the weak are unable either to beat off their aggressors when insulted, or to get the better of their victims if they choose to insult. Hence it seems to me that my accuser was not serious in speaking of my insolence, but was only jesting; his purpose was, not to persuade you that such is my nature, but to set me in a comic light, as a fine stroke of fancy.

He further asserts that my shop is the meeting place of a number of rogues who have spent their own money and hatch plots against those who wish to preserve theirs. But you must all take note that these statements of his are no more accusations against me than against anyone else who has a trade, nor against those who visit my shop any more than those who frequent other men of business.

For each of you is in the habit of paying a call at either a perfumer's or a barber's or a shoemaker's shop, or wherever he may chance to go,—in most cases, it is to the tradesmen who have set up nearest the marketplace, and in fewest, to those who are farthest from it. So if any of you should brand with roguery the men who visit my shop, clearly you must do the same to those who pass their time in the shops of others; and if to them, to all the Athenians: for you are all in the habit of paying a call and passing your time at some shop or other.

But really I see no need for me to be so very particular in rebutting each one of the statements that he has made, and to weary you any longer. For if I have argued the principal points, what need is there to dwell seriously on trifles in the same way as he does? But I beg you all, gentlemen of the Council, to hold the same views concerning me as you have held till now.

Do not be led by this man to deprive me of the sole benefit in my country of which fortune has granted me a share, nor let this one person prevail on you to withdraw now what you all agreed to grant me in the past. For, gentlemen, since Heaven had deprived us of the chiefest things, the city voted us this pension, regarding the chances of evil and of good as the same for all alike.

Surely I should be the most miserable of creatures if, after being deprived by my misfortune of the fairest and greatest things, the accuser should cause me the loss of that which the city bestowed in her thoughtful care for men in my situation. No, no, gentlemen; you must not vote that way. And why should I find you thus inclined?

Because anyone has ever been brought to trial at my instance and lost his fortune? There is nobody who can prove it.

Well, is it that I am a busybody, a hot head, a seeker of quarrels?

That is not the sort of use I happen to make of such means of subsistence as I have. That I am grossly insolent and savage? Even he would not allege this himself, except he should wish to add one more to the series of his lies. Or that I was in power at the time of the Thirty, and oppressed a great number of the citizens? But I went into exile with your people to Chalics, and when I was free to live secure as a citizen with those persons I chose to depart and share your perils.

I therefore ask you, gentlemen of the Council, not to treat me, a man who has committed no offence, in the same way as those who are guilty of numerous wrongs, but to give the same vote as the other Councils did on my case, remembering that I am neither rendering an account of State moneys placed in my charge, nor undergoing now an inquiry into my past proceedings in any office, but that the subject of this speech of mine is merely an obol.

In this way you will all give the decision that is just, while I, in return for that, will feel duly grateful to you; and this man will learn in the future not to scheme against those who are weaker than himself, but only to overreach his equals.

Source: Lamb, W. R. M., trans. 1930. *Lysias, with an English Translation.* Cambridge, MA: Harvard University Press.

▣ Herodotus (5th c. BCE)

Herodotus is known as the "father of history," and his work, from the fifth century BCE, is indeed the earliest complete history that survives. Herodotus weaves fact and fancy; among his reports and tall tales we can find clues to the lives of people with disabilities. In his tale of the Babylonian marriage market, for example, we see that deformed women were considered ugly, but not unmarriageable. The blind Scythian slaves are examples of blind people with professions, in contrast to the common ancient image of blind people as bards and beggars. The tale of King Darius and his injury reflects a world in which a simple fall can result in permanent disability, even for the most powerful person on earth. Darius's cruelty is highlighted in the following selection, but also highlighted is the ability of a group of disabled men to guard a camp. (See Barry

Baldwin. 1967. "Medical Grounds for Exemptions from Military Service at Athens." Classical Philology 62: 42–43.) Finally, we see the individual, nonmedicalized nature of prosthetic devices in the tale of Hegesistratus and his makeshift (and highly unlikely) prosthetic foot.

1.196

This is the equipment of their persons. I will now speak of their established customs. The wisest of these, in our judgement, is one which I have learned by inquiry is also a custom of the Eneti in Illyria. It is this: once a year in every village all the maidens as they attained marriageable age were collected and brought together into one place with a crowd of men standing around. Then a crier would display and offer them for sale one by one, first the fairest of all; and then, when she had fetched a great price, he put up for sale the next most attractive, selling all the maidens as lawful wives. Rich men of Assyria who desired to marry would outbid each other for the fairest; the ordinary people, who desired to marry and had no use for beauty, could take the ugly ones and money besides; for when the crier had sold all the most attractive, he would put up the one that was least beautiful, or crippled, and offer her to whoever would take her to wife for the least amount, until she fell to one who promised to accept least; the money came from the sale of the attractive ones, who thus paid the dowry of the ugly and the crippled. But a man could not give his daughter in marriage to whomever he liked, nor could one that bought a girl take her away without giving security that he would in fact make her his wife. And if the couple could not agree, it was a law that the money be returned. Men might also come from other villages to buy if they so desired. This, then, was their best custom; but it does not continue at this time; they have invented a new one lately [so that the women not be wronged or taken to another city]; since the conquest of Babylon made them afflicted and poor, everyone of the people that lacks a livelihood prostitutes his daughters.

3.129–130

Not long after this, it happened that Darius twisted his foot in dismounting from his horse while hunting so violently that the ball of the ankle joint was dislocated from its socket. Darius called in the best physicians of Egypt, whom he had until now kept near his person. But by violently twisting the foot they made the injury worse; and for seven days and nights the king could not sleep because of the pain. On the eighth day, when he was doing poorly, someone who had heard in Sardis of the skill of Democedes of Croton told Darius of him; and he told them to bring him as quickly as possible. When they found him among the slaves of Oroetes, where he was forgotten, they brought him along, dragging his chains and dressed in rags.

Darius asked him when he was brought in if he were trained in medicine. He refused to admit it, for he was afraid that if he revealed himself he would be cut off from Hellas for good. It was clear to Darius, however, that he was trained in deceit, and he ordered those who had brought him to bring along scourges and goads. Then he confessed, saying that his training was not exact, but that he had associated with a physician and had a passing acquaintance with medicine. But when Darius turned the case over to him and Democedes applied Greek remedies and used gentleness instead of the Egyptians' violence, he enabled him to sleep and in a short time had him well, although Darius had had no hope of regaining the use of his foot.

4.2

Now the Scythians blind all their slaves, because of the milk they drink; and this is how they get it; taking tubes of bone very much like flutes, they insert these into the genitalia of the mares and blow into them, some blowing while others milk. According to them, their reason for doing this is that blowing makes the mare's veins swell and her udder drop. When done milking, they pour the milk into deep wooden buckets, and make their slaves stand around the buckets and shake the milk; they draw off what stands on the surface and value this most; what lies at the bottom is less valued. This is why the Scythians blind all prisoners whom they take: for they do not cultivate the soil, but are nomads.

4.135

This was Gobryas' advice, and at nightfall Darius followed it. He left the men who were worn out, and those whose loss mattered least to him, there in the camp, and all the asses, too, tethered. His reasons for leaving the asses, and the infirm among his soldiers,

were the following; the asses, so that they would bray; the men, who were left because of their infirmity, he pretended were to guard the camp while he attacked the Scythians with the fit part of his army. Giving this order to those who were left behind, and lighting campfires, Darius made all haste to reach the Ister. When the asses found themselves deserted by the multitude, they brayed the louder for it; and the Scythians heard them and assumed that the Persians were in the place.

9.37

Mardonius' sacrifices also foretold an unfavorable outcome if he should be zealous to attack first, and good if he should but defend himself. He too used the Greek manner of sacrifice, and Hegesistratus of Elis was his diviner, the most notable of the sons of Tellias. This man had been put in prison and condemned to die by the Spartans for the great harm which he had done them. Being in such bad shape inasmuch as he was in peril of his life and was likely to be very grievously maltreated before his death, he did something which was almost beyond belief; made fast in iron-bound stocks, he got an iron weapon which was brought in some way into his prison, and straightway conceived a plan of such courage as we have never known; reckoning how best the rest of it might get free, he cut off his own foot at the instep.

This done, he tunneled through the wall out of the way of the guards who kept watch over him, and so escaped to Tegea. All night he journeyed, and all day he hid and lay hidden in the woods, till on the third night he came to Tegea, while all the people of Lacedaemon sought him. The latter were greatly amazed when they saw the half of his foot which had been cut off and lying there but were unable to find the man himself.

This then is the way in which he escaped the Lacedaemonians and took refuge in Tegea, which at that time was unfriendly to Lacedaemon. After he was healed and had made himself a foot of wood, he declared himself an open enemy of the Lacedaemonians. Yet the enmity which he bore them brought him no good at the last, for they caught him at his divinations in Zacynthus and killed him.

Source: Rawlinson, George, trans. 1858–1860. *The History of Herodotus*. Republished 1910. London: J. M. Dent.

▣ Hippocrates (ca. 400 BCE)

The Hippocratic corpus is a compilation of material that spans the fifth through the second centuries BCE. It includes writings by the author credited with the discovery of rational medicine, Hippocrates himself, although nothing is identified securely. The corpus also includes writings by the students of Hippocrates and other medical writers. The corpus is especially valuable in that it provides vivid descriptions of people with what we would call physical disability. Classical art in general portrayed mathematically perfect bodies, with the exception of comedic and mythological figures. The examples from the corpus that follow show the experimental, itinerant, and occasionally charlatan nature of the medical profession. Some documents suggest that the ancient physician might be more likely to cause permanent disability than to prevent it. Note also that amputation appears to be a passive matter (i.e., the limbs fall off of their own accord); that limb dislocations and other complications were common enough to be categorized; and that variants of gait are described thoroughly (in "On Joints"). "On the Sacred Disease" discusses the disease we now know as epilepsy, which was termed the sacred disease in Hippocrates' time and was believed to result from divine causes. In his discussion of the disease, Hippocrates expounds his conviction that all diseases, even epilepsy, resulted from natural mechanisms.

"On Fractures"

Part 1

In treating fractures and dislocations, the physician must make the extension as straight as possible, for this is the most natural direction. But if it incline to either side, it should rather turn to that of pronation, for there is thus less harm than if it be toward supination. Those, then, who act in such cases without deliberation, for the most part do not fall into any great mistake, for the person who is to have his arm bound, presents it in the proper position from necessity, but physicians who fancy themselves learned in these matters, are they who commit blunders. There is no necessity for much study, then, in order to set a broken arm, and in a word, any ordinary physician can perform it; but I am under the necessity of giving the longer directions on this subject, because I know physicians who have the reputation of being skilled in giving the proper positions to the arm in binding it up, while in reality they are only showing

their own ignorance. But many other things in our art are judged of in this manner, for people rather admire what is new, although they do not know whether it be proper or not, than what they are accustomed to, and know already to be proper; and what is strange, they prefer to what is obvious. I must now state what the mistakes of medical men are, which I wish to unteach, and what instructions I have to give as the management of the arm; for what I have to say regarding it, will apply to the other bones in the body.

Part 2

The arm, then, for that is the subject we were treating of, was presented in the prone position to be bound, but the physician forced his patient to hold it as the archers do when they project the shoulder, and in this position he bound it up, thinking within himself that he was acting according to Nature, and in proof of this he pointed out that all the bones in the fore-arm were thus in a straight line, and that the integuments both inside and outside, were also in a straight line, and that the flesh and nerves (tendons?) were thus put in their natural position, and he appealed to what happens in archery, as a proof of this. And so saying, and so doing, he is looked up to as a sage; and yet he forgets that in all the other arts and performances, whether executed by strength or dexterity, what is reckoned the natural position is not the same, and that in the same piece of work it may happen that the natural position of the right arm is not the same as that of the left. For there is one attitude in throwing the javelin, and another in slinging, another in casting stones, another in boxing, and another in a state of repose. And whatever arts one examines, it will be found that the natural position of the arms is not the same in each, but that in every case the arms are put into the attitude which suits best with the instrument that is used, and the work to be performed.

Part 9

The human foot is composed of several small bones like the hand. These bones therefore are scarcely ever broken, unless the skin at the same time be wounded by some sharp and heavy body. The treatment of such injuries, therefore, will be delivered under the head of wounds. But if any bone be moved from its place, or a joint of the toes be luxated, or any of the bones of the part called the tarsus be displaced, it must be forced back again to its place as described with regard to the hand; and is to be treated with cerate, compresses, and bandages, like the fractures, with the exception of the splints; and is to be secured tightly in the same way, and the bandages renewed on the third day; and the patient thus bandaged should return the same answers as in fractures, as to the bandages feeling tight or slack. All these bones recover perfectly in twenty days, except those that are connected with the bones of the leg, and are in a line with them. It is advantageous to lie in bed during the whole of this time; but the patients, thinking light of the complaint, have not perseverance to do this, and they walk about before they get well; wherefore many of these do not make a perfect recovery. And often the pain puts them in mind of the injury; and deservedly, for the feet sustain the weight of the whole body. When, therefore, they walk about before they are whole, the joints which have been luxated are cured incompletely; and, on that account, while walking about, they have pains in the leg from time to time.

Part 11

In persons who jumping from any high object pitch upon their heel with great force, the bones are separated, and the veins pour forth their contents, owing to the contusion of the flesh surrounding the bone, and hence a swelling and much pain supervene. For this bone (os calcis) is not a small one, protrudes beyond the line of the leg, and is connected with important veins and tendons; from the back tendon of the leg is inserted into this bone.

Part 13

Sometimes the bones connected with the foot are displaced, sometimes both bones with their epiphysis; sometimes the whole epiphysis is slightly moved, and sometimes the other bone. These cases are less troublesome than the same accidents at the wrist, if the patients will have resolution to give them rest. The mode of treatment is the same as that of the other, for the reduction is to be made, as of the other, by means of extension, but greater force is required, as the parts of the body concerned are stronger in this case. But, for the most part, two men will be sufficient, by making extension in opposite directions, but, not withstanding, if they are not sufficiently strong, it is easy to make more powerful extension in the following way: having fixed in the ground either the nave of a wheel, or any such object, something soft is to be bound round the foot,

and then some broad thongs of ox-skin being brought round it, the heads of the thongs are to be fastened to a pestle or any other piece of wood, the end of which is to be inserted into the nave, and it, the pestle, is to be pulled away, while other persons make counterextension by grasping the shoulders and the ham. It is also sometimes necessary to secure the upper extremity otherwise; this if you desire to effect, fasten deeply in the ground a round, smooth piece of wood, and place the upper extremity of the piece of wood at the perineum, so that it may prevent the body from yielding to the pulling at the foot, and, moreover, to prevent the leg while stretched, from inclining downward; some person seated at this side should push back the hip, so that the body may not turn round with the pulling, and for this purpose, if you think fit, pieces of wood may be fastened about the armpits on each side. . . .

Part 15

And when both bones of the leg are broken without a wound of the skin, stronger extension is required. We may make extension by some of the methods formerly described, provided the bones ride over one another to a considerable degree. But extension by men is also sufficient, and for the most part two strong men will suffice, by making extension and counterextension. Extension must naturally be made straight in a line with the leg and thigh. And in both cases they are to be bandaged while in a state of extension, for the same position does not suit with the leg and the arm. For when the fractured bones of the arm or fore-arm are bandaged, the fore-arm is suspended in a sling, and if you bind them up while extended, the figures of the fleshy parts will be changed in bending the arm at the elbow, for the elbow cannot be kept long extended, since persons are not in the custom of keeping the joint long in this form, but in a bent position, and persons who have been wounded in the arm, and are still able to walk about, require to have the arm bent at the elbow-joint. But the leg, both in walking and standing, is habitually extended, either completely or nearly so, and is usually in a depending position from its construction, and in order that it may bear the weight of the rest of the body. Wherefore it readily bears to be extended when necessary, and even when in bed the limb is often in this position. And when wounded, necessity subdues the understanding, since the patients become incapable of raising themselves up, so that they neither think of bending the limb nor of getting up erect, but remaining lying in the same position.

"On the Sacred Disease"

But this disease seems to me to be no more divine than others; but it has its nature such as other diseases have, and a cause whence it originates, and its nature and cause are divine only just as much as all others are, and it is curable no less than the others, unless when, the form of time, it is confirmed, and has become stronger than the remedies applied. Its origin is hereditary, like that of other diseases. For if a phlegmatic person be born of a phlegmatic, and a bilious of a bilious, and a phthisical of a phthisical, and one having spleen disease, of another having disease of the spleen, what is to hinder it from happening that where the father and mother were subject to this disease, certain of their offspring should be so affected also? As the semen comes from all parts of the body, healthy particles will come from healthy parts, and unhealthy from unhealthy parts. And another great proof that it is in nothing more divine than other diseases is, that it occurs in those who are of a phlegmatic constitution, but does not attack the bilious. Yet, if it were more divine than the others, this disease ought to befall all alike, and make no distinction between the bilious and phlegmatic.

But the brain is the cause of this affection, as it is of other very great diseases, and in what manner and from what cause it is formed, I will now plainly declare. The brain of man, as in all other animals, is double, and a thin membrane divides it through the middle, and therefore the pain is not always in the same part of the head; for sometimes it is situated on either side, and sometimes the whole is affected; and veins run toward it from all parts of the body, many of which are small, but two are thick, the one from the liver, and the other from the spleen. And it is thus with regard to the one from the liver: a portion of it runs downward through the parts on the side, near the kidneys and the psoas muscles, to the inner part of the thigh, and extends to the foot. It is called vena cava. The other runs upward by the right veins and the lungs, and divides into branches for the heart and the right arm. The remaining part of it rises upward across the clavicle to the right side of the neck, and is superficial so as to be seen; near the ear it is concealed, and there it divides; its thickest, largest, and most hollow part ends in the brain; another small vein goes to the right ear, another to the right eye, and another to the nostril. Such are the distributions of the hepatic vein. And a vein from the spleen is distributed on the left side, upward and downward, like that from the liver, but more slender and feeble. . . .

And the disease called the Sacred arises from causes as the others, namely, those things which enter and quit the body, such as cold, the sun, and the winds, which are ever changing and are never at rest. And these things are divine, so that there is no necessity for making a distinction, and holding this disease to be more divine than the others, but all are divine, and all human. And each has its own peculiar nature and power, and none is of an ambiguous nature, or irremediable. And the most of them are curable by the same means as those by which any other thing is food to one, and injurious to another. Thus, then, the physician should understand and distinguish the season of each, so that at one time he may attend to the nourishment and increase, and at another to abstraction and diminution. And in this disease as in all others, he must strive not to feed the disease but endeavor to wear it out by administering whatever is most opposed to each disease, and not that which favors and is allied to it. For by that which is allied to it, it gains vigor and increase, but it wears out and disappears under the use of that which is opposed to it. But whoever is acquainted with such a change in men, and can render a man humid and dry, hot and cold by regimen, could also cure this disease, if he recognizes the proper season for administering his remedies, without minding purifications, spells and all other illiberal practices of a like kind.

Source: Adams, Francis, trans. 1849. *On Fractures, by Hippocrates.* London. Available at http://classics.mit.edu/Hippocrates/fractur.1.1.html

Source: Adams, Francis, trans. 1849. *On the Sacred Disease, by Hippocrates.* London. Available at http://classics.mit.edu/Hippocrates/sacred.html

▣ Sophocles, from *Philoctetes* (Performed in 409 BCE)

After being bitten by an asp at a ceremonial altar, Philoctetes develops a festering wound and lives in extreme pain. His fellow sailors decide to abandon him on an island on the way to war at Troy. As the war begins to go badly, Neoptolemus is sent back to retrieve Heracles' bow, which had been given to Philoctetes as a gift. The weapon turns out to be the key that ensures the Athenians' success against the Trojans.

Chorus I have heard a rumor, but never seen with my eyes, how the man who once approached the bed of *Zeus* was bound upon a swift wheel by the almighty son of *Cronus*. But of no other mortal do I know, either by hearsay or by sight, that has encountered a doom so repugnant as this of *Philoctetes*. For though he had wronged no one by force or thievery, but conducted himself fairly towards the fair, he was left to perish so undeservedly. I truly marvel how—how in the world—as he listened in solitude to the breakers rushing around him, he kept his hold upon a life so full of grief. . . .

Neoptolemus Please, come on. Why so silent with no apparent cause? And why are you paralyzed?

Philoctetes Ai, ai!

Neoptolemus What is the matter?

Philoctetes Nothing serious—go on, son.

Neoptolemus Are you in pain from the disease that frequents you?

Philoctetes No, indeed no. I think it is better now.—Gods, oh!

Neoptolemus Why do you groan like this and call on the gods?

Philoctetes That they may come to me with power to save and soothe.—Ai! Ai!

Neoptolemus What troubles you? Speak, do not keep so silent. It is plain enough that you are suffering somehow.

Philoctetes I am destroyed, boy—I can never conceal my suffering when you are close. Ah! Ah! It shoots through me, shoots straight through! Oh, the pain, the misery! I am destroyed, boy—I am devoured! Ah, by the gods I beg you, if you have a sword ready to hand, strike at my ankle—cut it off now! Do not spare my life! Quick, boy, quick!

Neoptolemus What new thing has come on you so suddenly that you wail for yourself with these loud shrieks?

Philoctetes You know, son.

Neoptolemus What is it?

Philoctetes You know, boy.

Neoptolemus What ails you? I do not know.

Philoctetes How could you not know? Oh, oh!

Neoptolemus Yes, terrible is the burden of your disease.

Philoctetes Terrible beyond telling! Oh, pity me!

Neoptolemus What shall I do?

Philoctetes Do not betray me because of fear. This plague comes only now and then,—perhaps when she has been sated with her roamings elsewhere.

Neoptolemus Ah, poor wretch! Poor man, truly for all your sufferings! Shall I support you, or somehow offer a helping hand?

Philoctetes No, no. But take this bow of mine—as you earlier asked of me—and keep it in your care and safe until this present bout with my disease is past. For indeed sleep takes me as soon as this pain passes away, nor can it cease before then. But you must allow me to sleep in peace. And if those men come in the meantime, then by the gods I forbid you willingly or unwillingly, or by any skilled trickery, to give up this bow to them, lest you bring destruction at once on yourself and on me, who am your suppliant.

Neoptolemus Have no fears as to my caution. The bow shall pass into no hands but yours and mine. Give it to me, and may good luck accompany it!

Philoctetes There, take it boy. And humble yourself before the jealous gods, so that the bow may not prove baneful for you, as it did for me and for him who owned it before me.

Neoptolemus O gods, grant this to the two of us! And grant us a voyage prosperous and unimpeded, to whatever goal the god may deem right and that our mission provides!

⊡ Sophocles, *Oedipus the King*
(Performed ca. 421 BCE)

In one of Sophocles' best-known works, Oedipus discovers that he has inadvertently killed his father and married his mother, Jocasta, in order to ascend the throne of Thebes. The first excerpt below demonstrates his anguish at this knowledge and his self-destructive pursuit of the truth of his heritage. The scene ends with Oedipus's blinding as a metaphor for the disastrous insight he has acquired. The second excerpt consists of the final lines of the tragedy. Blindness is portrayed at its most dramatic: it is sudden, horrifying, divine retribution. Oedipus will now be forced into exile, newly blinded, his life worse than death. The drama of blindness appears frequently in Greek literature and other media, but it hardly represents the lives of the ordinary blind people. The gradual onset of blindness from cataracts or other disease does not make for a tale of high drama, nor do tales of villagers who adjusted to failing sight.

Oedipus   He says that I am Laius' murderer.

Jocasta   Of his own knowledge, or by some one taught?

Oedipus   Yon scoundrel seer suborning. For himself,
He takes good care to free his lips from blame.

Jocasta   Leave now thyself, and all thy thoughts of this,
And list to me, and learn how little skill
In arts prophetic mortal man may claim;
And of this truth I'll give thee proof full clear.
There came to Laius once an oracle
(I say not that it came from Phœbus' self,
But from his servants) that his fate was fixed
By his son's hand to fall—his own and mine:
And him, so rumour runs, a robber band
Of aliens slew, where meet the three great roads.
Nor did three days succeed the infant's birth,
Before, by other hands, he cast him forth,
Maiming his ankles, on a lonely hill.
Here, then, Apollo failed to make the boy
His father's murderer; nor did Laius die
By his son's hand. So fared the oracles;
Therefore regard them not. Whate'er the God
Desires to search he will himself declare.

Oedipus   *[trembling]* O what a fearful boding! thoughts disturbed

Thrill through my soul, my queen, at this thy tale.

Jocasta   What means this shuddering, this averted glance?

Oedipus   I thought I heard thee say that Laius died,
Slain in a skirmish where the three roads meet?

Jocasta   So was it said, and still the rumours hold.

Oedipus   Where was the spot in which this matter passed?

Jocasta   They call the country Phocis, and the roads
From Delphi and from Daulia there converge.

Oedipus   And time? what interval has passed since then?

Jocasta   But just before thou camest to possess
And rule this land the tidings were proclaimed.

Oedipus   Great Zeus! what fate hast thou decreed for me?

Jocasta   What thought is this, my Œdipus, of thine?

Oedipus   Ask me not yet, but tell of Laius' frame,
His build, his features, and his years of life.

Jocasta   Tall was he, and the white hairs snowed his head,
And in his face not much unlike to thee.

Oedipus   Woe, woe is me! so seems it I have plunged
All blindly into curses terrible.

Jocasta   What sayest thou? I shudder as I see thee.

Oedipus   Desponding fear comes o'er me, lest the seer
Has seen indeed. But one thing more I'll ask.

Jocasta   I fear to speak, yet what thou ask'st I'll tell.

Oedipus   Went he in humble guise, or with a troop
Of spearmen, as becomes a man that rules?

Jocasta   Five were they altogether, and of them
One was a herald, and one chariot had he.

Oedipus   Woe! woe! 'tis all too clear.

Antistrophe A

Oedipus   Ah, friend,
You are my steadfast servant still,
You still remain to care for me, blind.

Alas! Alas!
You are not hid from me;
I know you clearly,
And though in darkness,
still I hear your voice.

Chorus O dreadful doer,
how did you so endure
To quench your eyes? What
daimon drove you on?

Strophe B

Oedipus Apollo it was,
Apollo, friends
Who brought to pass these
evil, evil woes of mine.
The hand of no one struck
my eyes but wretched me.
For why should I see,
When nothing sweet there
is to see with sight?

Chorus This is just as
you say.

Oedipus What more is
there for me to see,
My friends, what to love,
What joy to hear a greet-
ing?
Lead me at once away from
here,
Lead me away, friends,
wretched as I am,
Accursed, and hated most
Of mortals to the gods.

Chorus Wretched alike
in mind and in your fortune,
How I wish that I had never
known you.

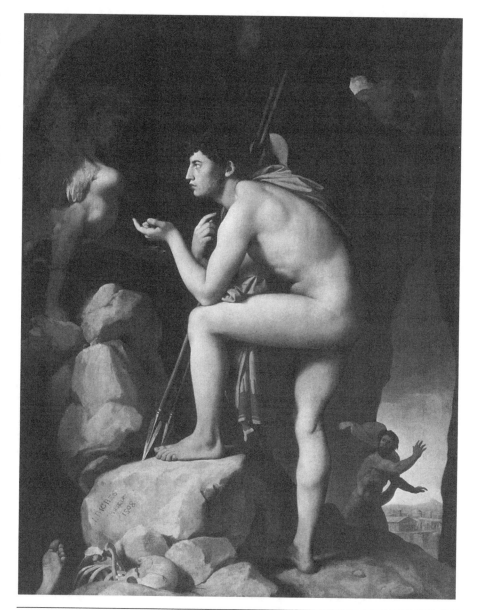

Oedipus and the Sphinx *(1808), by Jean Auguste Ingres (1780–1867). Oedipus, who was disabled as an infant when his father pinned his ankles and had him left on a hillside to die of exposure, walked with a limp. In this portrait, he is poised to answer the sphinx's riddle: "What walks on four legs in the morning, two legs at noon, and three legs in the evening?" As one who uses a cane, Oedipus realizes the answer is "Man," who crawls as a baby, walks upright in his youth and adulthood, and eventually needs assistive aids as he ages. The sphinx's designation as monstrously feminine leads her to commit suicide when her riddle is unraveled. Oil on canvas, 189 144 cm.*

Source: Louvre, Paris. Photo credit: Scala/Art Resource, New York.

Antistrophe B

Oedipus May he perish, whoever freed me
From fierce bonds at my feet,
Snatched me from death and saved me, doing me
no joy.

For if then I had died, I should not be
So great a grief to friends and to myself.

Chorus This also is my wish.

Oedipus I would not have come to murder my father,

Nor have been called among men
The bridegroom of her from whom I was born.
But as it is I am godless, child of unholiness,
Wretched sire in common with my father.
And if there is any evil older than evil left,
Is it the lot of Oedipus.

Chorus   I know not how I could give you good advice,
For you would be better dead than living blind.

Oedipus   That how things are was not done for the best—
Teach me not this, or give me more advice.
If I had sight I know not with what eyes
I could ever face my father among the dead,
Or my wretched mother. What I have done to them
Is too great for a noose to expiate.
Do you think the sight of my children would be a joy
For me to see, born as they were to me?
No, never for these eyes of mine to see.
Nor the city, nor the tower, nor the sacred
Statues of gods; of these I deprive myself,
Noblest among the Thebans, born and bred,
Now suffering everything. I tell you all
To exile me as impious, shown by the gods
Untouchable and of the race of Laius.
When I uncovered such a stain on me,
Could I look with steady eyes upon the people?
No, No! And if there were a way to block
The spring of hearing, I would not forbear
To lock up wholly this my wretched body.
I should be blind and deaf.—For it is sweet
When thought can dwell outside our evils.
Alas, Cithaeron, why did you shelter me?
Why did you not take and kill me at once, so I
Might never reveal to men whence I was born?
O Polybus, O Corinth, O my father's halls,
Ancient in fable, what an outer fairness,
A festering of evils, you raised in me.
For now I am evil found, and born of evil.
O the three paths! Alas the hidden glen,
The grove of oak, the narrow triple roads
That drank from my own hands my father's blood.
Do you remember any of the deeds
I did before you then on my way here
And what I after did? O wedlock, wedlock!
You gave me birth, and then spawned in return
Issue from the selfsame seed; you revealed
Father, brother, children, in blood relation,

The bride both wife and mother, and whatever
Actions are done most shameful among men.
But it is wrong to speak what is not good to do.
By the gods, hide me at once outside our land,
Or murder me, or hurl me in the sea
Where you shall never look on me again.
Come, venture to lay your hands on this wretched man.
Do it. Be not afraid. No mortal man
There is, except myself, to bear my evils.

Chorus   Here is Creon, just in time for what you ask
To work and to advise, for he alone
Is left in place of you to guard the land.

Oedipus   Alas, what word, then, shall I tell this man?
What righteous ground of trust is clear in me,
As in the past in all I have done with him evil?

Creon   Oedipus, I have not come to laugh at you,
Nor to reproach you for your former wrongs.
(To the attendants)
If you defer no longer to mortal offspring,
Respect at least the all-nourishing flame
Of Apollo, lord of the sun. Fear to display
So great a pestilence, which neither earth
Nor holy rain nor light will well receive.
But you, conduct him to the house at once.
It is most pious for the kin alone
To hear and to behold the family sins.

Oedipus   By the gods, since you have plucked me from my fear,
Most noble, facing the most vile man,
Hear me one word—I will speak for you, not me.

Creon   What desire do you so persist to get?

Oedipus   As soon as you can, hurl me from this land to where no mortal man will ever greet me.

Creon   I would do all this, be sure, but I want first
To find out from the god what must be done.

Oedipus   His oracle, at least, is wholly clear;
Leave me to ruin, an impious parricide.

Creon   Thus spake the oracle. Still, as we stand
It is better to find out sure what we should do.

Oedipus   Will you inquire about so wretched a man?

Creon   Yes. You will surely put trust in the god.

Oedipus   I order you and beg you, give the woman
Now in the house such a burial as you yourself
Would want. Do last rites justly for your kin.
But may this city never be condemned—
My father's realm—because I live within.
Let me live in the mountains where Cithaeron
Yonder has fame of me, which father and mother
When they were alive established as my tomb.
There I may die by those who sought to kill me.
And yet this much I know, neither a sickness
Nor anything else can kill me. I would not
Be saved from death, except for some dread evil.
Well, let my fate go wherever it may.
As for my sons, Creon, assume no trouble;
They are men and will have no difficulty
Of living wherever they may be.
O my poor grievous daughters, who never knew
Their dinner table set apart from me,
But always shared in everything I touched—
Take care of them for me, and first of all
Allow me to touch them and bemoan our ills.
Grant it, lord,
Grant it, noble. If with my hand I touch them
I would think I had them just as when I could see.
(Creon's attendants bring in Antigone and Ismene.)
What's that?
By the gods, can it be I hear my dear ones weeping?
And have you taken pity on me, Creon?
Have you had my darling children sent to me?
Do I speak right?

Creon   You do. For it was I who brought them here,
Knowing this present joy your joy of old.

Oedipus   May you fare well. For their coming
may the spirit
That watches over you be better than mine.
My children, where are you? Come to me, come
Into your brother's hands, that brought about
Your father's eyes, once bright, to see like this.
Your father, children, who, seeing and knowing
nothing,
Became a father whence he was got himself.
I weep also for you—I cannot see you—
To think of the bitter life in days to come
Which you will have to lead among mankind.
What citizens' gatherings will you approach?
What festivals attend, where you will not cry

When you go home, instead of gay rejoicing?
And when you arrive at marriageable age,
What man, my daughters, will there be to chance you,
Incurring such reproaches on his head,
Disgraceful to my children and to yours?
What evil will be absent, when your father
Killed his own father, sowed seed in her who bore
him,
From whom he was born himself, and equally
Has fathered you whence he himself was born.
Such will be the reproaches. Who then will wed you?
My children, there is no one for you. Clearly
You must decay in barrenness, unwed.
Son of Menoeceus—since you are alone
Left as a father to them, for we who produced them
Are both in ruin—see that you never let
These girls wander as beggars without husbands,
Let them not fall into such woes as mine.
But pity them, seeing how young they are
To be bereft of all except your aid.
Grant this, my noble friend, with a touch of your
hand.
My children, if your minds were now mature,
I would give you much advice. But pray this for me,
To live as the time allows, to find a life
Better than that your siring father had.

Creon   You have wept enough here, come, go
inside the house.

Oedipus   I must obey, though nothing sweet.

Creon   All things are good in their time.

Oedipus   Do you know in what way I go?

Creon   Tell me, I'll know when I hear.

Oedipus   Send me outside the land.

Creon   You ask what the god will do.

Oedipus   But to the gods I am hated.

Creon   Still it will soon be done.

Oedipus   Then you agree?

Creon   What I think not I would not say in vain.

Oedipus   Now lead me away.

Creon   Come then, but let the children go.

Oedipus   Do not take them from me.

Creon   Wish not to govern all,
For what you ruled will not follow you through life.

Chorus   Dwellers in native Thebes, behold this Oedipus
Who solved the famous riddle, was your mightiest man.
What citizen on his lot did not with envy gaze?
See to how great a surge of dread fate he has come!
So I would say a mortal man, while he is watching
To see the final day, can have no happiness
Till he pass the bound of life, nor be relieved of pain.

Source: Storr, F., trans. 1912–1913. Lines 730–780 in *Oedipus the King* by Sophocles. London. Available at http://www.underthe sun.cc/Classics/Sophocles/OedipusRex/OedipusRex3.html

▣ Diodorus of Sicily, Book XVII.69 (50 BCE)

In this excerpt, Diodorus sets up the "barbaric" nature of the Persians to contrast with the benevolence of Alexander the Great. While not unbiased journalism, the account offers insight into the connection between ability, disability, and identity in social and economic terms.

At this point in his advance [Alexander] was confronted by a strange and dreadful sight, one to provoke indignation against the perpetrators and sympathetic pity for the unfortunate victims. He was met by Greeks bearing branches of supplication. They had been carried away from their homes by previous kings of Persia and were about eight hundred in number, most of them elderly. All had been mutilated, some lacking hands, some feet, and some ears and noses. They were persons who had acquired skills or crafts and had made good progress in their instruction; then their other extremities had been amputated and they were left only those which were vital to their profession. All the soldiers, seeing their venerable years and the losses which their bodies had suffered, pitied the lot of the wretches. Alexander most of all was affected by them and unable to restrain his tears.

They all cried with one voice and besought Alexander to help them in their misfortunes. The king called their leaders to come forward and, greeting them with a respect in keeping with his own greatness of spirit, promised to make it a matter of utmost concern that they should be restored to their homes. They gathered to debate the matter, and decided that it would be better for them to remain where they were rather than to return home. If they were brought back safely, they would be scattered in small groups and would find their abuse at the hands of Fortune an object of reproach as they lived on in their cities. If, however, they continued living together, as companions in misfortune, they would find a solace in their mutilation in the similar mutilation of the others. So they again appeared before the king, told him of their decision, and asked him to give them help appropriate to this proposal. Alexander applauded their decision and gave each of them three thousand drachmae, five men's robes and the same number for women, two yoke of oxen, fifty sheep, and fifty bushels of wheat. He made them also exempt from all royal taxes and charged his administrative officials to see that they were harmed by no one.

Source: Welles, C. Bradford, trans. 1983. [Vol. VIII, pp. 315–319]. Cambridge, MA: Harvard University Press.

The Ancient World: Rome

▣ Julius Caesar, *Civil Wars* (ca. 1st c. BCE)

Caesar, whose assassination in 44 BCE signaled the end of the Roman Republic, wrote about his military exploits in the third person. This excerpt offers a glimpse of the permanent physical disabilities that men would have experienced as the result of warfare, which was the expected state of affairs in almost all phases of Roman history.

Book 3, Chapter 53

Thus six engagements having happened in one day, three at Dyrrachium, and three at the fortifications, when a computation was made of the number of slain, we found that about two thousand fell on Pompey's side, several of them volunteer veterans and centurions. Among them was Velerius, the son of Lucius Flaccus, who as praetor had formerly had the government of Asia, and six military standards were taken. Of our men, not more than twenty were missing in all the action. But in the fort, not a single soldier escaped without a wound; and in one cohort, four centurions lost their eyes. And being desirous to produce testimony of the fatigue they under went, and the danger they sustained, they counted to Caesar about thirty thousand arrows which had been thrown into the effort; and in the shield of the centurion Scaeva, which was brought to him, were found two hundred and thirty holes. In reward for this man's services, both to himself and the public, Caesar presented to him two hundred thousand pieces of coppery money, and declared him promoted from the eighth to the first centurion. For it appeared that the fort had been in a great measure saved by his exertions; and he afterward very amply rewarded the cohorts with double pay, corn, clothing, and other military honors.

Source: McDevitte, W. A., & W. S. Bohn, trans. 1869. *The Civil Wars by Julius Caesar.* New York: Harper & Brothers.

▣ Plutarch on Cicero (2nd c. CE)

Plutarch cared more about portraying the internal characteristics of great Greek and Roman men than about portraying their historical contexts. His commentaries demonstrate the Roman penchant for equating appearance with character and for interpreting nature as providing physical "deformities" as warnings. The name "Cicero" has become a byword for rhetoric, yet Plutarch explains that his name comes from a physical peculiarity, not a grand tradition.

He who first of that house was surnamed Cicero seems to have been a person worthy to be remembered; since those who succeeded him not only did not reject, but were fond of the name, though vulgarly made a matter of reproach. For the Latins call a vetch Cicer, and a nick or dent at the tip of his nose, which resembled the opening in a vetch, gave him the surname of Cicero.

Cicero, whose story I am writing, is said to have replied with spirit to some of his friends, who recommended him to lay aside or change the name when he first stood for office and engaged in politics, that he would make it his endeavor to render the name of Cicero more glorious than that of the Scauri and Catuli. And when he was quæstor in Sicily, and was making an offering of silver plate to the gods, and had inscribed his two names, Marcus and Tullius, instead of the third

65

he jestingly told the artificer to engrave the figure of a vetch by them. Thus much is told us about his name.

Of his birth it is reported, that his mother was delivered without pain or labor, on the third of the new Calends, the same day on which now the magistrates of Rome pray and sacrifice for the emperor. It is said, also, that a vision appeared to his nurse, and foretold the child she then suckled should afterwards become a great benefit to the Roman States.

Source: Dryden, John, trans. Reprinted 1909–1914. *Plutarch's Lives.* New York: P. F. Collier & Son Company.

▣ Juvenal, Excerpts from *Satire 2* (2nd c. CE)

Juvenal and Martial were Roman satirists of the early imperial period (Juvenal died ca. 130 CE). Juvenal writes stinging barbs against what he perceives as corrupt Roman society. No one is immune from his bitter commentary, and it is interesting to note that people with what we would call disabilities are not in any special category. Rather, they are mocked side by side with ugly people, smelly people, and pretentious people. While Juvenal makes fun of people whom we would categorize as disabled today, he is equally likely to jeer at anyone who crosses the hierarchical social boundaries of early imperial Rome. (See Walters, Jonathan. 1998. "Making a Spectacle: Deviant Men, Invective, and Pleasure." Arethusa ["Vile Bodies: Roman Satire and Corporeal Discourse"] 31:355–367.)

They don't talk so much; their passion is rather for silence; They keep their hair cut short, but oh, those wonderful eyebrows! I like Peribomius better; at least he's honest about it, Shows what he is by his walk and his glances, so I can excuse him, Him and his likes, whose urge is frank enough for forgiveness. Worse, much worse, are the ones who denounce, with a Hercules' anger, Vice, and waggle their tongues about Virtue, and waggle their rear ends. Sextus does things that Varillus observes and remarks, "How disgusting!" Yet he does them himself. A white man can sneer at a Negro, A cripple's a joke to the sound, but this is too much, that the Gracchi Scream to high heaven against people they call rabble rousers. This is confusion confounded, Verres denouncing a robber, Milo opposed to assassins, Catiline chiding Cethegus, Clodius damning adulterers, the second triumvirate shouting "down with proscription"! We had, and not long since, such a fellow Who, in true tragic style, joined fornication with incest, Then re-enacted the code which would horrify all human beings, Not to say Venus and Mars, and while he was doing so, Julia Rid her fertile womb of blobs that resembled her uncle. Is it not perfectly right, therefore, that the vilest of sinners Hate these hypocrites? If they snap at you, turn on them, bite them!. . .

Umbricius has much on his mind. "Since there's no place in the city," He says, "For an honest man, and no reward for his labors, Since have less today than yesterday, since by tomorrow That will have dwindled still more, I have made my decision. I'm going To the place where, I've heard, Daedalus put off his wings, While my white hair is still new, my old age in the prime of its straightness, While my fate spinner still has yarn on her spool, while I'm able Still to support myself on two good legs, without crutches. Rome, good-bye! Let the rest stay in the town if they want to, Fellows like A, B, and C, who make black white at their pleasure, Finding it easy to grab contracts for rivers and harbors, Putting up temples, or cleaning out sewers, or hauling off corpses, Or, if it comes to that, auctioning slaves in the market . . . Rubrius, looking no better, came next. He wasn't a noble. That may have been reassuring, but then, he had been convicted Of an old offense, and one that is better not mentioned. Worse than the sodomite Nero, who lashed other pathics with satire. Montanus was there. He was late because of the size of his belly. Curly the Cur was there, who reeks, in the morning, with odors That would outsink the smell of at least two funeral parlors. Pompey was there, an informer whose whisper could cut your throat, Fuscus, whose battles were planned in hallways of Parian marble, Tactics just the right sort to suit the vultures of Poland. Careful Veiento came, and with him the deadly Catullus Burning with love for a girl he had never seen. What a portent, Even for times like these! He was blind, but a flattering fawner, Sinister, one who belonged with the beggars infesting the bridges, Swarming out to the wheels, or blowing the richer ones kisses. No one was more amazed at the fish than he was; he gestured Toward the left as he spoke; it happened to be on his right. That was always his way, if he praised some Cilician bruiser Or the stage machines that lift the boys to the awnings. Veiento was almost as bad; carried away by his frenzy Almost into a trance, he presently vaticinated: "Omens of triumph I see, my Lord. Thou wilt capture a monarch Foreign-born like this turbot, Arviragus of the Britons.

This I can tell by the spiky fins erect on the backbone." Fabricius went on and on; the only thing he omitted Was the place where the fish spawned and the actual date of its birthday. . . .

Cheer when they find, for once, a citizen rare and distinguished. True nobility lies in more than a name and a title. We call somebody's dwarf an Atlas; his black boy is Swansdown, We label some ugly lopsided girl Europa; and mongrels, Mangy and worthless, the kind that try to lick oil from dry vessels, We call Lion, or Tiger, or Pard, or whatever roars loudest. So, beware lest your title is given in any such spirit, (that one's title be assigned as an opposite and therefore a spiteful joke)—Lest "The Victor of Crete" means Crete's where you took such a beating.

Sources: Ramsay, G. G., ed. and trans. 1918. Juvenal, *Satires*. London: Loeb Classical Library.

◙ Martial, *Epigrams 12.93; 14.210, 212, 213* (1st c. CE)

Like Juvenal, Martial was also a Roman satirist of the early imperial period (Martial died ca. 104 CE). Martial's epigrams, quite vile by today's standards, also highlight various physical characteristics as amusing or distasteful, but also on an individual basis, not an institutionalized one. Martial's epigrams on disabled people are interspersed with others that mock golddiggers, liars, and sycophants.

Sexualization of Dwarfs

Labulla has found a way to kiss her lover in her husband's presence. She keeps on kissing her dwarf fool. The lover immediately catches hold of him while he is still damp with many kisses and sends him back charged with his own kisses to the smiling lady of the house. How much greater a fool is the husband!

Idiot

His stupidity does not lie, is not feigned by wily art. He that is witless to excess has his wits.

Dwarf

If you looked only at the man's head, you would believe him Hector; if you saw him standing, you would think him Astyanax.

Buckler

Wont often to be defeated and to be victorious rarely, this will be to you a buckler, but the shield of a dwarf.

Polyphemus, slave of my friend Severus, your size and aspect are such that the cyclops himself might be amazed at you. But Scylla is no smaller. If you put the two savage monsters together, each will become the terror of the other.

Unwilling any longer to bear and suffer the coursings hither and thither, the early morning rounds, and the haughty salutations of the powerful, Caelius started to feign the gout. In his anxiety to prove it genuine, he anoints and bandages his healthy feet and walks with laboring tread. See what the cultivation and art of pain can do. Caelius stopped feigning the gout.

Source: Davis, William Stearns, ed. 1912–1913. *Readings in Ancient History: Illustrative Extracts from the Sources*. 2 Vols. Boston: Allyn & Bacon.

◙ Seneca the Younger, Excerpt from *Apocolocyntosis* (1st c. CE)

Seneca the Younger, the Stoic politician and philosopher who had the misfortune of serving as tutor to Emperor Nero, composed this lighthearted satire that mocks the deification of Nero's predecessor, Claudius. Emperor Claudius was known for his limp and his indistinct speech, perhaps a stutter, which is the subject of the mockery in the Apocolocyntosis, sometimes translated as the "Pumpkinification of Claudius." (See Braund, Susanna Morton, and Paula James. 1998. "Quasi Homo: Distortion and Contortion in Seneca's Apocolocyntosis." Arethusa ["Vile Bodies: Roman Satire and Corporeal Discourse"] 31:285–311.)

[1] I wish to record an occurrence which took place in heaven on the third day before the Ides of October, in the new year which began our fortunate era. I am not going to be diverted by either fear or favor. I shall tell the unvarnished truth. If anybody asks me where I got my information, I say at once, I'll not answer if I don't want to. Who is going to make me? I know I have been free to do as I like since the day when he died who had made the proverb true: One must be born either king or fool. If I please to answer, I shall say what comes to my tongue. Who ever demanded affidavits from an historian? Still, if I must produce my

authority, apply to the man who saw Drusilla going heavenward; he will say he saw Claudius limping along in the same direction. Willy-nilly, he has to see everything that happens in heaven; for he is the superintendent of the Appian road, by which you know both the divine Augustus and Tiberius Caesar went to join the gods. If you ask this man he will tell you privately; in presence of more than one he'll never speak a word. For since the day when he took oath in the Senate that he had seen Drusilla going up to heaven and in return for such good news nobody believed him, he has declared in so many words that he'll not testify about anything, not even if he should see a man murdered in the middle of the Forum. What I have heard from him, then, I state positively and plainly, so help him!

> [2] Now was come the season when Phoebus
>   had narrowed the daylight,
> Shortening his journey, while sleep's dim
>   hours were left to grow longer;
> Now victorious Cynthia was widening the
>   bounds of her kingdom;
> Ugly-faced Winter was snatching away the
>   rich glories of Autumn,
> So that the tardy vintager, seeing that Bacchus
>   was aging,
> Hastily, here and there, was plucking the clus-
>   ters forgotten.

I presume I shall be better understood if I say that the month was October and the day October thirteenth; the exact hour I cannot tell you—it's easier to get philosophers to agree than timepieces—but it was between noon and one o'clock.

"Too clumsily put!" you will say. "All the poets are unsatisfied to describe sunrises and sunsets, so that they are even tackling the middle of the day: are you going to neglect so good an hour?"

> Phoebus already had passed the highest point
>   of his circuit,
> Wearily shaking the reins as his car drew
>   nearer the evening,
> Leading away the half-spent light on [his]
>   down-dipping pathway.

[3] Claudius began to give up the ghost, but couldn't find a way out for it. Then Mercury, who had always had a fancy for his character, led aside one of the three Fates and said: "Why, O hard-hearted woman, do you let the wretched man be tormented?

Isn't he ever to have a rest, after being tortured so long? It is the sixty-fourth year that he has been afflicted with life. What grudge have you got against him and the nation? For once let the prophets tell the truth, who have been taking him off every year, every month even, since he was made emperor. And still it's no wonder if they go wrong and nobody knows his hour; for nobody ever made any account of his being born. Do what is necessary:

> 'Give him over to death: let a better man reign
>   in his place.'"

But Clotho remarked, "I swear I intended to give him a trifle more time, till he should make citizens out of the few that are left outside—for he had made up his mind to see everybody, Greeks, Gauls, Spaniards, Britons, wearing togas. However, since it is perhaps a good thing to have a few foreigners left as a nucleus, and since you wish it, it shall be attended to." Then she opened a bandbox and brought out three spindles; one was that of Augurinus, the next was Baba's, the third Claudius.' "I will have these three die at short intervals within a year," she said, "and not send him off unattended. For it isn't right that one who has been in the habit of seeing so many thousands of people following him about, going ahead of him, and all around him, should all of a sudden be left alone. For a while he will be satisfied with these boon-companions."

> [4] Thus having spoken she wound up the
>   thread on his spindle neglected,
> Breaking off the royal days of his stupid
>   existence.
> Lachesis, waiting meanwhile, with tresses
>   charmingly ordered,
> Crowning the locks on her brow with a wreath
>   of Pierian laurel,
> Drew from a snowy fleece white strands
>   which, cleverly fashioned,
> Under her artful fingers began with new colors
>   to glisten:—
> Spun to a thread that drew the admiring gaze
>   of her sisters.
> Changed was the common wool, until as a
>   metal most precious,
> Golden the age that was winding down in that
>   beautiful fillet.
> Ceaselessly they too labored; and bringing the
>   finest of fleeces,
> Gayly they filled her hands, for sweet was the
>   duty allotted.

She, in her eagerness, hastened the work, nor
    was conscious of effort;
Lightly the soft strands fell from the whirling
    point of her spindle,
Passing the life of Tithonus, passing the life-
    time of Nestor.
Phoebus came with his singing, and, happy in
    anticipation,
Joyously plied the plectrum, or aided the work
    of the spinners:
Kept their hearts intent, with his song beguil-
    ing their labor.
While beyond thought they rejoiced in their
    brother's music, their hands spun,
Busily twining a destiny passing all human
    allotment,
Wrought through the spell of Phoebus' lyre
    and his praise, as he bade them:
"Stay not your hands, O Fateful Sisters, but
    make him a victor
Over the barriers that limit the common life-
    time of mortals;
Let him be blessed with a grace and a beauty
    like mine, and in music
Grant him no meaner gifts. An age of joy shall
    he bring men
Weary for laws that await his restoring. Like
    Lucifer comes he,
Putting the scattered stars to flight, or like
    Hesper at nightfall,
Rising when stars return; or e'en as the Sun,—
    when Aurora
First has dispelled the dark and blushingly led
    forth the morning,—
Brightly gleams on the world and renews his
    chariot's journey,
So cometh Caesar; so in his glory shall Rome
    behold Nero.
Thus do his radiant features gleam with a
    gentle effulgence,
Graced by the flowing locks that fall
    encircling his shoulders."

Thus Apollo. But Lachesis, who herself, too, had a fondness for the handsomest of men, wrought with generous hand, and bestowed upon Nero many years from her own store. As for Claudius, however, everybody gave orders

With joy and great content to send him out of doors.[1]

And indeed he did go up the flume, and from that moment ceased to appear to be alive. He expired,

moreover, while listening to comic actors, so you understand it isn't without reason that I am afraid of those fellows. His last words that were heard among men were these, after a louder utterance in the locality where he expressed himself the more easily: "Oh, dear! I think I have hurt myself."[2] Whether he had, I don't know; at any rate he was in the habit of hurting everything.

[5] What happened afterward on earth it is superfluous to describe. For you know very well, and there is no danger that things which the universal joy had impressed upon the memory will slip from it; no one forgets his own good fortune. Listen to what happened in heaven: it is on the authority of the narrator. The news was brought to Jupiter that somebody had come, a rather tall man, quite gray-headed; that he was threatening something or other, for he kept shaking his head; and that he limped with his right foot. The messenger said he had asked of what nation he was, but his answer was mumbled in some kind of an incoherent noise; he didn't recognize the man's language, but he wasn't either Greek or Roman or of any known race. Then Jupiter told Hercules, who had traveled all over the world and was supposed to be acquainted with all the nations, to go and find out what sort of a man it was. Hercules at the first sight was a good deal disturbed, even though he was one who didn't fear any sort of monsters. When he beheld the aspect of this unknown specimen, its extraordinary gait, its voice belonging to no earthly creature but more like that of the monsters of the deep, hoarse and inarticulate, he thought that a thirteenth labor had come to him. When he looked more carefully, however, it appeared to be a man. He approached him and thus spoke, as was easiest for a Greek chap:

Who and whence art thou, and where are thy city and
    parents?

Claudius was delighted to find literary people there, hoping there would be some place for his histories. So he, too, in a Homeric verse, indicating himself to be Caesar, said:

Hence from Ilium the winds have among the Cicones
    cast me.

But the following verse would have been truer, and equally Homeric:

There their city I wasted; the people I slaughtered.

[6] And he would have imposed upon the guileless Hercules, had not Fever been there, who alone had left her shrine and come with him. All the other divinities he had left behind at Rome. She said, "It is simple nonsense that he is giving you. I tell you—I who have lived with him for so many years—he was born at Lugudunum; you behold one of Marcus' citizens. As I'm telling you, he was born sixteen miles from Vienna, a genuine Gaul. And so as a Gaul ought to do, he captured Rome. Take my word for it, he was born at Lugudunum, where Licinus reigned for many years. But you, who have tramped more lands than any wandering muleteer, ought to know men from Lugudunum and that there are a good many miles between the Xanthus and the Rhone." At this point Claudius fired up and angrily grumbled as loudly as he could. What he was saying, nobody understood, except that he commanded Fever to be led away to punishment. With the familiar gesture of his limp hand, that was steady enough for the one purpose of decapitating people as he was accustomed, he had ordered her head to be struck off. You would suppose all those present were his freedmen, so little attention did any one pay him. [7] Then Hercules said, "Listen to me and stop talking nonsense. You have come to a place where the mice gnaw iron. Tell me the truth, quick, or I'll knock the silliness out of you." And in order to be more terrifying, he struck the attitude of a tragedian and said:

> "Declare at once the place you call your natal
>   town,
> Or else, by this tough cudgel smitten, down
>   you go!
> This club has slaughtered many a mighty
>   potentate.
> What's that, that in a muffled voice you're
>   trying to say?
> Where is the land or race to own your shaky
>   head?
> Speak out. Oh, I remember when afar I sought
> The triple-bodied king's domains, whose
>   famous herd
> From the western sea I drove to the city of
>   Inachus,
> I saw a hill above two rivers, towering high
> In face of Phoebus rising each day opposite,
> Where the broad Rhone pours by in swiftly
>   moving flood,
> And Arar, pausing ere it lets its waters go,
> Silently laves the borders of its quiet pools.
> Is that the land that nursed you when you first
>   drew breath?"

These things he said with spirit, and boldly enough. All the same, he was inwardly a good deal afraid of the *madman's blow*. Claudius, seeing the mighty hero, forgot his nonsense and perceived that while no one had been a match for him at Rome, here he didn't have the same advantage; a cock is master only on his own dunghill. So, as well as could be made out, this is what he appeared to say: "I did hope that you, Hercules, bravest of the gods, would stand by me before the others, and if any one had asked me who could vouch for me, I should have named you, who know me best. For if you recall, I was the one who held court before your temple all day long during the months of July and August. You know how many troubles I had there, listening to the lawyers day and night; and if you had fallen among those fellows, though you may think that you are pretty courageous, you would have preferred to clean Augeas' stables. I have cleaned out much more filth. But since I want"—[3]

[8] "It's no wonder you have made an assault upon the senate-house; nothing is closed to you. Only tell us what sort of a god you want him to be made. He cannot be an *Epicurean god, neither having himself any care nor causing any to others.* A Stoic? How can he be 'round,' as Varro says, 'without head or prepuce'? Yet there is something in him of the Stoic god, now I see. He has neither heart nor head. By Hercules, though, if me had asked this favor of Saturn, whose festival month the Saturnalian prince kept going the whole year long, he wouldn't have got it; and surely he wouldn't of Jove, whom so far as he possibly could he convicted of incest. For he put to death Silanus his son-in-law, just because the man preferred that his sister, prettiest of all the girls, so that everybody called her Venus, should be called his Juno. 'Why his sister?' you say,—in fact, I ask it. Think, you blockhead. At Athens that sort of thing is halfway allowed; at Alexandria altogether. 'But since at Rome,' you say, 'the mice live on dainties.' He's going to straighten our crooked ways! He doesn't know what goes on in his own chamber, and now 'he searches the regions of heaven.' He wants to become a god. Isn't he satisfied that he has a temple in Britain; that the barbarians worship him and beseech him as a god that they may *find him a merciful madman?*"

[9] At length it occurred to Jove that while ordinary persons are staying in the senate-house it is not permitted to express an opinion nor to argue. "I had allowed you to ask questions, Conscript Fathers," he said, "but you have brought out simply rubbish. I want

you to observe the rules of the Senate. What will this person, whoever he is, think of us?"

When the said individual had been sent out, Father Janus was the first to be asked his opinion. He had been elected afternoon consul for the first of July, being a very shrewd man, who always sees *at once both forward and backward.* He spoke at some length, and fluently, because he lives in the Forum; but the stenographer could not follow, and therefore I do not report him, for fear of misquoting what he said. He said a good deal about the importance of the gods, and that this honor ought not to be given commonly. "Once," said he, "it was a great thing to be made a god, but now you have made the distinction a farce. And so lest my remarks seem to be dealing with personalities rather than with the case, I move that from this day forward no one shall be made a god, from among all those who *eat the fruit of the corn-land* or those whom the *fruitful corn-land* feeds. Whoever contrary to this decree of the Senate shall be made, called, or depicted as a god, is to be given to the hobgoblins, and to get a thrashing among the newly hired gladiators at the next show."

The next to be asked his opinion was Diespiter the son of Vica Porta, who was himself also a consul-elect, and a money-changer; by this business he supported himself, and he was accustomed to sell citizenships in a small way. Hercules approached him politely and gave him an admonitory touch on the ear. Accordingly he expressed his opinion in these words: "Whereas the divine Claudius is by blood related to the divine Augustus and no less also to the divine Augusta, his grandmother, who was made a goddess by his own orders, and whereas he far surpasses all mortals in wisdom, and it is for the public interest that there be some one who can join Romulus in 'eating of boiling hot-turnips,' I move that from this day the divine Claudius be a god, with title equally as good as that of any one who has been made so before him, and that this event be added to the Metamorphoses of Ovid."

The opinions were various, and Claudius seemed to be winning the vote. For Hercules, who saw that his iron was in the fire, kept running to this one and that one, saying, "Don't go back on me; this is my personal affair. And then if you want anything, I'll do it in my turn. One hand washes the other."

[10] Then the divine Augustus arose at the point for expressing his opinion, and discoursed with the utmost eloquence. "I call you to witness, Conscript Fathers," said he, "that since I was made a god, I have never addressed you; I always mind my own business. And I can no longer disguise my feelings nor conceal the distress that shame makes all the greater. Was it for this that I secured peace on land and sea? For this did I make an end of civil wars? For this did I found the city on a basis of law, adorn it with monuments, that—what to say, Conscript Fathers, I cannot discover. All words are beneath my indignation. So in desperation I must take to the phrase of that most clever man, Messala Corvinus, 'I am ashamed of my authority.' This fellow, Conscript Fathers, who doesn't seem to you as if he could disturb a fly, used to kill people as easily as a dog stops to rest. But why should I enumerate the many great men? I have no heart to lament public calamities when I behold those of my own family. And so I will pass over the former and describe these. For I know, even if my sister doesn't know [as they say in Greek], *my knee is nearer than my shin.* That fellow whom you see there, hiding under my name for so many years, has shown his gratitude to me by slaying the two Julias, my great-granddaughters, one by the sword, the other by starvation, and L. Silanus, one of my great-great-grandsons. We shall see, Jupiter, whether in a bad case, and one which is certainly your own, you are going to be just. Tell me, divine Claudius, why you condemned any one of the men and women whom you put to death before you understood their cases, or even listened to them. Where is this kind of thing customary? [11] It's not the way in heaven. Here is Jupiter, now, who has been ruling for so many years. One person's leg he has broken, Vulcan's whom

Snatching him by the foot, he hurled from the heavenly threshold;

and he got angry at his wide and hung her up, but he didn't kill her, did he? But you have put to death Messalina, to whom I was as much a great-uncle as I was to you. 'I don't know,' you say? May the gods be hard on you! It is more shameful that you didn't know it than that you killed her. He has never ceased to follow up the dead-and-gone C. Caesar. The latter had killed his father-in-law; Claudius here, his son-in-law besides. Gaius forbade the sons of Crassus to be called Magnus; this man returned him the name, but took off his head. He killed in one household Crassus, Magnus, Scribonia, the Tristionias, and Assario; and they were aristocrats too, and Crassus besides so stupid that he was even qualified to reign. Now do you want to make this man a god? Look at his body, born when the gods were angry. And finally, if he can say three consecutive words together, he can have me as his slave. Who will worship this god? Who will believe in him? As long as you make such gods as he, nobody will believe that you are gods yourselves. In short, Conscript Fathers, if I have behaved myself honorably among you, if I have not answered anybody in an ungentlemanly manner, avenge my injuries. This is the resolution which I have to offer;" and he read as follows from his tablet: "Since the divine Claudius has killed his father-in-law Appius Silanus, his two sons-in-law Magnus Pompeius and L. Silanus, his daughter's father-in-law Crassus Frugi, a man as like himself as one egg is to another, Scribonia his daughter's mother-in-law, his wife Messalina, and others too numerous to mention, I propose that strict punishment be meted out to him, that he be granted no rest from adjudicating cases, and that he be got out of the way as soon as possible, departing from heaven within thirty days and from Olympus within three."

There was a division of the house, and this resolution was carried. Without delay the Cyllenian dragged him by the nape of his neck off from heaven toward the lower regions,

"Whence they say no man returns."

[12] While they were going down the Via Sacra, Mercury inquired what such a crowd of people could mean: whether it was Claudius' funeral. And indeed it was a most elegant and elaborate display, so that you would easily recognize that a god was being carried off to burial. There was so great a crowd of trumpeters, hornblowers, and players upon every kind of brass instruments, so great a concord, that even Claudius could hear it. Everybody was joyful and in high spirits. The Roman people walked about like free men. Only Agatho and a few pettifoggers were weeping, but their grief was plainly heartfelt. The real lawyers were coming out of their hiding-places, pale and thin, scarcely drawing breath, like people who were just coming to life again. One of them, when he had seen the pettifoggers getting their heads together and lamenting their calamity, came up and said, "I told you the Saturnalia wouldn't last forever." Claudius, when he saw his own funeral, understood that he was dead. For in a mighty *great chorus* they were chanting a dirge in anapests:

"Pour forth your tears, lift up woful voices;
Let the Forum echo with sorrowful cries.
Nobly has fallen a man most sagacious,
Than whom no other ever was braver,
Not in the whole world.
He in the quick-sped race could be victor
Over the swiftest; he could rebellious
Parthians scatter, chase with his flying
Missiles the Persian, steadiest-handed,
Bend back the bow which, driving the foeman
Headlong in flight, should pierce him afar, while
Gay-coated Medes turned their backs to disaster.
Conqueror he of Britons beyond the
Shores of the known sea:
Even the dark-blue-shielded Brigantes
Forced he to bend their necks to the fetters
That Romulus forged, and Ocean himself
To tremble before the Roman dominion.
Mourn for the man than whom no one more
    quickly
Was able to see the right in a lawsuit,
Only at hearing one side of the quarrel,—
Often not either. Where is the judge now
Willing to listen to cases the year through?
Thou shalt be given the office resigned thee
By him who presides in the court of the shades,
The lord of a hundred cities Cretaean.
Smite on your breasts, ye shysters forsaken,
With hands of despair, O bribe-taking crew;
Ye too, half-fledged poets, now should bewail;
And ye above all, who lately were able
To gather great gains by shaking the dice-box."

[13] Claudius was delighted with his praises, and desired to stay longer to look on. But the Talthybius of the gods laid a hand on him and pulled him away, with his head covered so that nobody could recognize him, across the Campus Martius, and between the Tiber and the Arcade went down to the lower world. The freedman Narcissus had already gone ahead by a short cut to be ready to receive his patron, and as the latter was approaching he ran up, all sleek from the bath, and said: "What's this? Gods, among men?" "Hurry up," said Mercury, "and announce that we are coming." In less time than it takes to tell it, Narcissus skipped out. All the way being down hill, the descent was easy. And so, in spite of his gout, he came in twinkling to Pluto's door, where lay Cerberus, or as Horace says, "the beast with the hundred heads." Narcissus was a trifle scared—he had been accustomed to have a white dog as a pet—when he saw that huge, hairy black dog, which, on my word, is one that you wouldn't like to meet in the dark. And with a

loud voice he said, "Claudius is coming." Then a crowd began to come forward with clapping of hands and chanting: *"We have got him; let us rejoice!"* Among them were C. Silius the consul-elect, Iuncus the ex-praetor, Sextus Traulus, M. Helvius, Trogus, Cotta, Vettius Valens, and Fabius, Roman knights whom Narcissus had ordered to execution. In the middle of this company of singers was Mnester the dancer, whom Claudius had made shorter for the sake of appearances. To Messalina—the report that Claudius had come quickly spread—they gathered; first of all, the freedmen Polybius, Myron, Harpocras, Amphaeus, and Pheronactus, all of whom Claudius had sent ahead in order that he might not be anywhere unprepared; then the two prefects Justus Catonius and Rufrius Pollio; then the Emperor's friends Saturnius Lusius and Pedo Pompeius and Lupus and Celer Asinius, of consular rank; finally his brother's daughter, his sister's daughter, his sons-in-law, his father-in-law, his mother-in-law, in fact all his relatives; and forming in line they came to meet Claudius. When he had seen them, he exclaimed: *"Plenty of friends, everywhere!* How did you come here?" Then said Pedo Pompeius: "What are you talking about, you cruel villain? 'How?' did you ask? Well, who else but you has sent us here, you murderer of all your friends? Come to the court of justice. I'll show you where our tribunal is."

[14] He led him to the bar of Aeacus, who conducted the trial under the Cornelian law against assassins. He asked that the court would enter the name, and recorded the accusation: Senators killed, thirty-five; Roman knights, two hundred and twenty-one; other persons, as many as the sands on the seashore. No one was found as counsel for the accused until at length P. Petronius came forward, an old boon companion of his, a man skilled in the Claudian tongue, and asked for a postponement. It was not granted. Pedo Pompeius spoke for the prosecution with loud shouts. The attorney for the defense wanted to begin his reply. Aeacus, most equitable of persons, forbade him and condemned Claudius after hearing only one side, saying: *"Right will be done him if he be treated as he treated others."* Then there was a tremendous silence. Everybody was struck dumb by the novelty of the procedure. They said the thing never happened before. To Claudius it seemed more unjust than new. Over the nature of the penalty there was a long discussion, as to what would be an appropriate sentence for him. Various ones said that if they made Tantalus' suffering too long he would perish of thirst unless somebody came to his rescue; and that poor Ixion's wheel ought at last to be stopped. But it was decided that no release should be given to any of the old ones, lest Claudius should sometime hope for the same in his turn. It was decided that a new punishment ought to be arranged, that for him must be devised some vain task and the hope of gratifying some desire, without end or consummation. Then Aeacus commanded him to gamble with a bottomless dice-box. And already he had begun to search for his constantly escaping dice and to accomplish nothing; for

[15] Every time when he wanted to throw
　　from his clattering dice-box,
Both of the dice escaped him by way of the
　　hole in the bottom.
Then when he gathered them up and once
　　more ventured to play them,
Over again they gave him the slip, and kept
　　him pursuing,
Constantly baffling his hopes by skipping
　　away through his fingers,
Always trickily sliding through with the same
　　old deception,—
Tiresome as when poor Sisyphus reaches the
　　top of his mountain
Vainly to feel his burden go rolling back from
　　his shoulders.

Suddenly C. Caesar appeared and began to claim him as a slave. He produced witnesses who had seen Claudius getting thrashed by him with whips, with rods, and with his fists. The man was adjudged to C. Caesar; Caesar presented him to Aeacus; the latter delivered him to Menander his freedman, to be his law-clerk.

Notes

1. Greek quotations in the original are in the translation indicated by italics.

2. Camden's note: This is euphemistic to the point of incomprehensibility. The actual Latin (*'vae me, puto, concacavi me'*) should instead be translated as "Oh, dear! I think I have soiled myself."

3. Perhaps here Claudius begins the persuasion which proved effective with Hercules. The break which follows in the MSS., if due, as is supposed, to the loss of even only one leaf from the archetype from which they are all derived, would seem to have included in the gap more incidents than have been suggested in the various attempts to fill it.

Source: Ball, Allan Perley, trans. 1902. *Apocolocyntosis.* New York: Columbia University Press. Available at http://www.forumromanum.org/literature/apocolocyntosis.html

▣ Livy, Excerpts from *The History of Rome* (1st c. BCE)

The official historian of Rome under Augustus, Livy (died 17 CE) looked to the Golden Age of Rome for precedents and examples of its grandeur and right to rule the world. These excerpts from his writings are accounts of bad omens, formulaic in tone. Interestingly, a child whose sex cannot be determined is as horrifying as speaking oxen and rivers of blood. (See Bloom, Amy. 2002. Normal. *New York: Random House, for a commentary on the modern horror of ambiguously sexed people; see pp. 101–102, 119–120 in Garland, Robert. 1995.* The Eye of the Beholder. *Ithaca, NY: Cornell University Press, for a discussion of the ancient interpretations.)*

It was further decided that before the consul left the City certain portents should be expiated. Various places had been struck by lightning: the statue of Jupiter on the Alban Mount and a tree near his temple, a grove at Ostia, the city wall and temple of Fortune at Capua and the wall and one of the gates at Sinuessa. Some people asserted that the water at Alba had run blood and that in the sanctuary of the temple of Fors Fortuna in Rome a statuette in the diadem of the goddess had fallen of itself on to her hand. It was confidently believed that at Privernum an ox had spoken and that a vulture had flown down on to a booth in the crowded forum. At Sinuessa it was reported that a child was born of doubtful sex, these are commonly called androgyni—a word like many others borrowed from the Greek, a language which readily admits compound words—also that it had rained milk and that a boy had been born with an elephant's head. These portents were expiated by sacrifices of full-grown victims, and a day was appointed for special intercessions at all the shrines. . . .

Prior to the departure of the consuls religious observances were kept up for nine days owing to the fall of a shower of stones at Veii. As usual, no sooner was one portent announced than reports were brought in of others. At Menturnae the temple of Jupiter and the sacred grove of Marica were struck with lightning, as were also the wall of Atella and one of the gates. The people of Menturnae reported a second and more appalling portent; a stream of blood had flowed in at their gate. At Capua a wolf had entered the gate by night and mauled one of the watch. These portents were expiated by the sacrifice of full-grown victims, and special intercessions for the whole of one day were ordered by the pontiffs. Subsequently a second nine days' observance was ordered in consequence of a shower of stones which fell in the Armilustrum. No sooner were men's fears allayed by these expiatory rites than a fresh report came, this time from Frusino, to the effect that a child had been born there in size and appearance equal to one four years old, and what was still more startling, like the case at Sinuessa two years previously, it was impossible to say whether it was male or female. The diviners who had been summoned from Etruria said that this was a dreadful portent, and the thing must be banished from Roman soil, kept from any contact with the earth, and buried in the sea. They enclosed it alive in a box, took it out to sea, and dropped it overboard. . . .

Whatever money was discovered was to be replaced, and the deficit made up; and should it be thought necessary expiatory sacrifices were to be offered in accordance with the instructions of the pontiffs on the previous occasions. Their anxiety to atone for the violation of the temple was made all the keener by the simultaneous announcements of portents from numerous localities. In Lucania it was alleged that the heavens had been on fire; at Privernum the sun had been glowing red through the whole of a cloudless day; at the temple of Juno Sospita in Lanuvium a terrible noise was heard in the night. Numerous monstrous births were also reported amongst the Sabines a child was born of doubtful sex; another similar case was discovered where the child was already sixteen years old; at Frusino a lamb was yeaned with a head like a pig; at Sinuessa a pig was littered with a human head, and on the public domain-land in Lucania a foal appeared with five feet. These were all regarded as horrid and monstrous products of a nature which had gone astray to produce strange and hybrid growths; the hermaphrodites were looked upon as of especially evil omen and were ordered to be at once carried out to sea just as quite recently in the consulships of C. Claudius and M. Nero similar ill-omened births had been disposed of.

Source: Roberts, Canon, trans. 1905. *Livy: The History of Rome, Vol. 4.* London: J. M. Dent & Sons. Excerpts are from 27.11.1–6; 27.37.1–7; 31.12.5–10 in the original work.

Pliny the Elder (23–79 CE), Excerpts from *Natural History*

Pliny the Elder, who lived in the first century CE, wrote his Natural History, from which the following excerpts are taken, to compile thousands of facts, observations, and historical data. These include fanciful ethnographic data about peculiar physical features from little-known places, and, within the known world, reports of hermaphrodites, the transmission of disabling conditions from parent to child, and commentary on human stature. Perhaps the most interesting selection is Pliny's brief mention of Quintus Pedius, "born dumb." (See Gourevitch, Danielle. 1991. "Un enfant muet de naissance s'exprime par le dessin: à propos d'un cas rapporté par Pline l'Ancien." L'Evolution Psychiatrique 56:889–893.)

Book 6, Chapter 35

At the present day there are reported to be forty-five other kinds of Ethiopians. But the whole race was called Aetheria, and then Atlantia, and finally it took its name from Aethiops the son of Vulcan. It is by no means surprising that the outermost districts of this region produce animal and human monstrosities, considering the capacity of the mobile element of fire to mould their bodies and carve their outlines. It is certainly reported that in the interior on the east side there are tribes of people without noses, their whole face being perfectly flat, and other tribes that have no upper lip and others no tongues. Also one section has the mouth closed up and has no nostrils but only a single orifice through which it breathes and sucks in drink by means of oat straws, as well as grains of oat, which grows wild there, for food. Some of the tribes communicate by means of nods and gestures instead of speech; and some were unacquainted with the use of fire before the reign of King Ptolemy Lathyrus in Egypt. Some writers have actually reported a race of Pygmies living among the marshes in which the Nile rises. On the coast, in a region that we shall describe later, there is a range of mountains of a glowing red color, which have the appearance of being on fire.

Book 7, Chapter 2

Beyond the Nasamones and adjacent to them Calliphanes records the Machlyes, who are Androgyni and perform the function of either sex alternately. Aristotle adds that their left breast is that of a man and their right breast that of a woman. Isogonus and Numphodorus report that there are families in the same part of Africa that practice sorcery, whose praises cause meadows to dry up, trees to wither and infants to perish. Isogonus adds that there are people of the same kind among the Triballi and the Illyrians, who also bewitch with a glance and who kill those they stare at for a longer time, especially with a look of anger, and that their evil eye is most felt by adults; and that what is more remarkable is that they have two pupils in each eye. Apollonides also reports women of this kind in Scythia, who are called the Bitia, and Phylarchus also the Thibii tribe and many others of the same nature in Pontus, whose distinguishing marks he records as being a double pupil in one eye and the likeness of a horse in the other, and he also says that they are incapable of drowning. . . .

Indians have union with wild animals and the offspring is of mixed race and half animal; that among the Calingi, a tribe of the same part of India, women conceive at the age of five and do not live more than eight years, and that in another part men are born with a hairy tail and extremely swift, while others are entirely covered by their ears.

Book 7, Chapter 3

Recently on the day of the obsequies of his late Majesty Augustus a certain woman of the lower orders named Fausta at Ostia was delivered of two male and two female infants, which unquestionably portended the food shortage that followed. We also find the case of a woman in the Peloponnese who four times produced quintuplets, the greater number of each birth surviving. In Egypt also Trogus alleges cases of seven infants born at a single birth.

Persons are also born of both sexes combined—what we call Hermaphrodites, formerly called androgyny and considered as portents, but now as entertainments. Pompey the Great among the decorations of his theatre placed images of celebrated marvels, made with special elaboration for the purpose by the talent of eminent artists; among them we read of Eutychis who at Tralles was carried to her funeral pyre by twenty children and who had given birth 30 times, and Alcippe who gave birth to an elephant—although it is true that the latter case ranks among portents, for one of the first occurrences of the Marsian War was that a maidservant gave birth to a snake, and also monstrous births of various kinds are recorded among the ominous things that happened. Claudius Caesar writes that a hippo-centaur was born in Tessaly and died the same day; and in his reign we actually saw one that was brought here for him from Egypt preserved in honey. One case is that of an infant at Saguntum that at once went back into the womb, in the year in which that city was destroyed by Hannibal.

Book 7, Chapter 12

It is also well known that sound parents may have deformed children and deformed parents sound children or children with the same deformity, as the case may be; that some marks and moles and even scars reappear in the offspring, in some cases a birthmark on the arm reappearing in the fourth generation (we are told that in the Lepidus family three children were born, though not all in succession, with a membrane over the eyes); and indeed that other children have resembled their grandfather, and that also there has been a case of twins of which one resembled the father and the other the mother, and one of a child who resembled his brother like a twin although born a year later. . . .

A fisherman in Sicily not only resembled the proconsul Sura in appearance but actually reproduced his gape while speaking and his tongue-tied stammering utterance.

Book 7, Chapter 16

It is known that at the age of three a person's measurement is half his future stature. But it is almost a matter of observation that with the entire human race the stature on the whole is becoming smaller daily, and that few men are taller than their fathers as the conflagration that is the crisis towards which the age is now verging is exhausting the fertility of the semen. When a mountain in Crete was cleft by an earthquake a body 69 feet in height was found, which some people thought must be that of Orion and others of Otus. The records attest that the body of Orestes dug up at the command of an oracle measured 10 ft. 6 in. Moreover, the famous bard Homer nearly 1000 years ago never ceased to lament that mortals were smaller of stature than in the old days. In the case of Naevius Pollio the annals do not record his height, but they show that it was deemed portentous, because he was almost killed by the people flocking

round him. The tallest person our age has seen was a man named Gabbara brought from Arabia in the principate of his late Majesty Claudius who was 9 feet in height. Under his late Majesty Augustus there were two persons 6 inches taller, whose bodies on account of this remarkable height were preserve[d] in the tomb in Sallust's Gardens; their names were Pusio and Secundilla. When the same emperor was head of the state the smallest person was a dwarf 2 feet 5 inches high named Conopas, the pet of his granddaughter Julia, and the smallest female was Andromeda, a freedwoman of Julia Augusta. Marcus Varro states that the Knights of Rome Manius Maximus and Marcus Tullius were 3 feet high, and we have ourselves seen their bodies preserved in coffins. It is a matter of common knowledge that persons are born 18 inches high and some taller, who complete their life's course at the age of three.

We find in the records that at Salamis the son of Euthymenes grew to 4 feet 6 inches in his third year; he walked slowly, was dull of sense, became sexually quite mature, had a bass voice, and was carried off by a sudden attack of paralysis when he turned three. We ourselves recently saw almost all these features except sexual maturity in a son of the Knight of Rome Cornelius Tacitus, Deputy Finance Minister in Belgic Gaul. The Greeks call these cases "perverts," but in the Latin country there is no name for them.

Book 11, Chapter 37

Man is the only animal whose eyes are liable to distortion, which is the origin of the family names Squint-eye and Blinky. From the eyes also came the name of One-eye that used to be given to persons born blind in one eye, and that of eyelet given to persons both of whose eyes were small; the One-eye family received the name of an injury done to one of them.

Book 11, Chapter 52

When animals are born with extra limbs these are useless, as is always the case when a human being is born with a sixth finger. In Egypt it was decided to rear a monstrosity, a human being with another pair of eyes at the back of the head, though he could not see with these.

For my own part I am surprised that Aristotle not only believed but also published his belief that our bodies contain premonitory signs of our career. But although I think this view unfounded, and not proper to be brought forward without hesitation lest everybody should anxiously seek to find these auguries in himself, nevertheless I will touch upon it, because so great a master of the sciences as Aristotle has not despised it. Well then, he puts down as signs of a short life few teeth, very long fingers, a leaden complexion and an exceptional number of broken creases in the hand; and on the other side he says that those people are long-lived who have sloping shoulder, one or two long creases in the hand, more than thirty-two teeth, and large ears. Yet he does not, I imagine, note all these attributes present in one person, but separately, trifling things, as I consider them, though nevertheless commonly talked about. In a similar manner among ourselves Trogus, himself also one of the most critical authorities, has added some outward signs of character which I will append in his own words: 'When the forehead is large it indicates that the mind beneath it is sluggish; people with a small forehead have a nimble mind, those with a round forehead . . .'

Book 28, Chapter 10

The blood let from any part of the patient himself makes, we are told by Orpheus and Archelaus, a very efficacious application for quinsy; efficacious too if applied to the mouth of those who have fainted in an epileptic fit, for they rise up immediately. Some say the big toes should be pricked and the drops of blood applied to the face, or that a virgin should touch it with her right thumb; hence their conclusion that epileptics should eat virgin meat. Aeschines the Athenian used the ash of excrements for quinsy, sore tonsils, sore uvula, and carcinomata. This medicament he called botryon.

Book 34, Chapter 6

Nor are people ashamed to buy these at a price equal to the pay of a military tribune, although they clearly take even their name from the lighted candles they carry. At the sale of a chandelier of this sort by the instructions of the auctioneer (named Theon) selling it there was thrown in as part of the bargain the fuller Clesippus a humpback and also of a hideous appearance in other respects besides, the lot being bought by a woman named Gegania for 50,000 Sesterces. This woman gave a party to show off her purchases, and for the mockery of the guests the man appeared with no clothes on; his mistress conceiving an outrageous passion for him admitted him to her bed and later gave him

a place in her will thus becoming excessively rich he worshipped the lampstand in question as a divinity and so caused this story to be attached to Corinthian lampstands in general, thought the claims of morality were vindicated by his erecting a noble tombstone to perpetuate throughout the living world for all time the memory of Gegania's shame.

Book 35, Chapter 7

There was also a celebrated debate on the subject of painting held between some men of eminence which must not be omitted, when the former consul and winner of a triumph Quintus Pedius, who was appointed by the Dictator Caesar as his joint heir with Augustus, had a grandson Quintus Pedius who was born dumb; in this debate the orator Messala, of whose family the boy's grandmother had been a member, gave the advice that the boy should have lessons in painting, and his late lamented Majesty Augustus also approved of the plan. The child made great progress in the art, but died before he grew up.

Source: Bostock, John, and H. T. Riley, trans. 1855. *Pliny the Elder: The Natural History.* London: Henry G. Bohn.

▣ Tacitus, Excerpts from the *Annals* (1st/2nd c. CE)

The historian Tacitus, who wrote the Annals in the first century CE, compares his beloved fallen Republic (in which he never lived) with the Augustan principate, which he perceives as corrupt and dangerous. In these excerpts, Tacitus paints a picture of a failed Augustus by pointing to his old age and "sickly frame." Augustus's successor, Tiberius, is characterized by his taciturn gloominess. Tacitus continues to disparage Augustus's successors by reporting their own physical and mental characteristics and by reporting the company they kept, including people who were deformed in both physique and etiquette. (See Robert Garland's third chapter, "The Roman Emperor in his Monstrous World." 1995. Pp. 45–58 in The Eye of the Beholder, Ithaca, NY: Cornell University Press, for further discussion.)

Annals 1.4.1

Thus the State had been revolutionized, and there was not a vestige left of the old sound morality. Script of equality, all looked up to the commands of a sovereign without the least apprehension for the present, while Augustus in the vigour of life, could maintain his own position, that of his house, and the general tranquility. When in advanced old age, he was worn out by a sickly frame, and the end was near and new prospects opened, a few spoke in vain of the blessings of freedom, but most people dreaded and some longed for war.

Annals 1.76.12

Drusus presided over a show of gladiators which he gave in his own name and in that of his brother Gaermanicus, for he gloated intensely over bloodshed, however cheap its victims. This was alarming to the populace, and his father had, it was said, rebuked him. Why Tiberius kept away from the spectacle was variously explained. According to some, it was his loathing of a crowd, according to others, his gloomy temper, and a fear of contrast with the gracious presence of Augustus. I cannot believe that he deliberately gave his son the opportunity of displaying his ferocity and provoking the people's disgust, although even this was said.

Annals 12.49.1

Julius Pelignus was then procurator of Cappadocia, a man despised alike for his feebleness of mind and his grotesque personal appearance. He was however very intimate with Claudius, who, when in private life, used to beguile the dullness of his leisure with the society of jesters.

Annals 15.34–35

There an incident occurred, which many thought unlucky, though to the emperor it seemed due to the providence of auspicious deities. The people who had been present, had quitted the theatre, and the empty building then fell in without harm to anyone. Thereupon Nero in an elaborate ode thanked the gods, celebrating the good luck which attended the late downfall, and as he was on his way to cross the sea of Hadria, he rested awhile at Beneventum, where a crowded gladiatorial show was being exhibited by Vatinius. The man was one of the most conspicuously infamous sights in the imperial court, bred as he had

been, in a shoemaker's shop, of a deformed person and vulgar wit, originally introduced as a butt. After a time he grew so powerful by accusing all the best men, that in influence, wealth, and ability to injure, he was pre-eminent even in that bad company.

Source: Church, Alfred John, and William Jackson Brodribb, trans. ca. 1888. Tacitus, P. Cornelius. *The Annals.* Available at http://classics.mit.edu//Tacitus/annals.html

▣ Suetonius, Excerpts from the *Lives* (110 CE)

On one hand, Suetonius (born 69 CE) had access to imperial primary source material and was a contemporary of many of his biographical subjects. On the other hand, he wrote not only to inform but also to entertain, and his accounts of the Roman rulers are lurid and exaggerated. Still, we can find clues about how Suetonius's audience might have perceived disability. Alongside Julius Caesar's epilepsy, Caligula's mental and physical sickness, and Claudius's and Domitian's various characteristics, we see the sort of imperial disdain for physical variation that Suetonius's contemporary, Tacitus, also reports.

The Deified Julius, Chapter 43

Caesar is said to have been tall, fair, and well-built, with a rather broad face and keen, dark-brown eyes. His health was sound, apart from sudden comas and a tendency to nightmares which troubled him towards the end of his life; but he twice had epileptic fits while on campaign. He was something of a dandy, always keeping his head carefully trimmed and shaved; and had been accused of having certain other hairy parts of his body depilated with tweezers. His baldness was a disfigurement which his enemies harped upon, much to his exasperation; he used to comb the thin strands of hair forward from his poll, and of all the honors voted him by the Senate and People, none pleased him so much as the privilege of wearing a laurel wreath on all occasions—he constantly took advantage of it.

His dress was, it seems, unusual: he had added wrist-length sleeves with fringes to his purple-striped senatorial tunic, and the belt which he wore over it was never tightly fastened—hence Sulla's warning to the aristocratic party: "Beware of that boy with the loose clothes!"

The Deified Augustus

Chapter 43

None of Augustus' predecessors had ever provided so many, so different, or such splendid public shows. He records the presentation of four Games in his own name and twenty-three in the names of other city magistrates who were either absent or could not afford the expense. Sometimes plays were shown in all the various city districts, and on several stages, the actors speaking the appropriate local language; and gladiators fought not only in the Forum or the Amphitheatre, but in the Circus and Enclosure as well; or the show might, on the contrary, be limited to a wild-beast hunt. He also held athletic competitions in the Campus Martius, for which he put up tiers of wooden seats; and dug an artificial lake beside the Tiber, where the present Caesarian Grove stands, for a mock sea-battle. On these occasions he posted guards in different parts of the city to prevent ruffians from turning the emptiness of the streets to their own advantage. Chariot-races and foot-races took place in the Circus, and among those who hunted the wild beasts were several volunteers of distinguished family. Augustus also ordered frequent performances of the Troy Game by two troops, of older and younger boys; it was an admirable tradition, he held, that the scions of noble houses should make their public debut in this way. When Nonius Asprenas fell from his horse at one performance and was crippled, Augustus comforted him with a golden torque and the hereditary surname of 'Torquatus.' Soon afterwards, however, he discontinued the Troy Game, because Asinius Pollio the orator attacked it bitterly in the House; his grandson, Aeserninus, having broken a leg too.

Chapter 67

Augustus behaved strictly but graciously and kindly towards his dependants and slaves, and honored some of his freedmen, such as Licinus, Celadus, and others, with his close intimacy. A slave named Cosmus, who had complained of him in the vilest terms, was punished merely by being put in irons. Once, when Augustus and his steward Diomedes were out walking together and a wild boar suddenly charged at them, Diomedes took fright and dodged behind his master. Augustus later made a joke of the incident, though he had been in considerable danger, preferring to call Diomedes a coward than anything worse—after all, his action had not been premeditated. Yet, when one Polus, a favorite freedman, was convicted of adultery with Roman matrons, Augustus ordered him to commit suicide; and sentenced Thallus, an imperial secretary to have his legs broken for divulging the contents of a letter—his fee had been twenty-five gold pieces. And because Gaius Caesar's tutor and attendants used their master's sickness and subsequent death as an excuse for arrogant, greedy behavior in his province, Augustus had them flung into a river with weights tied around their necks.

Chapter 83

As soon as the Civil Wars were over Augustus discontinued his riding and fencing exercises on the Campus Martius and used, instead, to play catch with two companions, or hand-ball with several. But soon he was content to go riding, or take walks, muffled in a cloak or blanket, that ended with a sprint and some jumping. Sometimes he went fishing as a relaxation; sometimes he played at dice, marbles, or nuts in the company of little boys, and was always on the lookout for ones with pretty faces and cheerful chatter, especially Syrians and Moors–he loathed people who were dwarfish or in any way deformed, regarding them as freaks of nature and bringers of bad luck.

The Life of Tiberius, Chapter 61

Soon Tiberius broke out in every sort of cruelty and never lacked for victims: these were, first, his mother's friends and even acquaintances; then those of his grandsons and daughter-in-law; finally, those of Sejanus. With Sejanus out of the way his savageries increased; which proved that Sejanus had not, as some thought, been inciting him to commit them, but merely providing the opportunities that he demanded. Nevertheless, in Tiberius' brief and sketchy autobiography we find him daring to assert that Sejanus had been killed because he had found him persecuting Nero and Drusus, the sons of Germanicus; the fact being that he had himself put Nero to death when Sejanus was already an object of suspicion, and Drusus after he had fallen from power. A detailed list of Tiberius' barbarities would take a long time to compile; I shall content myself with a few samples. Not a day, however holy, passed without an execution; he even desecrated New Year's Day. Many of his men victims were accused and punished with their children—some actually by their children—and the relatives forbidden to go into mourning. Special awards were voted to the informers who had denounced them and, in certain circumstances, to the witnesses too. An informer's word was always believed. Every crime became a capital one, even the utterance of a few careless words. A poet found himself accused of slander—he had written a tragedy which presented King Agamemnon in a bad light—and a historian had made the mistake of describing Caesar's assassins, Brutus and Cassius, as 'the last of the Romans.' Both these authors were executed without delay, and their works—though once publicly read before Augustus, and accorded general praise—were called in and destroyed. Tiberius denied those who escaped a prison sentence not only the solace of reading books, but the privilege of talking to their fellow-prisoners. Some of the accused, on being warned to appear in court, felt sure that the verdict would be 'guilty' and, to avoid the trouble and humiliation of a trial, stayed at home and severed an artery; yet Tiberius' men bandaged their wounds and hurried them, half-dead, to prison. Others obeyed their summons and then drank poison in full view of the Senate. The bodies of all executed persons were flung on the Stairs of Mourning, and dragged to the Tiber with hooks—as many as twenty a day, including women and children. Tradition forbade the strangling of virgins; so, when little girls had been condemned to die in this way, the executioner began by violating them. Tiberius used to punish with life those who wished to die. He regarded death as a comparatively light affliction, and on hearing that a man named Carnulus had forestalled his execution by suicide, exclaimed: 'Carnulus has got away!' Once, during a gaol inspection, a prisoner begged to be put out of his misery; Tiberius replied: 'No, we are not yet friends again.' An ex-consul has recorded in his memoirs that he attended a banquet at which Tiberius was suddenly asked loudly by a dwarf, standing among a group of jesters near the table: 'What of Paconius? Why is he still alive after being charged with treason?' Tiberius told him to hold his saucy tongue; but a few days later requested the Senate to make a quick decision about Paconius' execution.

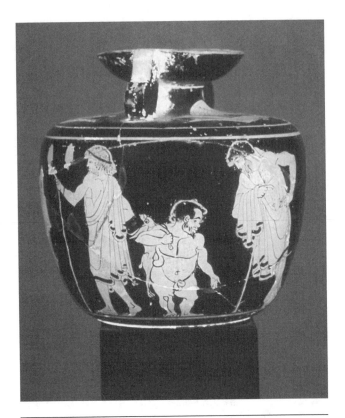

Doctor bleeding a patient and dwarf carrying a hare. The scene on this vase details common medical treatments in ancient Greece for various illnesses. The person of short stature may demonstrate some integration of disabled people into the medical arts. Ceramic, red figure aryballos, 480–470 BCE.

Source: Louvre, Paris. Photo credit: Réunion des Musées Nationaux/Art Resource, New York.

Aretaeus of Cappadocia, "The Wandering Womb" (2nd c. CE)

Aretaeus of Cappadocia, a contemporary of Galen, accepts the basic Hippocratic doctrines about hysteria but adds dramatic analogy to his account.

In the middle of the flanks of women lies the womb, a female viscus, closely resembling an animal; for it is moved of itself hither and thither in the flanks, also upwards in a direct line to below the cartilage of the thorax, and also obliquely to the right or to the left, either to the liver or spleen; and it likewise is subject to prolapsus downwards, and, in a word, it is altogether erratic. It delights, also, in fragrant smells, and advances towards them; and it has an aversion to fetid smells, and flees from them; and, on the whole, the womb is like an animal within an animal.

When, therefore, it is suddenly carried upwards, and remains above for a considerable time, and violently compresses the intestines, the woman experiences a choking, after the form of epilepsy, but without convulsions. For the liver, diaphragm, lungs and heart are quickly squeezed within a narrow space; and therefore loss of breathing and of speech seems to be present. And, moreover, the carotids are compressed from sympathy with the heart, and hence there is heaviness of head, loss of sensibility, and deep sleep.

And in women there also arises another affection resembling this form, with sense of choking and loss of speech, but not proceeding from the womb; for it also happens to men, in the manner of catalepsy. But those from the uterus are remedied by fetid smells, and the application of fragrant things to the female parts; but in the others these things do no good; and the limbs are moved about in the affection from the womb, but in the other affection not at all. Moreover, voluntary and involuntary tremblings . . . but from the application of a pessary to induce abortion, powerful congelation of the womb, the stoppage of a copious haemorrhage, and such like.

If, therefore, upon the womb's being moved upwards, she begins to suffer: there is sluggishness in the performance of her offices, prostration of strength, atony, loss of the faculties of her knees, vertigo (and the limbs sink under her), headache, heaviness of the head, and the woman is pained in the veins on each side of the nose.

But if they fall down they have heartburn . . . in the hypochondriac regions; flanks empty, where is the seat of the womb; pulse intermittent, irregular, and failing; strong sense of choking; loss of speech and of sensibility; respiration imperceptible and indistinct; a very sudden and incredible death, for they have nothing deadly in their appearance; in color like that of life, and for a considerable time after death they are more ruddy than usual; eyes somewhat prominent, bright, not entirely fixed, but yet not very much turned aside.

But if the uterus be removed back to its seat before the affection comes to a conclusion, they escape the suffocation. When the belly rumbles there is moisture about the female parts, respiration thicker and more distinct, a very speedy rousing up from affection, in like manner as death is very sudden; for as it readily ascends to the higher regions, so it readily recedes. For the uterus is buoyant, but the membranes, its supporters, are humid, and the place is humid in which the uterus lies; and, moreover, it flees from fetid things. And seeks after sweet; wherefore it readily

inclines to this side and to that, like a log of wood, and floats upwards and downwards. For this reason the affection occurs in young women, but not in old. For in those in whom the age, mode of life, and understanding is more mobile, the uterus also is of a wandering nature; but in those more advanced in life, the age, mode of living, understanding, and the uterus are of a steady character. Wherefore this suffocation from the womb accompanies females alone.

But the affections common to men happen also to the uterus, such as inflammation and haemorrhage, and they have the common symptoms, namely, fever, asphyxia, coldness, loss of speech. But in haemorrhage the death is even more sudden, being like that of a slaughtered animal.

Source: Adams, F., trans. 1856. *Aretaeus, On the Causes and Symptoms of Acute Diseases 2, Excerpts. London:* Sydenham Society.

▣ Soranus, *Gynecology* (2nd c. CE)

Soranus of Ephesus wrote a treatise on gynecology that influenced medical practice for centuries. He is generally admired for his efforts to dispel superstitious beliefs about the female reproductive system. In the selection excerpted here, his ideas regarding what women should do to avoid bearing "misshapen" children illustrate the familiar efforts to determine the causes of physical disability.

1.36 The best time for fruitful intercourse is when menstruation is ending and abating, when urge and appetite for coitus are present, when the body is neither in want nor too congested and heavy from drunkenness and indigestion, and after the body has been rubbed down and a little food been eaten and when a pleasant state exists in every respect. 'When menstruation is ending and abating,' for the time before menstruation is not suitable, the uterus already being overburdened and in an unresponsive state because of the ingress of material and incapable of carrying on two motions contrary to each other, one for the excretion of material, the other for receiving.

1.39.2 In order that the offspring may not be rendered misshapen, women must be sober during coitus because in drunkenness the soul becomes the victim of strange fantasies; this, furthermore, because the offspring bears some resemblance to the mother as well not only in body but in soul.

Source: Temkin, Oswei, trans. 1991. *Soranus' Gynecology.* Baltimore, MD: Johns Hopkins University Press.

◙ Galen on Psychological Origins of Hysteria (2nd c. CE)

In this rare case history of elegant deductive analysis, the Greek physician and philosopher Galen of Pergamum observes that apparently physical ailments can sometimes have psychological causes. This idea was not rediscovered until the twentieth century.

I was called to see a woman who was stated to be sleepless at night and to lie tossing about from one position to another. Finding she had no fever, I made a detailed inquiry into everything that had happened to her especially considering such factors as we know to cause insomnia. But she either answered little or nothing at all, as if to show that it was useless to question her. Finally, she turned away, hiding herself completely by throwing the bedclothes over her whole body, and laying her head on another small pillow, as if desiring sleep.

After leaving I came to the conclusion that she was suffering from one of two things: either from a melancholy dependent on black bile, or else trouble about something she was unwilling to confess. I therefore deferred till the next day a closer investigation of this. Further, on first arriving, I was told by her attendant maid that she could not at present be seen; and on returning a second time, I was told the same again. So I went yet a third time, but the attendant asked me to go away, as she did not want her mistress disturbed. Having learned, however, that when I left she had washed and taken food in her customary manner, I came back the next day and in a private conversation with the maid on one subject and another I found out exactly what was worrying the patient. And this I discovered by chance.

After I had diagnosed that there was no bodily trouble, and that the woman was suffering from some mental uneasiness, it happened that, at the very time I was examining her, this was confirmed. Somebody came from the theatre and said he had seen Pylades dancing. Then both her expression and the color of her face changed. Seeing this, I applied my hand to her wrist, and noticed that her pulse had suddenly become extremely irregular. This kind of pulse indicates that the mind is disturbed; thus it occurs also in people who are disputing over any subject. So on the next day I said to one of my followers that, when I paid my visit to the woman, he was to come a little later and announce to me, 'Morphus is dancing today.' When he said this, I found that the pulse was unaffected. Similarly also on the next day, when I had an announcement made about the third member of the troupe, the pulse remained unchanged as before. On the fourth evening I kept very careful watch when it was announced that Pylades was dancing, and noticed that the pulse was very much disturbed. Thus I found out that the woman was in love with Pylades, and by very careful watch on the succeeding days my discovery was confirmed.

Similarly too I diagnosed the case of a slave who administered the household of another wealthy man, and who sickened in the same way. He was concerned about having to give an account of his expenses, in which he knew that there was a considerable sum wanting; the thought of this kept him awake, and he grew thin with anxiety. I first told his master that there was nothing physically wrong with the old man, and advised an investigation to be made as to whether he feared his master was about to ask an account of the sums he had entrusted to him and for this reason was worried, knowing that a considerable amount would be found wanting. The master told me I had made a good suggestion, so in order to make the diagnosis certain I advised him to do as follows: he was to tell the slave to give him back all the money he had in hand, lest, in the event of his sudden death, it should be lost, owing to the administration passing into the hands of some other servant whom he did not know: for there would be no use asking for an account from such a one. And when the master said this to him, he felt sure he would not be questioned. So he ceased to worry, and by the third day had regained his natural physical condition.

Now what was it that escaped the notice of previous physicians when examining the aforesaid woman and the aforesaid slave? For such discoveries are made by common inductions if one has even the smallest acquaintance with medical science. I suppose it is because they have no clear conception of how the body tends to be affected by mental conditions. Possibly also they do not know that the pulse is altered by quarrels and alarms that suddenly disturb the mind.

Source: Brock, A. J., trans. 1916. *Galen, On Prognosis 6.* Loeb Classical Library Series.

▣ Justinian, *Institutes* (535 CE)

During his reign in the sixth century, the Byzantine emperor Justinian codified centuries of Roman law. The excerpts here show that disability was categorized pragmatically, not medically. From the legal perspective, insanity was an issue of marriage and inheritance; deafness (along with the status of female, child, or slave) was an issue of the ability to give legal testimony. Physical disability directly linked to financial consequence.

Book 1, Section 10. Marriage

Roman citizens are bound together in lawful matrimony when they are united according to law, the males having attained the age of puberty, and the females a marriageable age, whether they are fathers or sons of a family; but, of the latter, they must first obtain the consent of their parents, in whose power they are. For both natural reason and the law require this consent; so much so, indeed, that it ought to precede the marriage. Hence the question has arisen, whether the daughter of a madman could be married, or his son marry? And as opinions were divided as to the son, we decided that as the daughter of a madman might, so may the son of a madman marry without the intervention of the father, according to the mode established by our *constitutio.*

Book 1, Section 23. Curatorship

Males arrived at the age of puberty, and females of a marriageable age, receive curators, until they have completed their twenty-fifth year; for, although they have attained the age of puberty, they are still of an age which makes them unfit to protect their own interests.

1. Curators are appointed by the same magistrates who appoint tutors. A curator cannot be appointed by testament, but if appointed, he may be confirmed in his office by a decree of the praetor of *praeses.*

2. No adolescent is obliged to receive a curator against his will, unless in case of a lawsuit, for a curator may be appointed for a particular special purpose.

3. Madmen and prodigals, although past the age of twenty-five, are yet placed under the curatorship of their *agnati* by the law of the Twelve Tables. But, ordinarily, curators are appointed for them, at Rome, by the prefect of the city or the praetor: in the provinces, by the *praesides,* after inquiry into the circumstances has been made.

4. Persons who are of unsound mind, or who are deaf, mute, or subject to any perpetual malady, since they are unable to manage their own affairs, must be placed under curators.

Book 2, Section 10. The Making of Wills

5. All the witnesses may seal the testament with the same seal; for, as Pomponius says, what if the engraving on all seven seals were the same? And a witness may use a seal belonging to another person.

6. Those persons can be witnesses with whom there is *testamenti factio.* But women, persons under the age of puberty, slaves, madmen, dumb persons, deaf persons, prodigals restrained from having their property in their power, and persons declared by law to be worthless and incompetent to witness, cannot be witnesses.

Book 3, Intestate Succession

3. *Sui heredes* may become heirs, without their knowledge, and even though insane; for in every case in which inheritances may be acquired without our knowledge, they may also be acquired by the insane. At the death of the father, ownership in an inheritance is at once continued; accordingly, the authority of a tutor is not necessary, as inheritances may be acquired by *sui heredes* without their knowledge: neither does an insane person acquire by assent of his curator, but by operation of law.

Book 4, Section 3. The Lex Aquilia

9. The words above quoted "the greatest value the thing has possessed at any time within a year previously," mean that if your slave is killed, being at the time of his death lame, maimed, or one-eyed, but having been within a year quite sound and of considerable value, the person who kills him is bound to pay not his actual value, but the greatest value he ever possessed within the year. Hence, this *action* may be said to be penal, as a person is bound under it not only for the damage he has done, but for much more; and, therefore, the *action* does not pass against his heir, as it would have done if the condemnation had not exceeded the amount of the actual damage.

Source: Moyle, J. B., trans. 1913. *The Institutes of Justinian.* Available at http://www.thelatinlibrary.com/law/institutes

The Bible:
Hebrew Scriptures—Old Testament

⊡ Isaac's Blindness: Jacob Takes the Blessing

The story of the deception of Isaac and the theft of his blessing by Jacob is generally attributed to the Yahwist source and dated to the mid-tenth century BCE. Here, Isaac's blindness is the result of the natural aging process. Isaac's blindness is mentioned only in this passage, where it provides the context for Jacob's deception. While the deception is possible because of Isaac's blindness, Jacob finds it necessary to deceive his father for his purposes since his father retains all the social status and familial power of the patriarch, which remain intact when he becomes disabled. While the reader is led to pity Isaac, it is because of his dysfunctional family rather than because of his age and disability.

Genesis 27:1–45

27:1 Isaac had grown old and his eyesight was fading. He summoned his elder son Esau.

'My son.'

'Yes.'

27:2 'I am old and I have no idea when I will die.

27:3 Now take your equipment, your dangler and bow, and go out in the field to trap me some game.

27:4 Make it into a tasty dish, the way I like it, and bring it to me to eat. My soul will then bless you before I die.'

27:5 Rebecca had been listening while Isaac was speaking to Esau, his son. Esau went out to the field to trap some game and bring it home.

27:6 Rebecca said to her son Jacob, 'I just heard your father speaking to your brother Esau. He said,

27:7 'Bring me some game and prepare it into something tasty. I will eat it and bless you in God's presence before I die.'

27:8 Now, my son, listen to me. Heed my instructions carefully.

27:9 Go to the sheep and take two choice young kids. I will prepare them with a tasty recipe, just the way your father likes them.

27:10 You must then bring it to your father, so that he will eat it and bless you before he dies.'

27:11 'But my brother Esau is hairy,' replied Jacob. 'I am smooth-skinned.

27:12 Suppose my father touches me. He will realize that I am an impostor! I will gain a curse rather than a blessing!'

27:13 'Let any curse be on me, my son,' said the mother. 'But listen to me. Go, bring me what I asked.'

27:14 [Jacob] went and fetched what his mother had requested. She took [the kids] and prepared them, using the tasty recipe that [Jacob's] father liked best.

27:15 Rebecca then took her older son Esau's best clothing, which she had in her keeping, and put them on her younger son Jacob.

27:16 She [also] placed the young goats' skins on his arms and on the hairless parts of his neck.

27:17 Rebecca handed to her son Jacob the delicacy, and the bread she had baked.

27:18 He came to his father. 'Father.'

'Yes. Who are you, my son?'

27:19 'It is I, Esau, your first-born,' said Jacob. 'I have done as you asked. Sit up, and eat the game I trapped, so that your soul will bless me.'

27:20 'How did you find it so quickly, my son?' asked Isaac.

'God your Lord was with me.

27:21 'Come closer to me,' said Isaac to Jacob. 'Let me touch you, my son. Are you really Esau or not?'

27:22 Jacob came closer to his father Isaac, and [Isaac] touched him. He said, 'The voice is Jacob's voice, but the hands are the hands of Esau.'

27:23 He did not realize who it was because there was hair on [Jacob's] arms, just like those of his brother Esau. [Isaac] was about to bless him.

27:24 'But are you *really* my son Esau?'

'I am.'

27:25 'Then serve me [the food]. I will eat the game that my son trapped, so that my soul may bless you.'

[Jacob] served it, and [Isaac] ate. He then brought [Isaac] some wine, and he drank it.

27:26 His father Isaac said to him, 'Come closer and kiss me, my son.'

27:27 [Jacob] approached and kissed him. [Isaac] smelled the fragrance of his garments, and blessed him.

He said, 'See, my son's fragrance is like the perfume of a field blessed by God.

27:28 'May God grant you the dew of heaven and the fat of the earth, much grain and wine.

27:29 Nations will serve you; governments will bow down to you. You shall be like a lord over your brother; your mother's children will prostrate themselves to you. Those who curse you are cursed, and those who bless you are blessed.'

27:30 Isaac had finished blessing Jacob, and Jacob had just left his father Isaac, when his brother Esau came back from his hunt.

27:31 He had also prepared a delicacy and brought it to his father. 'Let my father get up and eat his son's venison,' he said, 'so that your soul may bless me.'

27:32 'Who are you?' asked his father Isaac.

'I am your first-born, Esau,' he replied.

27:33 Isaac was seized with a violent fit of trembling. 'Who . . . where . . . is the one who trapped game and just served it to me? I ate it all before you came and I blessed him. The blessing will remain his.'

27:34 When Esau heard his father's words, he let out a most loud and bitter scream. 'Bless me too, Father,' he pleaded.

27:35 'Your brother came with deceit, and he already took your blessing.'

27:36 'Isn't he truly named Jacob (*Ya'akov*)! He went behind my back (*akav*) twice. First he took my birthright, and now he took my blessing!'

[Esau] pleaded, 'Couldn't you have saved me a blessing too?'

27:37 Isaac tried to answer. 'But I made him like a lord over you,' he said. 'I have given him all his brothers as slaves. I have associated him with the grain and the wine. Where . . . what . . . can I do for you, my son?'

27:38 Esau said to his father, 'Is there only one blessing you have, my father? Father! Bless me too!' Esau raised his voice and began to weep.

27:39 His father Isaac then replied and said, 'The fat places of the earth can still be your dwelling, and [you can still have] the dew of heaven.

27:40 But you shall live by your sword. You may have to serve your brother, but when your complaints mount up, you will throw his yoke off your neck.'

27:41 Esau was furious at Jacob because of the blessing that his father had given him. He said to himself, 'The days of mourning for my father will be here soon. I will then be able to kill my brother Jacob.'

27:42 Her older son's plans were reported to Rebecca. She sent word and summoned her younger son Jacob. 'Your brother Esau is consoling himself by planning to kill you,' she said.

27:43 'Now, my son, listen to me. Set out and flee to my brother Laban in Charan.

27:44 Remain with him awhile until your brother's anger has subsided.

27:45 When your brother has calmed down from his rage against you, and has forgotten what you have done to him, I will send word and summon you home. But why should I lose you both on the same day?'

Source: Landsberg, Max, trans. 1917. Book of Genesis. In *The Hebrew Bible in English*. Jewish Publication Society. Available at http://www.mechon-mamre.org/e/et/et0.htm

▣ Jacob's Limp

The story of Jacob wrestling with a supernatural being at the Jabbok River is generally attributed to the Yahwist source and dated to the mid-tenth century BCE. While the nature of the creature that confronts Jacob remains uncertain, it is clearly perceived by Jacob (and reflected in his new name, Israel) that his true struggle has been with God. Jacob becomes disabled in this struggle, not by a blow, but by a touch. Both the new name and the limp are signs not only of the blessing Jacob receives but the renewal of the patriarchal covenant with the ancestor of the nation Israel. As a sign of the covenant, later generations of Israel participate symbolically in Jacob's disability by not eating the meat of the thigh muscle. Jacob's disability is mentioned only in this passage.

Genesis 32:22–32

32:22 He sent the gifts ahead of him, and spent the night in the camp.

32:23 In the middle of the night he got up, and took his two wives, his two handmaids, and his eleven sons, and sent them across the Jabbok River shallows.

32:24 After he had taken them and sent them across, he also sent across all his possessions.

32:25 Jacob remained alone. A stranger [appeared and] wrestled with him until just before daybreak.

32:26 When [the stranger] saw that he could not defeat him, he touched the upper joint of [Jacob's] thigh. Jacob's hip joint became dislocated as he wrestled with [the stranger].

32:27 'Let me leave!' said [the stranger]. 'Dawn is breaking.'

'I will not let you leave unless you bless me.'

32:28 'What is your name?'

'Jacob.'

32:29 'Your name will no longer be said to be Jacob, but Israel (*Yisra'el*). You have become great (*sar*) before God and man. You have won.'

32:30 Jacob returned the question. 'If you would,' he said, 'tell me what *your* name is.'

'Why do you ask my name?' replied [the stranger]. He then blessed [Jacob].

32:31 Jacob named the place Divine Face (*Peniel*). [He said,] 'I have seen the Divine face to face, and my soul has withstood it.'

32:32 The sun rose and was shining on him as he left Peniel. He was limping because of his thigh.

Source: Landsberg, Max, trans. 1917. Book of Genesis. In *The Hebrew Bible in English.* Jewish Publication Society. Available at http://www.mechon-mamre.org/e/et/et0.htm

▣ Purity Laws

The Priestly Purity Laws are attributed to the Priestly source, which dates to the time of the Babylonian Exile, from the mid-sixth to mid-fifth centuries BCE. Leviticus 13 and 14 deal with visible skin blemishes and apply to the whole community. Anyone who has a

blemish is institutionally marginalized from the community until he or she can provide proof that the blemish is gone. Leviticus 21:16–23 deals with the full range of disabilities and applies only to the Aaronide priestly caste. Here the prohibition applies only to serving in the priestly office. Aaronides who are unable to serve are still guaranteed all the benefits of the Aaronide priestly status. In all cases, the prohibitions are concerned with ritual purity rather than community health.

Leviticus 13

The Leprous Curse

13:1 God spoke to Moses and Aaron, saying:

13:2 If a person has a [white] blotch, discoloration or spot on the skin of his body, and it [is suspected] of being a mark of the leprous curse on his skin, he shall be brought to Aaron, or to one of his descendants, who are the priests.

13:3 The priest shall examine the mark on [the person's] skin, and if the hair on the mark has turned white, and the mark appears to have penetrated the skin, then it is the leprous curse. As soon as the priest sees it, he shall declare it unclean.

13:4 However, if there is a [white] spot on the skin, but it does not appear to have penetrated the skin and its hair has not turned white, then the priest shall quarantine the affected person for seven days.

13:5 The priest shall examine [the person] on the seventh day and if the mark has not increased in size, the priest shall quarantine [the victim] for an additional seven days.

13:6 The priest shall examine [him again] on the seventh day, and if the mark has faded or if it has not spread, the priest shall declare [the person] clean, since it is merely a white discoloration. [The person] must immerse [his body and] clothing, and he is then clean.

13:7 However, if the white discoloration increases in size on the skin after it was shown to the priest, who purified it, [the person] must show it to the priest again.

13:8 If the priest sees that the rash has increased in size on the skin, [he] shall declare [the person] unclean, since it is the leprous curse.

Healthy Skin in a Spot

13:9 When a person [is suspected of] having the leprous curse, he shall be brought to the priest.

13:10 If the priest sees that there is a white blotch on the skin, and it has turned the hair white or that there is an area of healthy skin inside the blotch,

13:11 then it is a chronic leprosy in his skin, and the priest must declare it unclean. He shall not quarantine it, since it is obviously unclean.

13:12 [This is the law] if the leprous area spreads over the skin, so that it covers all the skin of the afflicted person from head to foot, wherever the priest can see it.

13:13 When the priest sees that the leprous discoloration has covered all [the person's] skin, he shall declare the afflicted person clean. As long as he has turned completely white, he is clean.

13:14 However, on the day that healthy skin appears on [the person] he is unclean.

13:15 When the priest sees the healthy skin, he shall declare [the person] unclean. The healthy skin is a sign of uncleanness, since it is the leprous curse.

13:16 If the healthy skin turns white again, [the person] shall come back to the priest.

13:17 When the priest sees that the afflicted person has turned [completely] white, the priest shall declare him clean, and he is then ritually pure.

Leprosy on an Infection

13:18 [This is the law] when there is an infection on the body and it heals.

13:19 If a white blotch or bright pink spot then develops where the infection was, it must be shown to the priest.

13:20 The priest shall examine it, and if it appears to have penetrated the skin and its hair has turned white, it is the leprous curse that has erupted over the infection.

13:21 However, if the priest examines it, and it does not have white hair, nor does it appear to have penetrated the skin since it is a dull white, the priest shall quarantine the person for seven days.

13:22 If this spot then increases in size on the skin, the priest shall declare it unclean, since it is the curse.

13:23 However, if the spot remains stable and does not expand, it is scar tissue from the infection, and the priest shall declare it clean.

Leprosy on a Burn

13:24 [This is the law] when there is a burn on the body, and a bright pink or white spot appears where the burn has healed.

13:25 The priest shall examine it, and if the hair on the spot has turned white, and [the spot] appears to have penetrated the skin, it is the leprous curse breaking out on the burn. Since it is the leprous curse, the priest shall declare it unclean.

13:26 However, if the priest examines it, and the spot does not have white hair, and it is a dull white which does not appear to have penetrated the skin, then the priest shall quarantine it for seven days.

13:27 On the seventh day, the priest shall examine it, and if it has increased in size on the skin, the priest shall declare it unclean, since it is the leprous curse.

13:28 However, if the spot remains stable and does not increase in size, or if it has faded, then it is a discoloration due to the burn. Since it is merely scar tissue from the burn, the priest shall declare it clean.

Bald Patches

13:29 [This is the law] if a man or woman has an affliction on the head or beard.

13:30 The priest shall examine the affliction, and if it appears to have penetrated the skin and has fine blond hairs in it, the priest shall declare it unclean. Such a bald mark is a sign of the leprous curse on the head or beard.

13:31 However, if, when the priest examines the bald patch, [the affliction] does not appear to have penetrated the skin, but it does not have black hair in it, the priest shall quarantine the person afflicted by the bald patch for seven days.

13:32 On the seventh day, the priest shall examine the mark. If the bald mark has not increased in size, and if there is no blond hair in it so that the mark does not appear to have penetrated the skin,

13:33 [the person] shall shave himself, without shaving off the bald patch. The priest shall then quarantine [the person having] the bald patch for a second seven day period.

13:34 The priest shall examine the bald patch on the seventh day, and if the area of fallen hair has not increased in size, or if [the affliction] does not appear to have penetrated the skin, the priest shall declare it clean. [The person] must then immerse his [body and] clothing, and he is clean.

13:35 However, if the bald patch increases in size after he has cleansed himself,

13:36 the priest must examine it [again]. If the bald patch has increased in size, the priest need not look for blond hairs, since it is [automatically] unclean.

13:37 But if the bald patch remains the same, or if the black hair grows on it, then the bald patch has healed and it is clean. The priest shall declare [the person] clean.

Dull White Spots

13:38 If the skin of a man's or woman's body becomes covered with white spots,

13:39 the priest shall examine it. If the skin is [merely] covered with dull white spots, it is a simple rash breaking out on the skin, and it is clean.

Baldness

13:40 If a man loses the hair on his head, it is simple baldness, and he is clean.

13:41 Similarly, if he loses hair near his face, it is merely a receding hairline and he is clean.

13:42 However, if he has a bright pink mark on his bald spot or where his hairline has receded, it may be a sign of the leprous curse on his bald spot or hairless forehead.

13:43 The priest shall examine it, and if the blotch on his bald spot or hairless forehead is bright pink, then [it is] like leprosy on the skin of his body.

13:44 The person is considered afflicted by the leprous curse, and he is unclean. Since he is unclean, and the mark is on his head, the priest must declare him unclean.

13:45 When a person has the mark of the leprous curse, his clothing must have a tear in it, he must go without a haircut, and he must cover his head down to his lips. 'Unclean! Unclean!' he must call out.

13:46 As long as he has the mark, he shall remain unclean. Since he is unclean, he must remain alone, and his place shall be outside the camp.

Discoloration of Garments

13:47 [This is the law] when a garment has the mark of the leprous curse. It can be woolen cloth, linen cloth,

13:48 linen or wool [threads meant for] the warp or woof, leather, or anything made of leather.

13:49 If a bright green or bright red area appears in the cloth, leather, warp or woof [thread], or in any leather article, [it may be] the mark of the leprous curse, and it must be shown to the priest.

13:50 The priest shall examine the mark, and quarantine the affected [article] for seven days.

13:51 On the seventh day, he shall examine the affected area, and if the mark has increased in size on the cloth, the warp or woof [thread], the leather, or the article crafted from leather, then it is a malignant leprous mark, and it is unclean.

13:52 The cloth, the warp or woof [thread], whether wool or linen, or the leather article containing the spot must be burned. Since it is a malignant leprosy, it must be burned in fire.

13:53 However, if, when the priest examines it, the mark has not expanded in the garment, the warp or woof [thread], or the leather article,

13:54 the priest shall order the article having the mark to be scrubbed and then quarantined for a second seven-day period.

13:55 After the mark has been scrubbed [and quarantined], the priest shall examine the article, and if the mark has not changed in appearance, then [even if] it has not expanded, it is unclean and must be burned. It is a mark of decay [that can be] on the smooth or fluffy side [of the cloth].

13:56 If the priest examines it after it has been scrubbed [and quarantined], and the mark has faded from the cloth, then he shall tear off [the mark] from the cloth, the leather, or from the warp or woof [threads].

13:57 If [the mark] then appears again in the [same] cloth, warp or woof [thread] or leather item, it is infected, and [the article] having the mark must be burned in fire.

13:58 If the mark is removed when the cloth, warp or woof [thread] or leather article is scrubbed, [the article] shall be immersed this second time, and it is clean.

13:59 This is the [entire] law concerning the mark of the leprous curse in wool or linen cloth, in warp or woof [thread], or in any leather item, through which it is rendered clean or unclean.

Leviticus 14

Purification of a Leper

14:1 God spoke to Moses, saying:

14:2 This is the law concerning the leper when he is purified and placed under the jurisdiction of the priest.

14:3 The priest shall go outside the camp, where he shall examine the leper to determine that the leprous mark has healed.

14:4 The priest shall then order that for the person undergoing purification there be taken two live kosher birds, a piece of cedar, some crimson [wool], and a hyssop branch.

14:5 The priest shall give orders that one bird be slaughtered over fresh spring water in a clay bowl.

14:6 He shall then take the live bird together with the piece of cedar, the crimson wool, and the hyssop. Along with the live bird, he shall dip [the other articles] into the spring water mixed with the blood of the slaughtered bird.

14:7 He shall then sprinkle [this mixture] seven times on the person undergoing purification from the leprous curse, thus rendering him clean. He shall send the living bird away toward the fields.

14:8 The person undergoing purification shall then immerse his clothing, and [the priest] shall shave off all the person's hair. He shall then immerse in a mikvah and thus complete [the first part] of the purification process. He may return to the camp, but he must remain outside his tent for seven days.

14:9 On the seventh day, [the priest] shall shave off all [the person's] hair. His head, beard, eyebrows and other [body] hair must all be shaved off. He shall then immerse his clothing and body in a mikvah and he is clean.

14:10 On the eighth day, he shall take two unblemished [male] sheep, one unblemished yearling female sheep, three-tenths [of an ephah] of the best grade wheat flour mixed with oil as a meal offering, and one log of [olive] oil.

14:11 The priest tending to the purification process shall stand [all these items] and the person undergoing purification before God at the Communion Tent entrance.

14:12 The priest shall take one [male] sheep and present it as a guilt offering along with the log of oil. He shall wave them in the manner prescribed for a wave offering before God.

14:13 He shall then slaughter the sheep in the same place where burnt offerings and sin offerings are slaughtered, in a holy place. This guilt offering is holy of holies, and it is just like a sin offering to the priest.

14:14 The priest shall take some of the guilt offering's blood and place it on the right ear lobe, right thumb, and right big toe of the person undergoing purification.

14:15 The priest shall take some of the log of oil and pour it into the palm of [another] priest's hand.

14:16 [This second] priest shall then dip his right forefinger into the oil in his left hand, and with his finger, sprinkle some oil before God seven times.

14:17 The priest shall place some of the oil in his hand on the right ear, right thumb, and right big toe of the person undergoing purification, over the guilt offering's blood.

14:18 The priest shall then place the rest of the oil in his hand on the head of the person undergoing purification. In this manner, the priest shall make atonement for him before God.

14:19 The priest shall then sacrifice the sin offering to remove the defilement for the person undergoing purification. After that, he shall slaughter the burnt offering,

14:20 and the priest shall present the burnt offering and the meal offering on the altar. The priest shall thus make atonement for him, and [the person] is then ritually clean.

The Poor Leper's Offering

14:21 If [the leper] is poor and cannot afford [the above sacrifices], he shall take one [male] sheep as a guilt offering. This shall be the wave offering to atone for him. [He shall also take] one-tenth [ephah] of the best grade wheat meal mixed with oil as a meal offering, and a log of olive oil.

14:22 [In addition, he shall bring] two turtle doves or two young common doves, as he can afford, one for a sin offering, and one for a burnt offering.

14:23 On the eighth day of his purification, he shall bring them to the priest, to the Communion Tent entrance, before God.

14:24 The priest shall take the guilt offering sheep and the log of oil, and wave them in the motions prescribed for a wave offering before God.

14:25 He shall slaughter the guilt offering sheep. The priest shall take the blood of the guilt offering and place it on the right ear lobe, the right thumb, and the right big toe of the person undergoing purification.

14:26 The priest shall then pour some of the oil onto the left hand of [another] priest.

14:27 With his right finger, [this second] priest shall sprinkle some of the oil on his left hand seven times before God.

14:28 The priest shall place some of the oil from his hand on the right ear lobe, right thumb and right big toe of the person undergoing purification, right over the place where the blood of the guilt offering [was put].

14:29 The priest shall then place the rest of the oil that is in his hand on the head of the person undergoing purification. [With all this] he shall make atonement for [the person] before God.

14:30 He shall then prepare one of the turtle doves or young common doves that [the person] was able to afford.

14:31 [Taking this offering] that the person could afford, [the priest] shall sacrifice one [bird] as a sin offering and one as a meal offering, [and then present] the meal offering. The priest shall thus make atonement before God for the person undergoing purification.

14:32 The above is the [entire] law concerning the person who has the mark of the leprous curse on him, and who cannot afford [more] for his purification.

Discoloration in Houses

14:33 God spoke to Moses and Aaron, saying:

14:34 When you come to the land of Canaan, which I am giving to you as an inheritance, I will place the mark of the leprous curse in houses in the land you inherit.

14:35 The owner of the house shall come and tell the priest, 'It looks to me as if there is [something] like a [leprous] mark in the house.'

14:36 The priest shall give orders that the house be emptied out before [any] priest comes to see the mark, so that everything in the house will not become unclean. Only then shall a priest come to see the house.

14:37 He shall examine the mark [to determine if] the mark on the wall of the house consists of penetrating streaks that are bright green or bright red, which appear to be below [the surface of] the wall.

14:38 [If they are,] the priest shall leave the house [and stand just outside] the entrance of the house. The priest shall then quarantine the house for seven days.

14:39 On the seventh day, he shall return and examine [it to determine] whether or not the mark has expanded on the wall of the house.

14:40 [If it has], the priest shall give orders that [people] remove the stones having the mark, and that they throw [the stones] outside the city in an unclean place.

14:41 He shall then have the inside of the house scraped off all around [the mark], and [the people doing it] shall discard the removed dust outside the city in an unclean place.

14:42 [The people] shall take other stones to replace the [removed] stones. [The owner] shall then plaster the [entire] house with new clay.

14:43 If, after the stones have been removed and the house has been scraped and replastered, the mark comes back

14:44 the priest shall return and examine it. If the mark has spread in the house [again], it is a malignant leprous mark which is unclean.

14:45 [The priest] must [order that] the house be demolished, and its stones, wood and all the clay from the house shall be brought outside the city to an unclean place.

14:46 As long as the house is in quarantine, anyone entering it shall be unclean until evening.

14:47 If one [remains in the house long enough to] relax, he must immerse [both his body and] his clothing. [However] he must immerse his clothing [only if he has remained] in the house [long enough] to eat [a small meal].

14:48 However, if the priest returns [at the end of the seven days] after the house has been replastered, and he sees that the mark has not reappeared in the house, then the mark has gone away and the priest shall declare the house clean.

14:49 To purify the house, he shall order two birds, a piece of cedar, some crimson wool, and a hyssop branch.

14:50 He shall slaughter one bird over fresh spring water in a clay bowl.

14:51 He shall then take the piece of cedar, the hyssop, the crimson wool, and the live bird, dip them in the blood of the slaughtered bird and fresh spring water and sprinkle it on the house seven times.

14:52 Thus, with the bird's blood and spring water, along with the live bird, cedar wood, hyssop and crimson wool, he shall purify the house.

14:53 He shall then send the live bird outside the city toward the fields. [In this manner] he shall make atonement for the house, and it is then clean.

14:54 The above is the [entire] law for every leprous mark, bald patch,

14:55 leprous mark in a garment or house,

14:56 and [white] blotch, discoloration or spot [on the skin],

14:57 so that decisions can be rendered as to the day one is rendered clean and the day one is rendered unclean. This is the [entire] law concerning the leprous curse.

Leviticus 21: 16–23: Priestly Purity

21:16 God spoke to Moses, telling him to

21:17 speak to Aaron as follows:

Anyone among your descendants who has a blemish may not approach to present his God's food offering.

21:18 Thus, any blemished priest may not offer sacrifice.

[This includes] anyone who is blind or lame, or who has a deformed nose or a misshapen limb.

21:19 [Also included] is anyone who has a crippled leg, a crippled hand,

21:20 who is a hunchback or a dwarf, who has a blemish in the eye, who has severe eczema or ringworm, or who has a hernia.

21:21 Any descendant of Aaron the priest who has a blemish may not approach to present God's fire offering. As long as he has a blemish, he may not approach to present his God's food offering.

21:22 [Still] he may eat the food offerings of his God, both from the holy of holies and from the holy.

21:23 But he may not come to the cloth partition [in the sanctuary], and he may not approach the altar if he has a blemish. He shall thus not defile that which is holy to Me, since I am God [and] I sanctify it.

Source: Dembitz, L. N., trans. 1917. Book of Leviticus. In *The Hebrew Bible in English.* Jewish Publication Society. Available at http://www.mechon-mamre.org/e/et/et0.htm

▣ Mephibosheh: The Prince with a Disability

The story of Mephibosheth (or Meribbaal— 1 Chronicles 8:34, 9:40) is part of the Deuteronomic history dated to the seventh and sixth centuries BCE. The events of the narrative are set in the tenth century BCE. Although Mephibosheth's disability results from an accident following the judgment of God on his grandfather Saul, Mephibosheth's disability is never portrayed as part of that judgment. He is disabled because of a childhood accident, which is explanation enough (4:4). On first reading, it appears that David takes pity on Mephibosheth, the prince with a disability, in 9:1–13. However, if the passage is read in parallel to the encounter between Saul and David in 1 Samuel 24:8–22, we see that Mephibosheth has become the threat to David's throne that David had been to the throne of Saul. David is bound by covenant to Jonathan, Mephibosheth's father, and by promise to Saul to show loyalty to Mephibosheth, and so he cannot raise his hand against Mephibosheth. David's call of Jonathan to his own table is an act of control, not

of charity. Mephibosheth's neutral stance during the revolt of Absalom must be interpreted in light of his claim to the throne and the possible fall of the House of David and the return of the House of Saul. It is interesting to note that Mephibosheth has no qualms about using his disability—and poor attendant care— as an excuse for his actions.

2 Samuel 4:4; 9:1–13; 16:1–4; 19:24–30

4:4 Now Jonathan, Saul's son, had a son that was lame of his feet. He was five years old when the tidings came of Saul and Jonathan out of Jezreel, and his nurse took him up, and fled; and it came to pass, as she made haste to flee, that he fell, and became lame. And his name was Mephibosheth.

9:1 And David said: 'Is there yet any that is left of the house of Saul, that I may show him kindness for Jonathan's sake?'

9:2 Now there was of the house of Saul a servant whose name was Ziba, and they called him unto David; and the king said unto him: 'Art thou Ziba?' And he said: 'Thy servant is he.'

9:3 And the king said: 'Is there not yet any of the house of Saul, that I may show the kindness of God unto him?' And Ziba said unto the king: 'Jonathan hath yet a son, who is lame on his feet.'

9:4 And the king said unto him: 'Where is he?' And Ziba said unto the king: 'Behold, he is in the house of Machir the son of Ammiel, in Lo-debar.'

9:5 Then king David sent, and fetched him out of the house of Machir the son of Ammiel, from Lo-debar.

9:6 And Mephibosheth, the son of Jonathan, the son of Saul, came unto David, and fell on his face, and prostrated himself. And David said: 'Mephibosheth!' And he answered: 'Behold thy servant!'

9:7 And David said unto him: 'Fear not; for I will surely show thee kindness for Jonathan thy father's sake, and will restore thee all the land of Saul thy father; and thou shalt eat bread at my table continually.'

9:8 And he bowed down, and said: 'What is thy servant, that thou shouldest look upon such a dead dog as I am?'

9:9 Then the king called to Ziba, Saul's servant, and said unto him: 'All that pertained to Saul and to all his house have I given unto thy master's son.

9:10 And thou shalt till the land for him, thou, and thy sons, and thy servants; and thou shalt bring in the fruits, that thy master's son may have bread to eat; but

Mephibosheth thy master's son shall eat bread continually at my table.' Now Ziba had fifteen sons and twenty servants.

9:11 Then said Ziba unto the king: 'According to all that my lord the king commandeth his servant, so shall thy servant do; but Mephibosheth eateth at my table as one of the king's sons.'

9:12 Now Mephibosheth had a young son, whose name was Mica. And all that dwelt in the house of Ziba were servants unto Mephibosheth.

9:13 But Mephibosheth dwelt in Jerusalem; for he did eat continually at the king's table; and he was lame on both his feet.

16:1 And when David was a little past the top, behold, Ziba the servant of Mephibosheth met him, with a couple of asses saddled, and upon them two hundred loaves of bread, and a hundred clusters of raisins, and a hundred of summer fruits, and a bottle of wine.

16:2 And the king said unto Ziba: 'What meanest thou by these?' And Ziba said: 'The asses are for the king's household to ride on; and the bread and summer fruit for the young men to eat; and the wine, that such as are faint in the wilderness may drink.'

16:3 And the king said: 'And where is thy master's son?' And Ziba said unto the king: 'Behold, he abideth at Jerusalem; for he said: To-day will the house of Israel restore me the kingdom of my father.'

16:4 Then said the king to Ziba: 'Behold, thine is all that pertaineth unto Mephibosheth.' And Ziba said: 'I prostrate myself; let me find favour in thy sight, my lord, O king.'

19:24 And the king said unto Shimei: 'Thou shalt not die.' And the king swore unto him.

19:25 And Mephibosheth the son of Saul came down to meet the king; and he had neither dressed his feet, nor trimmed his beard, nor washed his clothes, from the day the king departed until the day he came home in peace.

19:26 And it came to pass, when he was come to Jerusalem to meet the king, that the king said unto him: 'Wherefore wentest not thou with me, Mephibosheth?'

19:27 And he answered: 'My lord, O king, my servant deceived me; for thy servant said: I will saddle me an ass, that I may ride thereon, and go with the king; because thy servant is lame.

19:28 And he hath slandered thy servant unto my lord the king; but my lord the king is as an angel of God; do therefore what is good in thine eyes.

19:29 For all my father's house were deserving of death at the hand of my lord the king; yet didst thou set thy servant among them that did eat at thine own table. What right therefore have I yet? or why should I cry any more unto the king?'

19:30 And the king said unto him: 'Why speakest thou any more of thy matters? I say: Thou and Ziba divide the land.'

Source: Drachman, Bernard, trans. 1917. Book of II Samuel. In *The Hebrew Bible in English.* Jewish Publication Society. Available at http://www.mechon-mamre.org/e/et/et0.htm

▣ David's Curse

The story of David's conquest of Jerusalem in the tenth century BCE *is part of the Deuteronomic history dated to the seventh and sixth centuries* BCE. *This is one of the most difficult passages in the Deuteronomic history to understand. Two interpretations predominate. One is that the Jebusites are so confident of their defenses that they taunt David, implying that those who are disabled can hold the city against him. The second interpretation is that this is sympathetic magic cursing with a disability anyone who attacks the city.*

2 Samuel 5:6–8

5:6 And the king and his men went to Jerusalem against the Jebusites, the inhabitants of the land, who spoke unto David, saying: 'Except thou take away the blind and the lame, thou shalt not come in hither'; thinking: 'David cannot come in hither.'

5:7 Nevertheless David took the stronghold of Zion; the same is the city of David.

5:8 And David said on that day: 'Whosoever smiteth the Jebusites, and getteth up to the gutter, and taketh away the lame and the blind, that are hated of David's soul—.' Wherefore they say: 'There are the blind and the lame; he cannot come into the house.'

Source: Drachman, Bernard, trans. 1917. Book of II Samuel. In *The Hebrew Bible in English.* Jewish Publication Society. Available at http://www.mechon-mamre.org/e/et/et0.htm

▣ God's Promise to Israel

Isaiah uses apocalyptic imagery in these passages to describe the hope of restoration that God is promising to a repentant Israel. That the "deaf shall hear," "the

blind shall see," "the lame shall leap," and "the speechless sing" stress apocalyptic paradox and reversal rather than healing of a medical condition. This stress on reversal is best seen in Isaiah 29:17, where the cedars of Lebanon are replaced by fertile fields and fertile fields are replaced by forests. Both cedars and fertile fields are desirable, so the stress is not on an improved condition but on the reversal where the impossible becomes possible. Isaiah 35:5–7, where the parallel is between arid and wet lands, may imply greater desirability of the reversal of the disability.

Isaiah 29:17–21

29:17 Is it not yet a very little while, and Lebanon shall be turned into a fruitful field, and the fruitful field shall be esteemed as a forest?

29:18 And in that day shall the deaf hear the words of a book, and the eyes of the blind shall see out of obscurity and out of darkness.

29:19 The humble also shall increase their joy in the Lord, and the neediest among men shall exult in the Holy One of Israel.

29:20 For the terrible one is brought to nought, and the scorner ceaseth, and all they that watch for iniquity are cut off;

29:21 That make a man an offender by words, and lay a snare for him that reproveth in the gate, and turn aside the just with a thing of nought.

Isaiah 35:5–7

35:5 Then the eyes of the blind shall be opened, and the ears of the deaf shall be unstopped.

35:6 Then shall the lame man leap as a hart, and the tongue of the dumb shall sing; for in the wilderness shall waters break out, and streams in the desert.

35:7 And the parched land shall become a pool, and the thirsty ground springs of water; in the habitation of jackals herds shall lie down, it shall be an enclosure for reeds and rushes.

Source: Book of Isaiah. 1917. In *The Hebrew Bible in English.* Jewish Publication Society. Available at http://www.mechon-mamre.org/e/et/et0.htm

The Bible: Apocrypha

▣ Tobit's Blindness

Tobit, dating to the third or second century BCE, tells the story of a righteous Jewish exile who loses his vision because of natural causes, complicated by medical treatment; however, his blindness is perceived as a sign of God's displeasure. Tobit's vision is restored through angelic intervention in the form of a magical, quasi-medical treatment.

Tobit 2:9–11

2:9 On the same night I returned from burying him, and because I was defiled I slept by the wall of the courtyard, and my face was uncovered.

2:10 I did not know that there were sparrows on the wall and their fresh droppings fell into my open eyes and white films formed on my eyes. I went to physicians, but they did not help me. Ahikar, however, took care of me until he went to Elymais.

2:11 Then my wife Anna earned money at women's work.

Tobit 3:7–17

3:7 On the same day, at Ecbatana in Media, it also happened that Sarah, the daughter of Raguel, was reproached by her father's maids,

3:8 Because she had been given to seven husbands, and the evil demon Asmodeus had slain each of them before he had been with her as his wife. So the maids said to her, "Do you not know that you strangle your husbands? You already have had seven and have had no benefit from any of them.

3:9 Why do you beat us? If they are dead, go with them! May we never see a son or daughter of yours!"

3:10 When she heard these things she was deeply grieved, even to the thought of hanging herself. But she said, "I am the only child of my father; if I do this, it will be a disgrace to him, and I shall bring his old age down in sorrow to the grave."

3:11 So she prayed by her window and said, "Blessed art thou, O Lord my God, and blessed is thy holy and honored name for ever. May all thy works praise thee for ever.

3:12 And now, O Lord, I have turned my eyes and my face toward thee.

3:13 Command that I be released from the earth and that I hear reproach no more.

3:14 Thou knowest, O Lord, that I am innocent of any sin with man,

3:15 and that I did not stain my name or the name of my father in the land of my captivity. I am my father's only child, and he has no child to be his heir, no near kinsman or kinsman's son for whom I should keep myself as wife. Already seven husbands of mine are dead. Why should I live? But if it be not pleasing to thee to take my life, command that respect be shown to me and pity be taken upon me, and that I hear reproach no more."

3:16 The prayer of both was heard in the presence of the glory of the great God.

3:17 And Raphael was sent to heal the two of them: to scale away the white films of Tobit's eyes; to give Sarah the daughter of Raguel in marriage to Tobias the son of Tobit, and to bind Asmodeus the evil demon, because Tobias was entitled to possess her. At that very moment Tobit returned and entered his house and Sarah the daughter of Raguel came down from her upper room.

Source: Book of Tobit. 1946. *Revised Standard Version of the Bible.* National Council of Churches of Christ in America. Available at http://www.piney.com/ApocTobit.html

The Bible:
Christian Scriptures—New Testament

▣ The Birth of John the Baptist

Luke 1:5–25 records the annunciation of the birth of John the Baptist, which comes to fruition in Luke 1:57–66. During the annunciation, Gabriel declares that Zechariah, John's father, will be mute "because you did not believe my words." While this is often interpreted as punishment, its function within the annunciation genre is as a "sign." Indeed, the pregnancy of his wife Elizabeth will serve as the "sign" in the better known annunciation to Mary in Luke 1:36 after her parallel questioning in Luke 1:34. It is interesting that in the birth narrative, as Zechariah's temporary disability comes to an end, either the author or his vocally normative characters make the assumption that because Zechariah is mute he must also be deaf in Luke 1:62.

Luke 1:5–25

1:5 In the time of Herod king of Judea there was a priest named Zechariah, who belonged to the priestly division of Abijah; his wife Elizabeth was also a descendant of Aaron.

1:6 Both of them were upright in the sight of God, observing all the Lord's commandments and regulations blamelessly.

1:7 But they had no children, because Elizabeth was barren; and they were both well along in years.

1:8 Once when Zechariah's division was on duty and he was serving as priest before God,

1:9 he was chosen by lot, according to the custom of the priesthood, to go into the temple of the Lord and burn incense.

1:10 And when the time for the burning of incense came, all the assembled worshipers were praying outside.

1:11 Then an angel of the Lord appeared to him, standing at the right side of the altar of incense.

1:12 When Zechariah saw him, he was startled and was gripped with fear.

1:13 But the angel said to him: "Do not be afraid, Zechariah; your prayer has been heard. Your wife Elizabeth will bear you a son, and you are to give him the name John.

1:14 He will be a joy and delight to you, and many will rejoice because of his birth,

1:15 for he will be great in the sight of the Lord. He is never to take wine or other fermented drink, and he will be filled with the Holy Spirit even from birth.

1:16 Many of the people of Israel will he bring back to the Lord their God.

1:17 And he will go on before the Lord, in the spirit and power of Elijah, to turn the hearts of the fathers to their children and the disobedient to the wisdom of the righteous—to make ready a people prepared for the Lord."

1:18 Zechariah asked the angel, "How can I be sure of this? I am an old man and my wife is well along in years."

1:19 The angel answered, "I am Gabriel. I stand in the presence of God, and I have been sent to speak to you and to tell you this good news.

1:20 And now you will be silent and not able to speak until the day this happens, because you did not believe my words, which will come true at their proper time."

1:21 Meanwhile, the people were waiting for Zechariah and wondering why he stayed so long in the temple.

1:22 When he came out, he could not speak to them. They realized he had seen a vision in the temple, for he kept making signs to them but remained unable to speak.

1:23 When his time of service was completed, he returned home.

1:24 After this his wife Elizabeth became pregnant and for five months remained in seclusion.

1:25 "The Lord has done this for me," she said. "In these days he has shown his favor and taken away my disgrace among the people."

Luke 1:57–66

1:57 When it was time for Elizabeth to have her baby, she gave birth to a son.

1:58 Her neighbors and relatives heard that the Lord had shown her great mercy, and they shared her joy.

1:59 On the eighth day they came to circumcise the child, and they were going to name him after his father Zechariah,

1:60 but his mother spoke up and said, "No! He is to be called John."

1:61 They said to her, "There is no one among your relatives who has that name."

1:62 Then they made signs to his father, to find out what he would like to name the child.

1:63 He asked for a writing tablet, and to everyone's astonishment he wrote, "His name is John."

1:64 Immediately his mouth was opened and his tongue was loosed, and he began to speak, praising God.

1:65 The neighbors were all filled with awe, and throughout the hill country of Judea people were talking about all these things.

1:66 Everyone who heard this wondered about it, asking, "What then is this child going to be?" For the Lord's hand was with him.

Source: Gospel of Luke. 1978. *New International Version of the Bible*. International Bible Society. Available at http://www.ibs.org/niv/index.php

▣ The Centurion's Faith in the Suffering Servant

Three accounts of healing take place in these verses: the man who was a leper, the servant with paralysis, and Peter's mother-in-law, who has a fever. These represent three different physical categories. While leprosy and paralysis might both be considered disabilities in contemporary society, they were seen as very different in ancient Israel and were treated very differently. While paralysis was a physical disability, leprosy was a physical impurity that required cleansing more than healing. Thus we have impaired purity, physical disability, and physical illness addressed in these passages. The faith of the centurion is not a condition for healing but is a motivation for healing. His faith's primary function is to prefigure the inclusion of Gentiles as followers of Christ. The primary purpose of these healings as stated in Matthew 8:17 is not to exhibit Jesus' power, as in many synoptic healings, but to identify him as the suffering servant of God fulfilling Isaiah 53:4, who does not erase disability but takes it upon himself.

Matthew 8:1–17

8:1 When he came down from the mountainside, large crowds followed him.

8:2 A man with leprosy came and knelt before him and said, "Lord, if you are willing, you can make me clean."

8:3 Jesus reached out his hand and touched the man. "I am willing," he said. "Be clean!" Immediately he was cured of his leprosy.

8:4 Then Jesus said to him, "See that you don't tell anyone. But go, show yourself to the priest and offer the gift Moses commanded, as a testimony to them."

8:5 When Jesus had entered Capernaum, a centurion came to him, asking for help.

8:6 "Lord," he said, "my servant lies at home paralyzed and in terrible suffering."

8:7 Jesus said to him, "I will go and heal him."

8:8 The centurion answered, "Lord, I'm not worthy for you to come under my roof. Just say the word, and my servant will be healed.

8:9 For I am also a man under authority, having under myself soldiers. I tell this one, 'Go,' and he goes; and tell another, 'Come,' and he comes; and tell my servant, 'Do this,' and he does it."

8:10 When Jesus heard it, he marveled, and said to those who followed, "Most certainly I tell you, I haven't found so great a faith, not even in Israel.

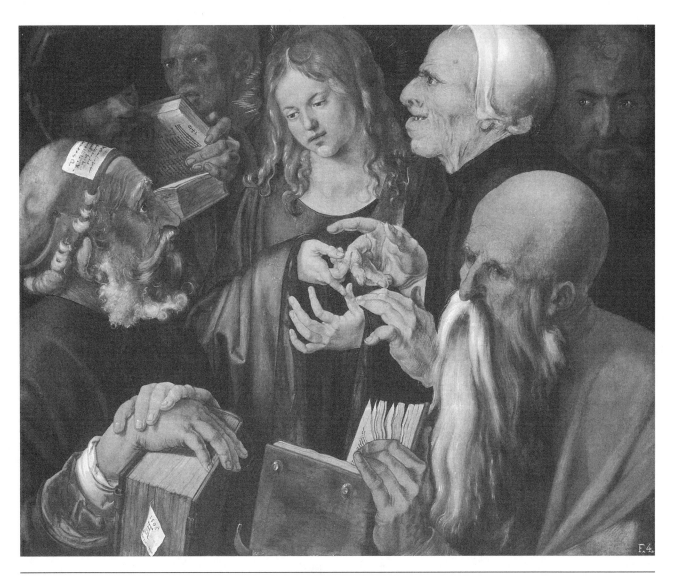

Christ among the Doctors, *by Albrecht Dürer (1471–1528). Here, the German artist Dürer portrays Christ arguing with a gathering of arrogant doctors who thrust their sacrosanct doctrines at him in refutation of his scriptural teachings. The work seems to hold up the idealism of youth against a malevolent portrait of the inflexibility of belief that accompanies old age and empirical dogma.*

Source: Fundacion Coleccion Thyssen-Bornemisza, Madrid. Photo credit: Scala/Art Resource, New York.

8:11 I tell you that many will come from the east and the west, and will sit down with Abraham, Isaac, and Jacob in the Kingdom of Heaven,

8:12 but the children of the Kingdom will be thrown out into the outer darkness. There will be weeping and gnashing of teeth."

8:13 Then Jesus said to the centurion, "Go! It will be done just as you believed it would." And his servant was healed at that very hour.

8:14 When Jesus came into Peter's house, he saw his wife's mother lying sick with a fever.

8:15 He touched her hand, and the fever left her. She got up and served him.

8:16 When evening came, they brought to him many possessed with demons. He cast out the spirits with a word, and healed all who were sick;

8:17 that it might be fulfilled which was spoken through Isaiah the prophet, saying: "He took our infirmities, and bore our diseases."

Source: Gospel of Matthew. 1978. *New International Version of the Bible.* International Bible Society. Available at http://www.ibs.org/niv/index.php

▣ Jesus and the Demoniac

These three passages identify demon possession as the cause of muteness and deafness. This etiology cannot be generalized to other cases of disability. These healing exorcisms pit Jesus against both the demonic forces and the religious opponents who claim he works his healings by demonic power. The demonic etiology of the disabilities in these few cases sets the stage for Jesus to declare "If Satan casts out Satan, he is divided against himself; how then will his kingdom stand? . . . But if it is by the Spirit of God that I cast out demons, then the kingdom of God has come to you" (Matthew 12:26, 12:28).

Matthew 9:32–33

32. While they were going out, a man who was demon-possessed and could not talk was brought to Jesus.

33. And when the demon was driven out, the man who had been mute spoke. The crowd was amazed and said, "Nothing like this has ever been seen in Israel."

Matthew 12:22–32

12:22 Then they brought him a demon-possessed man who was blind and mute, and Jesus healed him, so that he could both talk and see.

12:23 All the multitudes were amazed, and said, "Can this be the son of David?"

12:24 But when the Pharisees heard it, they said, "This man does not cast out demons, except by Beelzebul, the prince of the demons."

12:25 Knowing their thoughts, Jesus said to them, "Every kingdom divided against itself is brought to desolation, and every city or house divided against itself will not stand.

12:26 If Satan casts out Satan, he is divided against himself. How then will his kingdom stand?

12:27 If I by Beelzebul cast out demons, by whom do your children cast them out? Therefore they will be your judges.

12:28 But if I by the Spirit of God cast out demons, then the Kingdom of God has come upon you.

12:29 Or how can one enter into the house of the strong man, and plunder his goods, unless he first bind the strong man? Then he will plunder his house.

12:30 "He who is not with me is against me, and he who doesn't gather with me, scatters.

12:31 Therefore I tell you, every sin and blasphemy will be forgiven men, but the blasphemy against the Spirit will not be forgiven men.

12:32 Whoever speaks a word against the Son of Man, it will be forgiven him; but whoever speaks against the Holy Spirit, it will not be forgiven him, neither in this age, nor in that which is to come.

Luke 11:14–15

11:14 Jesus was driving out a demon that was mute. When the demon left, the man who had been mute spoke, and the crowd was amazed.

11:15 But some of them said, "By Beelzebub, the prince of demons, he is driving out demons."

Source: Gospels of Matthew and Luke. 1978. *New International Version of the Bible.* International Bible Society. Available at http://www.ibs.org/niv/index.php

▣ Jesus Heals a Man's Hand

This account is one of a series of accounts that describe a confrontation between Jesus and the Pharisees regarding the observance of the Law. In each account, Jesus uses rabbinic argumentation to justify his healing on the Sabbath. While there are variations between the method and content of the argument in the three accounts, all agree that the healing of the man's disability is a great enough "good" to justify the "work" of healing on the Sabbath.

Matthew 12:9–14

12:9 Going on from that place, he went into their synagogue,

12:10 And a man with a shriveled hand was there. Looking for a reason to accuse Jesus, they asked him, "Is it lawful to heal on the Sabbath?"

12:11 He said to them, "If any of you has a sheep and it falls into a pit on the Sabbath, will you not take hold of it and lift it out?

12:12 How much more valuable is a man than a sheep! Therefore it is lawful to do good on the Sabbath."

12:13 Then he said to the man, "Stretch out your hand." So he stretched it out and it was completely restored, just as sound as the other.

12:14 But the Pharisees went out and plotted how they might kill Jesus.

Mark 3:1–6

3:1 Another time he went into the synagogue, and a man with a shriveled hand was there.

3:2 Some of them were looking for a reason to accuse Jesus, so they watched him closely to see if he would heal him on the Sabbath.

3:3 Jesus said to the man with the shriveled hand, "Stand up in front of everyone."

3:4 Then Jesus asked them, "Which is lawful on the Sabbath: to do good or to do evil, to save life or to kill?" But they remained silent.

3:5 He looked around at them in anger and, deeply distressed at their stubborn hearts, said to the man, "Stretch out your hand." He stretched it out, and his hand was completely restored.

3:6 Then the Pharisees went out and began to plot with the Herodians how they might kill Jesus.

Luke 6:6–11

6:6 On another Sabbath he went into the synagogue and was teaching, and a man was there whose right hand was shriveled.

6:7 The Pharisees and the teachers of the law were looking for a reason to accuse Jesus, so they watched him closely to see if he would heal on the Sabbath.

6:8 But Jesus knew what they were thinking and said to the man with the shriveled hand, "Get up and stand in front of everyone." So he got up and stood there.

6:9 Then Jesus said to them, "I ask you, which is lawful on the Sabbath: to do good or to do evil, to save life or to destroy it?"

6:10 He looked around at them all, and then said to the man, "Stretch out your hand." He did so, and his hand was completely restored.

6:11 But they were furious and began to discuss with one another what they might do to Jesus.

Source: Gospels of Matthew, Mark, and Luke. 1978. *New International Version of the Bible.* International Bible Society. Available at http://www.ibs.org/niv/index.php

▣ The People Praise God for Healing

The gospels frequently use summary statements such at that found in Matthew 15:30–31 to verify the power

of Jesus in a general summary statement as the narrative transitions from one account to another. They serve to show that the healings reported in detail are only a sample of a much wider practice in the ministry of Jesus.

Matthew 15:30–31

15:30 Great crowds came to him, bringing the lame, the blind, the crippled, the mute and many others, and laid them at his feet; and he healed them.

15:31 The people were amazed when they saw the mute speaking, the crippled made well, the lame walking and the blind seeing. And they praised the God of Israel.

Source: Gospel of Matthew. 1978. *New International Version of the Bible.* International Bible Society. Available at http://www.ibs.org/niv/index.php

▣ The Son of David

The Gospel of Matthew, excluding the introduction of Jesus in Matthew 1:1, uses the title "Son of David" for Jesus only in relation to healing narratives, as seen in the two passages below and in Matthew 12:22–32. Matthew 21:14–17 is particularly significant in this regard. Only in Matthew is Jesus hailed as "Son of David" as he enters Jerusalem and proceeds to the Temple on Palm Sunday. Only in Matthew does he heal others once he reaches the Temple. Matthew portrays Jesus as greater than David by reversing and transcending the report of David's triumphal entry into Jerusalem in 2 Samuel 5:6–8, in which "the lame and the blind, those whom David hates" are banned from the Temple when David declares "The blind and the lame shall not come into the house."

Matthew 20:29–34

20:29 As Jesus and his disciples were leaving Jericho, a large crowd followed him.

20:30 Two blind men were sitting by the roadside, and when they heard that Jesus was going by, they shouted, "Lord, Son of David, have mercy on us!"

20:31 The crowd rebuked them and told them to be quiet, but they shouted all the louder, "Lord, Son of David, have mercy on us!"

20:32 Jesus stopped and called them. "What do you want me to do for you?" he asked.

20:33 "Lord," they answered, "we want our sight."

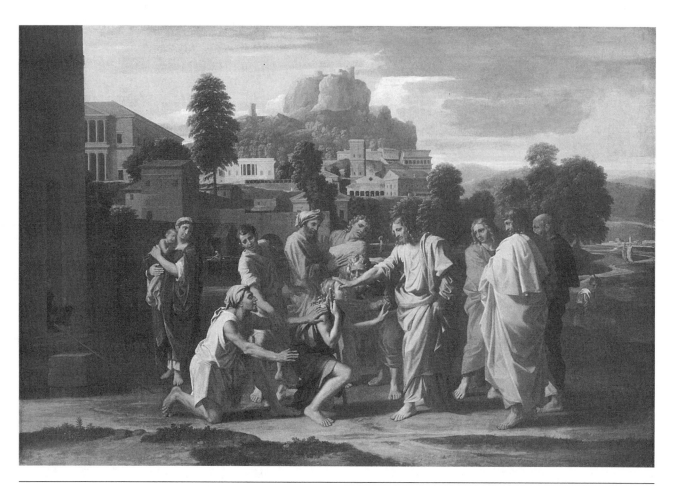

Christ Healing the Blind at Jericho, by Nicolas Poussin (1594–1665). St. Matthew (20:29–34) describes an incident of Jesus' miraculous cure of two blind men near Jericho.

Source: Louvre, Paris. Photo by R. G. Ojeda. Photo credit: Réunion des Musées Nationaux/Art Resource, New York.

20:34 Jesus had compassion on them and touched their eyes. Immediately they received their sight and followed him.

Matthew 21:14–17

21:14 The blind and the lame came to him at the temple, and he healed them.

21:15 But when the chief priests and the teachers of the law saw the wonderful things he did and the children shouting in the temple area, "Hosanna to the Son of David," they were indignant.

21:16 "Do you hear what these children are saying?" they asked him.

"Yes," replied Jesus, "have you never read, 'From the lips of children and infants you have ordained praise'?"

21:17 And he left them and went out of the city to Bethany, where he spent the night.

Source: Gospel of Matthew. 1978. *New International Version of the Bible.* International Bible Society. Available at http://www.ibs .org/niv/index.php

▣ Disability for the Sake of the Kingdom

This passage stresses that spiritual disability, specifically one that leads an individual to endanger another's spiritual life, is a far greater disability than one that is merely physical. It is better to be saved with a disability than to be damned with an able body. The

passage is parabolic, of course, and it relies for its dramatic impact on a normative abhorrence of disability.

Mark 9:43, 45, 47

9:43 If your hand causes you to sin, cut it off. It is better for you to enter life maimed than with two hands to go into hell, where the fire never goes out. . . .

9:45 And if your foot causes you to sin, cut it off. It is better for you to enter life crippled than to have two feet and be thrown into hell. . . .

9:47 And if your eye causes you to sin, pluck it out. It is better for you to enter the kingdom of God with one eye than to have two eyes and be thrown into hell.

Source: Gospel of Mark. 1978. *New International Version of the Bible.* International Bible Society. Available at http://www.ibs .org/niv/index.php

▣ Invitation to a Wedding Feast

Dinners play a crucial role in the Gospel of Luke, where Jesus is honored as a guest by the religious elite, who are in turn offended by his frequent dining with sinners. Such meals represent the ultimate of social acceptance. Jesus is the guest of one of these social and religious elite in Luke 14. Jesus tells his host that he should invite, and thus socially accept, "the poor, the crippled, the lame, and the blind." It is significant that these disability groups are grouped with "the poor" in this passage, since "the poor" are the exalted class in Luke. Jesus then tells a parable about the Kingdom of God where the socially acceptable elite refuse to come to the feast but the poor and those with disabilities will be invited and thus will be those who enter the Kingdom of God.

Luke 14:13–24

14:13 "But when you make a feast, ask the poor, the maimed, the lame, or the blind;

14:14 and you will be blessed, because they don't have the resources to repay you. For you will be repaid in the resurrection of the righteous."

14:15 When one of those who sat at the table with him heard these things, he said to him, "Blessed is he who will feast in the Kingdom of God!"

14:16 Jesus replied: "A certain man was preparing a great banquet and invited many guests.

14:17 At the time of the banquet he sent his servant to tell those who had been invited, 'Come, for everything is now ready.'

14:18 "But they all alike began to make excuses. The first said, 'I have just bought a field, and I must go and see it. Please excuse me.'

14:19 "Another said, 'I have just bought five yoke of oxen, and I'm on my way to try them out. Please excuse me.'

14:20 "Still another said, 'I just got married, so I can't come.'

14:21 "The servant came back and reported this to his master. Then the owner of the house became angry and ordered his servant, 'Go out quickly into the streets and alleys of the town and bring in the poor, the crippled, the blind and the lame.'

14:22 " 'Sir,' the servant said, 'what you ordered has been done, but there is still room.'

14:23 "Then the master told his servant, 'Go out to the roads and country lanes and make them come in, so that my house will be full.

14:24 I tell you, not one of those men who were invited will get a taste of my banquet.'"

Source: Gospel of Luke. 1978. *New International Version of the Bible.* International Bible Society. Available at http://www.ibs .org/niv/index.php

▣ Jesus Heals a Paralytic

The earliest account of the healing of the man with paralysis is probably that found in the Gospel of Mark (first century CE). Here a clear distinction is made between sin and disability. The Markan evangelist does not tell us why the man's friends brought him to Jesus. Jesus' act of compassion is the forgiveness of sins, which he sees as the man's true need. The act of healing, which is separate from the act of forgiveness, is meant solely as a sign of power for the religious leaders who are watching the event. The accounts of the same event in the Gospels of Matthew and Luke share this focus on the forgiveness of sins.

Mark 2:1–12

2:1 A few days later, when Jesus again entered Capernaum, the people heard that he had come home.

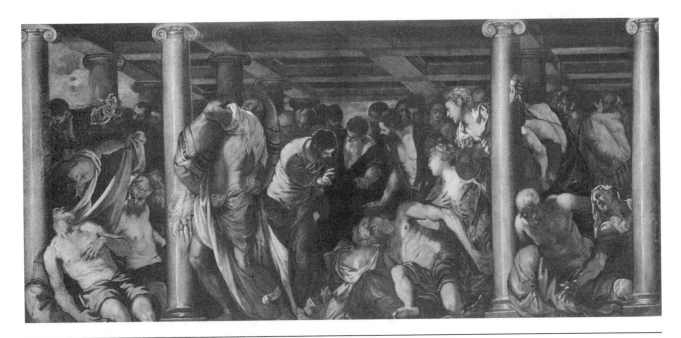

Christ Heals the Paralytic *(1579–1581), by Jacopo Robustic Tintoretto (1518–1594). Tintoretto's rendition of Jesus healing a man at the pool of Bethesda in Jerusalem who had been unable to walk for 38 years.*

Source: Scuola Grande di S. Rocco, Venice. Photo credit: Scala/Art Resource, New York.

2:2 So many gathered that there was no room left, not even outside the door, and he preached the word to them.

2:3 Some men came, bringing to him a paralytic, carried by four of them.

2:4 Since they could not get him to Jesus because of the crowd, they made an opening in the roof above Jesus and, after digging through it, lowered the mat the paralyzed man was lying on.

2:5 When Jesus saw their faith, he said to the paralytic, "Son, your sins are forgiven."

2:6 Now some teachers of the law were sitting there, thinking to themselves,

2:7 "Why does this fellow talk like that? He's blaspheming! Who can forgive sins but God alone?"

2:8 Immediately Jesus knew in his spirit that this was what they were thinking in their hearts, and he said to them, "Why are you thinking these things?

2:9 Which is easier: to say to the paralytic, 'Your sins are forgiven,' or to say, 'Get up, take your mat and walk'?

2:10 But that you may know that the Son of Man has authority on earth to forgive sins. . . ." He said to the paralytic,

2:11 "I tell you, get up, take your mat and go home."

2:12 He got up, took his mat and walked out in full view of them all. This amazed everyone and they praised God, saying, "We have never seen anything like this!"

Matthew 9:1–8

9:1 Jesus stepped into a boat, crossed over and came to his own town.

9:2 Some men brought to him a paralytic, lying on a mat. When Jesus saw their faith, he said to the paralytic, "Take heart, son; your sins are forgiven."

9:3 At this, some of the teachers of the law said to themselves, "This fellow is blaspheming!"

9:4 Knowing their thoughts, Jesus said, "Why do you entertain evil thoughts in your hearts?

9:5 Which is easier: to say, 'Your sins are forgiven,' or to say, 'Get up and walk'?

9:6 But so that you may know that the Son of Man has authority on earth to forgive sins. . . ." Then he said to the paralytic, "Get up, take your mat and go home."

9:7 And the man got up and went home.

9:8 When the crowd saw this, they were filled with awe; and they praised God, who had given such authority to men.

Luke 5: 17–26

5:17 One day as he was teaching, Pharisees and teachers of the law, who had come from every village of Galilee and from Judea and Jerusalem, were sitting there. And the power of the Lord was present for him to heal the sick.

5:18 Some men came carrying a paralytic on a mat and tried to take him into the house to lay him before Jesus.

5:19 When they could not find a way to do this because of the crowd, they went up on the roof and lowered him on his mat through the tiles into the middle of the crowd, right in front of Jesus.

5:20 When Jesus saw their faith, he said, "Friend, your sins are forgiven."

5:21 The Pharisees and the teachers of the law began thinking to themselves, "Who is this fellow who speaks blasphemy? Who can forgive sins but God alone?"

5:22 Jesus knew what they were thinking and asked, "Why are you thinking these things in your hearts?

5:23 Which is easier: to say, 'Your sins are forgiven,' or to say, 'Get up and walk'?

5:24 But that you may know that the Son of Man has authority on earth to forgive sins. . . ." He said to the paralyzed man, "I tell you, get up, take your mat and go home."

5:25 Immediately he stood up in front of them, took what he had been lying on and went home praising God.

5:26 Everyone was amazed and gave praise to God. They were filled with awe and said, "We have seen remarkable things today."

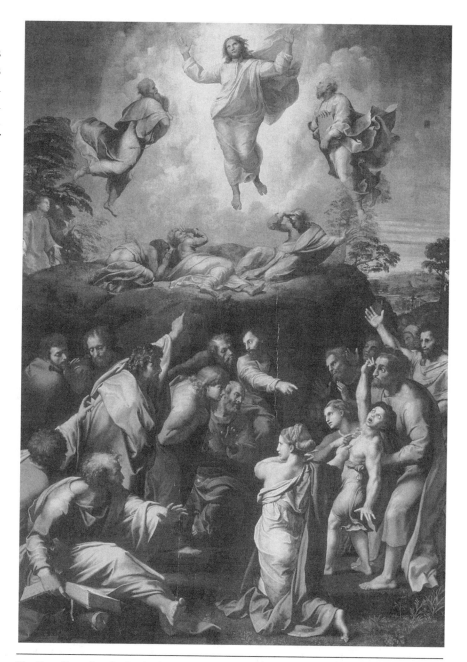

The Transfiguration, *by Raphael (1483–1520). The Italian painter Raphael died just before completing this version of Christ's ascension into Heaven. In the lower right corner parents and neighbors of a "lunatic boy" present him to the disciples seeking a miraculous cure. Without Christ they appear doubtful about their ability to fulfill the request. In the midst of the chaos around this contorted body, the body seems to be the only one aware of the events taking place in the top half of the painting.*

Source: Pinacoteca, Vatican Museums, Vatican State. Photo credit: Scala/Art Resource, New York.

Source: Gospels of Matthew, Mark, and Luke. 1978. *New International Version of the Bible.* International Bible Society. Available at http://www.ibs.org/niv/ index.php

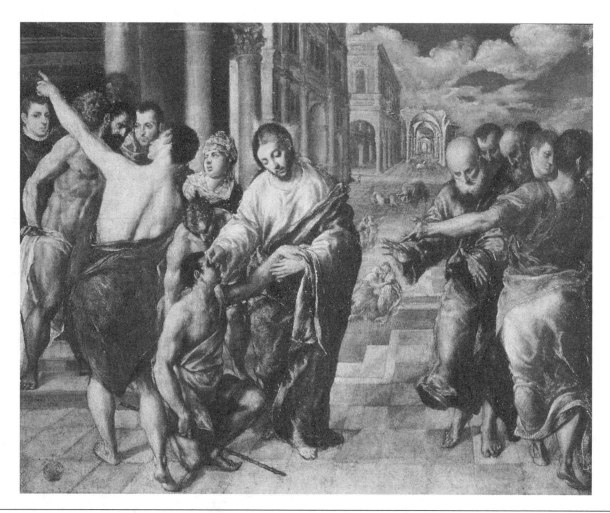

The Healing of the Blind Man, by El Greco (Domenikos Theotokopoulos, 1541–1614). Early Venetian paintings by the Spanish master El Greco (meaning "The Greek") such as this one demonstrate how the painter was influenced by Tintoretto's figural compositions and the use of deep spatial recesses. The theme of healing persons who were blind was an often rendered episode from Jesus' life. The story is interpreted to symbolize the revelation of faith through erasure of disability by the prophet. In the same way that the blind were given the faculty of sight by Jesus, so were the faithful supposed to be able to recognize the power of faith through the church.

Source: Galleria Nazionale, Parma, Italy. Photo credit: Scala/Art Resource, New York.

▣ Bartimaeus: A Blind Beggar Receives His Sight

The Gospels of Mark and Luke relate (first century CE) the story of the healing of a blind man named Bartimaeus ("Son of Timaeus"). Here Jesus rejects the attempt to socially marginalize the person with a disability, yet he does not presume that the disability is the source of the man's concern. Jesus asks what the man desires before he heals him.

Mark 10:46–52

10:46 Then they came to Jericho. As Jesus and his disciples, together with a large crowd, were leaving the city, a blind man, Bartimaeus (that is, the Son of Timaeus), was sitting by the roadside begging.

10:47 When he heard that it was Jesus of Nazareth, he began to shout, "Jesus, Son of David, have mercy on me!"

10:48 Many rebuked him and told him to be quiet, but he shouted all the more, "Son of David, have mercy on me!"

10:49 Jesus stopped and said, "Call him." So they called to the blind man, "Cheer up! On your feet! He's calling you."

10:50 Throwing his cloak aside, he jumped to his feet and came to Jesus.

10:51 "What do you want me to do for you?" Jesus asked him.

The blind man said, "Rabbi, I want to see."

18:41 "What do you want me to do for you?"

"Lord, I want to see," he replied.

18:42 Jesus said to him, "Receive your sight; your faith has healed you."

18:43 Immediately he received his sight and followed Jesus, praising God. When all the people saw it, they also praised God.

Source: Gospels of Mark and Luke. 1978. *New International Version of the Bible.* International Bible Society. Available at http://www.ibs.org/niv/index.php

Jesus Heals a Man Born Blind

The Gospel of John (first century CE) relates this account of the healing of a man with congenital blindness. Jesus rejects the association made by his disciples between the man's disability and sin. The passage is based on the inferred metaphorical contrast between the physical blindness of the healed man and the spiritual blindness of the synagogue leaders. The man's experience as the marginalized "other" frees him from the normative perspective of the visually able community.

John 9:1–41

9:1 As he went along, he saw a man blind from birth.

9:2 His disciples asked him, "Rabbi, who sinned, this man or his parents, that he was born blind?"

9:3 "Neither this man nor his parents sinned," said Jesus, "but this happened so that the work of God might be displayed in his life.

9:4 As long as it is day, we must do the work of him who sent me. Night is coming, when no one can work.

9:5 While I am in the world, I am the light of the world."

9:6 Having said this, he spit on the ground, made some mud with the saliva, and put it on the man's eyes.

9:7 "Go," he told him, "wash in the Pool of Siloam" (this word means Sent). So the man went and washed, and came home seeing.

9:8 His neighbors and those who had formerly seen him begging asked, "Isn't this the same man who used to sit and beg?"

9:9 Some claimed that he was.

Others said, "No, he only looks like him."

But he himself insisted, "I am the man."

9:10 "How then were your eyes opened?" they demanded.

9:11 He replied, "The man they call Jesus made some mud and put it on my eyes. He told me to go to

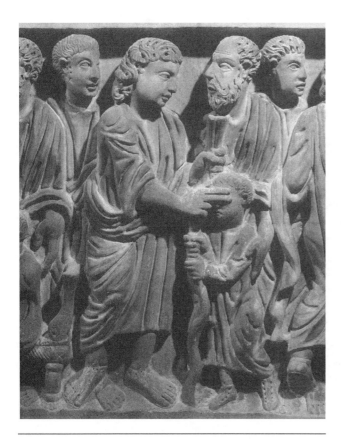

Christ Heals a Blind Man. *Relief (third century CE) on an early Christian sarcophagus. Like the paintings by El Greco and Lucas van Leyden, this relief depicts the healing of a man who is blind as a sign of Jesus' power as a prophet of God.*

Source: Mezzocamino, Via Ostiense, Rome. Cat. 41. Museo Nazionale Romano (Terme di Diocleziano), Rome. Photo credit: Erich Lessing/Art Resource.

10:52 "Go," said Jesus, "your faith has healed you." Immediately he received his sight and followed Jesus along the road.

Luke 18: 35–43

18:35 As Jesus approached Jericho, a blind man was sitting by the roadside begging.

18:36 When he heard the crowd going by, he asked what was happening.

18:37 They told him, "Jesus of Nazareth is passing by."

18:38 He called out, "Jesus, Son of David, have mercy on me!"

18:39 Those who led the way rebuked him and told him to be quiet, but he shouted all the more, "Son of David, have mercy on me!"

18:40 Jesus stopped and ordered the man to be brought to him. When he came near, Jesus asked him,

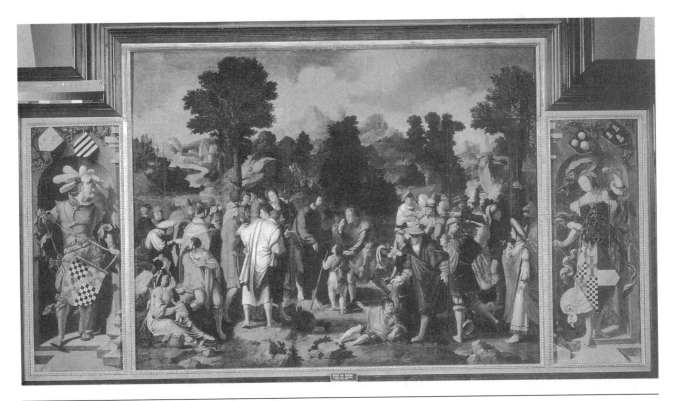

Christ Healing the Blind at Jericho, *by Lucas van Leyden (1494–1538). John (9:1–7) narrates how Christ restored the sight of a man blind from birth. The cure involved placing an ointment on the eyes of the man and then sending him to wash in a pool. Upon the man's return, the blindness was cured. Likewise, St. Matthew (20:29–34) describes a similar incident of miraculous cure for two blind men near Jericho.*

Source: Hermitage, St. Petersburg, Russia. Photo credit: Scala/Art Resource, New York.

Siloam and wash. So I went and washed, and then I could see."

9:12 "Where is this man?" they asked him.

"I don't know," he said.

The Pharisees Investigate the Healing

9:13 They brought to the Pharisees the man who had been blind.

9:14 Now the day on which Jesus had made the mud and opened the man's eyes was a Sabbath.

9:15 Therefore the Pharisees also asked him how he had received his sight. "He put mud on my eyes," the man replied, "and I washed, and now I see."

9:16 Some of the Pharisees said, "This man is not from God, for he does not keep the Sabbath."

But others asked, "How can a sinner do such miraculous signs?" So they were divided.

9:17 Finally they turned again to the blind man, "What have you to say about him? It was your eyes he opened."

The man replied, "He is a prophet."

9:18 The Jews still did not believe that he had been blind and had received his sight until they sent for the man's parents.

9:19 "Is this your son?" they asked. "Is this the one you say was born blind? How is it that now he can see?"

9:20 "We know he is our son," the parents answered, "and we know he was born blind.

9:21 But how he can see now, or who opened his eyes, we don't know. Ask him. He is of age; he will speak for himself."

9:22 His parents said this because they were afraid of the Jews, for already the Jews had decided that anyone who acknowledged that Jesus was the Christ would be put out of the synagogue.

9:23 That was why his parents said, "He is of age; ask him."

9:24 A second time they summoned the man who had been blind. "Give glory to God," they said. "We know this man is a sinner."

9:25 He replied, "Whether he is a sinner or not, I don't know. One thing I do know. I was blind but now I see!"

9:26 Then they asked him, "What did he do to you? How did he open your eyes?"

9:27 He answered, "I have told you already and you did not listen. Why do you want to hear it again? Do you want to become his disciples, too?"

9:28 Then they hurled insults at him and said, "You are this fellow's disciple! We are disciples of Moses!

9:29 We know that God spoke to Moses, but as for this fellow, we don't even know where he comes from."

9:30 The man answered, "Now that is remarkable! You don't know where he comes from, yet he opened my eyes.

9:31 We know that God does not listen to sinners. He listens to the godly man who does his will.

9:32 Nobody has ever heard of opening the eyes of a man born blind.

9:33 If this man were not from God, he could do nothing."

9:34 To this they replied, "You were steeped in sin at birth; how dare you lecture us!" And they threw him out.

Spiritual Blindness

9:35 Jesus heard that they had thrown him out, and when he found him, he said, "Do you believe in the Son of Man?"

9:36 "Who is he, sir?" the man asked. "Tell me so that I may believe in him."

9:37 Jesus said, "You have now seen him; in fact, he is the one speaking with you."

9:38 Then the man said, "Lord, I believe," and he worshiped him.

9:39 Jesus said, "For judgment I have come into this world, so that the blind will see and those who see will become blind."

9:40 Some Pharisees who were with him heard him say this and asked, "What? Are we blind too?"

9:41 Jesus said, "If you were blind, you would not be guilty of sin; but now that you claim you can see, your guilt remains.

Source: Gospel of John. 1978. *New International Version of the Bible.* International Bible Society. Available at http://www.ibs.org/niv/index.php

▣ The Healing at the Pool of Bethesda

The Gospel of John (first century CE) relates the account of a man who has waited for years to be healed at a miraculous pool. Jesus asks the man if he actually wants to be healed, and the man responds with an excuse. Jesus bypasses the excuse by healing the man directly. The account parallels the account of the man born blind in John 9:1–41. Here the man healed betrays Jesus to the religious leaders as opposed to defending him, as in John 9.

John 5:1–15

5:1 Some time later, Jesus went up to Jerusalem for a feast of the Jews.

5:2 Now there is in Jerusalem near the Sheep Gate a pool, which in Aramaic is called Bethesda and which is surrounded by five covered colonnades.

5:3 Here a great number of disabled people used to lie—the blind, the lame, the paralyzed.

5:4 From time to time an angel of the Lord would come down and stir up the waters. The first one into the pool after each such disturbance would be cured of whatever disease he had.

5:5 One who was there had been an invalid for thirty-eight years.

5:6 When Jesus saw him lying there and learned that he had been in this condition for a long time, he asked him, "Do you want to get well?"

5:7 "Sir," the invalid replied, "I have no one to help me into the pool when the water is stirred. While I am trying to get in, someone else goes down ahead of me."

5:8 Then Jesus said to him, "Get up! Pick up your mat and walk."

5:9 At once the man was cured; he picked up his mat and walked.

The day on which this took place was a Sabbath,

5:10 and so the Jews said to the man who had been healed, "It is the Sabbath; the law forbids you to carry your mat."

5:11 But he replied, "The man who made me well said to me, 'Pick up your mat and walk.'"

5:12 So they asked him, "Who is this fellow who told you to pick it up and walk?"

5:13 The man who was healed had no idea who it was, for Jesus had slipped away into the crowd that was there.

5:14 Later Jesus found him at the temple and said to him, "See, you are well again. Stop sinning or something worse may happen to you."

5:15 The man went away and told the Jews that it was Jesus who had made him well.

Source: Gospel of John. 1978. *New International Version of the Bible.* International Bible Society. Available at http://www.ibs.org/niv/index.php

◉ Jesus and John the Baptist

While in prison, John sends his disciples to Jesus to ask for verification of Jesus' messianic status. Jesus does not give a direct answer but through the symbolic action of healing claims to be fulfilling the promise of Isaiah 29:17–21 and Isaiah 35:5–7. The stress is not on Jesus' compassion on those perceived as less fortunate but on the sign of apocalyptic reversal.

Matthew 11:2–6

11:2 When John heard in prison what Christ was doing, he sent his disciples

11:3 to ask him, "Are you the one who was to come, or should we expect someone else?"

11:4 Jesus replied, "Go back and report to John what you hear and see:

11:5 The blind receive sight, the lame walk, those who have leprosy are cured, the deaf hear, the dead are raised, and the good news is preached to the poor.

11:6 Blessed is the man who does not fall away on account of me."

Luke 7:18–23

7:18 John's disciples told him about all these things. Calling two of them,

7:19 He sent them to the Lord to ask, "Are you the one who was to come, or should we expect someone else?"

7:20 When the men came to Jesus, they said, "John the Baptist sent us to you to ask, 'Are you the one who was to come, or should we expect someone else?'"

7:21 At that very time Jesus cured many who had diseases, sicknesses and evil spirits, and gave sight to many who were blind.

7:22 So he replied to the messengers, "Go back and report to John what you have seen and heard: The blind receive sight, the lame walk, those who have leprosy are cured, the deaf hear, the dead are raised, and the good news is preached to the poor.

7:23 Blessed is the man who does not fall away on account of me."

Source: Gospels of Matthew and Luke. 1978. *New International Version of the Bible*. International Bible Society. Available at http://www.ibs.org/niv/index.php

◉ The Disciples Heal at the Temple

The Lukan evangelist (first century CE) relates this account of the healing of the mobility-impaired beggar in order to show that the power and authority of Jesus now reside with Peter and the apostles. Jesus' disciples are presented here as his heirs by their exhibition of his healing power, which they perform "in the name of Jesus Christ of Nazareth." This is not presented as an act of one who is more powerful for one who is less fortunate. Peter's claim "Silver or gold I do not have" places him with the poor honored by the author of Acts. This is an act of shared empowerment by two equals who are socially marginalized but who are exalted in the power of the Gospel that Peter preaches. Whereas the community provides for the livelihood of the beggar through charity, the life he lives remains marginal. Peter provides for his reintegration into the community—seen in his entry into the temple—by means of healing. (See also Acts 9:32–35; see also a story of Paul's ability to heal in Acts 14:8–10.)

Acts 3:1–10

3:1 One day Peter and John were going up to the temple at the time of prayer—at three in the afternoon.

3:2 Now a man crippled from birth was being carried to the temple gate called Beautiful, where he was put every day to beg from those going into the temple courts.

3:3 When he saw Peter and John about to enter, he asked them for money.

3:4 Peter looked straight at him, as did John. Then Peter said, "Look at us!"

3:5 So the man gave them his attention, expecting to get something from them.

3:6 Then Peter said, "Silver or gold I do not have, but what I have I give you. In the name of Jesus Christ of Nazareth, walk."

3:7 Taking him by the right hand, he helped him up, and instantly the man's feet and ankles became strong.

3:8 He jumped to his feet and began to walk. Then he went with them into the temple courts, walking and jumping, and praising God.

3:9 When all the people saw him walking and praising God,

3:10 they recognized him as the same man who used to sit begging at the temple gate called Beautiful, and they were filled with wonder and amazement at what had happened to him.

───────────

Source: Acts of the Apostles. 1978. *New International Version of the Bible*. International Bible Society. Available at http://www.ibs .org/niv/index.php

◉ Followers in the Power of Christ

The summary of the work of Philip in Samaria found in Acts 8:5–8 recalls summary statements about the work of Jesus in such passages as Matthew 15:30–31. This parallel is intentional and serves to show that the power of Jesus is manifested in his follower as he proclaims him as the Messiah or Christ. This same sharing in the power of Christ is exhibited by Paul in Acts 14:8–18. Here, however, the mistaken conclusion that Paul and Barnabas are Hermes and Zeus provides the opportunity to clarify that this divine power does not originate with the followers but originates with God. The phrase "he had faith to be healed" in Acts 14:9 would probably be better translated "he had faith to be saved."

Acts 8:5–8

8:5 Philip went down to a city in Samaria and proclaimed the Christ there.

8:6 When the crowds heard Philip and saw the miraculous signs he did, they all paid close attention to what he said.

8:7 With shrieks, evil spirits came out of many, and many paralytics and cripples were healed.

8:8 So there was great joy in that city.

Acts 14:8–18

14:8 In Lystra there sat a man crippled in his feet, who was lame from birth and had never walked.

14:9 He listened to Paul as he was speaking. Paul looked directly at him, saw that he had faith to be healed.

14:10 and called out, "Stand up on your feet!" At that, the man jumped up and began to walk.

14:11 When the crowd saw what Paul had done, they shouted in the Lycaonian language, "The gods have come down to us in human form!"

14:12 Barnabas they called Zeus, and Paul they called Hermes because he was the chief speaker.

14:13 The priest of Zeus, whose temple was just outside the city, brought bulls and wreaths to the city gates because he and the crowd wanted to offer sacrifices to them.

14:14 But when the apostles Barnabas and Paul heard of this, they tore their clothes and rushed out into the crowd, shouting:

14:15 "Men, why are you doing this? We too are only men, human like you. We are bringing you good news, telling you to turn from these worthless things to the living God, who made heaven and earth and sea and everything in them.

14:16 In the past, he let all nations go their own way.

14:17 Yet he has not left himself without testimony: He has shown kindness by giving you rain from heaven and crops in their seasons; he provides you with plenty of food and fills your hearts with joy."

14:18 Even with these words, they had difficulty keeping the crowd from sacrificing to them.

───────────

Source: Acts of the Apostles. 1978. *New International Version of the Bible*. International Bible Society. Available at http://www.ibs .org/niv/index.php

◉ Blinding Power

While divine power in the New Testament is usually exhibited by healing disabilities, there are two events where divine power is shown through blinding rather than healing. These events are described in the accounts of the conversion of Saul of Tarsus (in Acts 9:1–19 as well as Paul's retelling of the event in Acts 22:4–16) and the blinding of Elymas Bar-Jesus by the Holy Spirit through that same Paul. While both of these blindings prove to be temporary, there is a significant difference. While Paul tells Bar-Jesus that he will be "blind for a while," Paul's own blindness seems to have been a permanent disability that required the healing intervention of Ananias, who proclaimed healing and the filling of the Holy Spirit in one sentence. In this instance, it is reported that "something like scales fell from his eyes, and his sight was restored."

Acts 9:1–19

9:1 Meanwhile, Saul was still breathing out murderous threats against the Lord's disciples. He went to the high priest

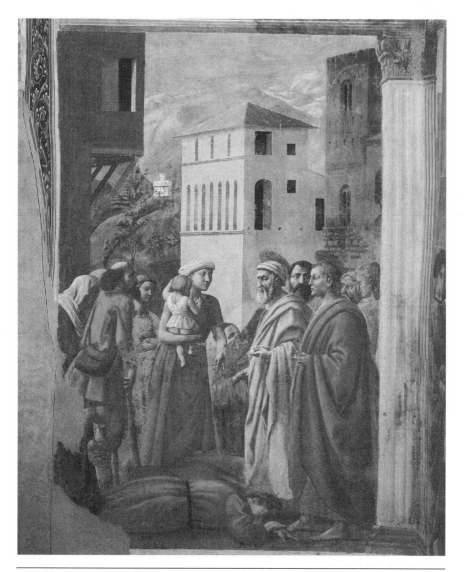

Distributing Alms and the Death of Ananias (Anonymous). In addition to Tabitha's resurrection and other tales of cure, the Book of Acts (9:32–43) provides an example of the cure of Ananias (also Aeneas): "And it came to pass, as Peter passed throughout all quarters, he came down also to the saints which dwelt at Lydda. And there he found a certain man named Aeneas, which had kept his bed eight years, and was sick of the palsy. And Peter said unto him, 'Aeneas, Jesus Christ maketh thee whole: arise, and make thy bed. And he arose immediately.'"

Source: Brancacci Chapel, S. Maria del Carmine, Florence, Italy. Photo credit: Erich Lessing/Art Resource, New York.

9:2 and asked him for letters to the synagogues in Damascus, so that if he found any there who belonged to the Way, whether men or women, he might take them as prisoners to Jerusalem.

9:3 As he neared Damascus on his journey, suddenly a light from heaven flashed around him.

9:4 He fell to the ground and heard a voice say to him, "Saul, Saul, why do you persecute me?"

9:5 "Who are you, Lord?" Saul asked.

9:6 "I am Jesus, whom you are persecuting," he replied. "Now get up and go into the city, and you will be told what you must do."

9:7 The men traveling with Saul stood there speechless; they heard the sound but did not see anyone.

9:8 Saul got up from the ground, but when he opened his eyes he could see nothing. So they led him by the hand into Damascus.

9:9 For three days he was blind, and did not eat or drink anything.

9:10 In Damascus there was a disciple named Ananias. The Lord called to him in a vision, "Ananias!"

"Yes, Lord," he answered.

9:11 The Lord told him, "Go to the house of Judas on Straight Street and ask for a man from Tarsus named Saul, for he is praying.

9:12 In a vision he has seen a man named Ananias come and place his hands on him to restore his sight."

9:13 "Lord," Ananias answered, "I have heard many reports about this man and all the harm he has done to your saints in Jerusalem.

9:14 And he has come here with authority from the chief priests to arrest all who call on your name."

9:15 But the Lord said to Ananias, "Go! This man is my chosen instrument to carry my name before the Gentiles and their kings and before the people of Israel.

9:16 I will show him how much he must suffer for my name."

9:17 Then Ananias went to the house and entered it. Placing his hands on Saul, he said, "Brother Saul, the Lord—Jesus, who appeared to you on the road as you were coming here—has sent me so that you may see again and be filled with the Holy Spirit."

9:18 Immediately, something like scales fell from Saul's eyes, and he could see again. He got up and was baptized,

9:19 and after taking some food, he regained his strength.

Acts 22:4–16

22:4 I persecuted the followers of this Way to their death, arresting both men and women and throwing them into prison,

22:5 as also the high priest and all the Council can testify. I even obtained letters from them to their brothers in Damascus, and went there to bring these people as prisoners to Jerusalem to be punished.

22:6 "About noon as I came near Damascus, suddenly a bright light from heaven flashed around me.

22:7 "I fell to the ground and heard a voice say to me, 'Saul! Saul! Why do you persecute me?'

22:8 "'Who are you, Lord?' I asked.

22:9 "'I am Jesus of Nazareth, whom you are persecuting,' he replied. My companions saw the light, but they did not understand the voice of him who was speaking to me.

22:10 "'What shall I do, Lord?' I asked.

22:11 "'Get up,' the Lord said, 'and go into Damascus. There you will be told all that you have been assigned to do.' My companions led me by the hand into Damascus, because the brilliance of the light had blinded me.

22:12 "A man named Ananias came to see me. He was a devout observer of the law and highly respected by all the Jews living there.

22:13 "He stood beside me and said, 'Brother Saul, receive your sight!' And at that very moment I was able to see him.

22:14 "Then he said: 'The God of our fathers has chosen you to know his will and to see the Righteous One and to hear words from his mouth.

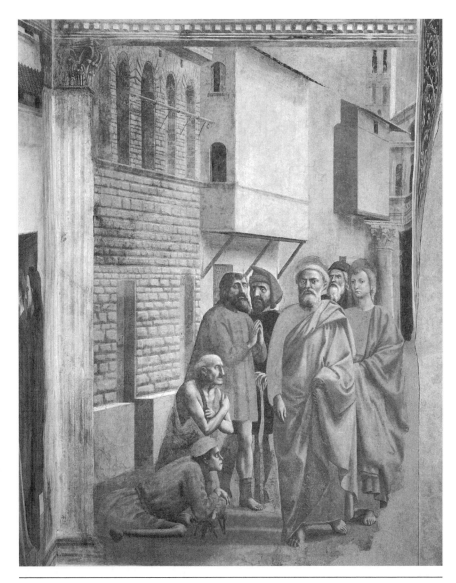

St. Peter Healing a Cripple with His Shadow *by Masaccio (1401–1428). In the Acts of the Apostles (5:12–14), this episode is recounted immediately after the story of Ananias, which is illustrated in the fresco* Distributing Alms and the Death of Ananias *in the same chapel.*
Source: Brancacci Chapel, S. Maria del Carmine, Florence, Italy. Photo credit: Scala/Art Resource, New York.

22:15 "'You will be his witness to all men of what you have seen and heard.

22:16 "'And now what are you waiting for? Get up, be baptized and wash your sins away, calling on his name.'"

Acts 13:6–12

13:6 They traveled through the whole island until they came to Paphos. There they met a Jewish sorcerer and false prophet named Bar-Jesus,

13:7 Who was an attendant of the proconsul, Sergius Paulus. The proconsul, an intelligent man, sent for Barnabas and Saul because he wanted to hear the word of God.

13:8 But Elymas the sorcerer (for that is what his name means) opposed them and tried to turn the proconsul from the faith.

13:9 Then Saul, who was also called Paul, filled with the Holy Spirit, looked straight at Elymas and said,

13:10 "You are a child of the devil and an enemy of everything that is right! You are full of all kinds of deceit and trickery. Will you never stop perverting the right ways of the Lord?

13:11 Now the hand of the Lord is against you. You are going to be blind, and for a time you will be unable to see the light of the sun."

13:12 Immediately mist and darkness came over him, and he groped about, seeking someone to lead him by the hand. When the proconsul saw what had happened, he believed, for he was amazed at the teaching about the Lord.

Source: Acts of the Apostles. 1978. *New International Version of the Bible.* International Bible Society. Available at http://www.ibs .org/niv/index.php

The Middle Ages

◉ Saint Augustine, *The City of God* (ca. 410 CE)

The Christian writers of the late Roman Empire incorporated familiar subject matter of earlier writers, often reshaping customary motifs to fit the Christian perspective. Augustine (354–430 CE) discusses peculiarities of the human body in much the same style as Pliny the Elder, but he goes beyond presenting them as ethnographic curiosities by placing them within the plan of the Christian God.

Book XVI, Chapter 8

Whether certain monstrous races of men are derived from the stock of Adam or Noah's sons.

It is also asked whether we are to believe that certain monstrous races of men, spoken of in secular history, have sprung from Noah's sons, or rather, I should say, from that one man from whom they themselves were descended. For it is reported that some have one eye in the middle of the forehead; some, feet turned backwards from the heel; some, a double sex, the right breast like a man, the left like a woman, and that they alternately beget and bring forth: others are said to have no mouth, and to breathe only through the nostrils; others are but a cubit high, and are therefore called by the Greeks "Pigmies": they say that in some places the women conceive in their fifth year, and do not live beyond their eighth. So, too, they tell of a race who have two feet but only one leg, and are of marvellous swiftness, though they do not bend the knee: they are called Skiopodes, because in the hot weather they lie down on their backs and shade themselves with their feet. Others are said to have no head, and their eyes in their shoulders; and other human or quasi-human races are depicted in mosaic in the harbor esplanade of Carthage, on the faith of histories of rarities. What shall I say of the Cynocephali, whose dog-like head and barking proclaim them beasts rather than men? But we are not bound to believe all we hear of these monstrosities. But whoever is anywhere born a man, that is, a rational, mortal animal, no matter what unusual appearance he presents in color, movement, sound, nor how peculiar he is in some power, part, or quality of his nature, no Christian can doubt that he springs from that one protoplast. We can distinguish the common human nature from that which is peculiar, and therefore wonderful.

The same account which is given of monstrous births in individual cases can be given of monstrous races. For God, the Creator of all, knows where and when each thing ought to be, or to have been created, because He sees the similarities and diversities which can contribute to the beauty of the whole. But He who cannot see the whole is offended by the deformity of the part, because he is blind to that which balances it, and to which it belongs. We know that men are born with more than four fingers on their bands or toes on their feet: this is a smaller matter; but far from us be the folly of supposing that the Creator mistook the number of a man's fingers, though we cannot account for the difference. And so in cases where the divergence from the rule is greater. He whose works no man justly finds fault with, knows what He has done. At Hippo-Diarrhytus there is a man whose hands are crescent-shaped, and have only two fingers each, and his feet similarly formed. If there were a race like him, it would be added to the history of the curious and wonderful. Shall we therefore deny that this man is descended from that one man who was first created? As for the Androgyni, or Hermaphrodites, as they are called, though they are rare, yet from time to time there appears persons of sex so doubtful, that it remains uncertain from which sex they take their name; though it is customary to give them a masculine name, as the more worthy. For no one ever called them Hermaphroditesses. Some years ago, quite within my own memory, a man was born in the East, double in his upper, but single in his lower half—having two heads, two chests, four hands, but one body and two feet like an ordinary man; and he lived so long that many had an opportunity of seeing him. But who could enumerate all the human births that have differed widely from their ascertained parents? As, therefore, no one will deny that these are all descended from that one man, so all the races which are reported to have diverged in bodily appearance from the usual course which nature generally or almost universally preserves, if they are embraced in that definition of man as rational and mortal animals, unquestionably trace their pedigree to that one first father of all. We are supposing these stories about various races who differ from one another and from us to be true; but possibly they are not: for if we were not aware that apes, and monkeys, and sphinxes are not men, but beasts, those historians would possibly describe them as races of men, and flaunt with impunity their false and vainglorious discoveries. But supposing they are men of whom these marvels are recorded, what if God has seen fit to create some races in this way, that we might not suppose that the monstrous births which appear among ourselves are the failures of that wisdom

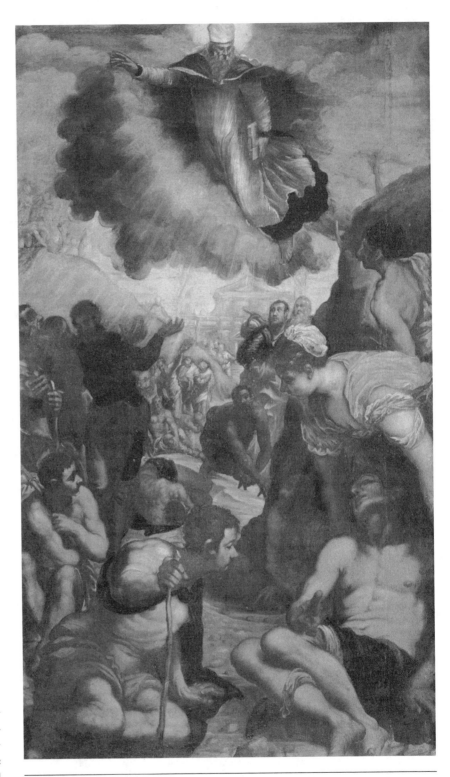

St. Augustine Healing the Plague Victims, *by Jacopo Robusti Tintoretto (1518–1594). Tintoretto portrays the devotion of St. Augustine to the victims of plague. The saints were most often invoked to ask for healing; to prevent shipwrecks, fires, and famines; or even to obtain material or spiritual help. In this respect, it seems that St. Anne was the most solicited of all saints, followed by the Holy Virgin Mary, St. Joseph, and St. Augustine.*

Source: Uffizi, Florence, Italy. Photo credit: Scala/Art Resource, New York.

whereby He fashions the human nature, as we speak of the failure of a less perfect workman? Accordingly, it ought not to seem absurd to us, that as in individual races there are monstrous births, so in the whole race there are monstrous races. Wherefore, to conclude this question cautiously and guardedly, either these things which have been told of some races have no existence at all; or if they do exist, they are not human races; or if they are human, they are descended from Adam.

Book X, Chapter 16

Whether those angels who demand that we pay them divine honour, or those who teach us to render holy service, not to themselves, but to God, are to be trusted about the way of life eternal.

What angels, then, are we to believe in this matter of blessed and eternal life?—those who wish to be worshipped with religious rites and observances, and require that men sacrifice to them; or those who say that all this worship is due to one God, the Creator, and teach us to render it with true piety to Him, by the vision of whom they are themselves already blessed, and in whom they promise that we shall be so? For that vision of God is the beauty of a vision so great, and is so infinitely desirable, that Plotinus does not hesitate to say that he who enjoys all other blessings in abundance, and has not this, is supremely miserable. Since, therefore, miracles are wrought by some angels to induce us to worship this God, by others, to induce us to worship themselves; and since the former forbid us to worship these, while the latter dare not forbid us to worship God, which are we to listen to? Let the Platonists reply, or any philosophers, or the theurgists, or rather, periurgists,—for this name is good enough for those who practise all such arts. In short, let all men answer,—if, at least, there survive in them any spark of natural perception which as rational beings, they possess when created,—let them, I say tell us whether we should sacrifice to the gods or angels who order us to sacrifice to them, or to that One to whom we are ordered to sacrifice by those who forbid us to worship either themselves or these others. If neither the one party nor the other had wrought miracles, but had merely uttered commands, the one to sacrifice to themselves, the other forbidding that, and ordering us to sacrifice to God, a godly mind would have been at no loss to discern which command proceeded from proud arrogance, and which from true

religion. I will say more. If miracles had been wrought only by those who demand sacrifice for themselves, while those who forbade this, and enjoined sacrificing to the one God only, thought fit entirely to forego the use of visible miracles, the authority of the latter was to be preferred by all who would use, not their eyes only, but their reason. But since God, for the sake of commending to us the oracles of His truth, has, by means of these immortal messengers, who proclaim His majesty and not their own pride, wrought miracles of surpassing grandeur, certainty, and distinctness, in order that the weak among the godly might not be drawn away to false religion by those who require us to sacrifice to them and endeavour to convince us by stupendous appeals to our senses, who is so utterly unreasonable as not to choose and follow the truth, when he finds that it is heralded by even more striking evidences than falsehood?

As for those miracles which history ascribes to the gods of the heathen,—I do not refer to those prodigies which at intervals happen from some unknown physical causes, and which are arranged and appointed by Divine Providence, such as monstrous births, and unusual meteorological phenomena, whether startling only, or also injurious, and which are said to be brought about and removed by communication with demons, and by their most deceitful craft,—but I refer to these prodigies which manifestly enough are wrought by their power and force, as, that the household gods which Aeneas carried from Troy in his flight moved from place to place; that Tarquin cut a whetstone with a razor; that the Epidaurian serpent attached himself as a companion to Aesculapius on his voyage to Rome; that the ship in which the image of the Phrygian mother stood, and which could not be moved by a host of men and oxen, was moved by one weak woman, who attached her girdle to the vessel and drew it, as proof of her chastity; that a vestal, whose virginity was questioned, removed the suspicion by carrying from the Tiber a sieve full of water without any of it dropping: these, then, and the like, are by no means to be compared for greatness and virtue to those which, we read, were wrought among God's people. How much less can we compare those marvels, which even the laws of heathen nations prohibit and punish,—I mean the magical and theurgic marvels, of which the great part are merely illusions practiced upon the senses, as the drawing down of the moon, "that," as Lucan says, "it may shed a stronger influence on the plants"? And if some of these do seem to equal those which are wrought by the godly, the end for which they are wrought distinguishes the two, and shows that ours are incomparably the more excellent. For those miracles commend the worship of a plurality of gods, who deserve worship the less the more they demand it; but these of ours commend the worship of the one God, who, both by the testimony of His own Scriptures, and by the eventual abolition of sacrifices, proves that He needs no such offerings. If, therefore, any angels demand sacrifice for themselves, we must prefer those who demand it, not for themselves, but for God, the Creator of all, whom they serve. For thus they prove how sincerely they love us, since they wish by sacrifice to subject us, not to themselves, but to Him by the contemplation of whom they themselves are blessed, and to bring us to Him from whom they themselves have never strayed. If, on the other hand, any angels wish us to sacrifice, not to one, but to many, not, indeed, to themselves, but to the gods whose angels they are, we must in this case also prefer those who are the angels of the one God of gods, and who so bid us to worship Him as to preclude our worshipping any other. But, further, if it be the case, as their pride and deceitfulness rather indicate, that they are neither good angels nor the angels of good gods, but wicked demons, who wish sacrifice to be paid, not to the one only and supreme god, but to themselves, what better protection against them can we choose than that of the one God whom the good angels serve, the angels who bid us sacrifice, not to themselves, but to Him whose sacrifice we ourselves ought to be?

Book XXI, Chapter 8

That it is not contrary to nature that, in an object whose nature is known, there should be discovered an alteration of the properties which have been known as its natural properties.

. . . For we say that all portents are contrary to nature; but they are not so. For how is that contrary to nature that happens by the will of God, since the will of so mighty a Creator is certainly the nature of each created thing? A portent, therefore, happens not contrary to nature, but contrary to what we know as nature. But who can number the multitude of portents recorded in profane histories? Let us then at present fix our attention on this one only that concerns the matter in hand. What is there so arranged by the

Author of the nature of heaven and earth as the exactly ordered course of the stars? What is there established by laws so sure and inflexible? And yet, when it pleased Him who with sovereignty and supreme power regulates all He has created, a star conspicuous among the rest by its size and splendor changed its color, size, form, and, most wonderful of all, the order and law of its course! . . .

For who that thoughtfully observes the countless multitude of men, and their similarity of nature, can fail to remark with surprise and admiration the individuality of each man's appearance, suggesting to us, as it does, that unless men were like one another, they would not be distinguished from the rest of the animals; while unless, on the other hand, they were unlike, they could not be distinguished from one another, so that those whom we declare to be like, we also find to be unlike? And the unlikeness is the more wonderful consideration of the two; for a common nature seems rather to require similarity. And yet, because the very rarity of things is that which makes them wonderful, we are filled with much greater wonder when we are introduced to two men so like, that we either always or frequently mistake in endeavoring to distinguish between them.

Source: Dods, Marcus, ed. and trans. 1948. *The City of God.* Vol. 1. New York: Hafner.

▣ Al-Jahiz, *The Book of Animals,* IV, 404–405 (776–868 CE)

Al-Jahiz lived at Basra (now in Iraq) and was among the most famous and prolific writers of the great Arab civilization. He was of unpleasant appearance, was "goggle-eyed" (=jahiz), and later in life suffered various disabling ailments. His remarks about different degrees of deafness, and the dispersal of sound, suggest that these points were well understood in the Arab centers of learning in the ninth century, a point seldom (if ever) mentioned by writers about medieval deafness.

Theologians say that your dumb man is deaf: his inability to speak is due not to any malformation of the tongue, but to the fact that having never heard sounds, articulated or otherwise, he does not know how to produce them. Not all deaf people are completely dumb, and there are also degrees of deafness.

[The text now provides some examples of loud noises that some deaf people can hear.]

Others can hear words if spoken in their ear, but otherwise they hear nothing, even if the speaker raises his voice; if the speaker positions himself so that the sound goes right into their ear, they understand perfectly, whereas if he speaks just as loudly into the air, the sound of his voice not being concentrated and conducted along a canal into the brain, they do not understand.

Source: Pellat, C., ed., and D. M. Hawke, trans. 1969. "Kitab al-Hayawan" [The life of animals]. In *The Life and Works of Jahiz*. London: Routledge & Kegan Paul.

▣ Al-Mas'udi (ca. 896–956 CE)

Al-Mas'udi provided more information on everyday life and humor than most historians do, including stories of disabled people, often in relation to the Caliph ruling at the time. Many of these present unexpected roles for disabled people.

[An intimate of Ma'mun related that the Caliph told him:] 'Nothing has ever left me so speechless as the answers given by three people.' [The third incident follows:] The inhabitants of Kufa had joined together to complain to me of their governor, a man whose policies and behaviour had my entire approval. I had this reply conveyed to them: 'Although I know all there is to know about this man, I have nevertheless resolved to grant you an audience tomorrow morning. Choose, therefore, a delegate who will speak for you, for I know how prolix you are.'

They answered me as follows:

'The only man whom we feel is worthy to carry on a discussion in the presence of the Caliph is afflicted with deafness. However, if the Commander of the Faithful will be kind enough to tolerate this, perhaps he will do us the honour of letting us know.'

I agreed to bear patiently with their delegate and, on the very next day, the deputation arrived. I had the deaf man brought in. I invited those present to sit and then I asked him what their grievances against the governor were.

'Commander of the Faithful,' he replied, 'he is the worst governor in the world. The year you appointed him, we had to sell our clothes and furniture; the next year, our savings and land; and now, in the third year, we are forced to leave our homes in order to beseech the Commander of the Faithful, that, touched by our sufferings, he may do us the great favour of ordering his removal.'

'You are lying, you bastard!' I cried. 'He is a man whose policies and behaviour I admire, as I honour his piety and wisdom. I chose him for you on purpose, because I know well how often you revolt against those who govern you.'

'My lord,' the speaker replied, 'what you say is true and it is I who lied, but since you so admire the piety, loyalty, integrity, justice and moderation of this governor, why have you left him exclusively with us all these years, to the prejudice of so many other cities, the interests of which Almighty God has confided to your care, as he has confided ours? Set him therefore over these other lands, that he may grant them, in their turn, the treasures of moderation and justice which he has lavished on us.'

'Get out!' I said, 'and may God refuse you His protection. I agree to dismiss your governor.'

[The wit of a blind man, Abu al-Ayna (d. 895), was much celebrated. Mas'udi gives some examples, but he notes also a shrewd reflection by Abu al-Ayna on his own disability. In 860, he had gone to see the Caliph Mutawakkil, who was charmed by his conversation. Mutawakkil asked Abu al-Ayna about his attitude to wine.]

'I would not be able to drink only a little,' replied Abu al-Ayna, 'and I make a fool of myself in public when I drink a lot.'

'Let your scruples alone,' went on Mutawakkil, 'and be our guest.'

Abu al-Ayna answered:

'I am blind. Now a man in my state makes sudden movements, he wanders out of his path and does not observe what others see in him. All those who are here lavish their attentions on you, but I need the care of another. Now it could be that you might look at me with a contented eye, yet be inwardly irritated; or you might appear irritated, hiding your inner satisfaction, and I, being unable to distinguish one state from the other, would be lost. I therefore prefer to hold tight to my safety rather than run the risk of danger.'

Source: Lunde, P., and C. Stone, ed. and trans. 1989. Pp. 193–194 in *The Meadows of Gold. The Abbasids, by Mas'udi*. London: Kegan Paul International.

▣ Anselm of Canterbury, *Proslogion* (ca. 1070–1100)

Anselm of Canterbury, a Benedictine monk who became archbishop of Canterbury, wrote several theological treatises that influenced the development of scholastic theology in the centuries after his death. The Proslogion aims to prove God's existence by means of the "ontological argument" that God can be understood as "that greater than which cannot be thought." This argument, however, depending as it does on intellect, seems to require an account of how a cognitively disabled person might come to know God. The Proslogion thus includes a discourse on the fool's ability to conceive of God, starting with the familiar verse from the Psalms, "The fool says in his heart, 'There is no God.'" Anselm's ideas were answered by the monk Gaunilo, whose rebuttal follows the selection from Anselm.

Chapter 4: How the Fool Managed to Say in His Heart That Which Cannot Be Thought

How in the world could he have said in his heart what he could not think? Or how indeed could he not have thought what he said in his heart, since saying it in his heart is the same as thinking it? But if he really thought it because he said it in his heart, and did not say it in his heart because he could not possibly have thought it—and that seems to be precisely what happened—then there must be more than one way in which something can be said in one's heart or thought. For a thing is thought in one way when the words signifying it are thought, and it is thought in quite another way when the thing signified is understood. God can be thought not to exist in the first way but not in the second. For no one who understands what God is can think that he does not exist. Even though he may say those words in his heart he will give them some other meaning or no meaning at all. For God is that greater than which cannot be thought. Whoever understands this also understands that God exists in such a way that one cannot even think of him as not existing.

Thank you, my good God, thank you, because what I believed earlier through your gift I now understand through your illumination in such a way that I would be unable not to understand it even if I did not want to believe you existed.

Gaunilo: How Someone Writing on Behalf of the Fool Might Reply to All This

To one who questions whether (or simply denies that) there exists something of such a nature that nothing greater can be imagined, it is said that its existence is proved in the first place by the fact that anyone denying it already has it in his thought, since upon hearing it said he understands what is said; and in the second place by the fact that what he understands necessarily exists not only in the mind but in reality as well. Thus its existence is proved, because it is a greater thing to exist in reality as well than to exist in the mind alone, and if it exists only in the mind, then what exists in reality as well will be greater, and thus that which is greater than all else will be less than something else and not greater than all else, which is nonsense. Thus what is greater than all else must necessarily exist, not only in the mind (which has already been acknowledged to be the case), in reality as well, or else it could not be greater than all else.

But perhaps the fool could reply that this thing is said to exist in my mind only in the sense that I understand what is said. For could I not say that all sorts of false and completely nonexistent things exist in my mind since when someone speaks of them I understand what is said? Unless perhaps what is being said here is that one entertains this particular thing in the mind in a completely different way than one thinks of false or doubtful things, and thus what is being said is that having heard this particular thing I do not merely think it but understand it, for I cannot think of this thing in any other way except by understanding it, and that means understanding with certainty that it actually exists. But if this is true, then in the first place there will be no difference between first entertaining that thing in the mind and then understanding that it exists. Imagine the case of that picture which is first in the painter's mind, then exists in reality. It seems unthinkable that, once such an object was spoken or the words heard, the object could not be thought not to exist in the same way God can be thought not to exist. For if God cannot be thought not to exist, then what is the point of launching this whole argument against someone who might deny that something of such a nature actually exists? And in the second place, this basic notion—that God is such that, as soon as he is thought of, he must be perceived by the mind as unquestionably existing—this notion, I say, must be proved to me by some unquestionable argument, but not by the one offered here, namely that this must be in my understanding because I understand what I'm hearing. For as far as I am concerned one might say the same thing about other things that are certain or even false, things about which I might be deceived (as I believe I often am).

Thus the example of the painter who already has in his mind the picture he is about to produce cannot be made to support this argument. For that picture, before it comes into being, exists in the art of the painter, and such a thing existing in the art of some painter is nothing other than a certain part of his understanding; for as Saint Augustine says, "If a craftsman is going to make a box, he first has it in his art. The box he actually produces is not life, but that in his art is life, because the artisan's soul, in which all such things exist before they are brought forth, is alive. And how are these things alive in the living soul of the artisan unless because [they] are nothing other than the knowledge or understanding of the soul itself? But leaving aside those things which are known to belong to the nature of the mind itself, in the case of those things which are perceived as true by the mind through hearing or thought, in this case there is a difference between the thing itself and the mind which grasps it. Thus even if it should be true that there is something greater than which cannot be thought, this thing, whether heard or understood, would not be like the as-yet-unmade picture in the painter's mind.

Moreover, there is the point already suggested earlier, namely that when [I] hear of something greater than all other things which can be thought of—and that something can be nothing other than God himself—I can no more entertain a thought of this being in terms of species or genera familiar to me than I can entertain such a thought of God himself, and for this

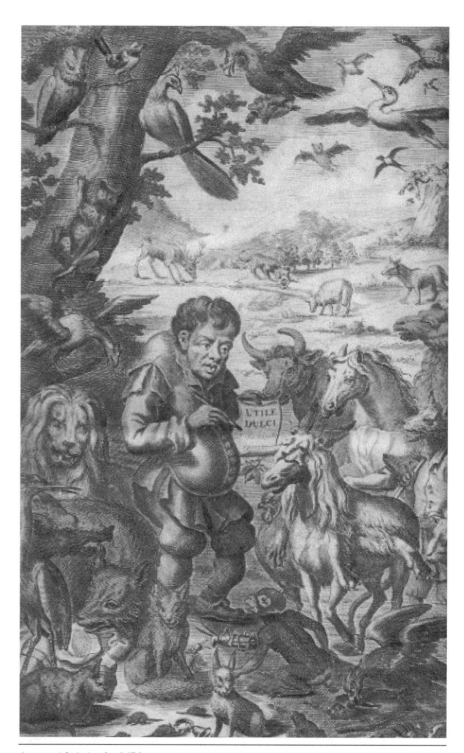

Aesop with Animals, 1476.
Source: Private library of Sharon Snyder and David Mitchell.

reason I am able to think he does not exist. For I have not known the thing itself and I cannot form a similitude of it from other things. For if I hear about some man completely unknown to me, whom I do not even know exists, I could at least think about him through that specific and generic knowledge by which I know what a man is or what men are like. Yet it could be true that, because the speaker was lying, the man I thought about actually did not exist at all, even though I had thought of him as an existing thing, my idea of him being based, not on knowledge of this particular man, but on knowledge of man in general. But when I hear someone say "God" or "something greater than everything else" I cannot think of it as I thought of that nonexistent man, for I was able to think of the latter in terms of some truly existing thing known to me, while in the former case I can think only of the bare words, and on this basis alone one can seldom or never gain any true knowledge. For when one thinks in this way, one thinks not so much of the word itself—which, insofar as it is the sound of letters or syllables is itself a real thing, but of what is signified by the sound heard. But a phrase like "that which is greater than everything else" is not thought of as one thinks about words when one knows what they mean. It is not thought of, that is, as one thinks about something he knows is true either in reality or in thought alone. It is thought of, instead, as one does when he does not really know what the words mean, but thinks of it only in terms of an affection produced by the words within his soul, yet tries to imagine what the words mean. On this basis, though, it would be amazing if he was ever able to penetrate to the truth of the thing. It is in this way and only in this way that this being is in my mind when I hear and understand someone saying there is something greater than everything else that can be thought of. So much for the claim that the supreme nature already exists in my mind.

Nevertheless, that this being must exist not only in my mind but in reality as well is proved to me by the following argument: If it did not, then whatever did exist in reality would be greater, and thus the thing which has already been proved to exist in my mind will not be greater than everything else. If it is said that this being, which cannot be conceived of in terms of any existing thing, exists in the mind, I do not deny that it exists in mine. But through this alone it can hardly be said to attain existence in reality. I will not concede that much to it unless convinced by some indubitable argument. For whoever says that it must

exist because otherwise that which is greater than all other beings will not be greater than all other beings, that person isn't paying careful enough attention to what he says. For I do not yet grant, in fact I deny it or at least question it, that the thing existing in my mind is greater than any real thing. Nor do I concede that it exists in any way except this: the sort of existence (if you can call it such) a thing has when the mind attempts to form some image of a thing unknown to it on the basis of nothing more than some words the person has heard. How then is it demonstrated to me that the thing exists in reality merely because it is said to be greater than everything else? For I continue to deny and doubt that this is established, since I continue to question whether this greater thing is in my mind or thought even in the way that many doubtful or unreal things are. It would first have to be proved to me that this greater thing really exists somewhere. Only then will we be able to infer from the fact that is greater than everything else that it also subsists in itself.

For example, they say there is in the ocean somewhere an island which, due to the difficulty (or rather the impossibility) of finding what does not actually exist, is called "the lost island." And they say that this island has all manner of riches and delights, even more of them than the Isles of the Blest, and having no owner or inhabitant it is superior in the abundance of its riches to all other lands which are inhabited by men. If someone should tell me that such is the case, I will find it easy to understand what he says, since there is nothing difficult about it. But suppose he then adds, as if he were stating a logical consequence, "Well then, you can no longer doubt that this island more excellent than all other lands really exists somewhere, since you do not doubt that it is in your mind; and since it is more excellent to exist not only in the mind but in reality as well, this island must necessarily exist, because if it didn't, any other island really existing would be more excellent than it, and thus that island now thought of by you as more excellent will not be such." If, I say, someone tries to convince me though this argument that the island really exists and there should be no more doubt about it, I will either think he is joking or I will have a hard time deciding who is the bigger fool, me if I believe him or him if he thinks he has proved its existence without having first convinced me that this excellence is something undoubtedly existing in reality and not just something false or uncertain existing in my mind.

In the meantime, this is how the fool answers. If it is asserted in the first place that this being is so great that its nonbeing is logically inconceivable (this in turn being proved by nothing except that otherwise it would not be greater than all other beings), then the fool can answer, "When did I say that such a being, namely one greater than all others, actually exists, thus allowing you to proceed from there to argue that it so really exists that its very nonexistence is inconceivable?" It should first be proved conclusively that some being superior to (that is, greater and better than) all others exists, so that on this basis we can go on to prove the attributes such a greater and better being must possess. When, however, it is said that this highest being cannot be thought of as not existing, perhaps it would have been better to say that its nonbeing or the possibility of its nonbeing is unintelligible. For strictly speaking false things are unintelligible even though they can be thought of in the same way the fool thought God did not exist. I am absolutely certain that I exist, although I nevertheless know that my nonexistence is possible. And I understand without doubting it that the highest thing there is, namely God, exists and cannot not exist. I do not know, however, whether I can think of myself as nonexistent when I know for certain that I exist. If it turns out that I can do so in this case, why should I not be able to do the same concerning other things I know with equal certainty? If I cannot, though, the impossibility of doing so will not be something peculiar to thinking about God.

The other parts of that book are argued with such veracity, brilliance and splendor, and filled with such value, such an intimate fragrance of devout and holy feeling, that they should in no way be condemned because of those things which, at the beginning, . . . [though] rightly intuited, [are] less firmly argued. Rather those things should be argued more robustly and the entire work thus received with great respect and praise.

Anselm's Reply to Gaunilo

Since whoever wrote this reply to me is not the fool against whom I wrote in my treatise but instead one who, though speaking on behalf of the fool, is a catholic Christian and no fool himself, I can speak to him as a catholic Christian.

You say—whoever you are who claim that the fool can say these things—that something greater than which cannot be thought of is in the mind only as something that cannot be thought of in terms of some [existent thing known to us]. And you say that one can no more argue, "since a being greater than which cannot be thought of exists in my mind it must also exist in reality," than one can argue, "the lost island certainly exists in reality because when it is described in words the hearer has no doubt that it exists in his mind." I say in reply that if "a being greater than which cannot be thought of" is neither understood nor thought of, nor is it in our understanding or our thought, then God either is not that greater than which cannot be thought of or he is not understood or thought of, nor is he in the understanding or mind. In proving that this is false I appeal to your faith and conscience. Therefore "a being greater than which cannot be thought of" is really understood and thought of and it really is in our understanding and thought. And that is why the arguments by which you attempt to prove the contrary either are not true or what you think follows from them does not follow from them at all.

Moreover, you imagine that although "a being greater than which cannot be thought of" is understood, it does not follow that it exists in our understanding nor does it follow that, since it is in our understanding, it must exist in reality. I myself say with certainty that if such a being can even be thought of as existing, it must necessarily exist. For "a being greater than which cannot be thought of" cannot be thought of except as having no beginning; but whatever can be thought of as existing yet does not actually exist can be thought of as having a beginning. Therefore "a being greater than which cannot be thought of" cannot be thought of yet not actually exist. Therefore, if it can be thought of, it necessarily exists.

Furthermore, if it can be thought of at all, it must necessarily exist. For no one who denies or doubts the existence of "a being greater than which cannot be thought of" denies or doubts that, if it did exist, it would be impossible for it not to exist either in reality or in the mind. Otherwise it would not be "a being greater than which cannot be thought of." But whatever can be thought of yet does not actually exist, could, if it did come to exist, not exist again in reality and in the mind. That is why, if it can even be thought of, "a being greater than which cannot be thought of" cannot be nonexistent.

But let us suppose that it does not exist (if it is even possible to suppose as much). Whatever can be thought of yet does not exist, even if it should come into existence, would not be "a being greater than which cannot be thought of." Thus "a being greater than which cannot be thought of" would not be "a being greater than which cannot be thought of," which is absurd. Thus if "a being greater than which cannot be thought of" can even be thought of, it is false to say that it does not exist; and it is even more false if such can be understood and exist in the understanding.

I will go even farther. Without doubt whatever does not exist somewhere or at some time, even if it does exist somewhere or at some time, can be thought of as capable of existing never and nowhere, just as it does not exist somewhere or at some time. For what did not exist yesterday and exists today can be thought of as never existing, just as it is thought of as not having existed yesterday. And what does not exist here but does exist somewhere else can be thought of as not existing anywhere. And it is the same with something some parts of which are absent at times. If that is the case, then all of its parts and thus the thing in its entirety can be thought of as existing never and nowhere. For if it is said that time always exists and the world is everywhere, it is nevertheless true that time as a whole does not exist forever, nor does the entire world exist everywhere. And if individual parts of time exist when other parts do not, they can be thought of as never existing at all. And just as particular parts of the world do not exist where other parts do, so they can be thought of as never existing at all, anywhere. And what is composed of parts can be broken up in the mind and be nonexistent. Thus whatever does not exist as a whole sometime or somewhere can be thought of as not existing, even if it actually exists at the moment. But "a being greater than which cannot be thought of," if it exists, cannot be thought of as not existing. Otherwise it is not "a being greater than which cannot be thought of," which is absurd. Thus it cannot fail to exist in its totality always and everywhere.

Do you not believe that the being of which these things are understood can be thought about or understood or be in the thought or understanding to some extent? For if he is not, then we cannot understand these things about him. If you say that he is not understood or in the understanding because he is not fully understood, say as well that one who cannot look directly at the sun does not see the light of day, which is nothing other than the light of the sun. Certainly "a being greater than which cannot be thought of" is understood and exists in the understanding at least to the extent that these statements about it are understood. . . .

You often picture me as offering this argument: Because what is greater than all other things exists in the understanding, it must also exist in reality or else the being which is greater than all others would not be such. Never in my entire treatise do I say this. For there is a big difference between saying "greater than all other things" and "a being greater than which cannot be thought of." If someone says "a being greater than which cannot be thought of" is not something actually existing or is something which could possibly not exist or something which cannot even be understood, such assertions are easily refuted. For what does not exist is capable of not existing, and what is capable of not existing can be thought of as not existing. But whatever can be thought of as not existing, if it does actually exist, is not "a being greater than which cannot be thought of." . . .

It is not, it seems, so easy to prove the same thing of "that which is greater than all other things," for it is not all that obvious that something which can be thought of as not existing is not nevertheless greater than all things which actually exist.

Source: Burr, David, trans. n.d. *St. Anselm of Canterbury, Proslogion.* Available at http://dburr.hist.vt.edu/Anselm.html

▣ Kai Kaus, *Qabus-nama* (1082–1083 CE)

The Cabous Namè (in English: Qabus-nama or Kabusnama) is written as an instruction manual for princes. A passage in Chapter 7 asserts that a child who is not exposed to language during infancy will grow up unable to speak, providing as proof the example of congenitally deaf children. This assertion may have been the source of the Emperor Akbar's infamous experiment in which he had infants reared by deaf-mute nurses in a locked house, so that they would not be exposed to language. He was curious to discover what language, if any, they would produce.

Make an effort to be an attentive listener, for when one knows how to listen one may acquire wisdom and good expression, as may be shown from the case of children.

Suppose for example that a child were confined in a cellar from birth, and there were given its milk and food, but had never a word or caress from its mother or nursemaid. Clearly, as it grew, it would remain dumb and unable to produce a word, unless [or until] it chanced to have some opportunity to hear [speech] and so to learn to speak. A further proof is the fact that all who are born deaf are also mute. Isn't it the case that all dumb people are deaf?

Source: English translation of Querry, A., trans. 1886. *Kai Kaus. Le Cabous Namè ou livre de Cabous.* Paris: Leroux.

▣ Ibn Khallikan, *Biographical Dictionary*

Ibn Khallikan produced this famous thirteenth-century collection of 865 biographies of well-known Muslims through six centuries, many also giving information on lesser-known persons. Over 100 entries mention some disability. A few among these were deaf people.

Thalab the Grammarian (Abu 'l-Abbas Ahmad Ibn Yahya Ibn Zaid Ibn Saiyar) (815–904), Vol. I: 85

[Thalab the Grammarian became deaf later in life, and lost his life in a traffic accident in Baghdad, apparently as a result of being unable to hear.]

The accident which caused his death happened in the following manner: he had left the mosque on Friday, when the afternoon-prayer was over; and some time before he had got a deafness, which prevented him from hearing unless with great difficulty; he was holding a book in his hand and reading it in the street, when a horse knocked against him and threw him into a deep pit, out of which he was taken nearly senseless. He was immediately borne to his house, complaining of his head, and he died the next day.

Imad ad-Dawlat (ca. 892–949), Vol. II: 333

[After capturing Shiraz, Imad ad-Dawlat found hidden wealth, which enabled him to consolidate his grip. He then had a further stroke of good luck, arising because a deaf tailor misunderstood the situation and thought that he had been betrayed.]

Imad ad-Dawlat . . . caused a dress to be cut out for his own use, and having inquired for a skilful tailor to make it up, they told him of a person who had served the former governor of the town in that capacity.

In pursuance of his orders, this man was brought to him; and the fellow, happening to be deaf, imagined that secret information had been lodged against him for retaining in his possession some property which his former master had confided in his care. Impressed with this belief, he swore, when spoken to by the prince, that he had only twelve chests in his house, and did not know what they contained. Surprised at such an answer, Imad ad-Dawlat sent for the chests, which were discovered to be filled with money and dresses to an immense amount.

Dibil Ibn Ali'l-Khuzai (765–860/861), Vol. I: 507–511

It is stated also that he was deaf and had a scrofulous swelling on the back of his neck. —Dibil was a good poet, but scurrilous and addicted to satire; always ready to slander men of merit, and sparing none, not even the khalifs. He lived (however) to an advanced age, and he used to say: 'For fifty years I have gone about with my cross on my shoulder, but could find none to crucify me on it.' [Some examples are given of prominent men who would happily have crucified Dibil for his satirical verses about them.]

[Dibil's conduct was sometimes eccentric:] 'Dibil' means 'a tall camel.' He used to relate that one day as he was passing along, he saw a man in a fit of epilepsy; on which he went up and shouted in his ear, as loud as he could, the word 'Dibil,' and that the man rose up and walked away as if nothing had happened.

Muhammad Ibn Sirin (653/654–729), Vol. II: 586–589

[Muhammad Ibn Sirin was a highly esteemed law lecturer of Basra who was also valued as an accurate and early transmitter of sayings and incidents ("traditions," or *hadiths*) from the life of the prophet Muhammad. As the hadiths were to become the major source of rules for everyday conduct among Muslims, second only to the Quran, the accuracy of oral transmission was a subject of intensive study. Doubt could be cast on a tradition if anything detrimental was known about the conduct or probity of any link in the chain of transmission, as appears in some comments below. It might be anticipated that a known, significant hearing impairment would be considered a serious defect in a transmitter; but evidently this was not so in the case of Ibn Sirin.]

Abu Bakr Muhammad Ibn Sirin was a native of Basra. His father was slave to Anas Ibn Malik [footnote: "one of the most eminent among the Companions" (of the prophet Muhammad)] . . . Muhammad Ibn Sirin delivered Traditions on the authority of Abu Huraira, Abd Allah Ibn Omar, Abd Allah Ibn az-Zubair, Imran Ibn Husain, and Anas Ibn Malik;

[To students of law] "As-Shabi used to say 'Stick to that deaf man!' meaning thereby Ibn Sirin; because he was dull of hearing. . . . Al-Asmai used to say:

'Al-Hasan al-Basri [was, in furnishing Traditions] a generous prince; but when the deaf man (meaning Ibn Sirin) furnishes Traditions, retain them carefully; as for Ka-ada, [he was, as a collector of Traditions, like] one who gathers fire-wood in the dark, [picking up both bad and good].'

Abu'l-Abbas Muhammad Ibn Yakub al-Asamm, Vol. 4: 397

Abu'l-Abbas Muhammad Ibn Yakub al-Asamm ('the deaf'), a mawla to the Omaiyide family, a native of Naisapur and the chief Traditionist of that age in Khorasan, taught during seventy-six years the knowledge which he had acquired. His death took place in . . . 957. He lost his hearing after having travelled and made his studies.

Abu'l-Aswad ad-Duwali (d. 688/689), Vol. I: 662–667

[Eminent and learned grammarian and poet of Basra. His remark about the need to appear in public even though disabled, if he were not to risk disappearing from anyone's notice, seems to transcend history and geography.]

It is related that Abu'l-Aswad had an attack of the palsy, and that he used to go to the market himself, although scarcely able to draw his leg after him, and yet he was rich and possessed both male and female slaves: a person who knew this accosted him one day and said: 'God has dispensed you from the necessity of moving about on your own business; why do you not remain seated at home?' To which he replied: 'No; I go in and out, and the eunuch says: "He is coming," and the boy says: "He is coming," whereas, were I to continue sitting in the house, the sheep might [pass] urine upon me without any person's preventing them.'

Katada Ibn Diama As-Sadusi (679/680–735/736), Vol. II: 513–514

[A learned man who had been born blind, at Basra.]

"'Katada,' said Abu Amr, 'was the most learned genealogist of his time, and, in his youth he met Daghfal. He used to go from one end of Basra to the other without a guide.'"

Source: de Slane, M. G., trans. 1842. *Ibn Khallikan's Biographical Dictionary Translated from the Arabic.* 4 vols. Paris; Oriental Translation Fund.

◉ Legend of Saint Wilgefortis (1100s–1400s)

Saint Wilgefortis (traditionally thought to be derived from virgo, "virgin," and fortis, "strong"), supposedly a Portuguese virgin martyr, is a fictional saint whose story resulted from the combination of several popular legends. She is known by a variety of alternate names in different countries. The legend demonstrates the use of masculine attributes as chosen deformity by women to escape the imprisonment of marriage.

A fabulous female saint known also as UNCUMBER, KUMMERNIS, KOMINA, COMERA, CUMERANA, HULFE, ONTCOMMENE, ONTCOMMER, DIGNEFORTIS, EUTROPIA, REGINFLEDIS, LIVRADE, LIBERATA, etc.

The legend makes her a Christian daughter of a pagan King of Portugal. In order to keep her vow of chastity, she prayed God to disfigure her body, that she might evade the command of her father to marry a pagan prince. God caused a beard to grow on her chin, whereupon her father had her crucified. Connected with this legend is the story of a destitute fiddler to whom, when he played before her image (or before her crucified body), she gave one of her golden boots. Being condemned to death for the theft of the boot, he was granted his request to play before her a second time, and, in presence of all, she kicked off her other boot, thus establishing his innocence.

The legend is not a Christian adaptation of the Hermaphroditus of Greek mythology or of other androgynous myths of pagan antiquity, as it cannot be traced back further than the fifteenth century. It rather originated from a misinterpretation of the famous "Volto Santo" of Lucca, a representation of the crucified Saviour, clothed in a long tunic, His eyes wide open,

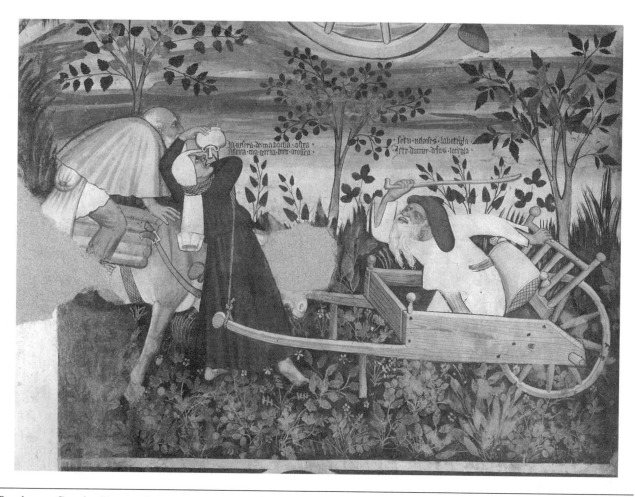

People on a Cart, *by Giacomo Jaquerio (fifteenth century). An example of medieval wheeled mobility for a man who cannot walk.*
Source: Castle, Manta, Italy. Photo credit: Scala/Art Resource, New York.

His long hair falling over His shoulders, and His head covered with a crown. This crucifix, popularly believed to be the work of Nicodemus, is preserved in the Basilica of Lucca and highly venerated by the people. In the early Middle Ages it was common to represent Christ on the cross clothed in a long tunic, and wearing a royal crown; but since the eleventh century this practice has been discontinued. Thus it happened that copies of the "Volto Santo" of Lucca, spread by pilgrims and merchants in various parts of Europe, were no longer recognized as representations of the crucified Saviour, but came to be looked upon as pictures of a woman who had suffered martyrdom.

The name Wilgefortis is usually derived from *Virgo fortis,* but recently Schnürer has shown that Wilgefortis is probably a corruption of *Hilge Vartz* (*Vartz, Fratz,* face), "Holy Face." This would corroborate the opinion that the legend originated in the

"Volto Santo." The old English name *Uncumber,* as also the German *Oncommer* and their equivalents in other languages, rose from the popular belief that every one who invokes the saint in the hour of death will die *ohne Kummer,* without anxiety. When the cult of St. Wilgefortis began to spread in the fifteenth and sixteenth centuries, her name found its way into various breviaries and martyrologies. Thus a breviary, printed at Paris for the Diocese of Salisbury in 1533, has a beautiful metric antiphon and prayer in her honour. Her feast is celebrated on 20 July. She is usually represented nailed to a cross: as a girl of ten or twelve years, frequently with a beard, or as throwing her golden boot to a musician playing before her, sometimes also with one foot bare.

Source: Ott, Michael. 1913. "Wilgefortis." In *Catholic Encyclopedia.* Available at http://www.newadvent.org/cathen/ 15622a.htm

▣ "Tomi" from *Samguk Sagi* (1145)

Samguk Sagi was put together by Kim Pusik in 1145; the work covers the history of the Three Kingdom period, roughly from the first century BCE *to the seventh century* CE. *Tomi's story shows that disablement was practiced as a form of punishment in ancient Korea. The story celebrates a wife's virtue in remaining faithful to her disabled husband.*

Tomi was a native of Paekche (B.C.18–A.D.678). He was a righteous man of humble birth, with a beautiful and chaste wife, and those who knew him spoke well of him. King Kaeru [128–166] heard of the couple and summoned Tomi. "Generally, women consider chastity and purity to be their foremost virtues," he said, "but if they are tempted with clever words in the dark when no one else is around, few will remain unmoved."

Tomi replied, "One cannot fathom another's mind, but your subject's wife would remain true even on pain of death."

Wishing to test the wife's virtue, the king detained Tomi on some pretext and sent a trusted attendant on horseback to Tomi's house to announce a royal visit. That night the king himself arrived and said to Tomi's wife, "I've long heard about your beauty and I like you. I won you from your husband in a wager. Tomorrow I'll make you my consort, so from now on you're mine."

"The king would not tell a lie, so how could I disobey you? Please enter the room first. I'll change my clothes and follow you," the wife said to the king. She then sent in a female slave disguised as herself.

Later, when the king realized that he had been deceived, he grew angry. On trumped-up charges the king had Tomi's eyes gouged out and had him dragged to a skiff and set adrift on the river. Then he had Tomi's wife sent in and tried to violate her. She declared, "Now that I've lost my husband, I cannot live alone. Still more, since I am to serve your majesty, how could I go against your will? But at the moment I am menstruating, and my body is unclean. Please allow me to wait another day, and then I'll be yours." The king believed her. The wife then seized the opportunity to escape and reached the shore, only to find that there was no boat. She cried to Heaven, and an empty skiff appeared. She jumped aboard and reached Ch'onso Island, where she found her husband. He was still alive, and the couple dug up tree roots to still their hunger. Eventually the couple boarded a boat that took them to the foot of Mount San in Koguryo. The people there took pity on them and provided them with clothes and food. They lived on, and eventually died far from home.

Source: *Samguk Sagi*, in the *Anthology of Korean Literature: From Early Times to the Nineteenth Century*. Compiled and edited by Peter H. Lee. Honolulu: The University Press of Hawaii, 1981, p. 25.

▣ Snorri Sturluson, *Saga of Harald Hardrade* (1179–1241)

The Saga of Harald Hardrade is part of the series Heimskringla, which chronicled the histories of the kings of Norway. Harald (1015–1066) was given the epithet Hardrade (i.e., "severe counsellor," "tyrant") by the Norwegians, perhaps in response to cruelties such as those detailed in the first selection, which describes Harald blinding the Greek emperor. The second selection, not specifically about Harald, describes the miraculous cure of a disabled man.

14. King Olaf's Miracle and Blinding the Greek Emperor

When Harald drew near to the prison King Olaf the Saint stood before him and said he would assist him. On that spot of the street a chapel has since been built and consecrated to Saint Olaf and which chapel has stood there ever since. The prison was so constructed that there was a high tower open above, but a door below to go into it from the street. Through it Harald was thrust in, along with Haldor and Ulf. Next night a lady of distinction with two servants came, by the help of ladders, to the top of the tower, let down a rope into the prison and hauled them up. Saint Olaf had formerly cured this lady of a sickness and he had appeared to her in a vision and told her to deliver his brother. Harald went immediately to the Varings, who all rose from their seats when he came in and received him with joy. The men armed themselves forthwith and went to where the emperor slept. They took the emperor prisoner and put out both the eyes of him. So says Thorarin Skeggjason in his poem:

"Of glowing gold that decks the hand
The king got plenty in this land;
But it's great emperor in the strife
Was made stone-blind for all his life."

So says Thiodolf, the skald, also:—

"He who the hungry wolf's wild yell
Quiets with prey, the stern, the fell,
Midst the uproar of shriek and shout
Stung the Greek emperor's eyes both out:
The Norse king's mark will not adorn,
The Norse king's mark gives cause to mourn;
His mark the Eastern king must bear,
Groping his sightless way in fear."

In these two songs, and many others, it is told that Harald himself blinded the Greek emperor; and they would surely have named some duke, count, or other great man, if they had not known this to be the true account; and King Harald himself and other men who were with him spread the account.

59. King Olaf's Miracle on a Cripple

West in Valland, a man had such bad health that he became a cripple, and went on his knees and elbows. One day he was upon the road, and had fallen asleep. He dreamt that a gallant man came up to him and asked him where he was going. When he named the neighbouring town, the man said to him, "Go to Saint Olaf's church that stands in London, and there thou shalt be cured." There-upon he awoke, and went straightway to inquire the road to Olaf's church in London. At last he came to London Bridge, and asked the men of the castle if they could tell him where Olaf's church was; but they replied, there were so many churches that they could not tell to whom each of them was consecrated. Soon after a man came up and asked him where he wanted to go, and he answered to Olaf's church. Then said the man, "We shall both go together to Olaf's church, for I know the way to it." Thereupon they went over the bridge to the shrine where Olaf's church was; and when they came to the gates of the churchyard the man mounted over the half-door that was in the gate, but the cripple rolled himself in, and rose up immediately sound and strong: when he looked about him his conductor had vanished.

Source: Laing, Samuel, trans. 1844. Snorri Sturluson. Heimskringla. Online Medieval and Classical Library Release #15b. Available at http://sunsite.berkeley .edu/OMACL/Heimskringla/

▣ Saint Francis of Assisi
(1181–1226)

The excerpt below begins with Francis's recovery after being locked up by his father for throwing away the household fortune as an act of material renunciation. In the later excerpt, which details events from around 1208, St. Francis of Assisi firmly renounces his possession of all worldly belongings, and puts on a coarse woolen tunic (a dress worn by some of the poorest Umbrian peasants), and takes up a spiritual life among them. During one trip on horseback across the Umbrian plain he came upon an individual with leprosy. In order to conquer his repulsion, he embraced the man and gave him all his remaining money. This is a common story of saintly sacrifice toward disabled individuals as a sign of religious devotion to socially rejected bodies.

Chapter 1: The Convalescent

There awoke one morning in Assisi a young man who was just recovering from a severe illness. It was seven hundred years ago. The hour was an early one. The window blinds were not yet opened. Out of doors the day's business was in full blast; the bells for mass had long ago rung out from St. Maria del Vescovado, which lay almost under the windows. The strong morning light streamed in through the crack where the window blinds met.

The young man knew it all so well—one morning after another the long weeks of his convalescence had passed thus. Soon his mother would come in and would draw the shutters aside, and the light would enter in dazzling brightness. Then he would get his morning draught, and his bed would be made over; he used to lie on one side of the wide bed while the other was made up for him. And so he would lie there, tired, but at peace, and look out on the blue cloudless autumn sky, listening to the splashing on the stones of the street as the people of the neighbourhood threw their waste water out of the windows. As the forenoon advanced the rays of the sun began to come in—first along the high wall of the window alcove—then right across the brick floor of the room, and when they approached the bed, it was time to take the midday meal. After midday the blinds were again closed, and he took his siesta in the quiet comfortable obscurity of the room. Then he awoke and the blinds were again

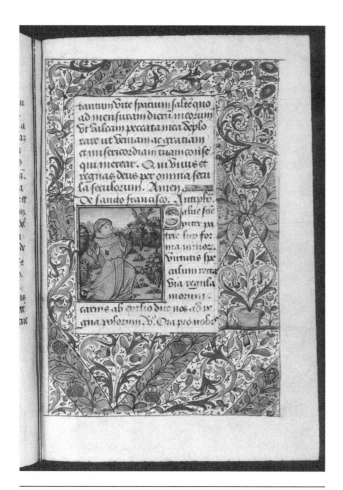

"Saint Francis Receiving the Stigmata: Suffrage to Saint Francis." Two years before his death, Saint Francis received the stigmata (the wounds of Christ) in his hands, feet, and side. Such bodily markings were often represented as a testimony of one's religious faithfulness. From the Playfair Book of Hours (Ms. L.475-1918, Fol. 167r. French [Rouen], late fifteenth century [CT13091]).

Source: Victoria and Albert Museum, London. Photo credit: Victoria and Albert Museum, London/Art Resource, New York.

thrown open to admit the light; the sun had left the window—but if he raised himself up in the bed, he could see the mountains under a blue veil on the other side of the plain, and soon the crimson evening red of the late autumn day burned in the western sky. As the darkness quickly fell, he heard the noise of sheep, which were driven bleating into the stable, and of peasants and peasant girls, who sang on their way home from the fields. They were the wonderful heart-gripping folk-songs of Umbria which the invalid heard—the songs which even to-day are in the people's mouths and whose slow, wonderfully melancholy tones fill the soul with sadness till it is ready to burst with helpless longing and melancholy.

At last the songs ceased and it was night. Over the distant mountains gleamed a single bright star. When that showed itself, it was time to close the shutters and to light the night-lamp—the lamp which in the long nights of fever had constantly burned through the long hours of his uneasy dreams.

To-day there was to be a change—to-day at last he was to have permission to leave his bed. How glad he was to go into the other rooms, to see and touch all the things he had so long missed, and had been so near losing forever. He must even venture down into the business, see the clerks measure the good Tuscan cloth with their yardsticks, and draw in the bright ringing coins.

Just as the young man was busy with these dreams the door opened. As on every morning of his illness, it was his mother who entered. As she threw the shutters aside he saw that she carried, as she brought his morning meal, a suit of man's clothes over her arm.

"I have had a new suit of clothes made for you, my Francis," said she as she laid them down at the foot of the bed.

And as he finished his meal she sat down by the window while he dressed himself.

"What a lovely morning it is," said she, almost as if she were talking to herself. "How brightly the sun shines! I see all the houses over in Bettona so clearly, although there is the whole extent of the broad plain between us, and out in the middle of the green vineyards, Isola Romanesca lies like an island in a lake. And smoke is rising straight up from all the chimneys—as if from a censer in a church. Ah, it seems to me, my Francis, that on such a morning as this, heaven and earth are as beautiful as a church on a feast-day, and that all creatures praise, love and thank God."

To these words Francis gave no answer but silence.

But a moment later he broke out, as he ceased his dressing:

"How weak I am!"

His mother changed the current of her remarks and their tone.

"It is always so, when one has been sick," she said brightly. "As long as you lie in bed you think that you can do anything, but as soon as you get your feet from under the covers you find that it is different. I know this from my own experience, and therefore I had the foresight to bring a stick for you."

And she went to the door and brought in a beautiful polished stick with an ivory handle. Soon after the mother and son together left the sick-room.

But first of all the poor were in his thoughts. To see them, to hear their troubles, to help them in their necessities—there were hereafter his principal concerns. And little by little the desire was firmly established within his heart: "if I could only find by personal experience how it felt to be poor—how it is to be, not one of those who go by and throw down a shilling, but to be the one who stands in rags and dirt, and humbly bowing, stretches out his faded hat for alms!" Many a time, we may think, he stood among the beggars at some church door—stood among them while they pitifully asked for a mite. But it was not like him to do only this. He himself must do the begging in order to understand poverty, and this could not be done in Assisi where everyone knew him.

For the lepers occupied a very particular position among the sick and poor of the Middle Ages. Based on a passage in the Prophet Isaiah (liii.4) the lepers were looked upon as an image of the Redeemer, more than all other sufferers. As early as the days of Gregory the Great we find the story of the monk, Martyrius, who met a leper by the wayside, who from pain and weariness was fallen to the ground and could drag himself no further. Martyrius wrapped the sick man in his cloak and carried him to his convent. But the leper changed in his arms to Jesus himself, who rose to heaven as he blessed the monk, and said to him: "Martyrius, thou wert not ashamed of me on earth; I will not be ashamed of thee in heaven!" A similar legend is told of St. Julian, of St. Leo IX, and of the Blessed Colombini.

And so the lepers were more than any others an object for pious care during the Middle Ages. For them was founded a special order of knights—Knights of Lazarus—whose whole office was to take care of the lepers. So too there were erected all over Europe the numerous houses of St. George, [of which] lepers' homes there were 19,000 in the thirteenth century. But in spite of everything the life of the leper was sad enough, they were repulsed by the rest of humanity, and they were hedged in by severe laws isolating them and hemming them in on all sides.

As with all other cities, there was also in the vicinity of Assisi a lepers' hospital—the lepers were in fact the first real hospital patients and in some languages their name expresses this fact. The hospital lay midway between Assisi and Portiuncula, near where the words *Casa Gualdi* appear over the entrance to a large estate. It was called San Salvatore delle Pareti, and was owned by an order of Crucigers, founded under Alexander III for the care of the lepers.

On his walks in this place, Francis now and then passed by the hospital, but the mere sight of it had filled him with horror. He would not even give an alms to a leper unless some one else would take it for him. Especially when the wind blew from the hospital, and the weak, nauseating odor, peculiar to the leper, came across the road, he would hurry past with averted face and fingers in his nostrils.

It was in this that he felt his greatest weakness, and in it he was to win his greatest victory.

For one day, as he was as usual calling upon God, it happened that the answer came. And the answer was this: "the flesh it is your duty to despise and hate, if you wish to know my will. And when you have begun thus, all that which now seems to you sweet and lovely will become intolerable and bitter, but all which you used to avoid will turn itself to great sweetness and exceeding joy."

These were the words which at last gave Francis a definite programme, which showed him the way he was to follow. He certainly pondered over these words in his lonely rides over the Umbrian plain and, just as he one day woke out of reverie, he found the horse making a sudden movement, and saw on the road before him, only a few steps distant, *a leper,* in his familiar uniform.

Francis started, and even his horse shared in the movement, and his first impulse was to turn and flee as fast as he could. But there were the words he had heard within himself, so clearly before him—"what you used to abhor shall be to you joy and sweetness." . . . And *what* had he hated more than the lepers? Here was the time to take the Lord at His word—to show his good will. . . .

And with a mighty victory over himself, Francis sprang from his horse, approached the leper, from whose deformed countenance the awful odor of corruption issued forth, placed his alms in the outstretched wasted hand—bent down quickly and kissed the fingers of the sick man, covered with the awful disease, whilst his system was nauseated with the action. . . .

When he again sat upon his horse, he hardly knew how he had got there. He was overcome by excitement, his heart beat, he knew not whither he rode. But the Lord had kept his word. Sweetness, happiness, joy streamed into his soul—flowed and kept flowing, although his soul seemed full and more full—like the clear stream which, filling an earthen vessel, keeps on pouring and flows over its rim, with an ever clearer, purer stream. . . .

The next day Francis voluntarily wandered down the road he had hitherto always avoided—the road to San Salvatore delle Pareti. And when he reached the gate he knocked, and when it was opened to him he entered. From all the cells the sick came swarming out—came with their half-destroyed faces, blind inflamed eyes, with club-feet, with swollen, corrupted arms and fingerless hands. And all this dreadful crowd gathered around the young merchant, and the odor from their unclean swellings was so strong that Francis against his will for a moment had to hold his breath to save himself from sickness. But he soon recovered control of himself, he drew out the well-filled purse he had brought with him, and began to deal out his alms. And on every one of the dreadful hands that were reached out to take his gifts he imprinted a kiss, as he had done the day before.

Thus it was that Francis won the greatest victory man can win—the victory over oneself. From now on he was master of himself, and not like the most of us—his own slave.

But even the greatest victor in the spiritual field must be ever on the watch for his always vigilant enemy. Francis had conquered in great things—the tempter tried now to bring him to defeat in small things.

Francis continued as before to go everyday to his oratory in the cave outside the city to pray there. Now it often happened that on the way there he met a humpbacked old woman—one of the common deformed creatures who, in the south, so willingly betake themselves to the sheltering obscurity of the churches. They can be seen there all day long, rattling their rosaries, or dozing in a corner, but the instant a stranger approaches, they draw the kerchief around their heads, limp out from their corner, and mutter piteously with outstretched hand: *Un soldo, signore! Un soldo, signorino mio!* (A penny, sir! A penny, sir!)

Such a pitiful old beggar was it who now every day limped across the young man's path. And it happened that in the newly converted young soul there rose a repugnance and a resistance—a repugnance to the dirt and misery of the old woman, a resistance to her troublesome ways and to her persistency. And as he went on his way, and the sun shone, and the fields were green, and the distant mountains showed grey-blue, a voice whispered within him: "And are you willing to give up all this—are you willing to abandon it all? You will give up light and sun, life and joy, the cheerful open-air feasts—and will shut yourself up in a cave and waste your best years in useless prayers, and finally become an old fool, shaking with the palsy, who pitifully wanders about from church to church, and, perhaps in secret, sighs and mourns over his wasted life?"

Thus the wicked enemy whispered into the young man's soul, and this was the moment when Francis's youth and light-loving eyes and knightly soul weakened. But as he reached his cave he always succeeded in conquering himself—and the harder the struggle had been, the deeper was the peace which followed—the joy and the hope—all in converse with God.

Source: O'Connor Sloane, T., trans. 1955. Johannes Jorgensen. *St. Francis of Assisi: A Biography.* Garden City, NY: Doubleday.

◙ Zeami, *Semimaru*
(ca. 1300s)

This version of the story of the fictional character Semimaru was written in fourteenth-century Japan by Zeami. Although many versions of the story exist, all revolve around Semimaru, a blind musician who plays the biwa *(a type of lute). In this version, Semimaru is the son of Emperor Daigo. The play provides a glimpse of how the Japanese viewed disability at the time of its writing. This excerpt begins with Semimaru's banishment—his father has commanded that he be abandoned on Mount Osaka, because his blindness is interpreted as his having failed in his religious obligations in a former life. Semimaru's mentally ill sister Sakagami, who lives as a wanderer, visits him, and they commiserate on how they have fallen from their royal origins.*

Kiyotsura and Attendants
Like lame-wheeled carriages
We creep forth reluctantly
On the journey from the Capital;
How hard it is to say farewell
As dawn clouds streak the east!
Today he first departs the Capital
When again to return? His chances are as fragile
As unraveled threads too thin to intertwine.
Friendless, his destination is unknown.
Even without an affliction
Good fortune is elusive in this world,
Like the floating log the turtle gropes for

Once a century: The path is in darkness
And he, a blind turtle, must follow it.
Now as the clouds of delusion rise
We have reached Mount Osaka
We have reached Mount Osaka.

[*Semimaru sits on a stool before the Chorus. Kiyotsura kneels at the shite-pillar. The Bearers exit through the slit door.*]

Semimaru

Kiyotsura!

Kiyotsura

I am before you.

[*From his kneeling position, he bows deeply.*]

Semimaru

Are you to leave me on this mountain?

Kiyotsura

Yes, your highness. So the Emperor has commanded, and I have brought you this far. But I wonder just where I should leave you.

Since the days of the ancient sage kings
Our Emperors have ruled the country wisely,
Looking after its people with compassion—
But what can his Majesty have had in mind?
Nothing could have caught me so unprepared.

Semimaru

What a foolish thing to say, Kiyotsura. I was born blind because I was lax in my religious duties in a former life.

That is why the Emperor, my father,
Ordered you to leave me in the wilderness,
Heartless this would seem, but it's his plan
To purge in this world my burden from the past,
And spare me suffering in the world to come.
This is a father's true kindness.
You should not bewail his decree.

Kiyotsura

Now I shall shave your head.
His Majesty has so commanded.

Semimaru

What does this act signify?

Kiyotsura

It means you have become a priest,
A most joyous event.

[*Semimaru rises. The stage assistant removes his nobleman's outer robe and places a priest's hat on his head.*]

Semimaru

Surely Seishi's poem described such a scene:
"I have cut my fragrant scented hair
My head is pillowed half on sandalwood."

Kiyotsura

Such splendid clothes will summon thieves, I fear.
Allow me to take your robe and give you instead
This cloak of straw they call a *mino*.

[*Semimaru mimes receiving the mino.*]

Semimaru

Is this the *mino* mentioned in the lines.
"I went to Tamino Island when it rained"?

Kiyotsura

And I give you this *kasa* rainhat
To protect you also from the rain and dew.

[*He takes a kasa from the stage assistant and hands it to Semimaru.*]

Semimaru

Then this must be the *kasa* of the poem
"Samurai—take a kasa for your lord."

[*Semimaru puts down the kasa.*]

Kiyotsura

And this staff will guide you on your way.
Please take it in your hands.

[*He takes a staff from the stage assistant and hands it to Semimaru.*]

Semimaru

Is this the staff about which Henjo wrote:
"Since my staff was fashioned by the gods
I can cross the mountain of a thousand years"?

[*Kiyotsura kneels at the shite-pillar.*]

Kiyotsura

His staff brought a thousand prosperous years,

Semimaru

But here the place is Mount Osaka,

Kiyotsura

A straw-thatched hut by the barrier;

Semimaru

Bamboo pillars and staff, my sole support.

Kiyotsura

By your father, the Emperor,

Semimaru

Abandoned,

Chorus

I meet my unsure fate at Mount Osaka.
You who know me, you who know me not
Behold—this is how a prince, Daigo's son,
Has reached the last extremity of grief.

[*He lowers his head to give a sad expression to his mask.*]

Travelers and men on horses
Riding to and from the Capital,
Many people, dressed for their journeys,
Will drench their sleeves in sudden showers

How hard it is to abandon him,
To leave him all alone—
How hard it is to abandon him,
To tear ourselves away.
[*Kiyotsura bows to Semimaru.*]
But even farewells must have an end;
By the light of the daybreak moon
Stifling tears that have no end, they depart.
[*Weeping, Kiyotsura goes to the bridgeway.*]
Semimaru, the Prince, left behind alone,
Takes in his arms his lute, his one possession,
Clutches his staff and falls down weeping.
[*Semimaru picks up the staff and kasa, comes forward, and turns toward the departing Kiyotsura. Kiyotsura stops at the second pine and looks back at him, then exits. Semimaru retreats, kneels, drops his kasa and staff, and weeps. Hakuga no Sammi enters and stands at the naming-place.*]

Hakuga

I am Hakuga no Sammi. I have learned that Prince Semimaru has been abandoned on Mount Osaka and it pains me so much to think of him at the mercy of the rain and dew that I have decided to build a straw hut where he may live.

[*He opens the door of the hut, then goes to Semimaru at the shite-pillar.*]

The hut is ready at last, I shall inform him of this.
[*He bows to Semimaru.*]

Pardon me, sir; Hakuga is before you. If you stay here in this way, you will be soaked by the rain. I have built you a straw hut and I hope you will live in it. Please, come with me.

[*He takes Semimaru's hand and leads him inside the hut, then steps back and bows.*]

If ever you need anything, you have only to summon me, Hakuga no Sammi. I shall always be ready to serve you. I take my leave of you for now.

[*He closes the door of the hut, then exits. Sakagami enters wearing the zo mask. Her robe is folded back from her right shoulder indicating that she is deranged. She stops at the first pine.*]

Sakagami

I am the third child of the Emperor Daigo,
The one called Sakagami, Unruly Hair.
Though born a princess, some deed of evil
From my unknown past in former lives
Causes my mind at times to act deranged.
And in my madness I wander distant ways.
My blueblack hair grows skywards;
Though I stroke it, it will not lie flat.
[*She smooths down her hair.*]

Those children over there—what are they laughing at?
[*She looks to the right as if watching passersby.*]
What? You find it funny that my hair stands on end? Yes,
I suppose hair that grows upside down is funny.
My hair is disordered, but much less than you—
Imagine, commoners laughing at me!
How extraordinary it is that so much before our eyes is upside down. Flower seeds buried in the ground rise up to grace the branches of a thousand trees. The moon hangs high in the heavens, but its light sinks to the bottom of countless waters.
[*She looks up and down.*]
I wonder which of all these should be said to go in the proper direction and which is upside down?
I am a princess, yet I have fallen,
And mingle with the ruck of common men;
[*She proceeds to the stage while chanting.*]
My hair, rising upward from my body,
Turns white with the touch of stars and frost:
The natural order or upside down?
How amazing that both should be within me!
[*She enters the stage.*]
The wind combs even the willows' hair
But neither can the wind untangle,
Nor my hand separate this hair.
[*She takes hold of her hair and looks at it.*]
Shall I rip it from my head? Throw it away?
I lift my sleeved hands—what is this?
The hair-tearing dance? How demeaning!
[*She begins to dance, in a deranged manner.*]

Chorus

As I set forth from the flowery Capital
From the flowery Capital,
At Kamo River what were those mournful cries?
The river ducks? Not knowing where I went
I crossed the river Shirakawa
And when I reached Awataguchi, I wondered,
"Whom shall I meet now at Matsuzaka?"
I thought I had yet to pass the barrier
But soon Mount Otowa fell behind me
How sad it was to leave the Capital!
Pine crickets, bell crickets, grasshoppers,
How they cried in the dusk at Yamashina!
I begged the villagers, "Don't scold me, too!"
I may be mad, but you should know
My heart is a pure rushing stream:
"When in the clear water
At Osaka Barrier
It sees its reflection

The tribute horse from Mochizuki
Will surely shy away."
Have my wanderings brought me to the same place?
In the running stream I see my reflection.
Though my own face, it horrifies me:
Hair like tangled briers crowns my head
Eyebrows blackly twist—yes, that is really
Sakagami's reflection in the water.
Water, they say, is a mirror,
But twilight ripples distort my face.

[*Sakagami sits at the stage assistant's position, indicating she has arrived at Mount Osaka. Semimaru, inside the hut, opens his fan and holds it in his left hand as if playing his lute.*]

Semimaru

The first string and the second wildly sound
The autumn wind brushes the pines and falls
With broken notes; the third string and the fourth
The fourth is myself, Semimaru,
And four are the strings of the lute I play
As sudden strings of rain drive down on me
How dreadful is this night!
"All things in life
In the end are alike;
Whether in a palace or a hovel
We cannot live forever."

[*While Semimaru is speaking Sakagami comes before the shite-pillar. Semimaru inclines his head toward her as she speaks.*]

Sakagami

How strange—I hear music from this straw-thatched hut,
The sounds of a *biwa,* elegantly plucked—
To think a hovel holds such melodies!
But why should the notes evoke this sharp nostalgia?
With steps silent, as the rain beating on the thatch
She stealthily approaches, stops and listens.

[*She silently comes to stage center. Semimaru folds his fan.*]

Semimaru

Who is there? Who's making that noise outside my hut?
Hakuga no Sammi, lately you've been coming
From time to time to visit me—is that you?

Sakagami

As I approach and listen carefully—that's the voice of my brother, the Prince!
It's Sakagami! I'm here!
Semimaru, is that you inside?

Semimaru

Can it be my sister, the Princess?

Amazed, he opens the door of his hut.

[*Taking his staff he rises and opens the door.*]

Sakagami

Oh—how wretched you look!

[*She comes up to Semimaru as he emerges from the hut.*]

Semimaru

They take each other hand in hand

[*They place their hands on each other's shoulders and kneel.*]

Sakagami

My royal brother,
is that indeed you?
Semimaru
My royal sister,
is that indeed you?

Chorus

They speak each other's names as in one voice.
Birds are also crying, here at Osaka,
Barrier of meeting—but no barrier
Holds back the tears that soak each other's sleeves.

[*Both weep. During the following passage Sakagami returns to the middle of the stage and kneels.*]

Chorus

They say that sandalwood reveals its fragrance
From the first two leaves—but how much closer still
Are we who sheltered beneath a single tree!
The wind rising in the orange blossoms
Awakens memories we shall preserve
We who flowered once on linking branches!
The love between brothers is told abroad:
Jozo and Jogen, Sori and Sokuri;
And nearer at hand, in Japan
The children of Emperor Ojin,
The princes Naniwa and Uji,
Who yielded the throne, each to the other:
All these were brothers and sisters
Bound in love, like us, like linking branches.

Sakagami

But did I imagine my brother
Would ever live in such a hovel?

Chorus

Had no music come from that straw-thatched hut
How should I have known? But I was drawn
By the music of those four strings,

Sakagami

Drawn like the water offered to the gods

Chorus

From deep wells of love and far-reaching ties.

The world may have reached its final phase
But the sun and moon have not dropped to the ground.
Things are still in their accustomed place, I thought,
But how can it be, then, that you and I
Should cast away our royalty and live like this,
Unable even to mingle with common men?
A mad woman, I have come wandering now
Far from the Capital girdled by clouds,
To these rustic scenes, a wretched beggar,
By the roads and forests, my only hope
The charity of rustics and travelers.
To think it was only yesterday you lived
In jeweled pavilions and golden halls;
You walked on polished floors and wore bright robes.
In less time than it takes to wave your sleeve,
Today a hovel is your sleeping-place.
Bamboo posts and bamboo fence, crudely fashioned
Eaves and door: straw your window, straw the roof,
And over your bed, the quilts are mats of straw:
Pretend they are your silken sheets of old.

Semimaru

My only visitors—how rarely they come—
Are monkeys on the peak, swinging in the trees;
Their doleful cries soak my sleeve with tears.
I tune my lute to the sound of the showers,
I play for solace, but tears obscure the sounds.
Even rain on the straw roof makes no noise.
Through breaks in the eaves moonlight seeps in.
But in my blindness, the moon and I are strangers.
In this hut I cannot even hear the rain—
How painful to contemplate life in this hut!
[*Both weep.*]

Sakagami

Now I must go; however long I stayed
The pain of parting never would diminish.
Farewell, Semimaru.
[*Both rise.*]

Semimaru

If sheltering under a single tree
Were our only tie, parting would still be sad;
How much sadder to let my sister go!
Imagine what it means to be alone!
[*Sakagami moves toward the shite-pillar.*]

Sakagami

Truly I pity you; even the pain
Of wandering may provide distraction,
But remaining here—how lonely it will be!
Even as I speak the evening clouds have risen,
I rise and hesitate; I stand in tears.

[*She weeps.*]

Semimaru

The evening crows call on the barrier road,
Their hearts unsettled

Sakagami

As my raven hair,
My longing unabated, I must go.

Semimaru

Barrier of Meeting, don't let her leave!

Sakagami

As I pass by the grove of cedars
[*She goes to the first pine.*]

Semimaru

Her voice grows distant . . .

Sakagami

By the eaves of the straw hut . . .

Semimaru

I stand hesitant.

Chorus

"Farewell," she calls to him, and he responds,
"Please visit me as often as you can."
[*Sakagami goes to the third pine and turns back to look at Semimaru.*]
Her voice grows faint but still he listens,
[*Sakagami starts to exit. Semimaru takes a few steps forward, stops and listens. His blind eyes gaze in her direction.*]
She turns a final time to look at him.
Weeping, weeping they have parted,
Weeping, weeping they have parted.
[*Sakagami exits, weeping. Semimaru also weeps.*]

Source: Matisoff, Susan, trans.; Keene, Donald, ed. 1970. *Semimaru: Twenty Plays of the No Theatre.* New York: Columbia University Press. Available at http://etext.lib.virginia.edu/japanese/noh/KeeSemi.html

◉ Bernard de Gordon, from *Lilium Medicinae* (1307)

Bernard de Gordon, a Scottish physician, devoted a chapter of his medical text Lilium Medicinae ("Lilies of Medicine") to the origins and treatment of leprosy. He described 11 different types of treatment for the disease; while acknowledging that the advanced form of the disease is incurable, he believed in the value of life-prolonging and palliative care. His description in this excerpt of a female patient with leprosy who was under his care indicates that at least some medieval leprosy patients did have access to medical care.

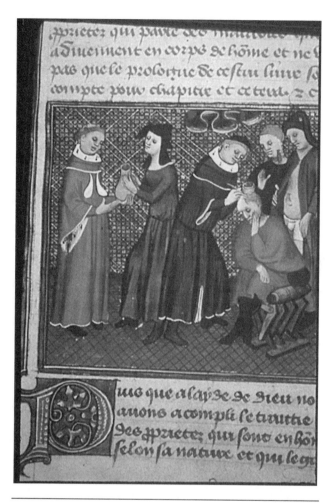

whose seed still remains in her womb. For, from coitus with a leper the woman is not infected unless she continues a long time, because of the density of the womb. But if a healthy man lies with a woman with whom a leper has lain, the leper's semen yet remaining in her womb, he will necessarily become leprous because the pores are loose in the male and the infection readily moves to the whole body. Therefore most extraordinary precaution is to be observed, and if some bad circumstance necessitates it, one should work to expel the seed from the womb by dancing, sneezing, bathing, and rinsing the womb with cleansing agents. Furthermore, such measures should be taken as far in advance as possible; and there are many other means, which need not be recited, of expelling the received semen. Without these, one should be prepared for the gourd [i.e., the beggar's cup], [life under] the stars, and everlasting disgrace. Everyone ought to guard against lying with a leprous woman, and I will tell what happened: a certain countess came leprous to Montpellier, and in the end she was under my treatment. A bachelor in medicine who attended to her, lay with her and impregnated her, and he was made completely leprous. Fortunate therefore is he who is made cautious by the dangers of others.

Source: Quoted in Holcomb, Richmond C. 1941. "The Antiquity of Congenital Syphilis." *Bulletin of the History of Medicine* 10:148–167.

Edward III, *Ordinance of Labourers* (1349)

In the Ordinance of Labourers, King Edward III attempted—unsuccessfully, as it turned out—to prevent wages from increasing because of the labor shortage caused by a recent outbreak of the bubonic plague. The ordinance is one of the first European poor laws that seeks to punish individuals for refusing to labor and return them to some form of work.

Because that many valiant beggars, as long as they may live of begging, do refuse to labor, giving themselves to idleness and vice, and sometime to theft and other abominations; none upon the said pain of imprisonment, shall under the color of pity or alms, give anything to such, which may labor, or presume to favor them towards their desires, so that thereby they may be compelled to labor for their necessary living.

Source: Edward III. 1349. *Ordinance of Labourers.* Available at http://www.britannia.com/history/ docs/ laborer1.html

Barthelemy l'Anglais, Livre des propriété des choses (Ms. 22532. France, fifteenth century). Patient giving urine sample during a medical examination. Medieval depiction of medical scrutiny of bodily fluids as mode of diagnosis and scrutiny of health.

Source: Bibliothèque Nationale, Paris. Photo credit: D.Y./Art Resource, New York.

Leprosy is either introduced from within the uterus, or after birth. If from within the uterus, it is because of conception at the time of menstruation, or because it is the child of a leper, or because a leper has had intercourse with a pregnant woman and thus the baby will be leprous, for leprosy is generated out of these great corruptions that befall the conception. If it should happen after birth, this can be because the air is bad, corrupted and pestilential, or because of prolonged use of melancholic foods, such as lentils and other legumes, and from such melancholic meats as that of foxes, bears, wild boars, hares and other quadrupeds such as asses and the like, since in some regions all wild animals are eaten. Leprosy also arises from too much company with lepers, and from coitus with a leprous woman. And also in him who lies with a woman who has lain with a leper

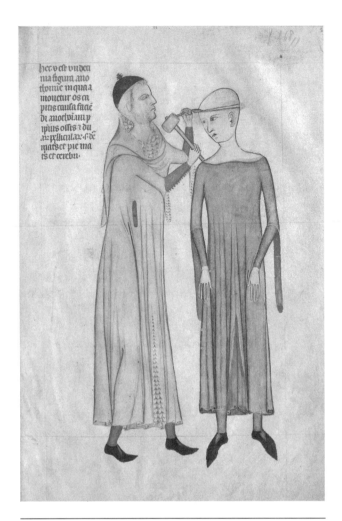

Guy de Pavia (fourteenth century), Doctor Operating on a Man's Skull (Liber notabilium Philippi septimi, francorum regis, a libris Galieni extractus, by Guy de Pavia. Italian manuscript, 1345. Ms. 333/562, fol. 11). A fourteenth-century example of medical intervention through the skull.

Source: Musée Condé, Chantilly, France. Photo credit: Giraudon/ Art Resource, New York.

▣ Saint Lidwina of Schiedam (1380–1433)

Saint Lidwina (Lydwine) lived in Schiedam (Holland). The text provides a glimpse of how illness and suffering provided a context for the experience of divine revelation. In particular, her story illustrates the strong tradition within Christianity of viewing suffering, if embraced willingly, as having the potential to lead to holiness and even to sensory experiences of God.

At the age of 15 Lidwina broke a rib while ice skating and remained bedridden for the rest of her life. She put her illness to a supernatural purpose. She was suffering voluntarily for the welfare of the Church. She fasted during this entire time when she was bedridden and was found often in ecstasy. It is interesting to note that the name Lidwina (a formalization of Lidie) comes from the Dutch word "lijden" which means to suffer. The aid of physicians were enlisted by Lidwina's parents to seek a cure for her disease. She was in intense pain, sobbed on her bed in a state of terrible abandonment, was given to constant vomiting, suffered burning fevers and could not hold down food of any kind. This situation lasted for three years . . .

Then followed a relatively blissful period but she was still confined to bed and could not get up. In the following years she still suffered greatly from abscesses, inflamed sores, and it was said she was near death twenty-two times. At the age of 28, the coldest winter ever experienced in Holland set in, when even the fish froze in the rivers, the tears she shed at night froze to her face. From the Third Order of Saint Francis in Schiedam she received a woolen shirt to wear, however she was not a member of that lay order.

Saint Lidwina . . . continued to suffer and the more she suffered, apparently, the more she was given God's Gift of contemplation and bilocation. She was given to be in two places at once, when Jesus asked her to be with him at Golgotha. In answer to His request, Lidwina replied: "O Saviour, I am ready to accompany you to that mountain and to suffer and die there with you!" (Huysmans, 1923)

"He took her with Him, and when she returned to her bed, which corporeally she had never left, they saw ulcers on her lips, wounds on her arms, the marks of thorns on her forehead and splinters on her limbs, which exhaled a very pronounced perfume of spices." A number of miraculous healings were reported. For example, Lidwina prayed for a woman, a friend of hers, who had a frightful toothache. The woman's pain ceased immediately. Also, another woman came to her to ask for her intercession for her child who was screaming with pain. When the child was placed on Lidwina's bed his troubles disappeared. When the child grew up, he became a priest in memory of Lidwina. Additional miracles continued after her death and she is not forgotten.

Source: Huysmans, J. K. 1979. *Saint Lidwina of Schiedam.* Hastings, Agnes, trans. Rockford, IL: Tan Books.

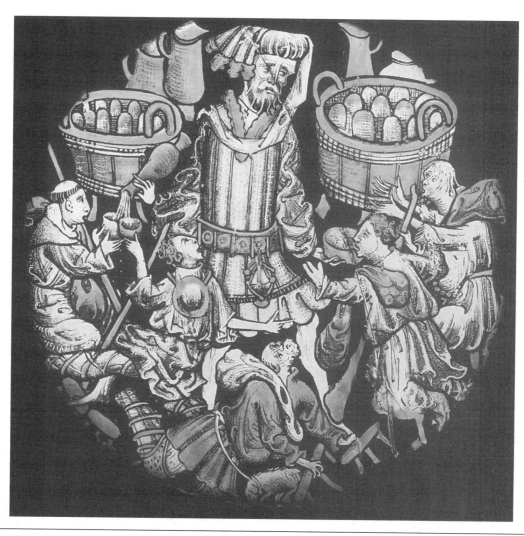

Distribution of Alms to Poor and Lame, fifteenth century. Stained glass depiction of organized efforts to give charity to disabled people unable to work or refused employment. The figure distributing help is literally mobbed by those seeking food and drink. English (Coventry?), stained glass.
Source: Victoria and Albert Museum, London. Photo credit: Victoria and Albert Museum, London/Art Resource, New York.

▣ *The Book of Margery Kempe,* Chapter 74 (ca. 1430)

Margery Kempe was a well-respected merchant-class wife and mother of 14 children in fifteenth-century England. Her comfortable position in the social hierarchy began to change, however, following the vision of Jesus she experienced after the birth of her first child. Thereafter, her increasing commitment to attaining holiness brought her into conflict with the hierarchy of her town, as her community tried to determine whether her holiness—which led her, for example, to succumb to fits of loud weeping during church services—was genuine. In the following excerpt, which echoes the selection about St. Francis of Assisi, Kempe is told by Jesus that if she truly loves him and his suffering, she must learn to overcome her revulsion from persons with leprosy. Accordingly, she visits two women with leprosy, kisses their sores, and tries to befriend and comfort them.

The sayd creatur on a day, heryng hir messe and revolvyng in hir mende the tyme of hir deth, sor syhyng and sorwyng for it was so long delayd, seyd on this maner, "Alasse, Lord, how long schal I thus wepyn and mornyn for thy lofe and for desyr of thy presens?" Owr Lord answeryd in hir sowle and seyd, "Al this fifteen yer." Than seyd sche, "A, Lord, I schal thynkyn many thowsend yerys." Owr Lord answeryd to hir, "Dowtyr, thu must bethynkyn the of my blissyd modyr that levyd aftyr me in erth fifteen yer, also Seynt John

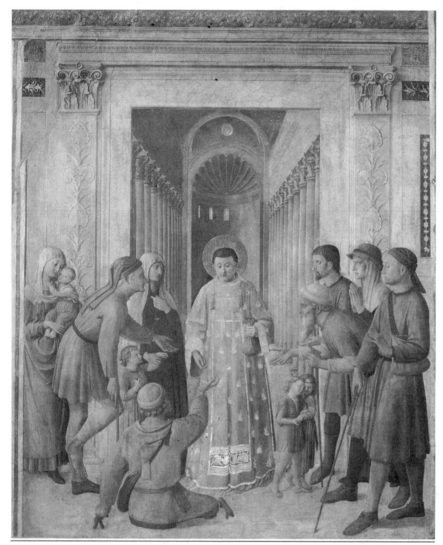

Saint Lawrence Distributing Alms to the Poor, by Fra Angelico (1387–1455). In order to thwart the greed of the prefect of Rome, who sought to raid the wealth of the church, St. Lawrence gathered up the poor and lame. On the appointed collection day he invited the prefect to accompany him to view the "wondrous riches of our God." Fresco.

Source: Cappella Niccolina, Vatican Palace, Vatican State. Photo credit: Scala/Art Resource, New York.

Lord Jhesu Crist wyth hys wowndys bledyng. And so sche dede in the syght of hir sowle, for thorw the beheldyng of the seke man hir mende was al takyn into owr Lord Jhesu Crist. Than had sche gret morning and sorwyng for sche myth not kyssyn the lazerys whan sche sey hem er met with hem in the stretys for the lofe of Jhesu. Now gan sche to lovyn that sche had most hatyd befor tyme, for ther was no thyng mor lothful ne mor abhomynabyl to hir whil sche was in the yerys of werldly prosperité than to seen er beheldyn a lazer, whom now thorw owr Lordys mercy sche desyryd to halsyn and kyssyn for the lofe of Jhesu whan sche had tyme and place convenyent. Than sche told hir confessowr how gret desyre sche had to kyssyn lazerys, and he warnyd hir that sche schulde kyssyn no men, but, yyf sche wolde algatys kyssyn, sche schuld kyssyn women. Than was sche glad, for sche had leve to kyssyn the seke women and went to a place wher seke women dwellyd whech wer ryth ful of the sekenes and fel down on hir kneys beforn hem, preyng hem that sche myth kyssyn her mowth for the lofe of Jhesu. And so sche kyssyd ther two seke women with many an holy thowt and many a devowt teer, and, whan sche had kyssyd hem and telde hem ful many good wordys and steryd hem to mekenes and pacyens that thei schulde not grutchyn wyth her sekenes but hyly thankyn God therfor and thei schulde han gret blysse in hevyn thorw the mercy of owr Lord Jhesu Crist, than the oo woman had so many temptacyons that sche wist not how sche myth best be governyd. Sche was so labowryd wyth hir gostly enmy that sche durst not blissyn hir ne do no worschep to God for dreed that the devyl schuld a slayn hir. And sche was labowryd wyth many fowle and horibyl thowtys, many mo than sche cowde tellyn. And, as sche seyd, sche was a mayde. Therfor the sayd creatur went to hir many tymys to comfortyn hir and preyd

the Evangelyst, and Mary Mawdelyn, the whech lovyd me rith hyly." "A, blysful Lord," seyd sche, "I wolde I wer as worthy to ben sekyr of thy lofe as Mary Mawdelyn was." Than seyd owr Lord, "Trewly, dowtyr, I love the as wel, and the same pes that I gaf to hir the same pes I geve to the. For, dowtyr, ther is no seynt in hevyn displesyd thow I love a creatur in erde as mech as I do hem. Therfor thei wil non otherwyse than I wil." Thus owr mercyful Lord Crist Jhesu drow hys creatur unto hys lofe and to mynde of hys passyon that sche myth not duryn to beheldyn a lazer er an other seke man, specialy yyf he had any wowndys aperyng on hym. So sche cryid and so sche wept as yyf sche had sen owr for hir, also ful specialy that God schulde strength hir ageyn hir enmye, and it is to belevyn that he dede so, blissyd mote he ben.

Source: Staley, Lynn, ed. 1996. *The Booke of Margery Kempe*. Kalamazoo, MI: Medieval Institute Publications.

▣ Sir Thomas Malory, *The Book of King Arthur and His Noble Knights of the Round Table* (ca. 1470)

In the following selection, clearly reminiscent of biblical healing accounts, we see Galahad performing two miraculous healings. This excerpt immediately follows the chapter in which Galahad and his followers were fed from the Sangreal (the Holy Grail) and thus is intended to illustrate the transmission of Jesus' healing power by means of the grail.

Book 17, Chapter 21

How Galahad Anointed with the Blood of the Spear the Maimed King, and Other Adventures

And Galahad went anon to the spear which lay upon the table, and touched the blood with his fingers, and came after to the maimed king and anointed his legs. And therewith he clothed him anon, and start upon his feet out of his bed as an whole man, and thanked Our Lord that He had healed him. And that was not to the world ward, for anon he yielded him to a place of religion of white monks, and was a full holy man. . . .

Truly, said Percivale, in the name of God, well hath my sister holden us covenant. Then took they out of the ship the table of silver, and he took it to Percivale and to Bors, to go to fore, and Galahad came behind. And right so they went to the city, and at the gate of the city they saw an old man crooked. Then Galahad called him and bade him help to bear this heavy thing. Truly, said the old man, it is ten year ago that I might not go but with crutches. Care thou not, said Galahad, and arise up and shew thy good will. And so he essayed, and found himself as whole as ever he was. Then ran he to the table, and took one part against Galahad. And anon arose there great noise in the city, that a cripple was made whole by knights marvellous that entered into the city.

Source: Eliot, Charles W., trans. 1909–1914. *The Holy Grail, by Sir Thomas Malory*. New York: P. F. Collier & Son, 1909–14.

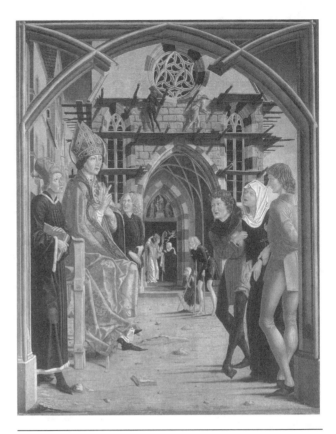

St. Wolfgang Heals the Possessed Woman Brought before Him, *by Michael Pacher (ca. 1434–1498) and Friedrich Pacher (1475–1481). In the background is the building of the church at St. Wolfgang. Closed Saint Wolfgang Altar (workday view). Examples of individuals with psychiatric disabilities were often treated as metaphysical signs of possession by the devil. In this illustration, some of the violence of exorcism is captured in the scene of restraint as the woman is dragged to the throne of St. Wolfgang.*

Source: St. Wolfgang Church, St. Wolfgang, Austria. Photo credit: Erich Lessing/Art Resource, New York.

▣ Christopher Columbus, from a Letter to Ferdinand and Isabella (1493)

In this excerpt from one of the early announcements of the "discovery" of the New World, taken from a letter to King Ferdinand and Queen Isabella of Spain, Columbus uses the absence of disease or deformity to create a utopian vision of native life on the islands around Hispaniola. In doing so, he participates in a common characteristic of European travel narrative writing, which constructs racialized societies as locations unfamiliar with conditions that ravaged Europe at the time.

The inhabitants of both sexes in this island, and in all the others which I have seen, or of which I have received information, go always naked as they were born, with the exception of some of the women, who use the covering of a leaf, or small bough, or an apron of cotton which they prepare for that purpose. None of them, as I have already said, are possessed of any iron, neither have they weapons, being unacquainted with, and indeed incompetent to use them, not from any deformity of body (for they are well-formed), but because they are timid and full of fear. They carry however in lieu of arms, canes dried in the sun, on the ends of which they fix heads of dried wood sharpened to a point, and even these they dare not use habitually; for it has often occurred when I have sent two or three of my men to any of the villages to speak with the natives, that they have come out in a disorderly troop, and have fled in

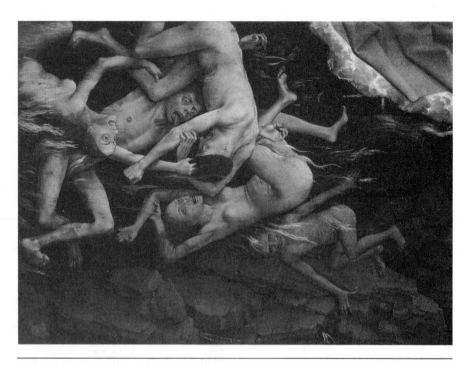

Last Judgment: Detail of the Damned in Hell, *by Rogier (Roger) van der Weyden (ca. 1399–1464). Representations of condemned individuals in the underworld often characterize them as having deformed bodies as a symbol of their torment and immorality.*

Source: Hotel-Dieu, Beaune, France. Photo credit: Giraudon/Art Resource, New York.

such haste at the approach of our men, that the fathers forsook their children and the children their fathers. This timidity did not arise from any loss or injury that they had received from us; for, on the contrary, I gave to all I approached whatever articles I had about me, such as cloth and many other things, taking nothing of theirs in return: but they are naturally timid and fearful. As soon however as they see that they are safe, and have laid aside all fear, they are very simple and honest, and exceedingly liberal with all they have; none of them refusing any thing he may possess when he is asked for it, but on the contrary inviting us to ask them.

Source: From a letter to Ferdinand and Isabella, King and Queen of Spain, in which Christopher Columbus describes his first voyage to the New World (1493). In Jehlen, Myra and Michall Warner, eds. 1997. P. 13 in *The English Literatures of America 1500–1800*. New York: Routledge.

▣ Erasmus of Rotterdam, *The Praise of Folly* (1511)

In The Praise of Folly, the Renaissance humanist Erasmus of Rotterdam used Folly (a personification of foolishness or stupidity) as the speaker in order to level real criticisms at his society. The work takes the form of a classical encomium, with Folly speaking her praise of herself, especially with reference to the many people and institutions (including governments and churches) that depend on her so much. In the selection excerpted here, Folly speaks in praise of "fools" and "madmen," but readers should keep in mind that Erasmus's heavy irony suggests anything but true praise of cognitively disabled and mentally ill individuals.

But to return to the happiness of fools, who when they have passed over this life with a great deal of pleasantness and without so much as the least fear or sense of death, they go straight forth into the Elysian field, to recreate their pious and careless souls with such sports as they used here. Let's proceed then, and compare the condition of any of your wise men with that of this fool. Fancy to me now some example of wisdom you'd set up against him; one that had spent his childhood and youth in learning the sciences and lost the sweetest part of his life in watchings, cares, studies, and for the remaining part of it never so much as tasted the least of pleasure; ever sparing, poor, sad,

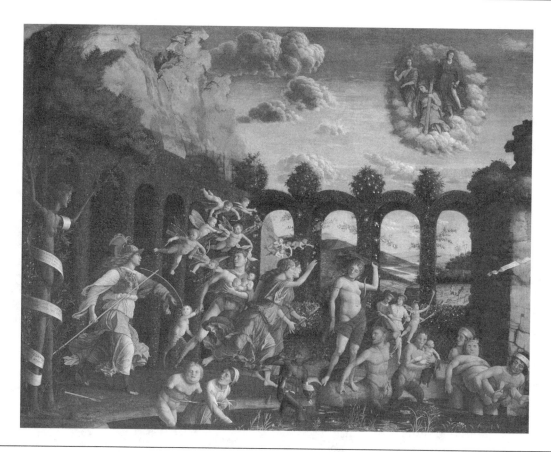

Minerva Chasing the Vices out of the Garden, *by Andreas Mantegna (1431–1506). The vices on exhibit in the lower left are identified with a variety of denigrated body types, including racialized and disability characteristics. Visual artists have often employed bodily difference as a sign of divine disfavor. Minerva, in full military regalia, dominates the scene by virtue of her own classical figure. Oil on canvas.*

Source: Louvre, Paris. Photo credit: Réunion des Musées Nationaux/Art Resource, New York.

sour, unjust, and rigorous to himself, and troublesome and hateful to others; broken with paleness, leanness, crassness, sore eyes, and an old age and death contracted before their time (though yet, what matter is it, when he die that never lived?); and such is the picture of this great wise man.

And here again do those frogs of the Stoics croak at me and say that nothing is more miserable than madness. But folly is the next degree, if not the very thing. For what else is madness than for a man to be out of his wits? But to let them see how they are clean out of the way, with the Muses' good favor we'll take this syllogism in pieces. Subtly argued, I must confess, but as Socrates in Plato teaches us how by splitting one Venus and one Cupid to make two of either, in like manner should those logicians have done and distinguished madness from madness, if at least they would be thought to be well in their wits themselves. For all madness is not miserable, or Horace had never called

his poetical fury a beloved madness; nor Plato placed the raptures of poets, prophets, and lovers among the chiefest blessings of this life; nor that sibyl in Virgil called Aeneas' travels mad labors. But there are two sorts of madness, the one that which the revengeful Furies send privily from hell, as often as they let loose their snakes and put into men's breasts either the desire of war, or an insatiate thirst after gold, or some dishonest love, or parricide, or incest, or sacrilege, or the like plagues, or when they terrify some guilty soul with the conscience of his crimes; the other, but nothing like this, that which comes from me and is of all other things the most desirable; which happens as often as some pleasing dotage not only clears the mind of its troublesome cares but renders it more jocund. And this was that which, as a special blessing of the gods, Cicero, writing to his friend Atticus, wished to himself, that he might be the less sensible of those miseries that then hung over the commonwealth.

Nor was that Grecian in Horace much wide of it, who was so far made that he would sit by himself whole days in the theatre laughing and clapping his hands, as if he had seen some tragedy acting, whereas in truth there was nothing presented; yet in other things a man well enough, pleasant among his friends, kind to his wife, and so good a master to his servants that if they had broken the seal of his bottle, he would not have run mad for it. But at last, when by the care of his friends and physic he was freed from his distemper and become his own man again, he thus expostulates with them, "Now, by Pollux, my friends, you have rather killed than preserved me in thus forcing me from my pleasure." By which you see he liked it so well that he lost it against his will. And trust me, I think they were the madder of the two, and had the greater need of hellebore, that should offer to look upon so pleasant a madness as an evil to be removed by physic; though yet I have not determined whether every distemper of the sense or understanding be to be called madness.

For neither he that having weak eyes should take a mule for an ass, nor he that should admire an insipid poem as excellent would be presently thought mad; but he that not only errs in his senses but is deceived also in his judgment, and that too more than ordinary and upon all occasions— he, I must confess, would be thought to come very near to it. As if anyone hearing an ass bray should take it for excellent music, or a beggar conceive himself a king. And yet this kind of madness, if, as it commonly happens, it turn to pleasure, it brings a great delight not only to them that are possessed with it but to those also that behold it, though perhaps they may not be altogether so mad as the other, for the species of this madness is much larger than the people take it to

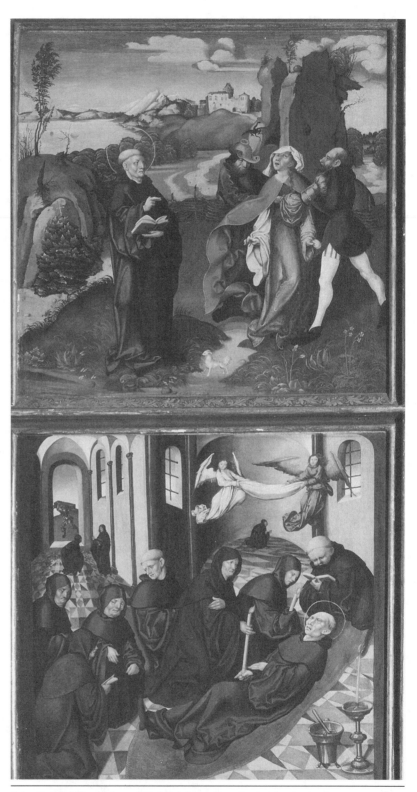

Saint Bernard Exorcising an Evil Spirit, *and* Death of Saint Bernard of Clairvaux, *by Joerg Breu, the Elder (1475–1537). Panel from the Altar of Saint Bernard. Tempera on wood. 1500, 74 × 74 cm. Another image in the long tradition of visual representations of the use of exorcism of evil spirits as an intervention for those with psychiatric conditions.*

Source: Sammlungen des Stiftes, Zwettl, Austria. Photo credit: Erich Lessing/Art Resource, New York.

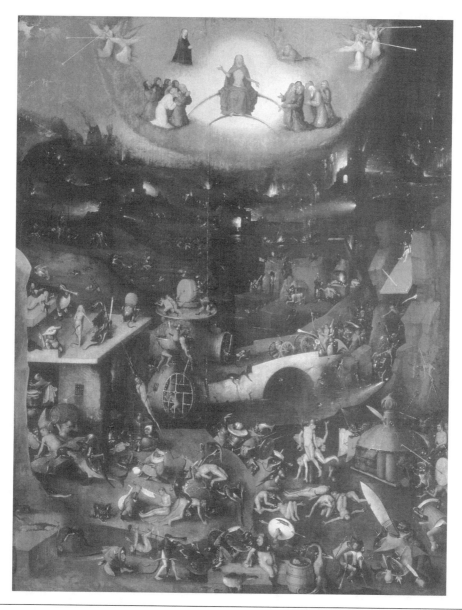

The Last Judgement *(ca. 1500), by Hieronymous Bosch (1450–1516). Central panel of triptych. Oil on oakwood, 164 × 127 cm. One of Bosch's most famous paintings, depicting the scene of judgment day as a chaos. As in the van Leyden painting on the same theme, many of the figures receiving punishment have visibly twisted, stunted, or defaced bodies that indicate their immoralilty. Disability has served as a form of artistic shorthand for human degeneration.*

Source: Akademie der Bildenden Kuenste, Vienna, Austria. Photo credit: Erich Lessing/Art Resource, New York.

be. For one mad man laughs at another, and beget themselves a mutual pleasure. Nor does it seldom happen that he that is the more mad, laughs at him that is less mad. And in this every man is the more happy in how many respects the more he is mad; and if I were judge in the case, he should be ranged in that class of folly that is peculiarly mine, which in truth is so large and universal that I scarce know anyone in all mankind that is wise at all hours, or has not some tang or other of madness.

Source: Erasmus, Desiderius. 1668. *The Praise of Folly*. John Wilson, trans. Available at http://etext.library.adelaide.edu.au/e/erasmus/praise/e65p.html

Part Two

Modernity and Normalization

◉ 1500–1800　◉ 1800–1945

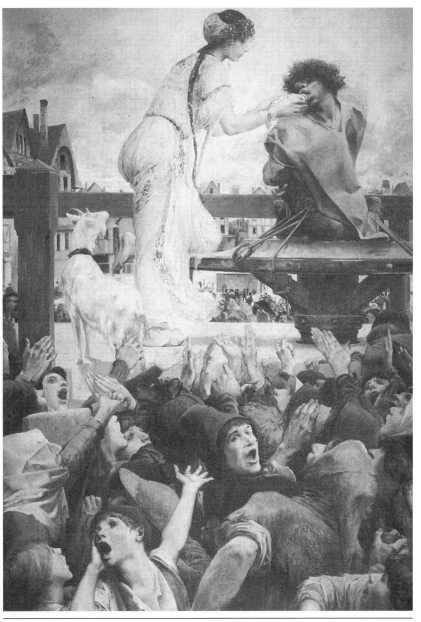

Illustration for The Hunchback of Notre Dame: *"Esmeralda Feeds Quasimodo," by Luc Olivier Merson (1846–1920). As the disabled Quasimodo is exhibited for public ridicule, the female protagonist, Esmeralda, experiences a moment of empathy and provides relief for his dehydration.*

Source: Art Resource, New York.

Modernity and Normalization: 1500–1800

▣ Busbecq on the Murder of Mustapha (1553)

The French diplomat Ogier Ghiselin de Busbecq was near at hand at the time, and soon after the event he weighed and sifted various accounts of the grim execution of Prince Mustapha and the subsequent death of Prince Jehangir to send a detailed and circumstantial report back to France. The excerpt provides a glimpse into the role played by mute servants in the sultan's court.

There was great uneasiness among the soldiers, when Mustapha arrived in the camp. He was brought to his father's tent, and there everything betokened peace. There was not a soldier on guard, no aide-de-camp, no policeman, nothing that could possibly alarm him and make him suspect treachery. But there were in the tent certain mutes—a favourite kind of servant among the Turks—strong and sturdy fellows, who had been appointed as his executioners. . . . As soon as he entered the inner tent, they threw themselves upon him, and endeavoured to put the fatal noose around his neck. Mustapha, being a man of considerable strength, made a stout defence, and fought. . . . Solyman felt how critical the matter was, being only separated by the linen hangings of his tent from the stage, on which this tragedy was being enacted. When he found that there was an unexpected delay in the execution of his scheme, he thrust out his head from the chamber of his tent, and glared on the mutes with fierce and threatening eyes; at the same time,

with signs full of hideous meaning, he sternly rebuked their slackness. Hereon the mutes, gaining fresh strength from the terror he inspired, threw Mustapha down, got the bowstring round his neck, and strangled him. [Editors' note: M. Miles (2000. "Signing in the Seraglio: Mutes, Dwarfs and Jestures at the Ottoman Court 1500–1700." *Disability & Society* 15:115–134) notes that Busbecq's original Latin reads: "at erant muti aliquot, quos Turcae habent in deliciis, validi & robustii homines, ad caedem ejus destinati" and comments that "in the translation, the word 'servant' seems to be an insertion based on the known history of service by deaf-mutes at the Ottoman court."]

Jehangir, the youngest [of Sultan Suleiman's sons] is dead. . . . The news of Mustapha's death, when it arrived at Constantinople, overwhelmed the young prince with terror and dismay. The poor lad, whose person was disfigured by a hump, had no strength of mind or body to enable him to resist the shock. . . . So great was his misery that it brought on an illness which terminated in his death.

[Editors' note: Busbecq had a good eye for local color and detail, much beyond the diplomatic scene. He may have liked to place on record his own goodness of heart in ransoming a Spanish captive, as we see in the following excerpt, yet he seems almost to admire the finely calibrated microexploitation by which a "complete cripple" could be rendered financially productive in Turkey.]

But the people who among us [i.e., in France] are beggars among them are slaves, for when a slave has lost the use of his limbs his master is still bound to maintain him; besides, however feeble a slave may be, they manage to get some service from him. I remember ransoming a Spanish gentleman, who had been an officer in his own army. Though he was completely crippled by his wounds, yet the Turk who had bought him managed to make some profit of him. He took him over to Asia, where flocks of geese are kept, and hired him out as goose-herd, by which he turned a nice little penny.

Source: Forster, C. T., and F. H. B. Daniell, ed. and trans. 1881. Vol. 1, pp. 117–118, 178–179, and 209–210 of *The Life and Letters of Ogier Ghiselin de Busbecq,* 2 Vols. London: Kegan Paul.

Albert Howe Lybyer on the Sultan Suleiman (1913)

At the Ottoman court at Istanbul in the early 1550s, power struggles were in full swing among those of the Sultan's women who had borne him sons or who had other highly placed strings to pull. When the Sultan died, the losers in such struggles could face an early death or lifelong house arrest. Further, this excerpt from a twentieth-century historian's account suggests that disability did not disqualify sons from the sultan's favor.

Roxelana had triumphed completely over the mother of Mustapha; her son-in-law Rustem, married to Suleiman's well-beloved daughter Mihrmah, had held the supreme office of grand vizier for nine years; her hump-backed son Jehangir was Suleiman's favorite child.

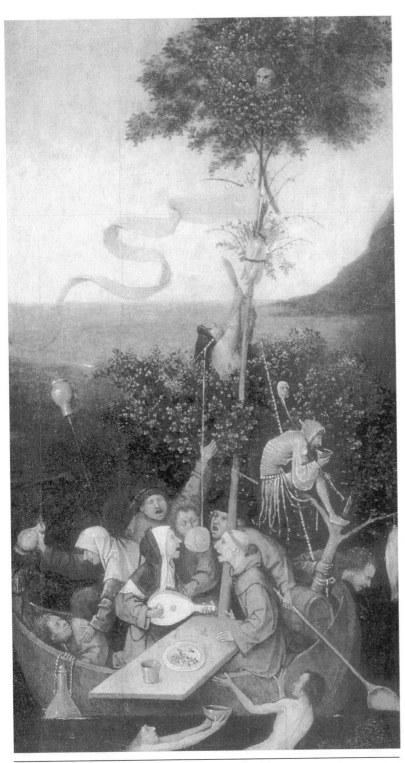

Ship of Fools, *by Hieronymous Bosch (1450–1516). The ship of fools was a method of sending those who could not or would not work away from towns and into the countryside. Here, Bosch situates authority figures in his ship instead of those considered insane, cognitively or physically disabled, or socially derelict in some other way.*

Source: Art Resource, New York.

Nevertheless, as late as the beginning of 1553 Suleiman seems to have intended still that Mustapha should occupy the throne.

Source: Lybyer, Albert Howe. 1913. P. 142 in *The Government of the Ottoman Empire in the Time of Suleiman the Magnificent.* Cambridge, MA: Harvard University Press.

◉ Bartolomej Georgijevic on the Murder of Mustapha (1569)

This report, another of the many accounts by European travel writers of the murder of Mustapha, contains a description of the sultan's fourth son, who was disabled but also recognized for his intellectual gifts.

[Speaking of Suleiman's sons] The fourth was sirnamed langir of the bunches, wher with he was both deformed before, & behinde in his backe, notwithstanding of a sharpe prudent and politike will.

Source: Georgijevic, Bartolomej, 1569. Gough, Hugh, trans. *The ofspring of the house of Ottomanno, etc.* London: Thomas Marshe.

◉ Descriptions of King James I of England (1566–1625)

King James I (he was James I of England, but James VI of Scotland), notorious persecutor of Puritans and Brownists in England, ruled with a condition similar to what would now be diagnosed as cerebral palsy. Many commentators have discussed the impact of his disability on private and public perceptions of his reign. The following excerpts demonstrate the wide range of commentary made upon his physical and psychological person by two of his contemporaries.

M. de Fontenoy, the envoy to James I's mother, reported to the secretary in 1584 that:

> His manners . . . are aggressive and very uncivil, both in speaking, eating, clothes, games . . . He never stays in one place, taking a singular pleasure in walking up and down, but his carriage is ungainly, his steps erratic and vagabond, even in his own chamber.

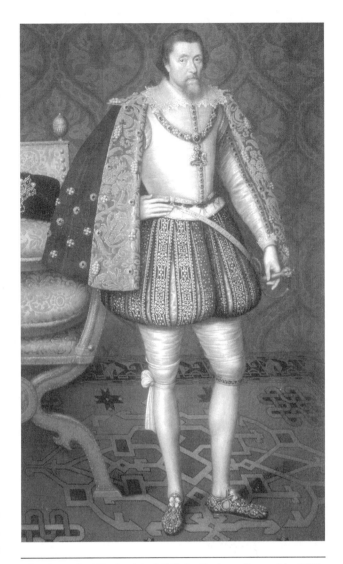

King James I of England *(c. 1619), by Paul van Somer I (c. 1576–1621). King James I, one of the persecutors of the Puritan and Brownist religious sects, had a disability akin to today's diagnosis of cerebral palsy. His disability was commonly referenced by his contemporaries—often to his detriment.*

In Anthony Weldon's book *The Court and Character of King James,* he describes James's demeanor and appearance in the following manner:

> The king's character is much easier to take than his picture, for he could never be brought to sit for the taking of that . . . He was of a middle stature, more corpulent through his cloathes than in his body, yet fat enough, his cloathes ever being made large and easie, the doublets quilted for steletto proofe, his breeches in great pleits and full stuffed: he was naturally

of a timorous disposition, which was the reason of his quilted doublets; his eyes large, ever rowling after any stranger that came in his presence, inasmuch as many for shame have left the roome, as being out of countenance; his beard was very thin: his tongue too large for his mouth, which ever made his speak full in the mouth, and made him drink very uncomely, as if eating his drink, which came out into the cup of each side of his mouth . . . his legs were very weake, having had (as was thought) some foul play in his youth, that weaknesse made him ever leaning on other mans shoulders; his walk was ever circular, his fingers ever in that walke fiddling about his codpiece.

Sources: *De Fontenay on James VI, 1584 (Aged 18 Years).* n.d. Available at: http://faculty.history.wisc.edu/sommerville/123/PF011.htm

Weldon, Anthony. 1650. *The Court and Character of King James.* London: John Wright.

◉ Ambroise Paré, from *Monsters and Marvels* (1575)

Ambroise Paré (1510–1590) was a well-recognized barber-surgeon in the courts of Charles IX, Henri III, and Catherine de Medici. In this excerpt from the opening of his work on human "monstrosity," the writer parses out distinctions between differences considered deviancy and those associated with the miraculous. In doing so, Paré created some early diagnostic categories that occupied the border between medical pathology and religious superstition.

Monsters are things that appear outside the course of Nature (and are usually signs of some forthcoming misfortune), such as a child who is born with one arm, another who will have two heads, and additional members over and above the ordinary.

Marvels are things which happen that are completely against Nature as when a woman will give birth to a serpent, or to a dog, or some other thing that is totally against Nature, as we shall show hereafter through several examples of said monsters and marvels which examples I have gathered along with the illustrations from several authors, such as the *Histories prodigieuses* of Pierre Boistuau, and from Claude Tiesserand, from Saint Paul, Saint Augustine, Esdras the Prophet, and from certain ancient philosophers, to wit from Hippocrates, Galen, Empedocles, Aristotle, Pliny, Lycosthenes, and others who will be quoted as deemed appropriate.

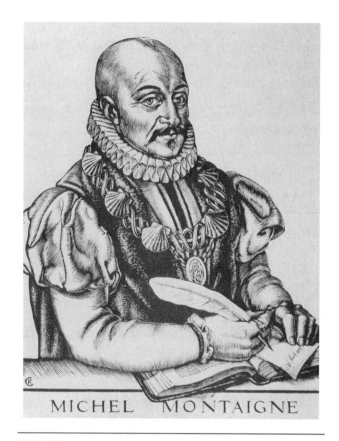

Michel de Montaigne (1533–1592) writing. Often referred to as the originator of the essay form, Montaigne wrote essays critical of the treatment of disabled people in France during the sixteenth century. He also inherited a painful gallbladder condition that resulted in a significant level of impairment.

Source: Art Resource, New York.

Maimed persons include the blind, the one-eyed, the hump-backed, those who limp or [have] arms too short, or the nose too sunken, as do the very flat-nosed; or those who have thick, inverted lips or a closure of the genitals in girls, because of the hymen; or because of a more than natural amount of flesh, or because they are hermaphrodites; or those having spots or warts or wens, or any other thing that is against Nature.

Source: Paré, Ambroise. 1982. Pallister, Janis L., trans. P. 3 in *Monsters and Marvels.* Chicago: University of Chicago Press. (Originally published 1575)

◉ Michel de Montaigne, from *Essays* (1575)

The sixteenth-century French philosopher Michel de Montaigne originated the essay form; the two essays

excerpted here show a more open-minded attitude toward disability than was common at the time. In the first excerpt, Montaigne ironically describes the many myths surrounding the sexual capacities of disabled people. He argues for a recognition that our beliefs about human differences are largely imagined and then detrimentally imposed upon individuals who appear outside of our expectations. The argument may also be a direct response to Ambroise Paré's metaphysical readings of human anomalies in Monsters and Marvels. In the second excerpt, Montaigne argues against the practice of displaying disabled children for money. His argument explicitly addresses the nonmonstrous spectacle represented by even extreme human differences while including disability in the continuum of divinely appointed diversity.

Chapter XI. Of Cripples

'Tis now two or three years ago that they made the year ten days shorter in France.—[By the adoption of the Gregorian calendar.]—How many changes may we expect should follow this reformation! it was really moving heaven and earth at once. Yet nothing for all that stirs from its place my neighbours still find their seasons of sowing and reaping, the opportunities of doing their business, the hurtful and propitious days, dust at the same time where they had, time out of mind, assigned them; there was no more error perceived in our old use, than there is amendment found in the alteration; so great an uncertainty there is throughout; so gross, obscure, and obtuse is our perception. 'Tis said that this regulation might have been carried on with less inconvenience, by subtracting for some years, according to the example of Augustus, the Bissextile, which is in some sort a day of impediment and trouble, till we had exactly satisfied this debt, the which itself is not done by this correction, and we yet remain some days in arrear: and yet, by this means, such order might be taken for the future, arranging that after the revolution of such or such a number of years, the supernumerary day might be always thrown out, so that we could not, henceforward, err above four-and-twenty hours in our computation. We have no other account of time but years; the world has for many ages made use of that only; and yet it is a measure that to this day we are not agreed upon, and one that we still doubt what form other nations have variously given to it, and what was the true use of it. What does this saying of some mean, that the heavens in growing old bow themselves down nearer towards us,

and put us into an uncertainty even of hours and days? and that which Plutarch says of the months, that astrology had not in his time determined as to the motion of the moon; what a fine condition are we in to keep records of things past.

I was just now ruminating, as I often do, what a free and roving thing human reason is. I ordinarily see that men, in things propounded to them, more willingly study to find out reasons than to ascertain truth: they slip over presuppositions, but are curious in examination of consequences; they leave the things, and fly to the causes. Pleasant talkers! The knowledge of causes only concerns him who has the conduct of things; not us, who are merely to undergo them, and who have perfectly full and accomplished use of them, according to our need, without penetrating into the original and essence; wine is none the more pleasant to him who knows its first faculties. On the contrary, both the body and the soul interrupt and weaken the right they have of the use of the world and of themselves, by mixing with it the opinion of learning; effects concern us, but the means not at all. To determine and to distribute appertain to superiority and command; as it does to subjection to accept. Let me reprehend our custom. They commonly begin thus: "How is such a thing done?" Whereas they should say, "Is such a thing done?" Our reason is able to create a hundred other worlds, and to find out the beginnings and contexture; it needs neither matter nor foundation: let it but run on, it builds as well in the air as on the earth, and with inanity as well as with matter:

"Dare pondus idonea fumo."
["Able to give weight to smoke."]

—Persius, v. 20.

I find that almost throughout we should say, "there is no such thing," and should myself often make use of this answer, but I dare not: for they cry that it is an evasion produced from ignorance and weakness of understanding; and I am fain, for the most part, to juggle for company, and prate of frivolous subjects and tales that I believe not a word of; besides that, in truth, 'tis a little rude and quarrelsome flatly to deny a stated fact; and few people but will affirm, especially in things hard to be believed, that they have seen them, or at least will name witnesses whose authority will stop our mouths from contradiction. In this way, we know the foundations and means of things that never were; and the world scuffles about a thousand questions, of which both the Pro and the Con are false.

"Ita finitima sunt falsa veris, ut in praecipitem locum non debeat se sapiens committere."

["False things are so near the true, that a wise man should not trust himself in a precipitous place."]

—Cicero, *Acad.*, ii. 21.

Truth and lies are faced alike; their port, taste, and proceedings are the same, and we look upon them with the same eye. I find that we are not only remiss in defending ourselves from deceit, but that we seek and offer ourselves to be gulled; we love to entangle ourselves in vanity, as a thing conformable to our being.

I have seen the birth of many miracles in my time; which, although they were abortive, yet have we not failed to foresee what they would have come to, had they lived their full age. 'Tis but finding the end of the clew, and a man may wind off as much as he will; and there is a greater distance betwixt nothing and the least thing in the world than there is betwixt this and the greatest. Now the first that are imbued with this beginning of novelty, when they set out with their tale, find, by the oppositions they meet with, where the difficulty of persuasion lies, and so caulk up that place with some false piece;

[Voltaire says of this passage, "He who would learn to doubt should read this whole chapter of Montaigne, the least methodical of all philosophers, but the wisest and most amiable."—*Melanges Historiques*, xvii. 694, ed. of Lefevre.]
besides that:

"Insita hominibus libido alendi de industria rumores."

["Men having a natural desire to nourish reports."]

—Livy, xxviii. 24.

we naturally make a conscience of restoring what has been lent us, without some usury and accession of our own. The particular error first makes the public error, and afterwards, in turn, the public error makes the particular one; and thus all this vast fabric goes forming and piling itself up from hand to hand, so that the remotest witness knows more about it than those who were nearest, and the last informed is better persuaded than the first.

'Tis a natural progress; for whoever believes anything, thinks it a work of charity to persuade another into the same opinion; which the better to do, he will make no difficulty of adding as much of his own invention as he conceives necessary to his tale to

encounter the resistance or want of conception he meets with in others. I myself, who make a great conscience of lying, and am not very solicitous of giving credit and authority to what I say, yet find that in the arguments I have in hand, being heated with the opposition of another, or by the proper warmth of my own narration, I swell and puff up my subject by voice, motion, vigour, and force of words, and moreover, by extension and amplification, not without some prejudice to the naked truth; but I do it conditionally withal, that to the first who brings me to myself, and who asks me the plain and bare truth, I presently surrender my passion, and deliver the matter to him without exaggeration, without emphasis, or any painting of my own. A quick and earnest way of speaking, as mine is, is apt to run into hyperbole. There is nothing to which men commonly are more inclined than to make way for their own opinions; where the ordinary means fail us, we add command, force, fire, and sword. 'Tis a misfortune to be at such a pass, that the best test of truth is the multitude of believers in a crowd, where the number of fools so much exceeds the wise:

"Quasi vero quidquam sit tam valde, quam nil sapere, vulgare."

["As if anything were so common as ignorance."]

—Cicero, *De Divin.*, ii.

"Sanitatis patrocinium est, insanientium turba."

["The multitude of fools is a protection to the wise."]

—St. Augustine, *De Civit. Dei*, vi. 10.

'Tis hard to resolve a man's judgment against the common opinions: the first persuasion, taken from the very subject itself, possesses the simple, and from them diffuses itself to the wise, under the authority of the number and antiquity of the witnesses. For my part, what I should not believe from one, I should not believe from a hundred and one: and I do not judge opinions by years.

'Tis not long since one of our princes, in whom the gout had spoiled an excellent nature and sprightly disposition, suffered himself to be so far persuaded with the report made to him of the marvellous operations of a certain priest who by words and gestures cured all sorts of diseases, as to go a long journey to seek him out, and by the force of his mere imagination, for some hours so persuaded and laid his legs asleep, as to obtain that service from them they had long time forgotten. Had fortune heaped up five or six such-like incidents, it had been enough to have brought this miracle into nature. There was afterwards discovered so much simplicity and so little art in the author of these performances, that he was thought too contemptible to be punished, as would be thought of most such things, were they well examined:

"Miramur ex intervallo fallentia."

["We admire after an interval (or at a distance) things that deceive."]

—Seneca, *Ep.*, 118, 2.

So does our sight often represent to us strange images at a distance that vanish on approaching near:

"Nunquam ad liquidum fama perducitur."

["Report is never fully substantiated."]

—Quintus Curtius, ix. 2.

'Tis wonderful from how many idle beginnings and frivolous causes such famous impressions commonly, proceed. This it is that obstructs information; for whilst we seek out causes and solid and weighty ends, worthy of so great a name, we lose the true ones; they escape our sight by their littleness. And, in truth, a very prudent, diligent, and subtle inquisition is required in such searches, indifferent, and not prepossessed. To this very hour, all these miracles and strange events have concealed themselves from me: I have never seen greater monster or miracle in the world than myself: one grows familiar with all strange things by time and custom, but the more I frequent and the better I know myself, the more does my own deformity astonish me, the less I understand myself.

The principal right of advancing and producing such accidents is reserved to fortune. Passing the day before yesterday through a village two leagues from my house, I found the place yet warm with a miracle that had lately failed of success there, where with first the neighbourhood had been several months amused; then the neighbouring provinces began to take it up, and to run thither in great companies of all sorts of people. A young fellow of the place had one night in sport counterfeited the voice of a spirit in his own house, without any other design at present, but only for sport; but this having succeeded with him better

than he expected, to extend his farce with more actors he associated with him a stupid silly country girl, and at last there were three of them of the same age and understanding, who from domestic, proceeded to public, preachings, hiding themselves under the altar of the church, never speaking but by night, and forbidding any light to be brought. From words which tended to the conversion of the world, and threats of the day of judgment (for these are subjects under the authority and reverence of which imposture most securely lurks), they proceeded to visions and gesticulations so simple and ridiculous that—nothing could hardly be so gross in the sports of little children. Yet had fortune never so little favoured the design, who knows to what height this juggling might have at last arrived? These poor devils are at present in prison, and are like shortly to pay for the common folly; and I know not whether some judge will not also make them smart for his. We see clearly into this, which is discovered; but in many things of the like nature that exceed our knowledge, I am of opinion that we ought to suspend our judgment, whether as to rejection or as to reception.

Great abuses in the world are begotten, or, to speak more boldly, all the abuses of the world are begotten, by our being taught to be afraid of professing our ignorance, and that we are bound to accept all things we are not able to refute: we speak of all things by precepts and decisions. The style at Rome was that even that which a witness deposed to having seen with his own eyes, and what a judge determined with his most certain knowledge, was couched in this form of speaking: "it seems to me." They make me hate things that are likely, when they would impose them upon me as infallible. I love these words which mollify and moderate the temerity of our propositions: "peradventure; in some sort; some; 'tis said, I think," and the like: and had I been set to train up children I had put this way of answering into their mouths, inquiring and not resolving: "What does this mean? I understand it not; it may be: is it true?" so that they should rather have retained the form of pupils at threescore years old than to go out doctors, as they do, at ten. Whoever will be cured of ignorance must confess it.

Iris is the daughter of Thaumas; [That is, of Admiration. She (Iris, the rainbow) is beautiful, and for that reason, because she has a face to be admired, she is said to have been "the daughter of Thamus."— Cicero, De Nat. Deor., iii. 20.] admiration is the foundation of all philosophy, inquisition the progress, ignorance the end. But there is a sort of ignorance, strong and generous, that yields nothing in honour and courage to knowledge; an ignorance which to conceive requires no less knowledge than to conceive knowledge itself. I read in my younger years a trial that Corras [a celebrated Calvinist lawyer, born at Toulouse; 1513, and assassinated there, 4th October 1572.], a councillor of Toulouse, printed, of a strange incident, of two men who presented themselves the one for the other. I remember (and I hardly remember anything else) that he seemed to have rendered the imposture of him whom he judged to be guilty, so wonderful and so far exceeding both our knowledge and his own, who was the judge, that I thought it a very bold sentence that condemned him to be hanged. Let us have some form of decree that says, "The court understands nothing of the matter" more freely and ingenuously than the Areopagites did, who, finding themselves perplexed with a cause they could not unravel, ordered the parties to appear again after a hundred years.

The witches of my neighbourhood run the hazard of their lives upon the report of every new author who seeks to give body to their dreams. To accommodate the examples that Holy Writ gives us of such things, most certain and irrefragable examples, and to tie them to our modern events, seeing that we neither see the causes nor the means, will require another sort-of wit than ours. It, peradventure, only appertains to that sole all-potent testimony to tell us. "This is, and that is, and not that other." God ought to be believed; and certainly with very good reason; but not one amongst us for all that who is astonished at his own narration (and he must of necessity be astonished if he be not out of his wits), whether he employ it about other men's affairs or against himself.

I am plain and heavy, and stick to the solid and the probable, avoiding those ancient reproaches:

> "Majorem fidem homines adhibent iis, quae
> non intelligunt;
> —Cupidine humani ingenii libentius obscura
> creduntur."

["Men are most apt to believe what they least understand: and from the acquisitiveness of the human intellect, obscure things are more easily credited." The second sentence is from Tacitus, *Hist.* 1. 22.]

I see very well that men get angry, and that I am forbidden to doubt upon pain of execrable injuries; a new way of persuading! Thank God, I am not to be cuffed into belief. Let them be angry with those who

accuse their opinion of falsity; I only accuse it of difficulty and boldness, and condemn the opposite affirmation equally, if not so imperiously, with them. He who will establish this proposition by authority and huffing discovers his reason to be very weak. For a verbal and scholastic altercation let them have as much appearance as their contradictors;

> "Videantur sane, non affirmentur modo;"

["They may indeed appear to be; let them not be affirmed (Let them state the probabilities, but not affirm.)"]

—Cicero, *Acad.*, n. 27.

but in the real consequence they draw from it these have much the advantage. To kill men, a clear and strong light is required, and our life is too real and essential to warrant these supernatural and fantastic accidents.

As to drugs and poisons, I throw them out of my count, as being the worst sort of homicides: yet even in this, 'tis said, that men are not always to rely upon the personal confessions of these people; for they have sometimes been known to accuse themselves of the murder of persons who have afterwards been found living and well. In these other extravagant accusations, I should be apt to say, that it is sufficient a man, what recommendation soever he may have, be believed as to human things; but of what is beyond his conception, and of supernatural effect, he ought then only to be believed when authorised by a supernatural approbation. The privilege it has pleased Almighty God to give to some of our witnesses, ought not to be lightly communicated and made cheap. I have my ears battered with a thousand such tales as these: "Three persons saw him such a day in the east three, the next day in the west: at such an hour, in such a place, and in such habit"; assuredly I should not believe it myself. How much more natural and likely do I find it that two men should lie than that one man in twelve hours' time should fly with the wind from east to west? How much more natural that our understanding should be carried from its place by the volubility of our disordered minds, than that one of us should be carried by a strange spirit upon a broomstaff, flesh and bones as we are, up the shaft of a chimney? Let not us seek illusions from without and unknown, we who are perpetually agitated with illusions domestic and our own. Methinks one is pardonable in disbelieving a miracle, at least, at all events where one can elude its verification as such, by means not miraculous; and

I am of St. Augustine's opinion, that, "'tis better to lean towards doubt than assurance, in things hard to prove and dangerous to believe."

'Tis now some years ago that I travelled through the territories of a sovereign prince, who, in my favour, and to abate my incredulity, did me the honour to let me see, in his own presence, and in a private place, ten or twelve prisoners of this kind, and amongst others, an old woman, a real witch in foulness and deformity, who long had been famous in that profession. I saw both proofs and free confessions, and I know not what insensible mark upon the miserable creature: I examined and talked with her and the rest as much and as long as I would, and gave the best and soundest attention I could, and I am not a man to suffer my judgment to be made captive by prepossession. In the end, and in all conscience, I should rather have prescribed them hellebore than hemlock;

> "Captisque res magis mentibus, quam conscel-eratis similis visa;"

> ["The thing was rather to be attributed to madness, than malice." ("The thing seemed to resemble minds possessed rather than guilty.")]

> —Livy, viii, 18.

justice has its corrections proper for such maladies. As to the oppositions and arguments that worthy men have made to me, both there, and often in other places, I have met with none that have convinced me, and that have not admitted a more likely solution than their conclusions. It is true, indeed, that the proofs and reasons that are founded upon experience and fact, I do not go about to untie, neither have they any end; I often cut them, as Alexander did the Gordian knot. After all, 'tis setting a man's conjectures at a very high price upon them to cause a man to be roasted alive.

We are told by several examples, as Praestantius of his father, that being more profoundly, asleep than men usually are, he fancied himself to be a mare, and that he served the soldiers for a sumpter; and what he fancied himself to be, he really proved. If sorcerers dream so materially; if dreams can sometimes so incorporate themselves with effects, still I cannot believe that therefore our will should be accountable to justice; which I say as one who am neither judge nor privy councillor, and who think myself by many degrees unworthy so to be, but a man of the common sort, born and avowed to the obedience of the public reason, both in its words and acts. He who should record my idle talk as being to the prejudice of the pettiest law, opinion, or custom of his parish, would do himself a great deal of wrong, and me much more; for, in what I say, I warrant no other certainty, but that 'tis what I had then in my thought, a tumultuous and wavering thought. All I say is by way of discourse, and nothing by way of advice:

> "Nec me pudet, ut istos fateri nescire, quod nesciam;"

> ["Neither am I ashamed, as they are, to confess my ignorance of what I do not know."]

> —Cicero, *Tusc.* Quaes., i. 25.

I should not speak so boldly, if it were my due to be believed; and so I told a great man, who complained of the tartness and contentiousness of my exhortations. Perceiving you to be ready and prepared on one part, I propose to you the other, with all the diligence and care I can, to clear your judgment, not to compel it. God has your hearts in His hands, and will furnish you with the means of choice. I am not so presumptuous even as to desire that my opinions should bias you—in a thing of so great importance: my fortune has not trained them up to so potent and elevated conclusions. Truly, I have not only a great many humours, but also a great many opinions, that I would endeavour to make my son dislike, if I had one. What, if the truest are not always the most commodious to man, being of so wild a composition?

Whether it be to the purpose or not, 'tis no great matter: 'tis a common proverb in Italy, that he knows not Venus in her perfect sweetness who has never lain with a lame mistress. Fortune, or some particular incident, long ago put this saying into the mouths of the people; and the same is said of men as well as of women; for the queen of the Amazons answered the Scythian who courted her to love, "Lame men perform best." In this feminine republic, to evade the dominion of the males, they lamed them in their infancy—arms, legs, and other members that gave them advantage over them, and only made use of them in that wherein we, in these parts of the world, make use of them. I should have been apt to think; that the shuffling pace of the lame mistress added some new pleasure to the work, and some extraordinary titillation to those who were at the sport; but I have lately learnt that ancient philosophy has itself determined it, which says that the legs and thighs of lame women, not receiving, by reason of their imperfection, their due aliment, it falls out that the genital parts above are fuller and better supplied and much more vigorous; or else that this defect, hindering exercise, they who are troubled with it less dissipate their strength, and come more entire to the sports of Venus; which also is the reason why the Greeks decried the women-weavers as being more hot than other women by reason of their sedentary trade, which they carry on without any great exercise of the body. What is it we may not reason of at this rate? I might also say of these, that the jaggling about whilst so sitting at work, rouses and provokes their desire, as the swinging and jolting of coaches does that of our ladies.

Do not these examples serve to make good what I said at first: that our reasons often anticipate the effect, and have so infinite an extent of jurisdiction that they judge and exercise themselves even on inanity itself and non-existency? Besides the flexibility of our invention to forge reasons of all sorts of dreams, our imagination is equally facile to receive impressions of falsity by very frivolous appearances; for, by the sole authority of the ancient and common use of this proverb, I have formerly made myself believe that I have had more pleasure in a woman by reason she was not straight, and accordingly reckoned that deformity amongst her graces.

Torquato Tasso, in the comparison he makes betwixt France and Italy, says that he has observed that our legs are generally smaller than those of the Italian gentlemen, and attributes the cause of it to our being continually on horseback; which is the very same cause from which Suetonius draws a quite opposite conclusion; for he says, on the contrary, that Germanicus had made his legs bigger by the continuation of the same exercise.

Nothing is so supple and erratic as our understanding; it is the shoe of Theramenes, fit for all feet. It is double and diverse, and the matters are double and diverse too. "Give me a drachm of silver," said a Cynic philosopher to Antigonus. "That is not a present befitting a king," replied he. "Give me then a talent," said the other. "That is not a present befitting a Cynic."

> "Seu plures calor ille vias et caeca relaxat
> Spiramenta, novas veniat qua succus in herbas
> Seu durat magis, et venas astringit hiantes;
> Ne tenues pluviae, rapidive potentia colic
> Acrior, aut Boreae penetrabile frigus adurat."

["Whether the heat opens more passages and secret pores through which the sap may be derived into the new-born herbs; or whether it rather hardens and binds the gaping veins that the small showers and keen influence of the violent sun or penetrating cold of Boreas may not hurt them."]

—*Virg., Georg., i. 89.*

"Ogni medaglia ha il suo rovescio."

["Every medal has its reverse."—Italian Proverb.]

This is the reason why Clitomachus said of old that Carneades had outdone the labours of Hercules, in having eradicated consent from men, that is to say, opinion and the courage of judging. This so vigorous fancy of Carneades sprang, in my opinion, anciently from the impudence of those who made profession of knowledge and their immeasurable self-conceit. AEsop was set to sale with two other slaves; the buyer asked the first of these what he could do; he, to enhance his own value, promised mountains and marvels, saying he could do this and that, and I know not what; the second said as much of himself or more: when it came to AEsop's turn, and that he was also asked what he could do; "Nothing," said he, "for these two have taken up all before me; they know everything." So has it happened in the school of philosophy: the pride of those who attributed the capacity of all things to the human mind created in others, out of despite and emulation, this opinion, that it is capable of nothing: the one maintain the same extreme in ignorance that the others do in knowledge; to make it undeniably manifest that man is immoderate throughout, and can never stop but of necessity and the want of ability to proceed further.

Chapter XXX. Of a Monstrous Child

This story shall go by itself; for I will leave it to physicians to discourse of. Two days ago I saw a child that two men and a nurse, who said they were the father, the uncle, and the aunt of it, carried about to get money by showing it, by reason it was so strange a creature. It was, as to all the rest, of a common form, and could stand upon its feet; could go and gabble much like other children of the same age; it had never as yet taken any other nourishment but from the nurse's breasts, and what, in my presence, they tried to put into the mouth of it, it only chewed a little and spat it out again without swallowing; the cry of it seemed indeed a little odd and particular, and it was just fourteen months old. Under the breast it was joined to another child, but without a head, and which had the spine of the back without motion, the rest entire; for though it had one arm shorter than the other, it had been broken by accident at their birth; they were joined breast to breast, and as if a lesser child sought to throw its arms about the neck of one something bigger. The juncture and thickness of the place where they were conjoined was not above four fingers, or thereabouts, so that if you thrust up the imperfect child you might see the navel of the other below it, and the joining was betwixt the paps and the navel. The navel of the imperfect child could not be seen, but all the rest of the belly, so that all that was not joined of the imperfect one, as arms, buttocks, thighs, and legs, hung dangling upon the other, and might reach to the mid-leg. The nurse, moreover, told us that it urined at both bodies, and that the members of the other were nourished, sensible, and in the same plight with that she gave suck to, excepting that they were shorter and less. This double body and several limbs relating to one head might be interpreted a favourable prognostic to the king,—[Henry III.]—of maintaining these various parts of our state under the union of his laws; but lest the event should prove otherwise, 'tis better to let it alone, for in things already past there needs no divination,

"Ut quum facts sunt, tum ad conjecturam aliqui interpretatione revocentur;"

["So as when they are come to pass, they may then by some interpretation be recalled to conjecture."]

—Cicero, *De Divin.*, ii. 31.

as 'tis said of Epimenides, that he always prophesied backward.

I have just seen a herdsman in Medoc, of about thirty years of age, who has no sign of any genital parts; he has three holes by which he incessantly voids his water; he is bearded, has desire, and seeks contact with women.

Those that we call monsters are not so to God, who sees in the immensity of His work the infinite forms that He has comprehended therein; and it is to be believed that this figure which astonishes us has relation to some other figure of the same kind unknown to man. From His all wisdom nothing but good, common; and regular proceeds; but we do not discern the disposition and relation:

"Quod crebro videt, non miratur, etiamsi, cur fiat, nescit. Quod ante non vidit, id, si evenerit, ostentum esse censet."

["What he often sees he does not admire, though he be ignorant how it comes to pass. When a thing happens he never saw before, he thinks that it is a portent."]

—Cicero, *De Divin.*, ii. 22.

Whatever falls out contrary to custom we say is contrary to nature, but nothing, whatever it be, is contrary to her. Let, therefore, this universal and natural reason expel the error and astonishment that novelty brings along with it.

Source: Cotton, Charles, trans., and William Carew Hazlitt, ed. 1877. *The Essays of Montaigne.* Available at: http://www.gutenberg.org/files/3598/old/mn18v10.txt (Chapter XI) and http://www.gutenberg.org/files/3592/old/mn12v10.txt (Chapter XXX).

◉ William Shakespeare, from *Richard III* (ca. 1591–1594)

Shakespeare's rendition of the story of King Richard III, often cited as the first "modern" protagonist, uses his torment by others on the basis of his disability as the impetus for courtly intrigue and brutal murder. The excerpt here is from his famous opening monologue, in which the future usurper of the throne of the two young heirs of King Edward IV contemplates his exclusion from peacetime merrymaking on the basis of his "deformities."

Act I, Scene i, Lines 1–40

London. A street. Enter Richard, Duke of Gloucester, solus

Gloucester:

Now is the winter of our discontent
Made glorious summer by this sun of York;
And all the clouds that lowered upon our house
In the deep bosom of the ocean buried.
Now are our brows bound with victorious wreaths,
Our bruised arms hung up for monuments,
Our stern alarums changed to merry meetings,
Our dreadful marches to delightful measures.
Grim-visaged war hath smoothed his wrinkled front,
And now, instead of mounting barbed steeds
To fright the souls of fearful adversaries,
He capers nimbly in a lady's chamber

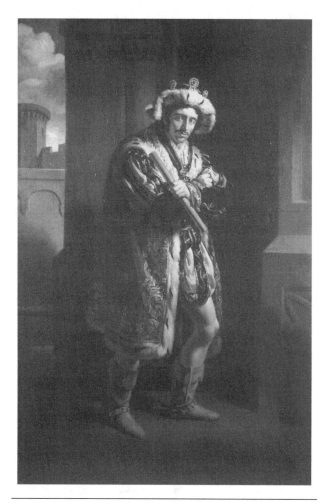

Edmund Kean as Richard III, *by John James Halls (19th c.). The renowned early nineteenth-century actor here portrays Shakespeare's Richard III, the "hump-backed king," as a physically deformed usurper of the British throne. The performance of the disabled avenger became one of the most commonly staged plays in Shakespeare's repertoire, and generations of actors have approached the dramatic role as a question of "to limp or not to limp."*

Source: Art Resource, New York.

To the lascivious pleasing of a lute.
But I, that am not shaped for sportive tricks
Nor made to court an amorous looking-glass;
I, that am rudely stamped, and want love's majesty
To strut before a wanton ambling nymph;
I, that am curtailed of this fair proportion,
Cheated of feature by dissembling nature,
Deformed, unfinished, sent before my time
Into this breathing world scarce half made up,
And that so lamely and unfashionable
That dogs bark at me as I halt by them—
Why I, in this weak piping time of peace,
Have no delight to pass away the time,
Unless to spy my shadow in the sun

And descant on mine own deformity
And therefore, since I cannot prove a lover
To entertain these fair well-spoken days,
I am determined to prove a villain
And hate the idle pleasures of these days.
Plots have I laid, inductions dangerous,
By drunken prophecies, libels, and dreams,
To set my brother Clarence and the king
In deadly hate the one against the other;
And if King Edward be as true and just
As I am subtle, false, and treacherous,
This day should Clarence closely be mewed up
About a prophecy which says that G
Of Edward's heirs the murderer shall be.

◉ Richard Wragg on the Ottoman Court (1590s)

The following excerpts from Mayes's book are based on the reports of Richard Wragg, the secretary to Edward Barton. In the autumn of 1593, Edward Barton, the Ambassador of Queen Elizabeth to the Ottoman Court, had been insulted by the acting Grand Vizier Ferhad Pasha. To bring this to the attention of Sultan Murad III, Barton adopted the local expedient of standing up in a boat near the seaside mosque where the Sultan went to pray.

1593 (Sept.) "Presently a dwarf who had helped Barton on other occasions beckoned to him to come to the shore" (P. 56). Later, when the Queen's presents to the Sultan were displayed, "The courtyard was crowded with dumb men and dwarfs," and Barton and his retinue "moved slowly through the exotic crowd of eunuchs, dwarfs and mutes till they came level with the kiosk" where the Sultan was seated (P. 58).

[Editors' note: After the death of Murad III and the accession of Sultan Mehmet III in 1595, there were great changes among the courtiers. To have any access to the Sultan, the European ambassadors were obliged to start again and make new contacts.]

1595 [After the death of Murad III and the accession of Sultan Mehmet III,] "There were changes among the pashas. Even the eunuchs, the dwarfs and the women of the harem he [Barton] had used in his diplomatic game were now swept away to the Old Seraglio like so much lumber" (P. 63).

Source: Mayes, Stanley. 1956. Pp. 54–63 in *An Organ for the Sultan.* London: Putnam.

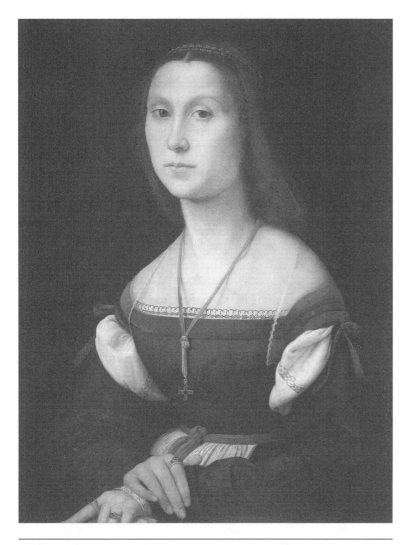

The Mute Woman, *by Raphael (1483–1520). Raphael, who included disabled figures in many of his works, identifies this woman as "mute" to deepen her mystery.*

Source: Art Resource, New York.

▣ John Sanderson's Travels in Constantinople (Late 16th c.)

In 1594, the year before Sultan Murad III died, the English traveler John Sanderson gleaned some statistics about people living in Constantinople (Istanbul). The total population was believed to be 1,231,207. The dwarfs and "dumb" men were listed among people offering various services:

1594 In Constantinople ar resident:

Solacks [*solaq*], his footemen 300

Falconers, dwarfs, and dome [i.e., dumb] men 300

Whores of all sorts, at least 1000

[Total] 1,231,207 (P. 82)

1595 (25 Jan.) Sultan Murad deceased the 7th of this moneth and was buryed the same day his sonne Sultan Mahemett arived, which was the 17th. That day his 19 sonns weare strangoled in thier brothers presence. . . . The 4 muti (thoughe by commandement) which murtherd them weare also strangoled. (P. 141)

1600 [After describing executions by impaling.] They strangle with a bowestring thier bretherin, bassaies, and other great men. (P. 87) [Footnote text: "Meaning the Sultan's brethren."]

[Editors' note: Sanderson remarked on the Grand Signior (the Sultan), the Bustanji bashi (Chief Gardener), and the Sultan's use of water transport on State barges (*qayiq* or caike).]

This Bustangiebassi is a man of accompt about the Turke, and the great (but not the common) executioner; for the Turke imploy{s} him in strangling viceroyes, throwing by night rebelliouse soldiers into the sea, and sutchlike. Chefe gardner is his office, havinge thowsands [of] jamoglaines and thier governors at his commaund. He kepethe the caikes, and always steereth when the Great Turke goeth uppon the water. . . . His [the Sultan's] court of dwarfs and dum men always folowe (except the very principall, who ar with him) in another caike; and many times also his women. (P. 89)

Source: Sanderson, John. 1931. Foster, William, ed. *The Travels of John Sanderson in the Levant 1584-1602 with His Autobiography and Selections from His Correspondence.* London: Hakluyt Society.

▣ Thomas Dallam, Account of an Organ Carryed to the Grand Seignor (1599)

Visiting the court of the Emperor Mehmet III at Constantinople, Thomas Dallam recorded a dazzling scene at the Sultan's court on September 25, 1599. An organ with chiming clock and mobile figures, designed and assembled by Dallam and his team on the orders of Queen Elizabeth, had been shipped to Constantinople and shown to the Sultan, with Dallam waiting outside. The organ was set to chime and play automatically, and the mobile figures had been through their motions, including a bush with birds that sang and opened their wings. The Sultan was pleased. He asked why the organ keys moved though nobody was playing them, and learned that the organ could be played using these keys. Dallam was brought in to demonstrate. He spent some minutes dazzled by the array of courtiers, among whom were 100 "dumb" men and 100 dwarfs, extremely short but thickset. Dallam was most impressed by the "dumb" men's sign language.

The Grand Sinyor satt still, behouldinge the presente which was befor him, and I stood daslinge my eyes with loukinge upon his people that stood behinde him, the which was four hundrethe persons in number.

Tow hundrethe of them weare his princepall padgis, the yongest of them 16 yeares of age, som 20, and som 30. They weare apparled in ritche clothe of goulde made in gowns to the mydlegge; . . . Those 200 weare all verrie proper men, and Christians borne. [They were slaves taken from Christian families of the empire. Some had become Muslims.]

The thirde hundrethe weare Dum men, that could nether heare nore speake, and theye weare likwyse in gouns of riche Clothe of gould and Cordivan buskins; . . . Som of them had haukes in theire fistes.

The fourthe hundrethe weare all dwarffs, bige-bodied men, but verrie low of stature. Everie Dwarfe did weare a simmeterrie (scimitar) by his side, and they weare also apareled in gowns of Clothe of gould.

I did moste of all wonder at those dumb men, for they lett me understande by theire perfitt sins (signs) all thinges that they had sene the presente dow by its motions.

Source: Bent, J. Theodore, ed. 1893. *Early Voyages and Travels in the Levant I. The Diary of Master Thomas Dallam 1599–1600.* London: Hakluyt Society.

▣ Stories from the *Ebisu Mandara* (ca. 1600–1950s)

The excerpts below represent brief biographies of notable Japanese disabled people, with some discussion of the occupations traditionally assigned to disabled people. They are intended as a beginning effort to construct a history of disabled people in Japan. The majority of these materials derive from the mythological figure Hiruko to the 1950s. Stories suggest that the disabled and rejected Hiruko was "rehabilitated" in popular imagination as Ebisu, the Japanese god of good fortune and fishermen. The texts are by a well-known writer, himself disabled.

6. Foster Parents of Iwakura

There is a piece of Haiku poem by famous poet Buson Yosano in the middle of the Edo period (1600–1868): "In Iwakura, Fall in Love Mad Women, Little Cuckoo." [It is] a fantastic work matching impending voice of little cuckoo and passionate love of women. There might be many cuckoos in villages of northern Kyoto in mountains leading to Mt. Kurama. There was a special relation between the place Iwakura and mad women, that is to say, those who became insane, suffered neurosis, or dementia. It went back some hundreds years, from the time the poem was composed in the Heian period (794–1185). Once a noble woman had a nervous breakdown but completely recovered by standing under the waterfall of Iwakura. The rumor spread out. More nobles visited Iwakura. Some brought children who were mentally retarded. However, they could not expect prompt recovery. The nobles asked nearby families to take care of these children for a long period, then some of them finally arranged adoption for lifelong care taking. Such a custom continued for more than one thousand years. Those families who adopted the children could expect good protection by the aristocracy.

8. Throng!! Japanese Gypsy

The gypsy is famous in Europe. In Japan also there were supposedly people who lived like them. [These were] aborigines who were subjugated, relatives of a ruling clan that had been defeated, driven away from their homeland, started a wandering life. Among them, it seems there were singers and players of flutes, drums, Chinese fiddles, biwa (lute) to earn the daily food; also Prologue Speaker for the drama, clowns to crack jokes, acrobats of tight-rope walking. It could be a lively group. Such a group was named Kugutsu. There is evidence that blind people and so-called midgets and hunchbacks showed their unique arts in the group. They might be original members, others might join asking protection after leaving villages due to difficulties to engage in agriculture or fishery with physical disability. According to legend, Yoshitsune Minamoto hid among the throng of Kugutsu when he went from Mount Kurama to Oshu by stealth.

9. Founder of Biwa by the Blind Semimaru

Oosaka no seki is the first checkpoint from Kyoto (capital city in those days) to eastern cities, going down from Higashiyama (East Mount) to Omi, [a] famous place from ancient days. Its name 'Oosaka' has connotation of 'hope to meet again', along with sorrow of parting. In the mount Oosaka near the checkpoint, word had spread that [an] exquisite melody was heard every night, nobody knew from what time. Whether it was the pastime of a Tengu (long-nosed goblin) or god of the mount, once people listened they were fascinated with the music. One full moon night it turned out who it was. A master hand of cross flute from the capital encountered a blind person playing biwa (lute) sitting on a rock facing [the] river. He gave only the name Semimaru, supposed to be [a] court servant or the fourth prince of the Emperor Daigo. The flute musician visited Mount Oosaka every night afterwards, [and] eventually was initiated the secret tune of biwa Ryusen Takuboku according to the record. The story was disseminated all over the country, reportedly, and many blind people [and] aspiring musicians came to ask lectures. Biwa, once monopolized by the aristocracy, was thus popularized by the blind.

10. Caretaking and Camping Car

The Kamakura period (1185–1333) was one of the periods when religion in Japan was most prosperous. New schools not only for the nobles but for general public appeared one after another. Nichirenshu school and Jodoshinshu school were among them, [and] Jishu school by Ippen shonin (a holy priest) was representative one. At this school was performed Odori Nenbutsu (dance and chant Buddhist prayer), which may have had power to induce people into religious ecstasy. He advocated Buddhist prayer throughout Japan, and was accompanied by [a] good many people. Ippen shonin hijiri-e (holy pictures of Ippen shonin) and Ippen shonin e-den (picture of life of Ippen shonin) are scrolls with paintings describing his life and we can see such scenes in them. Among various people there were persons with different impairments. Some seem to be on boards with small wooden

wheels, some use wooden getas (clogs) on their hands. . . . Moreover there was also a person whose female caretaker provided him with foods. It is interesting that a hut with wheels appeared also. In modern terms it is camping car. We can only guess how it was used but it is probable that the wheeled hut is for the sick and the disabled.

11. Foundation of Kengyo System—Akashi Kengyo

The Conflict of South and North Courts was the turbulent period when warriors and people throughout the country were split between the South Court of Yoshino and the North Court of Kyoto and battled in many regions. However, everybody alike wished the union of Japan, peace as the result of victory of one's own side. The Taiheiki (Record of Peace) is a full-length piece dealing with the riotous time, whose title seems to express such a wish better than its content. In those days, there was a man who unified the world regardless of military power, authority, hatred and betrayal, then firmly built up his position. It was Kengyo AKASHI (the Kengyo was a blind official responsible for welfare of blind people). He was an excellent player of Heike biwa (chanting of Heike warrior tales, with elements of courtly and religious music, which blind monks played on the lute), and began Ichikata School after unifying several schools existing in each region. He also put various narrations of Heike monogatari (Stories of Taira Clan) together. His reputation spread irrespective of South and North Courts, and his followers increased. He played at both courts when invited. Finally he was awarded a purple [permit?] [bowl?] as proof that he could go to the courts whenever he liked. Thus he founded the basis of Kengyo system for all blind people.

12. Prominent Activity of Biwa Hoshi (Lute-Playing Buddhist Friar)

There are magnificent dramas of prosperity and vicissitudes between Genji (Minamoto Clan) and Heik (Taira Clan), as almost all Japanese people know. They include episodes of Yoshitsune and Benkei at Gojo bridge, a folding fun target of Yoichi Nasu, a flute of Aoba and the death Atsumori, sincere loves of Tomoe Gogen, Heike Clan submerged themselves into the sea of Dannoura. Heroic battles and beautiful love stories scattered among them. It was blind biwa hoshi who popularized and let the original work Heike

Monogatari (Stories of Heike Clan) sink deeply into people's minds. They earned their daily food by narrating each paragraph of stories accompanied with the much-loved biwa at cities or on occasion of festive days of shrines and temples in front of many people. Without such activities of wandering from place to place and reciting them, the melancholic stories might not have been so widely known all over Japan. It was also those biwa hoshi that added flavour and made them more sophisticated while chanting. Those biwa hoshi appear often in literature of [the] Muromachi period (1333–1568), [and] also in well-known Choju Giga (Comic of birds and animals).

13. Strategists in the Age of Wars

Kansuke Yamamoto, the brains of the invincible Takeda army, reportedly was in reality a man who dragged his shorter leg, missing one of [his] eyes, with innumerable wounds on body, small and ugly. As he made himself the tactician of a feudal lord, after he had come adrift from another region, we can infer how intelligent he must have been. By the way, Hideyoshi Toyotomi who later obtained the ruling power of Japan, had the No. 1 strategist of the age, Hanbei Takenaka beside him. He was said to be worthy of aiming at the whole country. He suffered from a disease in the chest and planned recuperative life, then changed his mind, moved by passion of Hideyoshi even [if] it might shorten his lifespan. These two passed away accomplishing their purpose of life; on the other hand, Josui Kuroda (Kanbei) lived long and left a prosperous family behind him. Once [when] he was confined in the Itami Castle when he visited there as messenger of Hideyoshi, one of his knees became unstretchable. They say that he took the command of battles at the front line on a palanquin carried on [the] shoulders of subjects. There were other men, Kiyomasa Kato and Ukon Takayama, some say that they had suffered Hansen's disease (leprosy). The age of wars produced many disabled people, sacrificed their lives, but on other hand, even disabled people were given some importance depending on their ability.

15. The Blind with Shamisen at Hand

Now [the] shamisen is regarded as one of the most popular music instrument[s] but it was originally jabisen (lute using skin of snake) of Ryukyu (now

Okinawa) that was introduced at the end of Muromachi period (1333–1568). Like various commodities brought from overseas, jabisen must have arrived at the Sakai port, [the] most flourishing town of the day, and awaited buyers (and players). Those who became interested in such a new foreign music culture at first were feudal lords becoming wealthy and men of culture protected by lords, besides blind persons [who] also got in touch with it fairly soon. As Sakai town prospered, many biwa hoshi probably came in there. They knew how to play stringed instruments using bachi (plectrum) so it would be easier for them to get used to jabisen. The atmosphere of seeking something new in port town would be suitable for them to cast off attachment for biwa without much ado. The choice of the blind changed drastically the course of mainstream . . . popular Japanese music afterwards.

16. Patron of Basho—Sanpu Sugiyama

It is well known that Basho Matsuo, one of the most representative literary men of [the] Genroku period, enhanced the Haikai from a sort of word game to an art form. He had many pupils all over the country. Sanpu Sugiyama was among them, the most reliable person throughout his life, starting from [the] days before Basho had become famous. Sanpu was a powerful merchant named Koiya (house of camps), [and] was patron for Basho during his stay in Edo. Bashoan (hermitage of Basho) in Fukagawa was the source of his pseudonym as there was a big Basho (Japanese banana) in the garden, which was believed to be a watch house of fish reserve of Koiya to keep fish alive temporarily. Sanpu's life seems without any trouble, but in truth, he had [a] heavy hearing impairment. Reportedly Basho never composed Haiku poem about hearing troubles, showing consideration for Sanpu.

17. Koto (Japanese Harp) and Yatsuhashi Kengyo (The Highest Rank of Court Musician)

Shamisen and Koto were the most popular instruments played among [the] general public during the Edo era. These instruments were introduced by blind people who played them to earn their living. It was blind persons called Biwahoshi (blind religious minstrel) who Japanized [the] Jabisen (a snake-skin shamisen) of Ryukyu (now Okinawa prefecture). We cannot forget the fact of how the blind supported the music of Joruri (including Gidayubushi) accompanied with shamisen, although the reciter Takemoto Gidayu is the only well-known character of Gidayubushi, (Gidayu is a form of ballad-drama, Gidayubushi is its music accompaniment), which played on stage. It was written by Monzaemon Chikamatsu, one of the three most famous literati of [the] Genroku period. Even now, players of shamisen have names like Tsurusawa, Takesawa. These -sawa endings are derived from the founder Sawaoh Kengyo. [The] koto has long history, [being] originally played as musical instruments of Gagaku (ancient imperial court music). It is certain that Biwahoshi themselves, looking for new instruments other than biwa, improved koto and the way of performance so that ordinary people could enjoy it. We may say that Yatsuhashi Kengyo was the most important person who tried to spread koto. We can still enjoy his music nowadays, for example, instrumental music like Melody of 6-dan, Melody of 8-dan and vocal music of Kumiuta (included several pieces of Japanese poems of Kokinshu, etc.), accompanied by koto.

19. Sugiyama Kengyo, Worshipped at Shrine

It is said that Ieyasu Tokugawa, the founder of Edo Government who laid the basis of about 200 years of peaceful period, especially tried to protect the blind as there was a blind person among his own relatives. Kengyo Waich Sugiyama, kept close with the fifth Shogun (generalissimo) Tsuneyoshi, consolidated the system of Kengyo, placed chief kengyo not only in Kyoto but in Edo (now called Tokyo) to heighten the status of Edo. He also installed seminar house of acupuncture. He generalized acupuncture as a job of the blind, and initiated the Sugiyama school. In the beginning of Edo era, [the] Heike biwa was outdated, but neither [the] koto nor [the] shamisen had yet become popular, so the blind were looking for new types of work. Moreover, not all blind people could play music. Then acupuncture and massage became their important job. Sugiyama himself was once turned out by the first teacher of acupuncture because he showed little talent for it. On such an occasion, he supposedly devised [a] new method. It was to put a needle in a thin tube, different from [the] traditional way of tapping the end of needles or screwing the needles in. For his virtuous achievements, he is worshipped in the Sugiyama Shrine located in Chitose of the Sumida ward in Tokyo.

21. Akinari Ueda, with Cancroid Hands

We cannot forget the name of Akinari Ueda, author of Ugetsu Monogatari (Story of rain and moon), which is full of noble romantic scent and fantastic atmosphere, [a] rare masterpiece in Japanese literature before [the] modern ages. His grave is located in the garden of a subordinate temple in the precinct of Nanzenji Temple in Kyoto. The tomb stone was engraved with [a] crab, showing the epitaph "Tomb of Mucho" (without intestines). Mucho is the alias of crabs as they seem to have no bowels. He often used it as his pen name of Haiku poems, etc. Why did Akinari particularly stick to crabs? The reason was his fingers. He suffered smallpox and lost or shortened some fingers by the effects of the disease. When he wrote, he had to hold a pen with the remaining two fingers like a crab. A scholar of Akinari once wrote that a person with disability of legs may forget it while writing something even if he cannot walk. In the case of Akinari, however, he had to face up to his hands whenever he wrote. Using hands with disability, he created incomparable masterpieces.

22. Bakin Takizawa, Struggled Against

In the later half of the Edo period, the center of culture moved from the Kyoto-Osaka area to Edo, [and] publishing became active. Printing was done by carving a board for one entire page, not [a] word. They could print both pictures and phrases mixed with Chinese characters and Japanese letters without much trouble. To popularize printed matters, illustrations were very useful. Nanso Satomi Hakkenden, whose dramatis personae were 8 swordsmen that have the letter of Inu (dog) respective in their name, show various gallantry in the story. Chinsetsu Yumiharizuki is about the brave life of Tametomo Minamoto. Both works were written by Bakin Takizawa, published with the rise of printing culture. It took him more than 10 years to complete the works though, as they were very long stories of about tens of volumes. Encouragement by the readers might have renewed the source of energy for him. Suddenly a tragedy assaulted him. It was weakening eyesight by disease. Finally he totally lost sight, couldn't write a word. Ideas occurred to him, but he couldn't put them down. How vexatious it must be for an author! When he asked help from [his] daughter-in-law to dictate it, she was at a loss because phrases were mixed with difficult Chinese words and expressions.

24. Seibi Natsume, Suffered Gout

The Haiku poems, inspired artistic value by Basho Matsuo and rich poetic value by poets like Buson Yosa, were becoming popular as time went by. In modern terms, it can be described as [a] remarkable increase of [the] haiku population. Persons of excellent creativity of haiku with trustworthy personality were respected as leading figures of the field. Seibi Natsume was one of those reputable authorities. He possessed [a] tranquil, elegant style of haiku, commented on others' poems accurately, so he was adored by people. He wrote essays and studied senior haiku poets, too. It is said that he also took care of haiku poets from local cities or who were poor and relied upon him as *he* ran one of the biggest Fudasashi, which is equivalent to [a] pawnshop nowadays in Edo (now Tokyo). Issa Kobayashi, famous for the unique popular style of his works was also his guest while he was in Edo. He suffered severe gout throughout the life though. Not only [was he] unable to walk but also he was constantly agonized by intense pains. Once he retired from the business, but when his younger brother died early, he had to resume the responsibility of business again. He found relief only in composing haiku poems.

25. Origin of Wheel Chairs

We don't know when appeared Izariguruma, [the] prototype of wheelchairs. Supposedly it began to be used fairly early, in accordance with people's necessity. It was depicted in two different scenes in Hokusai Comic by Hokusai Katsushika in [the] Edo period. [The] lower picture shows [a] wheelchair with two levels, on which one can sit down. [The] upper picture shows a plain board with wheels made of wood. To move, they pushed with long poles against the ground, probably because it had smaller wheels than nowadays. The one man looks like a beggar, while the other seems to be an intelligent person with social status like master of haiku, etc., as he wears [a] special cap and respectable clothes. It is a good contrast that one uses only one pole, while the other uses two poles. It appeared, however, [that] the speed and operational technique of the wheelchair with one pole could be much superior to the other. Relaxed flexibility and shrewd toughness. It splendidly well expresses [the] difference of characters derived from respective lives.

26. Bokushi Suzuki of Hokuetsu Seppu

When the Tokugawa rule began to decay one of the most popular writers of the highly matured Edo Culture, Kyoden Santo, received a letter asking his assistance for . . . publishing a book. [The] sender's name was Bokushi Suzuki of Echigo (Niigata Prefecture now). Although Kyoden was a little acquainted with Bokushi as [a] haiku poet, the manuscript sent to him was not original haiku poem nor ordinary selected poems, nor a novel following the style of Kyoden to be famous like him. What was described scrupulously in it was the rural district of Echigo where Bokushi lived, snowbound almost half the year, and the life of people in heavy snow. The book 'Hokuetsu Seppu' was published by enthusiasm of Bokushi, and unexpectedly won so much popularity that a sequel to it was requested. In those days, there was boom of travel, so it might be regarded as variation of the travel guides introducing noted places and specialities of locality that were much published following the boom. The book, however, was the first scientific essay in Japan and work of ethnography in fact. The continuation was never written though. The author had serious problem of hearing and devoted himself to keeping diary which served as vent for his frustration and troubles among his family and family business (pawnshop) caused by the disability.

27. Famous Scholar, Hokiichi Hanawa

A boy who lost his eyesight at the age of six came up to Edo from [the] local town of Musashino with great hope, but he could not make progress in music with koto nor shamisen, nor was he good at acupuncture nor massage. He despaired of life, [and] thought to commit suicide by jumping into [the] Chidoriga-fuchi moat of Yotsuya; but his master encouraged him and said that he was allowed to do anything he was interested in for three years. Then if he couldn't succeed at anything, he must go back home. Following the advice, he decided to start studying. Fortunately a volunteer of so-called man-to-man tutor appeared next door to his house, his good luck bloomed all of a sudden. He became a pupil of Kamo no Mabuchi when he was 17, showed genius and finished 6 Japanese history books includ[ing] Nihon Shoki in short period. This is the famous episode of how Hokiichi Hanawa (1746–1821) made of himself a great scholar. Two years after he was promoted to be

Kengyo through his study, he assisted proofreading of Dai-Nihon Shi and received salary of 10 nin-buchi (amount on which 10 people could live for a year) by Mito-han (feudal clan). On the other hand, he gave periodical open lecture of Genji monogatari at his home. There was a senryu at that time who asked for directions to 'the blind man who can see' at Bancho. It might show how active was the private school held at his house in Bancho of Kojimachi town. He then initiated the great work of publishing Gunsho Ruiju (Collected Classics of Japanese Literature).

28. Terakoya (Private School) and Children with Disabilities

During [the] Edo period, almost all Han (feudal clans) installed schools to teach children of vassals. On the other hand, the number of Terakoya (private school at the local temple) for children of ordinary people increased rapidly as time went by. [There were] public schools for elites and private schools for general public. More precisely, we can think of the Terakoya as a private school with easygoing atmosphere, not aiming at higher education. The popularity of such terakoya in big cities like Edo and Osaka was surprisingly high near the end of [the] Edo shogunate. We can guess that it served as [the] basis of [the] rapid growth of [the] school system in [the] Meiji period. They taught mainly elementary Japanese, Chinese characters and calligraphy, mathematics with abacus as often said "reading, writing and abacus" without much formalities. There are records that among the pupils at Terakoya were some children with disability. It reveals the wish of parents for those children to learn writing so that they could earn money. Children with hearing problem[s] were, however, not accepted.

29. Kuzuhara Koto (Rank of Blind Court Musicians, Below Kengyo in Ancient Times), Folding Paper, and Wooden Printing

The wonder of art of Japanese paper folding that produces three-dimensional crane, tortoise and goldfish from a piece of paper became the topic in New York recently. The fact that a blind person demonstrated it caught further attention from people. One hundred and ten years ago, there was a blind man well known as an expert of paper folding, who lived in Yatsuhira village in Bingo (Kaminobe town, Aki-gun Hiroshima Prefecture now). Some exquisite masterpieces like a

crane with little chicks at the end of both wings were devised by him. His name was Kuzuhara Koto. He was a skilled player of the Japanese koto, became Koto when he was still young but couldn't achieve the rank of Kengyo until he died. It seemed he didn't need the position of Kengyo because he was born in [a] rich family in [a] local city where the life was not so busy as big city life. Besides, the authority of Kengyo decreased as people tended to buy the position with money more and more. To add to our surprise, Kuzuhara kept a diary for 33 years from [the] Edo period to [the] Meiji and it is still in existence. He wrote it using homemade block print. He set up types in a frame, recognising each different type [of] block by touch.

32. "Are You Going to Massage a Pine Tree?"

He lost eyesight when he was halfway through studies in school. Once he decided to die, but did not succeed. Then he awoke to the love of God and started the career as theologian. He went England to study, supported by good assistance and encouragement of his sister, then his name Takeo Iwahashi became better known abroad than in Japan. After returning to Japan, he dedicated himself to disseminate braille as he believed that study was necessary for blind people while advocating the love of God. It is a famous episode that he angrily said to those who were reluctant to acknowledge the need of study, "The day will come when you should have at least physical knowledge of human body to massage it. If not, you won't be admitted to massage anyone. It'll be too late to start studying. Are you going to massage a pine tree then?" He opened Light House in Osaka, issued newspapers and books in braille, [and] devoted himself to give assistance and improve [the] social status of the blind. He invited Ms. Helen Keller to Japan before and after the Second World War, [and] gave lectures throughout the country. It met with big response not only from the disabled but also from general public.

33. Hand Boy, Seisaku Noguchi

There was a boy teased with the nickname "Pole-hand". When he was a crawling baby, he fell in a fireplace and burnt one hand, eventually all fingers of the hand stuck together. It was a poor village at the lakeside of Inawashiro Lake in Aizu (Fukuoka prefecture now). His name was Seisaku Noguchi. As his family was strictly poor, he had to catch loaches and sell them in towns. Other children looked down on him and made fun of it. He had particularly strong competitive spirit with bright head. "Some day I'll pay it back to them!" His fighting spirit flared up in vexation and anger. After he graduated from elementary school, he worked as a substitute teacher. People around collected a fund for him to get operation of hand. Among them were those who had made fun of him. The operation succeeded and restored his fingers. Such a joy led him to medical science, then he changed his name to Hideyo Noguchi. This is the story of Dr. Noguchi, who was the first Japanese nominated [for] the candidacy of the Nobel Peace Prize.

34. 6-Shaku Sick Bed, Shiki Masaoka

"If I could stand up, I would eat snow on Mount Everest in the Himalayas in North India." This is one of eight series of poems with the phrase "If I could stand up". There are other pieces he composed as the inspiration hit him. For instance, I'd like to bath in the hot spring of Hakone, I'd like to float in a boat on a lake in the moonshine, etc. It is interesting that there exist comparable poems of traditional haiku and ones reflecting the thrust of the period Meiji when Japan opened the door to [the] world. The poet Shiki Matsuoka went to battlefield as journalist during Japan-China War (Nisshin War). On his coming back to Japan, he bled severely on the ship. Afterwards his illness worsened in the stomach, waist and hip and he was kept on a sick bed. As his disease was developing, needing medical treatment, we should call it sickness rather than disability. But we might classify him as one of disabled persons because he lived disabled daily life, not able to walk for a long time. Confined in sick bed of 6-shaku (about 2 square metres), he took his pen, facing the ceiling of his room, to infuse a new spirit into the traditional Japanese literature by accomplishing great works such as Renovation of haiku poems and then Renovation of tanka poems.

35. Cherry Blossoms, Japanese Harp (Koto) and Michio Miyagi

There might not be any Japanese who does not know melodies of koto like Variation of Sakura (Cherry blossom) known as 'Sakura Sakura', and the serenely delightful tune Spring Sea. Moreover, they are some of the most popular tunes abroad as music representing Japan and also symbolizing it. For that reason, the composer Michio Miyagi is regarded as a world famous musician. He was brought up in Korea, but had lost eyesight in his childhood. He returned to Japan alone and started professional training of koto. There might have been some hardships until he distinguished himself. But once his talent was approved and given adequate chances, his life became like a smooth sailing with favorable wind. As composer, he created several famous pieces including [the] formerly mentioned two tunes. As player, he contributed [to] the development of koto performance, tried to play ten koto in concert or play with other orchestral music, changed the instrument from merely [a] Japanese party accessory to the one that fits [a] large scale stage in the world. He fell from [a] night train and died, it was a mysterious accident. Only on that occasion do we notice that he was one of the disabled.

37. King of Joshu (Tochigi Prefecture)–Kijo Murakami

There lived a man in Takasaki city in Gunma prefecture who was moved by 'Papers for Poem Composers' by Shiki Masaoka and he found his real meaning of life in literature. He worked as Daisho (judicial scrivener now) and spent frustrated days due to disappointment he had met several times. It was caused by the disability of hearing. He failed [the] medical exam for entry to the Army officer school because of [his] hearing impairment, of which he had not been aware. Then he went to Tokyo by himself to study in [the] university aiming to be a lawyer, but the door was also shut because of the hearing problem. The condition worsened so much that even he himself realized at heart that he couldn't easily understand what others said. He found new life in literature facing the reality as it is, so he changed the course of [his] life and devoted himself to haiku poems. He made poems of mountains and rivers of the hometown Joshu with pride, and reflected the image of himself on wounded or disabled little animals. His name was Kijo Murakami (1870–1938), one of the representative haiku poets of [the] Taisho period.

Cool Spring Day,
A Blind Dog Goes Stumbling Under Moon,
There Lives the King in a Potato Field

38. New Age Woman with Crutch

It was just before the fascism [?] of the Showa period swallowed everything, when people sought for freedom, it was the so-called Taisho Democracy period in the early 20th century. The women's movement developed excitedly, women of various characteristics called New Age Women appeared spectacularly. Shizu Shiraki (1895–1918) was a new type woman representing the disabled. She was born in Sapporo, unhealthy from birth. Moreover, she suffered tubercular rheumatism after she fell down while climbing [a] mountain, it caused her to have the right leg amputated when she graduated from women's school. She enjoyed making Tanka poems and verses or trying to make occidental movies as [a] pastime in the hospital, then she made up her mind to be a writer making good use of her tragedy as fertilizer [for her imagination]. Her virgin work 'Woman with Crutch' and the second piece 'Death at the age thirty-three', both dealing with the agony of having one's limb cut off, received favorable assessment from the literary world. In real life, she got married with a painter Mr. Kiyotsugu Uenoyama in spite of objections by her relatives, [and] even . . . gave birth to a baby. She fulfilled the life with strong will to accomplish it, [and] died young at ten years earlier than predicted thirty-three. Her name is scarcely mentioned nowadays but she was a writer to set beside Ms. Yuriko Nakajo (called Miyamoto today).

39. Haiku Poet Moppo Tomita and His Best Friend Seifu

The great earthquake of Kanto in 1923 (Taisho 12) brought deaths to many people by earthquakes and the following fires. The poet Moppo Tomita was one of them, burnt to death at riverside of Higashi-Mukojima of Sumida River. He was born in Ele restaurant, and could not walk due to sickness suffered in infant days. People rumored that this came from a grudge of eels and he could not stay at the restaurant any more. He worked in Yuzenzome dyeing craftsman's, to be an in-house disciple overcoming the disability. Living together with mother and other brothers in a poor compound flat, he earned money by making dolls or cheap confectionery goods, doing his best to sustain living. [The] only relief he found in those days was haiku poems [which] he liked from . . . childhood. Then Seifu Arai appeared as real Messiah for his life. He was a rich man [a] running movie theater in Aaskusa town, [a] university student (Moppo didn't go to it) who had

[a] robust body. Those two had contrary characters but they made very close friends. Mr. Arai not only introduced Moppo's works to the literature world as a new wave but also took care of his living. Both in name and in real terms he was an excellent volunteer. Here is one of Moppo's masterpieces:

On Autumn Sunset,
a Spider Extends String on my Shoulder

40. First Night and Spring at Sanatorium

It was in 1936 (Showa 11) all judges of Literature World Award experienced deep shock. They encountered a devastatingly compassionate work. Its title was "The First Night of Life", depicting without reserve the agony of a person suffering Hansen's disease (leprosy). He had been driven to the extreme to live in a sanatorium shut out from outer world, completely away from his past, from the society he had lived in. In those days, there was no adequate medical treatment for Hansen's disease. Once caught, it led to a miserable death. Generally, people believed that it could be infected anywhere, anytime, so they extraordinarily feared the sickness. Anyone who caught it [had to] move to live separately in sanatoria compulsorily. The literary work was recommended for the Award not through fear or compassion but because it showed the keen critical eyes of the writer and his steady writing ability. His pen name was Tamio Hojo, his real name unknown. His past must have been so completely erased. "Spring of Little Bird" dealt similarly with the tragedy of separated life through [the] eyes and mind of a woman. It was once made into a movie and became well known. The author, Masako Ogawa, treated those sick people as nurse and is believed to have caught the disease later and died in a sanatorium in a small island in the Inland Sea.

41. Naked Wandering Painter, Kiyoshi Yamashita

In 1937 Children's shred drawing [i.e., collage] exhibition of Yawata Gakuen, institution for mentally disabled was held at Waseda University and became a hot topic. Especially [the] works of Kiyoshi Yamashita were remarkable in terms of quality and volume. In the exhibition at Seijusha Publishing Co. Ltd., 'Ginza ward' attracted the attention of many painters and Kiyoshi obtained [a] good reputation as [a] unique painter. Without seeing the original picture it can hardly be imagined how elaborately two or three mili colored papers were stuck and created vivid and delicate touch. Some praised his works as like Van Gogh's painting style in his Paris age. [The] following year, however, he had left the institution and started on wanderings. It may be true that the fear of a physical examination for conscription motivated him to wander but he was rather born to be a wanderer. Since then he repeatedly wandered around for several months or years and returned to the institution unexpectedly. The distance reached to the extent of travelling almost [the] whole [of] Japan. He expressed what he had seen and learned during his journeys in the form of shred drawing and wrote down his experience of wandering. The movie Hadaka no Taisho Hourouki (Story of Naked Big-Shot) describes his world in those days. Speaking of planned journeys, there was only once when he went to Europe accompanied by his teacher Ryuzaburo Sikiba. He truly encountered Van Gogh's world through this trip.

Source: Hanaka, Syuncho. 1998. *Ebisu Mandara* (Japanese and English texts). Available at the Japan Council on Disability website: http://www.jdnet.gr.jp/Ebisu/Index.en.html. Used by permission of the author.

◪ Wolfgang Büttner on the Fool Claus Narr (1572)

The author of this story, Wolfgang Büttner, uses the fool Claus Narr as a tool for his Protestant teachings. According to Protestant ethics, work and leisure should follow each other. Fun and joy are permissible, but neither should last too long.

XV, 32: Gemahlter Vogel [Painted Bird]

Er sahe einen gemahlten Vogel an der Wand stehen
den schewet vnd jechet er mit seinem Hute
daß er abflüge.
Als er aber nit auffliegen wolt
sprach er: Wolan der Vogel sitzt gewiß
er were recht gut zu schiessen
wenn der Wildtschütze hie were mit seinem zeuge.

Lehre.
Es taug noch wol wenn man kurtzweilt
Mit schimpfferey die zeit vertreibt
Doch wenn man sitzt zu lang vnd fest
So seynds nicht angeneme Gäst.
Von dem man sagen solt diß wort
Jhr sitzet gwiß an einem orth
Man möcht euch schiessen wie ein Wandt

An der ein gmahlter Vogel stand
Ein stetten Gast vnd nächtig Fisch
Wündscht ich mir nicht an meinem Tisch.

Account of the Source

Claus Narr saw a painted bird on the wall and attempted to shoo it away with his hat. When that did not succeed, he regretted that there was no hunter nearby who could shoot down the bird. In the paragraph entitled, "Lehre" (lesson), a reference is made to the fact that it is good when one can converse with jokes and fun. But it is not pleasant when guests have this opportunity and overstay their welcome. In this situation, these guests are like the painted bird on the wall, which one might gladly shoot. One does not desire to share his table with either a permanent guest or yesterday's fish.

Comments on the Lesson

The author of this story, Wolfgang Buettner, uses the fool as tool for the Protestant teachings. According to Protestant ethics, work and leisure should follow each other. Fun and joy are permissible, but neither should last too long. The painted bird, which the "natural" fool mistakes for a live bird, at first tries to chase away, and wishes to have shot, serves as an illustration of the unpleasantness that ensues when guests stay too long.

Source: Büttner, Wolfgang. 1572. Pp. 462–463 in *Von Claus Narren. Sechs hundert sieben vnd zwantzig Historien, etc.* Erstdruck: Eisleben.

◪ Richard Knolles, from *The Turkish History* (1603)

The 1553 murder of Mustapha inspired numerous accounts by Western observers, many of which mentioned the numerous disabled people at the court of the Emperor Suleiman, Mustapha's father. This account by Richard Knolles drew heavily on Hugh Gough's English translation of the account by Bartolomej Georgijevic. This excerpt begins after the Sultan's eldest son and heir apparent, Mustapha, having been summoned, arrives unarmed at an outer chamber of the tent of his father, the Emperor Suleiman.

So when he was come into the more inward roomes of the tent, he was with such honour as belonged to his state cheerfully received by his fathers Eunuchs. But

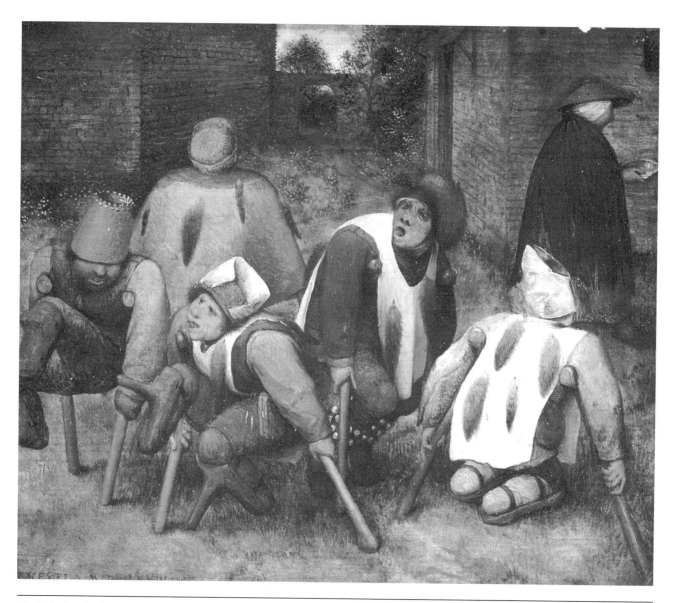

The Cripples, by Pieter Brueghel the Elder (1525–1569). In this work, Brueghel captures a group of disabled alms seekers preparing to head out to their street posts. The artist sardonically scribbled on the back of the painting: "Cripples go and be prosperous."

Source: Art Resource, New York.

seeing nothing else provided but one Seat whereon to sit himself alone, he perplexed in mind, stood still a while musing; at length asked where the Emperor his Father was? Whereunto they answered, That he should by and by see him; and with that casting his Eye aside, he saw seven Mutes (these are strong Men bereft of their Speech, whom the Turkish Tyrants have always in readiness, the more secretly to execute their bloody Butchery) coming from the other side of the Tent towards him; at whose sight strucken with a sudden terrour, said no more, but *Lo my death*; and with

that, arising, was about to have fled; but in vain, for he was caught hold on by the Eunuch and Mutes, and by force drawn to the place appointed for his death; where without further stay, the Mutes cast a Bowstring about his Neck, he poor Wretch still striving, and requesting that he might speak but two words to his Father before he died. [Suleiman in fact urged on the executioners with angry shouts.]

He [Suleiman] sent for *Tzihanger* the Crooked . . . in sporting wise . . . bid him go meet his Brother *Mustapha*. [Suleiman omitted to say that Jehangir would find only a corpse. He sent servants offering Mustapha's wealth and position to Jehangir. The latter refused, and died shortly afterwards. Knolles says that he stabbed himself.]

[Editors' note: Sultan Murad III (sometimes Murath, or Amurath), who reigned from 1574 to 1595, also had "mutes" among his servants, and engaged in vigorous and hazardous exercises with them, though he was subject to epileptic fits. In the following excerpt, Knolles quotes from a contemporary report by Johannes Leunclavius.]

This summer also, Amurath disporting himself with his Mutes, was almost dead. These Mutes are lusty strong Fellows, deprived of their Speech; who nevertheless certain by signs can both aptly express their own Conceits; and understand the meaning of others: these men for their Secrecie are the cruel Ministers of the Turkish Tyrants most horrible commands; and therefore of them had in great regard. With these Mutes mounted upon fair and fat, but heavy and unready Horses, was Amurath, upon a light and ready Horse, sporting himself (as the manner of the Turkish Emperours is) riding sometime about one, sometime about another; and striking now the Horse, now the Man, at his Pleasure, when suddenly he was taken with a fit of the falling Sickness, his old Disease; and so falling from his Horse, was taken up for dead. . . . Nevertheless, Amurath shortly after recovered again, and to appease that Rumor of his Death (openly upon their Sabbath, which is the Friday) rid from his Palace to the Temple of Sophia; where I with many others saw him (saith Leunclavius) his Countenance yet all pale and discoloured.

Source: Knolles, Richard. 1603. *The Turkish History, etc.* London: Adam Islip.

▣ Ottaviano Bon's Description of the Ottoman Court (1607)

The Italian diplomat Ottaviano Bon lived at Istanbul from 1604 to 1607, and some of his observations of the Ottoman Court were translated into English and published at various times in the seventeenth century. Of primary interest here are his descriptions of the signing system used by the many deaf individuals connected with the court.

[By cultivating a senior court official, Bon was able to tour some interior parts of the seraglio, when the Sultan was absent.] And in the Lake there was a little Boat, the which (as I was enformed) the Grand Signior did oftentimes goe into with his Mutes and Buffones, to make them row up and downe, and to sport with them, making them leape into the water; and many times as he walked with them above the sides of the Lake, he would throw them downe into it, and plunge them over head and eares. [p. 328]

[Bon made detailed notes about the education of pages for court service, and about other court servants.] Now, for the most part, they all stay at the least six yeeres in this Schoole, and such as are dull and hard of apprehension stay longer. [p. 355] Moreover, every one of them (according to his inclination and disposition) shall learne a Trade, necessary for the Service of the Kings person, to make up a Terbent, to shave, to paire nayles, to fold up Apparell handsomely, to keepe Landspaniels, to keepe Hawkes, to be Sewers, to be Quiries of the Stable, to be Targetbearers, and to waite at the Grand Signiors Table, and the like Services, as it is also used in the Courts of other Kings and Emperours. [p. 356]

Besides the Women, and Ajamoglans of this Seraglio, and the aforesaid Youths last spoken of; there are many and divers Ministers for all manner of necessarie services, and particular functions: there are also Buffons of all sorts, and such as shew trickes, Musicians, Wrestlers, many dumbe men both old and young, who have libertie to goe in and out with leave of the Capee Agha; And this is worthie the observation, that in the Serraglio, both the King and others can reason and discourse of any thing as well and as distinctly, alla mutesca, by nods and signes, as they can with words: a thing well befitting the gravitie of the better sort of Turkes, who care not for much babling. The same is also used amongst the Sultanaes, and other the Kings Women: for with them likewise there are divers dumbe women, both old and young. And this hath beene an ancient custome in the Serraglio: wherefore they get as many Mutes as they can possibly find: and chiefly for this one reason; that they hold it not a thing befitting the Grand Signior. Neither stands it with his greatnesse, to speake to any about him familiarly: but he may in that manner more tractably and domestically jest and sport with the Mutes, then with other that are about him. [pp. 362–363]

The Black-moore Girls, are no sooner brought into the Serraglio after their arrival at Constantinople, (for they come by Ship from Cairo and from thereabouts) but they are carryed to the Womens lodgings, where they are brought up and made fit for all services; and by how much the more uglie and deformed they are, by so much the more they are esteemed of, by the Sultanaes; wherefore the Bashaw of Cairo (who for the most part sends them all) is always diligent to get the most ill-favoured, cole-blacke, flat-nosed Girles that may bee had throughout all Egypt. [p. 369]

All the while that he [the Sultan] is at Table, he very seldome or never speakes to any man, albeit there stand afore him divers Mutes and Jesters, to make him merrie, playing trickes and sporting one with another Alla Mutescha, which the King understands very well, for by signes their meaning is easily conceived. Now whilst the Agha's are eating, the King passeth away the time with his Mutes and Buffones, not speaking (as I said) at all with his Tongue, but only by signes: and now and then he kicks and buffeteth them in sport, but forth-with makes them amends by giving them Money; for which purpose his pockets are aiwayes furnished. [pp. 374–375]

[Bon remarks on the sale of fruit from the Royal gardens. The gardeners] bring the money weekely to the Bustangee Bashee who afterwards gives it to his Majestie, and it is called the Kings Pocket-money; for he gives it away by handfuls, as he sees occasion, to his Mutes and Buffons. [p. 380]

[While the Sultan was being conveyed by boat,] Now the Bustangee Bashee, by reason the King talkes much with him in the Barge, (at which time, least any one should heare what they say, the Mutes fall a howling like little Dogs) may benefit or prejudice whom he pleaseth. [p. 385]

Source: Purchas, Samuel. 1607. Pp. 322–406 in *Hakluytus Posthumus or Purchas His Pilgrimes,* Vol. IX. Republished 1905. Glasgow, Scotland: MacLehose.

George Sandys, from *A Relation of a Journey* . . . (1615)

George Sandys, an English gentleman and a shrewd observer, visited Istanbul in 1610 and recorded what he saw and heard at the court of Sultan Ahmed I, who reigned from 1603 to 1617. Like many earlier observers, he remarked with wonder on the sign language used within the court.

[Of the Sultan] Yet he is an unrelenting punisher of offences, even in his owne houshold: having caused eight of his Pages, at my being there, to be throwne into

the Sea for Sodomy (an ordinary crime, if esteemed a crime, in that nation) in the night time. [p. 73]

Fifty Mutes he [the Sultan] hath borne deafe and dumbe, whereof some few be his daily companions; the rest are his Pages. It is a wonderfull thing to see how readily they can apprehend, and relate by signes, even matters of great difficultie. [p. 74]

Source: Sandys, George. 1615. *A Relation of a Iourney . . . Containing a Description of the Turkish Empire, etc.* London: W. Barrett.

Michel Baudier on the Ottoman Empire (1624)

Michel Baudier's work draws heavily on other writers and summarizes some aspects of Ottoman court life under Sultan Ahmed I. When Ahmed I died in 1617, his brother Mustafa I briefly acceded to the throne. But Mustafa seems to have been weak-minded and unable to assert any grip on the court. He earned the courtiers' contempt by speaking to people just as any ordinary person would do, rather than maintaining the distance, dignity, and mystique expected of the Sultan.

c. 1600–1620: Other men which are of his Family, speake not unto him but by signes, and this dumbe language is practised, and understood as readily in the Serrail, as a distinct and articulate voice among us. For which cause they use the service of as many dumbe men as they can find; who having accustomed others to their signes and gestures make them to learne their Language. The Sultana's doe the like. The gravitie of his person, and the custome of the Empire forbids him to speake to any. The Sultana's his women practise it, they have many dumbe slaves in their serrail. Sultan Mustapha Uncle to Osman, who in the end of the yeare 1617 held the scepter of the Turkish Empire, for that he could not accustome himselfe to this silent gravitie, gave occasion to the Councell of State to complaine of him, and to say that to speake freely unto his people as Mustapha did, was more fit for a lanizarie or a Turkish Merchant did, then for their Emperour. They contemned him, and held his freedome and familiaritie unworthy of the Empire.

[Baudier gleaned the following report of the demise in 1606 of Dernier, the Chief Gardener, which suggests that ad hoc executions did not always proceed smoothly.] He will defend his life couragiously, and

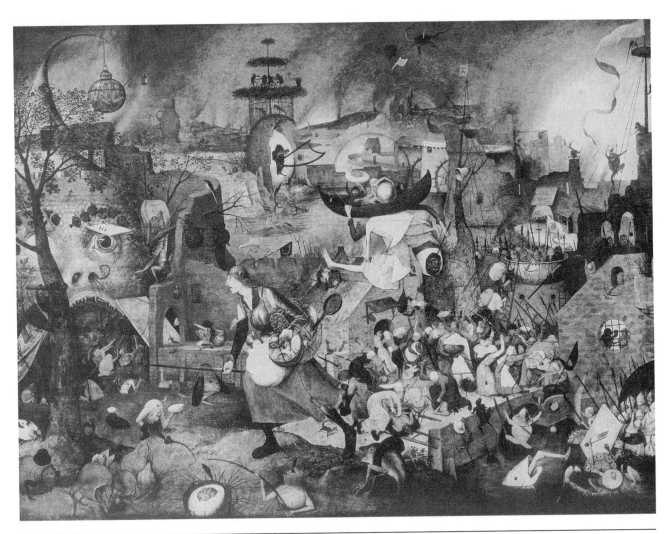

Dulle Griet [Mad Meg] *(1562–1566), by Pieter Brueghel the Elder (1525–1569). In this painting, Brueghel portrays an image of psychiatric disability at the heart of chaos and social destruction. The image foregrounds longstanding associations of cognitive difference with immorality.*

Source: Art Resource, New York.

let them see that a man, which hath long time handled a Spade and a Mattocke, is not soe easily mastered. *Achmat* sends for *Dernier* to the *Serrail*; he comes and is scarce entred when he suspects the partie which was made against him; he goes into the *Grand Seigneurs* quarter, being there, this troupe of *Capigis* fall upon him to seaze on him, and to put the Halter about his necke; he frees himself from them, and stands upon his defence although he had nothing in his hands, and with his fists scatters them bravely; hee beats one of their Noses flat, puts out the eye of another, and strikes out his teeth that held the Halter, and puts him out of breath which had taken hold of his Arme, and remaines free in the midst of al them which did inviron him, and durst not take him. [Eventually, more fearful of the Sultan's wrath than of Dernier's fist, they overpower and strangle him.] This thing happened at Constantinople in the year 1606. [pp. 178–180]

Source: Baudier, Michel. 1635. Grimeston, Edward, trans. *The history of the imperiall estate of the grand seigneurs their habitations, liues, titles . . . gouernment and tyranny.* London: Richard Meighen.

◉ Francis Bacon, from *Essayes or Counsels* (1625)

In this analysis of deformity, Francis Bacon, often referred to as the "father of empiricism," argues that the ridicule heaped upon deformed members of the court causes them to seek revenge against those who would malign them. Further, Bacon also counsels suspicion toward these seemingly "helpless" individuals, for their differences may serve as a disguise for loftier political ambitions. Rather than referring to living persons, the analysis could serve as a pointed piece of literary criticism about the ruses of Shakespeare's Richard III.

XLIV. Of Deformity

Deformed persons are commonly even with nature, for as nature hath done ill by them, so do they by nature, being for the most part (as the Scripture saith) *void of natural affection*; and so they have their revenge of nature. Certainly there is a consent between the body and the mind, and where nature erreth in the one, she ventureth in the other. *Ubi peccat in uno, periclitatur in altero.* But because there is in man an election touching the frame of his mind and a necessity in the frame of his body, the stars of natural inclination are sometimes obscured by the sun of discipline and virtue. Therefore it is good to consider of deformity, not as a sign, which is more deceivable, but as a cause, which seldom faileth of the effect. Whosoever hath anything fixed in his person that doth induce contempt hath also a perpetual spur in himself to rescue and deliver himself from scorn. Therefore all deformed persons are extreme bold. First, as in their own defence, as being exposed to scorn, but in process of time by a general habit. Also it stirreth in them industry, and especially of this kind, to watch and observe the weakness of others, that they may have somewhat to repay. Again, in their superiors it quencheth jealousy towards them, as persons that they think they may at pleasure despise; and it layeth their competitors and emulators asleep, as never believing they should be in possibility of advancement, till they see them in possession. So that upon the matter, in a great wit deformity is an advantage to rising. Kings in ancient times (and at this present in some countries) were wont to put great trust in eunuchs, because they that are envious towards all are more obnoxious and officious towards one. But yet their trust towards them hath rather been as to good spials and good whisperers than good magistrates and officers. And much like is the reason of deformed persons. Still the ground is, they will, if they be of spirit, seek to free themselves from scorn, which must be either by virtue or malice; and therefore let it not be marveled if sometimes they

prove excellent persons, as was Agesilaus, Aanger the son of Solyman, Aesop, Gasca, President of Peru; and Socrates may go likewise amongst them, with others.

Source: Bacon, Francis. 1625. T*he essayes or counsels, ciuill and morall, of Francis Lo. Verulam, Viscount St. Alban.* London: Hanna Barret. Available at: http://www.classicallibrary.org/bacon/essays/45.htm

▣ Witch Trial of Jane Hawkins (1638–1641)

The New England magistrates restricted and then expelled Jane Hawkins for her cultivation of the medical arts and religious authority as a woman. Women's efforts to occupy public positions of authority reserved for men prompted severe punishments from the Puritan patriarchy. These transgressions of gendered social roles often prompted accusations of witchcraft.

Jane Hawkins, the wife of Richard Hawkins, had liberty till the beginning of the third month, called May, and the magistrates (if she did not depart before) to dispose of her; and in the meantime she is not to meddle in surgery, or physic, drinks, plasters, or oils, nor to question matters of religion, except with the elders for satisfaction. March 12, 1638.

Jane Hawkins is enjoined to depart away tomorrow morning, and not to return again hither, upon pain of severe whipping and such other punishment as the court shall think meet; and her sons bound . . . to carry her away, according to order: June 2, 1641.

Source: Hall, David. 1991. *Witch-Hunting in Seventeenth Century New England: A Documentary History: 1638–1692.* Boston: Northwestern University Press.

▣ Evliya Efendi, from *Narrative of Travels in Europe, Asia, and Africa* (1635)

Evliya Efendi (also known as Evliya Celebi) served in the Seraglio under the Sultan Murad IV, who reigned from 1623 to 1640. Evliya is best known for his highly descriptive travel writing, but as a young man he spent a year as a page under Murad IV. He first met the Sultan in 1635. His account includes descriptions of fools, dwarfs, and mutes; discussion of female circumcision; and an analysis of the thoughts of the father of a hydrocephalic child.

On the day I was dressed as above related, with the splendid turban, two mutes came, and with many curious motions led me into the Khás oda (inner chamber), to Melek Ahmed Aghá and his predecessor Mustafá. [Vol. 1 (1) 133]

[In 1640 Evliya noted how Sultan Ibrahim (who reigned 1640–1648 and became known as Ibrahim the Mad) exchanged a man who would have given him good counsel for a pack of wolves who would lead him to his doom.] Kara Mustafá Páshá, the brave and sagacious vezir, being put to death, the Sultan [Ibrahim] fell into the hands of all the favourites and associates of the harem, the dwarfs, the mutes, the eunuchs, the women, particularly Jinjí Khoájeh. [Vol. 1 (1) 149]

[In a list of buildings in Constantinople, Evliya states that he has "preferred assigning each of the principal baths to a certain class of men in the following amusing way." Towards the end of a long list, there appear:] for the infirm (Maatúh), that of Koja Mohammed Páshá; for buffoons, that of Shengel; . . . for dwarfs, that of Little Aghá. [p. 180; *Ma'tuh* is a term historically used in Islamic Civil Law in Turkey to mean a person of unsound mind, sometimes "feebleminded."]

[In a list of baths in suburbs of Constantinople:] The bath of Kúlákis with good servants, nice waiters, who however are deaf as is implied by the name (Kúlákis, no ears). [Vol. 1 (ii) 45]

[Evliya gave a hugely detailed description of the vast and colourful procession of the guilds or fraternities of Constantinople:] (48) The Sheikhs of the beggars (Dilenjí), number seven thousand . . . some blind, some lame, some paralytic, some epileptic, some having lost a hand or foot, some naked and bare-foot, and some mounted on asses. [Vol. 1 (ii) 115] (254) The Sword-cutlers. . . . The most celebrated sword cutler is deaf David. Sultan Murád IV., who so well understood the worth and use of the sword, never used any but blades of Isfahán, or of deaf David. He made him by an Imperial rescript Chief of the sword-cutlers. [Vol. 1 (ii) 178]

Source: Efendi, Evliya. 1834. Ritter, Joseph von Hammer, trans. *Narrative of Travels in Europe, Asia, and Africa.* London: Oriental Translation Fund. (Originally published 1635)

▣ Henry Blount, from *A Voyage into the Levant* (1636)

Sir Henry Blount, who travelled through the Levant in the early 1630s, provided a few comments on the welfare of poor and disabled people in Turkey. He also wrote of some who pretended to be mad in order to eat without the need to work.

[On the Sultan's Janissaries in the 1630s:] They are never cast off for when old or maimed, they are kept in Garrison. [p. 116]

There are very few beggars in Turkey, by reason of the great plenty of Victuals; only one sort I wondered at, that is, their Santones who are able cunning Rogues much like our Tom of Bedlams; ever with some such disguise to pretend a crazed Brain. [p. 195]

Source: Blount, Henry. 1664. *A Voyage into the Levant,* 5th ed. London: Andrew Crooke. (Originally published 1636)

▣ John Milton, from *Paradise Lost* (1674)

In his invocation of the Muse at the beginning of the third book of his epic, the blind poet John Milton equates light with God and dark with formlessness. His blindness seems to become a metaphor when he likens his earlier description of night to being "Taught by the Heavenly Muse to venture down / The dark descent, and up to re-ascend." Although he can feel the "lamp," his eyes will never see again, because "so thick a drop serene hath quenched their orbs." He asks for an implanted inner eye, mentions and invokes predecessors, and asks for inner vision of report, imagining "things invisible to mortal sight" that can turn deprivation into a value.

Hail, holy Light, offspring of Heaven first-born!
Or of the Eternal coeternal beam
May I express thee unblamed? since God is light,
And never but in unapproached light
Dwelt from eternity, dwelt then in thee,
Bright effluence of bright essence increate!
Or hear'st thou rather pure Ethereal Stream,
Whose fountain who shall tell? Before the Sun,
Before the Heavens, thou wert, and at the voice
Of God, as with a mantle, didst invest
The rising World of waters dark and deep,
Won from the void and formless Infinite!

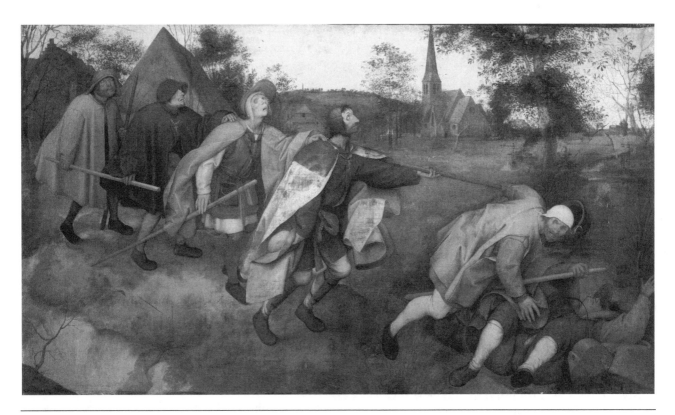

Parable of the Blind Leading the Blind, *by Pieter Brueghel the Elder (1525–1569). As with his paintings* The Cripples *and* Mad Meg, *Brueghel uses blindness as a metaphor for ineptitude. Ironically, the theme has become one of the most reproduced themes in visual artistic traditions.*

Source: Scala/Art Resource, New York.

Thee I revisit now with bolder wing,
Escaped the Stygian Pool, though long detained
In that obscure sojourn, while in my flight,
Through utter and through middle Darkness borne,
With other notes than to the Orphean lyre
I sung of Chaos and eternal Night,
Taught by the Heavenly Muse to venture down
The dark descent, and up to re-ascend,
Though hard and rare. Thee I revisit safe,
And feel thy sovran vital lamp; but thou
Revisit'st not these eyes, that rowl in vain
To find thy piercing ray, and find no dawn;
So thick a drop serene hath quenched their orbs,
Or dim suffusion veiled. Yet not the more
Cease I to wander where the Muses haunt
Clear spring, or shady grove, or sunny hill,
Smit with the love of sacred song; but chief
Thee, Sion, and the flowery brooks beneath,
That wash thy hallowed feet, and warbling flow,
Nightly I visit: nor sometimes forget
Those other two equalled with me in fate,
(So were I equalled with them in renown!)
Blind Thamyris and blind Maeonides,

And Tiresias and Phineus, prophets old:
Then feed on thoughts that voluntary move
Harmonious numbers; as the wakeful bird
Sings darkling, and, in shadiest covert hid,
Tunes her nocturnal note. Thus with the year
Seasons return; but not to me returns
Day, or the sweet approach of even or morn,
Or sight of vernal bloom, or summer's rose,
Or flocks, or herds, or human face divine;
But cloud instead and ever—during dark
Surrounds me, from the cheerful ways of men
Cut off, and, for the book of knowledge fair,
Presented with a universal blank
Of Nature's works, to me expunged and rased,
And wisdom at one entrance quite shut out.
So much the rather thou, Celestial Light,
Shine inward, and the mind through all her powers
Irradiate; there plant eyes; all mist from thence
Purge and disperse, that I may see and tell
Of things invisible to mortal sight.

Source: Milton, John. 1674. *Paradise Lost,* III.1–55. Available at: http://eir.library.utoronto.ca/rpo/display/poem2652.html

▣ Anne Bradstreet, "The Author to Her Book" (1678)

Bradstreet's book The Tenth Muse *was published in London in 1650. It is thought that she wrote this poem in 1666, when a second edition seemed to have been considered, although the poem was not published until 1678, after Bradstreet's death. In this prefatory poem, Bradstreet likens her presumed diminished skill as a woman writer to the birth of a deformed child. One may witness its various deficiencies and yet embrace the child as one's own.*

Thou ill-form'd offspring of my feeble brain,
Who after birth did'st by my side remain,
Till snatcht from thence by friends, less wise than true,
Who thee abroad, expos'd to publick view,
Made thee in rags halting to th' press to trudge,
Where errors were not lessened (all may judge).
At thy return my blushing was not small,
My rambling brat (in print) should mother call,
I cast thee by as one unfit for light,
They visage was so irksome in my sight;
Yet being mine own, at length affection would
Thy blemishes amend, if so I could:
I wash'd thy face, but more defects I saw,
And rubbing off a spot, still made a flaw.
I stretch thy joints to make thee even feet,
Yet still thou run'st more hobbling than is meet;
In better dress to trim thee was my mind,
But nought save homespun cloth i' th' house I find;
In this array, 'mongst vulgars may'st thou roam,
In critics hands, beware thou dost not come;
And take thy way where yet thou art not known,
If for thy father askt, say thou had'st none:
And for thy mother, she alas is poor,
Which caus'd her thus to send thee out of door.

Source: Bradstreet, Anne. 1678. "The Author to Her Book." Available at: http://www.vcu.edu/engweb/webtexts/Bradstreet/bradpoems.htm

▣ Sir Paul Rycaut, from *The History of the Present State of the Ottoman Empire* (1686)

The English diplomat Sir Paul Rycaut served at the Ottoman Court from 1661 to 1665, during the long reign of Sultan Mehmed IV (1648–1687). Among many people who left an account of their time in Istanbul and at the Ottoman court in the seventeenth century, Rycaut was one of very few who stated his sources for matters of which he was not personally a witness.

[Under Sultan Mehmet IV, reigned 1648–1687] Chap. VIII of the Mutes and Dwarfs. Besides the Pages, there is a sort of Attendants to make up the Ottoman Court, called *Bizebani*, or *Mutes*, men naturally born deaf, and so consequently for want of receiving the sound of words are dumb: These are in number about 40, who by night are lodged amongst the Pages in the two Chambers, but in the day time have their stations before the *Mosque* belonging to the Pages, where they learn and perfect themselves in the language of the *Mutes*, which is made up of several signs, in which by custome they can discourse and fully express themselves; not onely to signifie their sense in familiar questions, but to recount Stories, understand the Fables of their own Religion, the Laws and Precepts of the *Alchoran*, the name of *Mahomet*, and what else may be capable of being expressed by the Tongue. The most ancient amongst them, to the number of about eight or nine, are called the Favourite Mutes, and are admitted to attendance in the *Haz Oda*; who onely serve in the place of *Buffons* for the Grand Signior to sport with, whom he sometimes kicks, sometimes throws in the Cisterns of Water, sometimes makes fight together like the combat of *Clineas* and *Dametas*. But this language of the *Mutes* is so much in fashion in the *Ottoman* Court, that none almost but can deliver his sense in it, and is of much use to those who attend the Presence of the Grand Signior, before whom it is not reverent or seemly so much as to whisper. The Dwarfs are called *Giuge*; these also have their quarters amongst the Pages of the two Chambers, untill they have learned with due reverence and humility to stand in the Presence of the Grand Signior. And if one of these have that benefit, as by Natures fortunate error to be both a Dwarf, and an Eunuch, he is much more esteemed, than if Nature and Art had concurred together to make him the perfectest creature in the World; one of this sort was presented by a certain *Pasha*, to the Grand Signior, who was so acceptable to him and the Queen Mother, that he attired him immediately in clothe of Gold, and gave him liberty through all the Gates of the *Seraglio*. [pp. 62–64]

[Editors' note: This book includes an engraving showing a mute and a dwarf. They are full-figure, standing, adult males, dressed in full-length gowns, slippers, and hats, the dwarf being depicted as perhaps half height. The dwarf is not directly comparable with the mute, because he is shown standing behind and to one side of the mute.]

Source: Rycaut, Paul. 1686. *The history of the present state of the Ottoman Empire, etc.*, 6th ed. London: Clavell, Robinson, and Churchill. (Originally published 1666)

▣ Bobovi's Description of the Ottoman Court (1686)

The following excerpt describes the mute people who lived at the court of the Ottoman Empire during the seventeenth century. These observations, taken from Bobovius (Ali Bey), a senior interpreter at the court, briefly describe the use of sign language by the mute people. The work was translated into English from a French translation of 1686 (manuscript in the Bibliothèque Nationale, Paris), based on an Italian manuscript by Bobovius.

In the palace environs there are also fifty or sixty *dilsiz* or *zebani*. These are the mutes who sleep in the Great and Little Chambers, but sit before the Mosque of the pages of the Great Hall during the day, or are visited by other mutes who have left the Palace with pay and recompense of the sultan. They are expert in sign language and know the significance of everything by sign. They visit and converse with the young and help them to perfect their sign language by telling fables and histories, sayings and scriptures in sign. They teach them the names of the prophets and all sorts of other words. The eight or nine oldest mutes are housed in the *has oda* and are called *musahib* because they play and frolic with the sultan. He entertains himself by their fencing and somersaults in the water of the fountain and, when he is satisfied with their badinage, he throws them *akçes* or *sequins* and enjoys watching them pilfer and battle among themselves. When he wishes to have more diversity, he sometimes has both the dwarfs and the mutes come . . . . The dwarfs are called *cüce* and are lodged in the Great and the Little Hall of the pages until they are instructed and have perfected all of the requirements for living in the presence of the sultan with respect and charity. Truely, there are few things more highly valued than mutes,

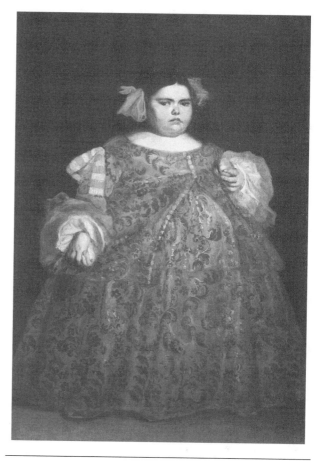

La Monstrua *(1680), by Juan Carreno de Miranda (1614–1685). The title of this painting of Eugenia Martinez Valleji means "the monster" and suggests a derogatory reading of the subject's size. Carreno de Miranda also objectified her sexual power by painting the same figure as a nude.*

Source: Art Resource, New York.

dwarfs and eunuchs altogether. The rarest present that one could give the sultan is a personage endowed with these three beautiful qualities. Once found, he lacked for nothing. He was dressed in precius vests and was extended the favor of the sultan and the Queen Mother. He passed freely in all quarters of the Palace. [p. 23]

While he [the sultan] eats, the mutes and dwarfs perform. He throws them morsels of the food served to him and watches the ensuing scuffle. [p. 63]

[Referring to a map of *Topkapi Sarayi*] 'C' is the *meşcit* in which the pages of the Great Hall pray five times a day. 'D' is the corner nook of the mutes, where they remain during the day with their elders. This is where one may come to learn the beauties of their language. [p. 75]

Pages of one chamber don't dare to mix with pages of another chamber. Indeed, they can communicate with those of other chambers only by speaking with the signs of the mutes. Those in the has oda are always forced to communicate by signs and gestures, maintaining a complete silence at all times in the sultan's presence. [p. 80]

Source: Fisher, C. G., & A. W. Fisher. 1987. *Topkapi Sarayi* in the Mid-Seventeenth Century: Bobovi's Description. *Archivum Ottomanicum* 10:5–81.

▣ Cotton Mather, from "The Wonders of the Invisible World" (1693)

Condemning testimony provided during the Salem witch trials often cited bodily torment as the sign of torture by women accused of witchcraft. Inexplicable pain and suffering of the afflicted, along with revelations of the accused person's own bodily differences, provided the proof of evildoing. The Puritan minister Cotton Mather provided this description of the trial of Bridget Bishop, the first woman to be tried and executed as a witch during the Salem witch trials.

I. She was indicted for bewitching of several persons in the neighborhood, the indictment being drawn up, according to the form in such cases usual. And pleading, not guilty, there were brought in several persons, who had undergone many kinds of miseries, which were preternaturally inflicted, and generally ascribed unto a horrible witchcraft. There was little occasion to prove the witchcraft; it being evident and notorious to all beholders. Now to fix the witchcraft on the prisoner at the bar; the first thing used was, the testimony of the bewitched; whereof, several testified, that the shape of the prisoner did oftentimes very grievously pinch them, choke them, bite them, and afflict them; urging them to write their names in a book, which the said specter called, ours. One of them did further testify, that it was the shape of the prisoner, with another, which one day took her from her wheel, and carrying her towards the riverside, threatened there to drown her; if she did not sign to the book mentioned; which yet she refused. Others of them did testify, that the said shape, did in her threats, brag to them, that she had been the death of sundry persons, then by her named; that she had ridden a man, then likewise named. Another testified, the apparition of ghosts under the specter of Bishop, crying out, you murdered us! About the truth whereof, there was in the matter of fact, but too much suspicion.

II. It was testified, that at the examination of the prisoner, before the magistrates, the bewitched were extremely tortured. If she did but cast her eyes on them, they were presently struck down; and this in such a manner as there could be no collusion in the business. But upon the touch of her hand upon them, when they lay in their swoons, they would immediacy revive; and not upon the touch of anyone's else. Moreover, upon some special actions of her body, as the shaking of her head, or the turning of her eyes, they precisely and painfully felt into the like postures. And many of the like accidents now fell out, while she was at the bar. One at the same time testifying, that she said, she could not be troubled to see the afflicted thus tormented.

III. There was testimony likewise brought in, that a man striking once at the place, where a bewitched person said, the shape of this Bishop stood, the bewitched cried out, that he had tore her coat, in the place then particularly specified; and the woman's coat, was found to be torn in that very place.

IV. One Deliverance Hobbs, who had confessed her being a witch, was now tormented by the specters, for her confession. And she now testified, that this bishop, tempted her to sign the book again, and to deny what she had confessed. She affirmed, that it was the shape of this prisoner, which whipped her with iron rods, to compel her thereunto. She affirmed, that this Bishop was at a general meeting of the witches, in a field at Salem Village, and there partook of a diabolical sacrament, in bread and wine then administered.

V. To render it further unquestionable, that the prisoner at the bar, was the person truly charged in *this* witchcraft, there were produced many evidences of *other* witchcrafts, by her perpetrated. For instance, John Cook testified, that about five or six years ago, one morning, about sunrise, he was in his chamber, assaulted by the shape of this prisoner: which looked on him, grinned at him, and very much hurt him, with a blow on the side of the head: and that on the same day, about noon, the same shape walked in the room where he was, and an apple strangely flew out of his hand, into the lap of his mother, six or eight foot from him.

VI. Samuel Gray, testified, that about fourteen years ago, he waked on a night, and saw the room where he lay, full of light; and that he then saw plainly a woman between the cradle, and the bedside, which looked upon him. He rose, and it vanished; though he found the doors all fast. Looking out at the entry door, he saw the same woman, in the same garb again; and said, *In God's name, what do you come for?* He went to bed, and had the same woman again assaulting him. The child in the cradle gave a great screech, and the woman disappeared. It was long before the child could be quieted; and though it were a very likely thriving child, yet from this time it pined away, and after divers months died in a sad condition. He knew not Bishop, nor her name; but when he saw her after this, he knew by her countenance, and apparel, and all circumstances, that it was the apparition of this Bishop, which had troubled him.

Source: Mather, Cotton. 1693. "The Wonders of the Invisible World." Available at: http://etext.lib.virginia.edu/etcbin/toccer-new2?id=Bur4Nar.sgm&images=images/modeng&data=/texts/english/modeng/parsed&tag=public&part=all

▣ Begging Laws (1697)

This excerpt provides an example of an early badging law used to identity "legitimate" disabled people, who were eligible to receive alms and permitted to beg within parishes.

Parliament directed that *all* people legitimately on relief . . . shall upon the shoulder of the right sleeve of the uppermost garment . . . in an open and visible manner, wear such badge or mark as is herein-after mentioned and expressed, that is to say, a large Roman P, together with the first letter of the name of the parish or place whereof such poor person is an inhabitant, cut either in red or blue cloth.

Source: "8 & 9 William 3, ch. 30." 1697. Reprinted in de Schweinitz, Karl. 1943. P. 87 in *England's Road to Social Security*. Philadelphia: University of Pennsylvania Press.

▣ John Dryden, from the Preface to *Fables, Ancient and Modern* (1700)

In this preface, John Dryden admits to some physical effects of his advancing age, but he declares that his mental acuity and "judgment" have persisted—indeed, have increased. His "faculties of soul" remain, even if his memory is fading slightly. He could "lawfully plead some part of the old gentleman's excuse" for any imperfections in the book, but he will not in this case, asking instead for a general allowance for mere human frailty.

By the mercy of God, I am already come within twenty years of his number, a cripple in my limbs; but what decays are in my mind, the reader must determine. I think myself as vigorous as ever in the faculties of my soul, excepting only my memory, which is not impair'd to any great degree; and if I lose not more of it, I have no great reason to complain. What judgment I had, increases rather than diminishes; and thoughts, such as they are, come crowding in so fast upon me, that my only difficulty is to choose or to reject; to run them into verse, or to give them the other harmony of prose. I have so long studied and practic'd both, that they are grown into a habit, and become familiar to me. In short, tho' I may lawfully plead some part of the old gentleman's excuse, yet I will reserve it till I think I have greater need, and ask no grains of allowance for the faults of this my present work, but those which are given of course to human frailty.

Source: Dryden, John. 1700. "Preface." *Fables, Ancient and Modern*. Available at: http://bartleby.school.aol.com/39/25.html

▣ "March's Ears" (1700)

This Welsh folktale touches upon a number of important themes, including the perceived importance of concealment to the disabled person as well as the fear of exposure and exhibition of the disability. This story emphasizes that disability affects the well-born and the low-born equally: no matter how many riches one possesses, a disability can ruin one's life.

March ab Meirchion was lord of Castellmarch, in Lleyn. He ruled over leagues of rich land, tilled by hundreds of willing and obedient vassals. He had great possessions, fleet horses, greyhounds, hawks; countless black cattle and sheep, and a great herd of swine. (But few possessed pigs at that time, and their flesh was esteemed better than the flesh of oxen. Arthur himself sought to have one of March's sows.) In his palace he had much treasure of gold, silver, and Conway pearls, and all men envied him. But March was not happy: he had a secret, and day and night he was torn with dread lest it should be discovered. *He had horse's ears!*

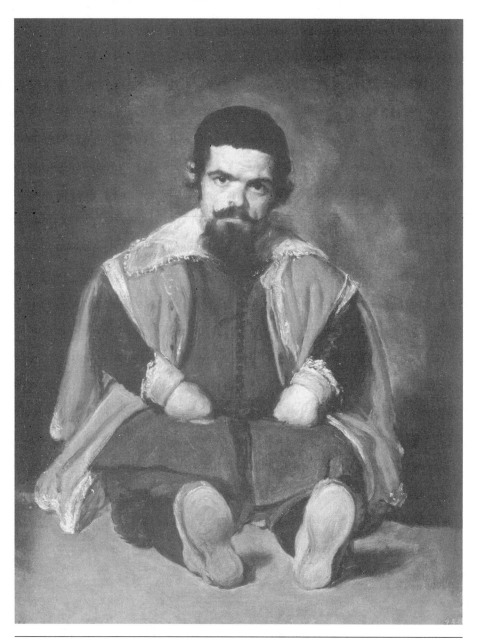

Portrait of the Jester Sebastian de Morra, *by Diego Rodriguez Velázquez (1599–1660). One of Spain's most famous painters, Velázquez dedicated himself to painting the "common things" in his environment. When not pursuing his livelihood as a portraitist of the upper classes, Velázquez shirked the classical tradition's emphasis on symmetry and conventional beauty by painting many of his acquaintances who were people with disabilities.*

Source: Art Resource, New York.

The barber became as unhappy as March: indeed his wretchedness was greater, because his fate would be worse if the secret were revealed. March would undergo ridicule, which is certainly a serious thing : but the barber would undergo decapitation, which is much more serious. The secret disagreed with his constitution so violently that he lost his appetite and his colour, and began to fall into a decline. So ill did he become that he had to call in a physician. This man was skilled in his craft, and he said to the barber, "You are being killed by a suppressed secret: unless you communicate it to someone you will soon be in your grave."

This announcement did not give the barber much consolation. He explained to the physician that if he did as he was directed he would lose his head. If in any event he had to come to the end of his earthly career, he preferred being interred with his head joined to, rather than separated from, his trunk. The physician then suggested that he should tell his secret to the ground. The barber thought there was not much danger to his cervical vertebrae (this is the learned name for neck bones) if he did this, and adopted the suggestion. He was at once

To no one was the secret known except his barber. This man he compelled to take a solemn oath that he would not reveal his deformity to any living soul. If he wittingly or unwittingly should let anyone know that March's ears were other than human, March swore that he would cut his head off.

relieved. His colour and appetite gradually came back, and before long he was as strong and well as he had ever been.

Now it happened that a fine crop of reeds grew on the spot where the barber whispered his secret to the ground. March prepared a great feast, and sent for one of Maelgwn Gwynedd's pipers, who was the best piper in the world, to make music for his guests. On his way to Castellmarch, the piper observed these fine reeds, and as his old pipe was getting worn out, he cut them and made an excellent new pipe. When his guests had eaten and drunk, March ordered the piper to play. What was the surprise of all when the pipe gave out no music, but only the words, "Horse's ears for March ab Meirchion, horse's ears for March ab Meirchion," over and over again. March drew his sword and would have slain the piper, but the hapless musician begged for mercy. He was not to blame, he said: he had tried to play his wonted music, but the pipe was charmed, and do what he would, he could get nothing out of it but the words, "Horse's ears for March ab Meirchion." March tried the pipe himself, but even he could not elicit any strains from it, but only the words, "Horse's ears for March ab Meirchion." So he forgave the piper and made no further effort to conceal his deformity.

Source: V. Wales. n.d. "March's Ears." In *Welsh Fairy Stories*. Available at: http://www.red4.co.uk/Folklore/fairytales/marchsears.htm

"The Story of the Barber's Sixth Brother" from *Arabian Nights* (1704–1717)

The plot of this tale from the Arabian Nights depends in part on the cultural ideas of difference regarding disabled people. The hunchback's body becomes not just an object of entertainment and merriment, but a literal object, as his apparently dead body is passed around, propped up, and examined before the discovery that his amazing "constitution" has made him only appear to be dead.

"This,"—continued the barber,—"is the tale I related to the Caliph, who, when I had finished, burst into fits of laughter."

"Well were you called 'the Silent,'" said he; "no name was ever better deserved. But for reasons of my own, which it is not necessary to mention, I desire you to leave the town, and never to come back."

"I had of course no choice but to obey, and travelled about for several years until I heard of the death of the Caliph, when I hastily returned to Bagdad, only to find that all my brothers were dead. It was at this time that I rendered to the young cripple the important service of which you have heard, and for which, as you know, he showed such profound ingratitude, that he preferred rather to leave Bagdad than to run the risk of seeing me. I sought him long from place to place, but it was only to-day, when I expected it least, that I came across him, as much irritated with me as ever"— So saying the tailor went on to relate the story of the lame man and the barber, which has already been told.

"When the barber," he continued, "had finished his tale, we came to the conclusion that the young man had been right, when he had accused him of being a great chatter-box. However, we wished to keep him with us, and share our feast, and we remained at table till the hour of afternoon prayer. Then the company broke up, and I went back to work in my shop."

"It was during this interval that the little hunchback, half drunk already, presented himself before me, singing and playing on his drum. I took him home, to amuse my wife, and she invited him to supper. While eating some fish, a bone got into his throat, and in spite of all we could do, he died shortly. It was all so sudden that we lost our heads, and in order to divert suspicion from ourselves, we carried the body to the house of a Jewish physician. He placed it in the chamber of the purveyor, and the purveyor propped it up in the street, where it was thought to have been killed by the merchant."

"This, Sire, is the story which I was obliged to tell to satisfy your highness. It is now for you to say if we deserve mercy or punishment; life or death?"

The Sultan of Kashgar listened with an air of pleasure that filled the tailor and his friends with hope. "I must confess," he exclaimed, "that I am much more interested in the stories of the barber and his brothers, and of the lame man, than in that of my own jester. But before I allow you all four to return to your own homes, and have the corpse of the hunchback properly buried, I should like to see this barber who has earned your pardon. And as he is in this town, let an usher go with you at once in search of him."

The usher and the tailor soon returned, bringing with them an old man who must have been at least ninety years of age. "O Silent One," said the Sultan, "I am told that you know many strange stories. Will you tell some of them to me?"

"Never mind my stories for the present," replied the barber, "but will your Highness graciously be pleased to explain why this Jew, this Christian, and this Mussulman, as well as this dead body, are all here?"

"What business is that of yours?" asked the Sultan with a smile; but seeing that the barber had some reasons for his question, he commanded that the tale of the hunch-back should be told him.

"It is certainly most surprising," cried he, when he had heard it all, "but I should like to examine the body." He then knelt down, and took the head on his knees, looking at it attentively. Suddenly he burst into such loud laughter that he fell right backwards, and when he had recovered himself enough to speak, he turned to the Sultan. "The man is no more dead than I am," he said; "watch me." As he spoke he drew a small case of medicines from his pocket and rubbed the neck of the hunchback with some ointment made of balsam. Next he opened the dead man's mouth, and by the help of a pair of pincers drew the bone from his throat. At this the hunch-back sneezed, stretched himself and opened his eyes.

The Sultan and all those who saw this operation did not know which to admire most, the constitution of the hunchback who had apparently been dead for a whole night and most of one day, or the skill of the barber, whom everyone now began to look upon as a great man. His Highness desired that the history of the hunchback should be written down, and placed in the archives beside that of the barber, so that they might be associated in people's minds to the end of time. And he did not stop there; for in order to wipe out the memory of what they had undergone, he commanded that the tailor, the doctor, the purveyor and the merchant, should each be clothed in his presence with a robe from his own wardrobe before they returned home. As for the barber, he bestowed on him a large pension, and kept him near his own person.

Source: Lang, Andrew, trans. 1898. "The Story of the Barber's Sixth Brother." *Arabian Nights*. Available at: http://www.wollamshram.ca/1001/Lang/lang.htm

◉ Joseph Addison, from *The Spectator* (1711)

The Spectator, a daily periodical issued by Joseph Addison and Richard Steele in 1711–1712 and by Addison alone in 1714, offered witty observations on manners and literature for a primarily middle-class audience. The excerpt from No. 58 provides a portion of Addison's invective against the many forms of what he calls "false wit" in literature. In the excerpt from No. 63, Addison draws on these examples to create a dream vision in which disabled human bodies serve as metaphors for false wit.

From No. 58

Ut pictura poesis erit

—Horace

Nothing is so much admired and so little understood as Wit. No Author that I know of has written professedly upon it; and as for those who make any Mention of it, they only treat on the Subject as it has accidentally fallen inn their Way, and that too in little short Reflections, or in general declamatory Flourishes, without entering into the Bottom of the Matter. I hope therefore I shall perform an acceptable Work to my Countrymen if I treat at large upon this Subject; which I shall endeavor to do in a Manner suitable to it, that I may not incur the Censure which a famous Critick bestows upon one who had written a Treatise upon *the Sublime* in a low groveling Stile. I intend to lay aside a whole Week for this Undertaking, that the Scheme of my Thoughts may not be broken and interrupted; and I dare promise my self, if my Readers will give me a Week's Attention, that this great City will be very much changed for the better by next *Saturday* Night. I shall endeavor to make what I say intelligible to ordinary Capacities; but if my Readers meet with any Paper that in some Parts of it may be a little out of their Reach, I would not have them discouraged, for they may assure themselves the next shall be much clearer.

As the great and only End of these my Speculations is to banish Vice and Ignorance out of the Territories of *Great Britain*, I shall endeavor as much as possible to establish among us a Taste of polite Writing. It is with this View that I have endeavored to set my Readers right in several Points relating to Operas and Tragedies; and shall from Time to Time impart my Notions of Comedy, as I think they may tend to its Refinement and Perfection. I find by my Bookseller that these Papers of Criticism, with that upon Humour, have met with a more kind Reception that indeed I could have hoped for from such Subjects; for which Reason I shall enter upon my present Undertaking with greater Cheerfulness.

In this and one or two following Papers I shall trace out the History of false Wit, and distinguish the several Kinds of it as they have prevailed in different Ages of the World. This I think the more necessary at present, because I observed there were Attempts on foot last Winter to revive some of those antiquated Modes of Wit that have been long exploded out of the Commonwealth of Letters. There were several Satyrs and Panegyricks handed about in Acrostick, by which Means some of the most arrant undisputed Blockheads about the Town began to entertain ambitious Thoughts, and to set up for polite Authors. I shall therefore describe at length those many Arts of false Wit, in which a Writer does not shew himself a Man of a beautiful Genius, but of great Industry.

The first Species of false Wit which I have met with is very venerable for its Antiquity, and has produced several Pieces which have lived very near as long as the *Iliad* itself: I mean those short Poems printed among the minor *Greek* Poets, which resemble the Figure of an Egg, a Pair of Wings, an Ax, a Shepherd's Pipe, and an Altar.

As for the first, it is a little oval Poem, and may not improperly be called a Scholar's Egg. I would endeavor to hatch it, or, in more intelligible Language, to translate it into *English*, did not I find the Interpretation of it very difficult; for the Author seems to have been more intent upon the Figure of his Poem, than upon the Sense of it.

The Pair of Wings consist of twelve Verses, or rather Feathers, every Verse decreasing gradually in its Measure according to its Situation in the Wing. The Subject of it (as in the rest of the Poems which follow) bears some remote Affinity with the Figure, for it describes a God of Love, who is always painted with Wings.

The Ax methinks would have been a good Figure for a Lampoon, had the Edge of it consisted of the most satirical Parts of the Work; but as it is in the Original, I take it to have been nothing else but the Posy of an Ax which was consecrated to *Minerva*, and was thought to have been the same . . .

From No. 63

Humano Capiti cervicem pictor Equinam
Jungere si velit et varias inducere plumas
Undique collatis membris, ut turpiter atrum
Desinat in piscem mulier Formosa superne;
Spectatum admissi risum teatis, amici?
Credite, Pisones, isti tabulae fore librum
Persimilen, cujus, velut aegri somnia, vanae
Finguntur species

—Horace

It is very hard for the Mind to disengage it self from a Subject in which it has been long employed. The Thoughts will be rising of themselves from time to time, tho' we give them no Encouragement; as the Tossings and Fluctuations of the Sea continue several hours after the Winds are laid.

It is to this that I impute my last Night's Dream or Vision which formed into one Continued Allegory the several Schemes of Wit, whether False, Mixed, or true, that have been the Subject of my late Papers.

Methoughts I was transported into a Country that was filled with Prodigies and Enchantments, Governed by the Goddess of Falsehood, and entitled the *Region of false Wit*. There was nothing in the Fields, the Woods, and the Rivers, that appeared natural. Several of the Trees blossom'd in Leaf-Gold, some of them produced Bone Lace, and some of them precious Stones, the Fountains bubbled in an Opera Tune, and were filled with Stags, Wild-Boars, and Mermaids, that lived among the Waters, at the same time that Dolphins and several kinds of Fish played upon the Banks, or took their Pastime in the Meadows. The Birds had many of them Golden beaks, and human Voices. The Flowers perfumed the Air with Smells of Incense, Amber-Greese and Pulvillios, and were so interwoven with one another, that they grew up in Pieces of Embroidery. The Winds were fill'd with Sighs and Messages of distant Lovers. As I was walking to and fro in this enchanted Wilderness, I could not forbear breaking out into Soliloquies upon the several Wonders which lay before me, when to my great Surprise I found there were artificial Ecchoes in every Walk, that by Repetitions of certain Words which I spoke, agreed with me, or contradicted me, in everything I said. In the midst of my Conversation with these invisible Companions, I discover'd in the Center of a very dark Grove a Monstrous Fabrick built after the Gothick manner, and covered with innumerable Devices in that barbarous kind of Sculpture. I immediately went up to it, and found it to be a kind of Heathen Temple consecrated to the God of Dullness. Upon my Entrance I saw the Deity of the Place dressed in the Habit of a Monk, with a Book in one Hand and a Rattle in the other. Upon his right Hand was Industry, with a Lamp burning before Her; and on his left Caprice, with a Monkey sitting on her Shoulder. Before his Feet there was shaped in that manner, to comply with the Inscription that surrounded it. Upon the Altar there lay several Offerings of Axes, Wings, and Eggs, cut in Paper, and inscribed with Verses. The Temple was filled with Votaries, who applied themselves to different Diversions, as their Fancies directed them. In one Part of it I saw a Regiment of Anagrams, who were continually in motion, turning to the Right or to the Left, facing about, doubling their Ranks, shifting their Stations, and throwing themselves into all the Figures and Counter-marches of the most changeable and perplexed Exercise.

Not far from these was a body of *Acrosticks*, made up of very disproportioned Persons. It was disposed into three Columns, the Officers planting themselves in a Line on the left Hand of each Column. The Officers were all of them at least Six Foot high, and made three Rows of very proper Men; but the Common Soldiers, who filled up the spaces between the Officers, were such Dwarfs, Cripples, and Scare-Crows, that one could hardly look upon them without laughing. There were behind the *Acrosticks* two or three files of *Chronograms*, which differed only from the former, as their Officers were equipped (like the Figure of Time) with an Hourglass in one Hand, and a Scythe in the other, and took their Posts promiscuously among the private Men whom they commanded.

In the Body of the Temple, and before the very Face of the Deity methoughts I saw the Phantom of *Tryphiodorus* the *Lipo-grammatist*, engaged in a Ball with four and twenty Persons, who pursued him by turns through all the Intricacies and Labyrinths of a Country Dance, without being able to overtake him.

Observing several to be very busie at the Western End of the *Temple*, I inquired into what they were doing, and found there was in that Quarter the great Magazine of *Rebus*'s. These were several things of the most different Natures tied up in Bundles. . . . One of the Workmen seeing me very much surprized, told me, there was an infinite deal of Wit in several of those Bundles, and that he would explain them to me if I pleased: I thanked him for his Civility, but told him I was in very great haste at that time. As I was going out of the Temple, I observed in one Corner of it a Cluster of Men and Women laughing very heartily, and diverting themselves at a Game of *Crambo*. I heard several *double Rhymes* as I passed by them, which raised a great deal of Mirth.

Not far from these was another Set of Merry People engaged at a Diversion, in which the whole Jest was to mistake one Person for another. To give occasion for these ludicrous Mistakes, they were divided into Pairs, every Pair being covered from Head to Foot

with the same kind of Dress, though, perhaps, there was not the least Resemblance in their Faces. By this means an old Man was sometimes mistaken for a Boy, a Woman for a Man, and a Black-a-moor for an *European*, which very often produced great Peals of Laughter. These I guess'd to be a Party of *Punns*. But being very desirous to get out of the World of Magick, which had almost turned my Brain, I left the Temple, and crossed over the Fields that lay about it with all the speed I could make. I was not gone far before I heard the Sound of Trumpets and Alarms, which seemed to proclaim the March of an Enemy; and, as I afterwards found, was in reality what I apprehended it. There appear'd at a great distance a very shining Light, and in the midst of it a Person of a most beautiful Aspect; her Name was TRUTH. On her Right Hand there marched a Male Deity, who bore several Quivers on his Shoulders, and grasped several Arrows in his Hand. His Name was *Wit*. The Approach of these two Enemies filled all the Territories of *False Wit* with an unspeakable Consternation, insomuch that the Goddess of those Regions Appear'd inn Person upon her Frontiers with the several inferior Deities, and the different Bodies of Forces which I had before seen in the Temple, who were now drawn up in Array, and prepared to give their Foes a warm Reception. As the March of the Enemy was very slow, it gave time to the several Inhabitants who border'd upon the *Regions of* FALSEHOOD to draw their Forces into a Body, with a Design to stand upon their Guard as Neuters, and attend the Issue of the Combat.

I must here inform my Reader, that the Frontiers of the Enchanted Region, which I have before described, were inhabited by the Species of MIXED WIT, who made a very odd Appearance when they were Mustered together in an Army. There were Men whose Bodies were stuck full of Darts, and Women whose eyes were burning Glasses: Men that had Hearts of Fire, and Women that had Breasts of Snow. It would be endless to describe several Monsters of the like Nature, that composed this great Army; which immediately fell asunder, and divided it self into two Parts; the one half throwing themselves behind the Banners of TRUTH, and the others behind those of FALSEHOOD.

The Goddess of FALSEHOOD was of a Gigantick Stature, and advanced some Paces before the front of her Army; but as the dazzling Light, which flowed from TRUTH, began to shine upon her, she faded insensibly; insomuch that inn a little space she looked rather like an huge Phantom, than a real Substance. At length, as the Goddess of TRUTH approached still nearer to her, she fell away entirely, and vanish'd amidst the Brightness of Place where she had been seen.

As at the rising of the Sun the Constellations grow thin, and the Stars go out one after another, 'till the whole Hemisphere is extinguish'd; such was the vanishing of the Goddess; and not only of the Goddess her self, but of the whole Army that attended her, which sympathized with their Leader, and shrunk into Nothing, in Proportion as the Goddess disappeared. At the same time the whole Temple sunk, the Fish betook themselves to the Streams, and thee wild Beasts to the Woods: The Fountains recover'd their Murmurs, the Birds their Voices, the Trees their Leaves, the Flowers their Scents, and the whole Face of Nature its true and genuine Appearance. Tho' I still continued asleep, I fancy'd my self as it were awaken'd out of a Dream, when I saw this Region of Prodigies restor'd to Woods and Rivers, Fields and Meadows.

Source: Addison, Joseph, and Richard Steele. 1711, May 7. *The Spectator*, 58. Available at: http://www.fullbooks.com/The-Spectator-Volume-17.html

Addison, Joseph, and Richard Steele. 1711, May 12. *The Spectator*, 63. Available at: http://www.fullbooks.com/The-Spectator-Volume-18.html

▣ Lady Mary Wortley Montagu, Poems (18th c.)

In 1716, Lady Mary Wortley Montagu accompanied her husband, Edward Wortley Montagu, when he was sent as ambassador to Constantinople. She had contracted smallpox the year before and had been left badly scarred. In Constantinople, she learned of the practice of inoculating people against smallpox, and she introduced the method upon her return to England. The first poem included here suggests the horror felt by women at this time at "losing their beauty" as a result of the scarring of smallpox. In the second poem, the speaker mourns her lost beauty most painfully at the moment when she finds someone she hopes can look beyond it. In the final poem, interestingly, we find that Wortley Montagu's experience of smallpox did not render her sympathetic to the disability of another; she uses Alexander Pope's body, deformed by tuberculosis of the spine, as the basis for some of her satire against him.

Satturday: The Small Pox. Flavia

The wretched Flavia, on her couch reclined,
Thus breath'd the anguish of a wounded mind,
A glass revers'd in her right hand she bore,
For now she shunn'd the face she sought before.
"How am I chang'd! alas! how am I grown
A frightful spectre to myself unknown!
Where's my complexion? where my radiant bloom,
That promis'd happiness for years to come?
Then with what pleasure I this face survey'd!
To look once more, my visits oft delay'd!
Charm'd with the view, a fresher red would rise,
And a new life shot sparkling from my eyes!
"Ah! faithless glass, my wonted bloom restore;
Alas! I rave, that bloom is now no more!
The greatest good the gods on men bestow,
Ev'n youth itself, to me is useless now.
There was a time (oh! that I could forget!)
When opera-tickets pour'd before my feet;
And at the Ring, where brightest beauties shine,
The earliest cherries of the spring were mine.
Witness, O Lilly; and thou, Motteux, tell,
How much japan these eyes have made ye sell.
With what contempt ye saw me oft despise
The humble offer of the raffled prize;
For at each raffle still each prize I bore,
With scorn rejected, or with triumph wore!
Now beauty's fled, and presents are no more!
"For me the patriot has the House forsook,
And left debates to catch a passing look:
For me the soldier has soft verses writ:
For me the beau has aim'd to be a wit.
For me the wit to nonsense was betray'd;
The gamester has for me his dun delay'd,
And overseen the card he would have play'd.
The bold and haughty, by success made vain,
Aw'd by my eyes have trembled to complain:
The bashful 'squire, touch'd by a wish unknown,
Has dar'd to speak with spirit not his own:
Fir'd by one wish, all did alike adore;
Now beauty's fled, and lovers are no more!
"As round the room I turn my weeping eyes,
New unaffected scenes of sorrow rise.
Far from my sight that killing picture bear,
The face disfigure, and the canvas tear:
That picture which with pride I us'd to show,
The lost resemblance that upbraids me now.
And thou, my toilette! where I oft have sat,

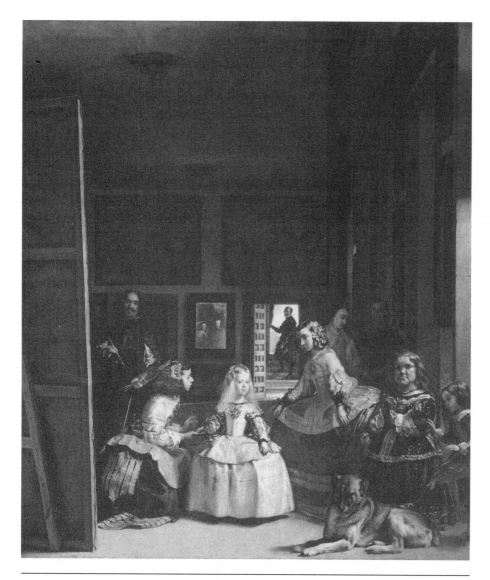

Las Meninas, or the Family of Phillip IV, *by Diego Rodriguez Velázquez (1599–1660). Building upon the role of individuals of short stature or with cognitive disabilities as those who were allowed to critique power openly, Velázquez allows the gaze of the disabled attendant in this work to meet that of the viewer. In doing so, the figure calls attention to the act of looking upon bodies as objects without self-awareness.*

Source: Art Resource, New York.

While hours unheeded pass'd in deep debate
How curls should fall, or where a patch to place;
If blue on scarlet best became my face:
Now on some happier nymph your aid bestow;
On fairer heads, ye useless jewels, glow!
No borrow'd lustre can my charms restore;
Beauty is fled, and dress is now no more!
"Ye meaner beauties, I permit ye shine;
Go, triumph in the hearts that once were mine:
But, 'midst your triumphs with confusion know,
'Tis to my ruin all your charms ye owe.

Would pitying Heav'n restore my wonted mien,
Ye still might move unthought of and unseen:
But oh, how vain, how wretched is the boast
Of beauty faded, and of empire lost!
What now is left but, weeping, to deplore
My beauty fled, and empire now no more!
"Ye cruel chemists, what withheld your aid?
Could no pomatum save a trembling maid?
How false and trifling is that art ye boast!
No art can give me back my beauty lost.
In tears, surrounded by my friends, I lay
Mask'd o'er, and trembled at the sight of day;
Mirmillio came my fortune to deplore
(A golden-headed cane well carv'd he bore),
Cordials, he cried, my spirits must restore!
Beauty is fled, and spirit is no more!
"Galen, the grave officious Squirt was there.
With fruitless grief and unavailing care;
Machaon too, the great Machaon, known
By his red cloak and his superior frown;
And why, he cried, this grief and this despair?
You shall again be well, again be fair;
Believe my oath (with that an oath he swore);
False was his oath; my beauty was no more!
"Cease, hapless maid, no more thy tale pursue,
Forsake mankind, and bid the world adieu!
Monarchs and beauties rule with equal sway:
All strive to serve, and glory to obey:
Alike unpitied when depos'd they grow,
Men mock the idol of their former vow.
"Adieu! ye parks—in some obscure recess,

Where gentle streams will weep at my distress,
Where no false friend will in my grief take part,
And mourn my ruin with a joyful heart;
There let me live in some deserted place,
There hide in shades this lost inglorious face.
Plays, operas, circles, I no more must view!
My toilette, patches, all the world adieu!"

This Once Was Me

This once was me, thus my complexion fair,
My cheek thus blooming, and thus curl'd my Hair,
This picture which with pride I us'd to show
The lost resemblance but upbraids me now,
Yet all these charms I only would renew
To make a mistrisse less unworthy you.
'Tis said, the Gods by ardent Bows are gain'd,
Iphis her wish (however wild) obtain'd,
Pygmalion warm'd to Life his Ivory maid,
Will no kind power restore my charms decaid?
With useless Beauty my first Youth was crown'd,
In all my Conquests I no pleasure found,
The croud I shunn'd, nor of Applause was vain
And Felt no pity for a Lover's pain.
The pangs of passion coldly I despised
And view'd with scorn the ravage of my Eyes.
Now that contempt too dearly is repaid,
Th'impetuous Fire does my whole Soul invade.
O more than Madness!—with compassion View
A Heart could only be enflam'd by You.
In that Lov'd Form there does at once unite
All that can raise Esteem, or give delight,
A Heart like mine is not below your care,
Artless and Honest, tender and sincere,
Where no mean thought has ever found a place
Look on my Heart, and you'll forget my Face.

Verses: Addressed to the Imitator of the First Satire of the Second Book of Horace

In two large columns on thy motley page
Where Roman wit is strip'd with English rage;
Where ribaldry to satire makes pretence,
And modern scandal rolls with ancient sense:
Whilst on one side we see how Horace thought,
And on the other how he never wrote;
Who can believe, who view the bad, the good
That the dull copyist better understood
That spirit he pretends to imitate,
Than heretofore that Greek he did translate?
Thine is just such an image of *his* pen,

As thou thyself art of the sons of men,
Where our own species in burlesque we trace,
A sign-post likeness of the human race,
That is at once resemblance and disgrace.
Horace can laugh, is delicate, is clear,
You only coarsely rail, or darkly sneer;
His style is elegant, his diction pure,
Whilst none thy crabbed numbers can endure;
Hard as thy heart, and as thy birth obscure.
If *he* has thorns, they all on roses grow;
Thine like thistles, and mean brambles show;
With this exception, that, though rank the soil,
Weeds as they are, they seem produc'd by toil.
Satire should, like a polish'd razor, keen,
Wound with a touch, that's scarcely felt or seen:
Thine is an oyster-knife, that hacks and hews;
The rage, but not the talent to abuse;
And is in *hate*, what *love* is in the stews.
'Tis the gross *lust* of hate, that still annoys,
Without distinction, as gross love enjoys:
Neither to folly, nor to vice confin'd,
The object of thy spleen is humankind:
It preys on all who yield, or who resist:
To thee 'tis provocation to exist.
But if thou seest a great and generous heart,
Thy bow is doubly bent to force a dart.
Nor dignity nor innocence is spar'd,
Nor age, nor sex, nor thrones, nor graves, rever'd.
Nor only justice vainly we demand,
But even benefits can't rein thy hand;
To this or that alike in vain we trust,
Nor find thee less ungrateful than unjust.
Not even youth and beauty can control
The universal rancour of thy soul;
Charms that might soften superstition's rage,
Might humble pride, or thaw the ice of age.
But how should'st thou by beauty's force be mov'd,
No more for loving made than to be lov'd?
It was the equity of righteous Heav'n,
That such a soul to such a form was giv'n;
And shows the uniformity of fate,
That one so odious should be born to hate.
When God created thee, one would believe
He said the same as to the snake of Eve;
To human race antipathy declare,
'Twixt them and thee be everlasting war.
But oh! the sequel of the sentence dread,
And whilst you *bruise their heel*, beware your head.
Nor think thy weakness shall be thy defence,
The female scold's protection in offence.
Sure 'tis as fair to beat who cannot fight,

As 'tis to libel those who cannot write.
And if thou draw'st thy pen to aid the law,
Others a cudgel, or a rod, may draw.
If none with vengeance yet thy crimes pursue,
Or give thy manifold affronts their due;
If limbs unbroken, skin without a stain,
Unwhipt, unblanketed, unkick'd, unslain,
That wretched little carcase you retain,
The reason is, not that the world wants eyes,
But thou'rt so mean, they see, and they despise:
When fretful *porcupine*, with ranc'rous will,
From mounted back shoots forth a harmless quill,
Cool the spectators stand; and all the while
Upon the angry little monster smile.
Thus 'tis with thee:—while impotently safe,
You strike unwounding, we unhurt can laugh.
Who but must laugh, this bully when he sees,
A puny insect shiv'ring at a breeze?
One over-match'd by every blast of wind,
Insulting and provoking all mankind.
Is this the *thing* to keep mankind in awe,
To make those tremble who escape the law?
Is this *the ridicule* to live so long,
The deathless satire and *immortal song?*
No: like the self-blown praise, thy scandal flies;
And, as we're told of wasps, it stings and dies.
If none do yet return th'intended blow,
You all your safety to your dulness owe:
But whilst that armour thy poor corse defends,
'Twill make thy readers few, as are thy friends:
Those, who thy nature loath'd, yet lov'd thy art,
Who lik'd thy head, and yet abhorr'd thy heart:
Chose thee to read, but never to converse,
And scorn'd in prose him whom they priz'd in verse
Ev'n they shall now their partial error see,
Shall shun thy writings like thy company;
And to thy books shall ope their eyes no more
Than to thy person they would do their door.
Nor thou the justice of the world disown,
That leaves thee thus an outcast and alone;
For though in law to murder be to kill,
In equity the murder's in the will:
Then whilst with coward-hand you stab a name,
And try at least t'assassinate our fame,
Like the first bold assassin's be thy lot,
Ne'er be thy guilt forgiven, or forgot;
But, as thou hat'st be hated by mankind,
And with the emblem of thy crooked mind

Mark'd on thy back, like Cain by God's own hand,
Wander, like him, accursed through the land.

———————

Source: Montagu, Lady Mary Wortley. 1993. Halsband, Robert, ed. *Essays and Poems and "Simplicity," a Comedy.* New York: Oxford University Press.

[Editors' note: This poem was probably written jointly by Lady Mary and Lord Hervey in 1733, in response to Alexander Pope's satire of Lady Mary.]

◉ Joseph Pitton de Tournefort, from *A Voyage into the Levant* (1717)

By the time Joseph Pitton de Tournefort was writing, in the early eighteenth century, an anti-Orientalist critique (that is, that Tournefort's treatment objectifies as exotic and radically different the people he describes) may be justified. Tournefort may have been reliable for some things, but often he gives signs of incorporating into his account material from earlier writers about things that he had not himself seen (and that quite possibly were no longer there to see). He also gives signs of embroidering and inflating events or practices.

The Pavilion which is toward the *Bosphorus*, is higher than that of the Port, and built on Arches which support three Salons terminated by gilded Domes. The Prince comes thither to sport with his Women and Mutes. [Vol. II, P. 185]

. . . the Palace therefore is fill'd only with a Train of Creatures intirely consecrated to him. They may be divided into five Classes; the *Eunuchs*, the *Ichoglans*, the *Azamoglans*, the *Women*, and the *Mutes*; to whom may be added the *Dwarfs* and the *Buffoons*, who deserve not to be accounted a distinct Class by themselves.

Besides the Officers already mention'd, the Sultans have also in their Palace two sorts of People, who serve to divert them; namely, the *Mutes*, and the *Dwarfs*. The Mutes of the Seraglio are a Species of rational Creatures by themselves: for, not to disturb the Prince's Repose, they have invented a Language among themselves, the Characters of which are express'd by Signs alone; and these Signs are understood by Night as well as by Day, by touching certain Parts of their Body. This Language is so much in fashion in the Seraglio, that they who would please there, and are oblig'd to be in the Prince's Presence, learn it very carefully: for it would be a want of the deep Respect they owe him, to whisper one another in the Ear before him. [Vol. II, P. 235]

Source: Tournefort, Joseph Pitton de. 1741. Ozell, J., trans. *A Voyage into the Levant, etc.* 3 Vols. London: Midwinter et al. (Originally published in French 1717)

◙ David Hume, "Of National Characters" (1748)

In the following excerpt, the Scottish philosopher David Hume comments on the innate biological and cognitive inferiority of "negroes." His writing participated in a late-eighteenth-century discourse of racial stigmatization based on the idea of inbuilt characteristics that could not be overcome.

I am apt to suspect the negroes and in general all other species of men (for there are four or five different kinds) to be naturally inferior to the whites. There never was a civilized nation of any other complexion than white, nor even any individual eminent either in action or speculation. No ingenious manufactures amongst them, no arts, no sciences. On the other hand, the most rude and barbarous of the whites, such as the ancient GERMANS, the present TARTARS, have still something eminent about them in their valour, form of government, or some other particular. Such a uniform and constant differences could not happen in so many countries and ages, if nature had not made an original distinction betwixt these breeds of men. Not to mention our colonies, there are Negroe slaves dispersed all over Europe, of which none ever discovered any symptoms of ingenuity, tho' low people, without education, will start up amongst us, and distinguish themselves in every profession. In JAMAICA indeed they talk of one negroe as a man of parts and learning; but 'tis likely he is admired for very slender accomplishments like a parrot, who speaks a few words plainly.

Source: Hume, David. 1748. "Of National Characters." In *Three Essays, Moral and Political.* Available at: http://www.engl.virginia.edu/enec981/dictionary/03humeK1.html

◙ David Hume, "Of the Standard of Taste" (1757)

In this discussion, Hume essentializes (and implicitly racializes) the idea of taste, the faculty of appreciating beauty and quality in its many forms, by connecting taste to superior health of sensory organs and a lack of taste to some defect therein. For Hume, therefore, taste results not from the superior education afforded to the few whose class, race, and gender status makes them eligible for it, but from inborn fineness of sensibility.

#12. It appears then, that, amidst all the variety and caprice of taste, there are certain general principles of approbation or blame, whose influence a careful eye may trace in all operations of the mind. Some particular forms or qualities, from the original structure of the internal fabric, are calculated to please, and others to displease; and if they fail of their effect in any particular instance, it is from some apparent defect or imperfection in the organ. A man in a fever would not insist on his palate as able to decide concerning flavours; nor would one, affected with the jaundice, pretend to give a verdict with regard to colours. In each creature, there is a sound and a defective state; and the former alone can be supposed to afford us a true standard of a taste and sentiment. If, in the sound state of the organ, there be an entire or considerable uniformity of sentiment among men, we may thence derive an idea of the perfect beauty; in like manner as the appearance of objects in daylight, to the eye of a man in health, is denominated their true and real colour, even while colour is allowed to be merely a phantasm of the senses.

#13. Many and frequent are the defects in the internal organs, which prevent or weaken the influence of those general principles, on which depends our sentiment of beauty or deformity. Though some objects, by the structure of the mind, be naturally calculated to give pleasure, it is not to be expected, that in every individual the pleasure will be equally felt. Particular incidents and situations occur, which either throw a false light on the objects, or hinder the true from conveying to the imagination the proper sentiment and perception.

#23. Thus, though the principles of taste be universal, and, nearly, if not entirely the same in all men; yet few are qualified to give judgment on any work of art, or establish their own sentiment as the standard of beauty. The organs of internal sensation are seldom so perfect as to allow the general principles their full play, and produce a feeling correspondent to those principles. They either labour under some defect, or are vitiated by some disorder; and by that means, excite a sentiment, which may be pronounced erroneous. When the critic has no delicacy, he judges without any distinction, and is only affected by the grosser and more palpable qualities of the object: The finer touches pass unnoticed and disregarded. Where he is not aided by practice, his verdict is attended with confusion and hesitation. Where no comparison has been employed, the most frivolous beauties, such as rather merit the name of defects, are the object of his admiration. Where he lies under the influence of prejudice, all his natural sentiments are perverted. Where good sense is wanting, he is not qualified to discern the beauties of design and reasoning, which are the highest and most excellent. Under some or other of these imperfections, the generality of men labour; and hence a true judge in the finer arts is observed, even during the most polished ages, to be so rare a character; Strong sense, united to delicate sentiment, improved by practice, perfected by comparison, and cleared of all prejudice, can alone entitle critics to this valuable character; and the joint verdict of such, wherever they are to be found, is the true standard of taste and beauty.

Source: Hume, David. 1757. "Of the Standard of Taste." In *Four Dissertations*. Available at: http://www.csulb.edu/~jvancamp/361r15.html

◉ Sarah Scott, from A *Description of Millenium Hall* (1762)

In this feminist utopia, bluestocking novelist Sarah Scott promulgates female separatism and self-sufficiency along with middle-class economic and moral virtue. Disability figures in this text as evidence of the pastoral charity of Scott's heroines, while also functioning as the novel's attempt at humane display of the kind of physical difference exploited at Bartholomew Fair.

Dear Sir,

Though, when I left London, I promised to write to you as soon as I had reached my northern retreat, yet,

I believe, you little expected instead of a letter to receive a volume; but I should not stand excused to myself, were I to fail communicating to you the pleasure I received in my road hither, from the sight of a society, whose acquaintance I owe to one of those fortunate, though in appearance trifling, accidents, from which sometimes arise the most pleasing circumstances of our lives for as such I must ever esteem the acquaintance of that amiable family, who have fixed their abode at a place which I shall nominate Millenium Hall, as the best adapted to the lives of the inhabitants, and to avoid giving the real name, fearing to offend that modesty which has induced them to conceal their virtues in retirement.

In giving you a very circumstantial account of this society, I confess I have a view beyond the pleasure, which a mind like yours must receive from the contemplations of so much virtue. Your constant endeavours have been to inculcate the best principles into youthful minds, the only probable means of mending mankind; for the foundation of most of our virtues, or our vices, are laid in that season of life when we are most susceptible of impression, and when on our minds, as on a sheet of white paper, any characters may be engraven; these laudable endeavours, by which we may reasonably expect the rising generation will be greatly improved, render particularly due to you, any examples which may teach those virtues that are not easily learnt by precept, and shew the facility of what, in mere speculation, might appear surrounded with a discouraging impracticability; you are the best judge, whether , by being made public, they may be conducive to your great end of benefiting the world. I therefore submit the future fate of the following sheets entirely to you, and shall not think any prefatory apology for the publication at all requisite; for though a man who supposes his own life and actions deserve universal notice, or can be of general use, may be liable to the imputation of vanity, yet as I have no other share than that of a spectator, and auditor, in what I purpose to relate, I presume no apology can be required; for my vanity must rather be mortified than flattered in the description of such virtues as will continually accuse me of my own deficiencies, and lead me to make an humiliating comparison between these excellent ladies and myself.

You may remember, Sir, that when I took leave of you with a design of retiring to my native country, there to enjoy the plenty and leisure for which a few years labour had furnished me with the necessary requisites, I was advised by an eminent physician to make a very extensive tour through the western part of this kingdom, in order, by frequent change of air, and continued exercise, to cure the ill effects of my long abode in the hot and unwholesome climate of Jamaica, where, while I increased my fortune, I gradually impaired my constitution; and though one, who like me, had dedicated all his application to mercantile gain, will not allow that he has given up the substance for the shadow, yet perhaps it would be difficult to deny, that I thus sacrificed the greater good in pursuit of the less.

The eagerness with which I longed to fix in my wished for retirement, made me imagine, that when I had once reached it, even the pursuit of health would be insufficient inducement to determine me to leave my retreat, I therefore chose to make the advised tour before I went into the north. As the pleasure arising from a variety of beautiful objects is but half enjoyed, when we have no one to share it with us, I accepted the offer Mr. Lamont (the son of my old friend) made of accompanying me in my journey. As this young gentleman has not the good fortune to be known to you, it may not be amiss, as will appear in the sequel, to let you into his character.

Mr. Lamont is a young man of about twenty-five years of age, of an agreeable person, and lively understanding; both perhaps have concurred to render him a coxcomb. The vivacity of his parts soon gained him such a degree of encouragement as excited his vanity, and raised in him an high opinion of himself. A very generous father enabled him to partake of every fashionable amusement, and the natural bent of his mind soon led him into all the dissipation which the gay world affords. Useful and improving studies were laid aside for such desultory reading, as he found most proper to furnish him with topics for conversation, in the idle societies he frequented. Thus that vivacity, which, properly qualified, might have become true wit, degenerated into pertness and impertinence. A consciousness of an understanding, which he never exerted, rendered him conceited; those talents which nature kindly bestowed upon him, by being perverted, gave rise to his greatest faults. His reasoning faculty, by a partial and superficial use, led him to infidelity,

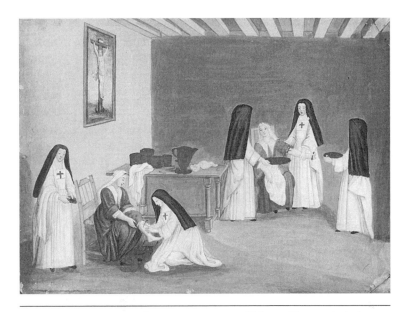

Nuns Attending at the Infirmary, *Anonymous (18th c.). This work depicts an example of an early hospital for the sick that catered primarily to those who were homeless or disabled. The bulk of the care sought to minister to the spiritual needs of patients.*

Source: Art Resource, New York.

and the desire of being thought superiorly distinguishing, established him an infidel. Fashion, not reason, has been the guide of all his thoughts and actions. But with these faults he is good-natured, and not unentertaining, especially in a tete a tete, where he does not desire to shine, and therefore his vanity lies dormant, and suffers the best qualifications of his mind to break forth. This induced me to accept of him as a fellow traveller.

We proceded on our journey as far as Cornwall, without meeting with any other than the usual incidents of the road, till one afternoon, when our chaise broke down. The worst circumstance attending this accident was our being several miles from a town, and so ignorant of the country, that we knew not whether there was any village within a moderate distance. We sent the postilion on my man's horse to the next town to fetch a smith, and leaving my servant to guard the chaise, Mr. Lamont and I walked towards an avenue of oaks, which we observed at a small distance. The thick shade they afforded us, the fragrance wafted from the woodbines with which they were encircled, was so delightful, and the beauty of the grounds so very attracting, that we strolled on, desirous of approaching the house to which this avenue led. It is a mile and a half in length, but the eye is so charmed with the remarkable verdure and neatness of the fields, with the beauty of the flowers which are planted all round them, and seem to mix with the quickest hedges, that time steals away insensibly.

When we had walked about half a mile in a scene truly pastoral, we began to think ourselves in the days of Theocritus, so sweetly did the sound of a flute come wafted through the air. Never did pastoral swain make sweeter melody on his oaten reed. Our ears now afforded us fresh attraction, and with quicker steps we proceeded, till we came within sight of the musician that had charmed us. Our pleasure was not a little heightened, to see, as the scene promised, in reality a shepherd, watching a large flock of sheep. We continued motionless, listening to his music, till a lamb straying from its fold demanded his care, and he laid aside his instrument, to guide home the little wanderer.

Curiosity now prompted us to walk on; the nearer we came to the house, the greater we found the profusion of flowers which ornamented every field. Some had no other defence than hedges of rose trees and sweet-briars, so artfully planted, that they made a very thick hedge, while at the lower part, pinks, jonquils, hyacinths, and various other flowers, seemed to grow under their protection. Primroses, violets, lilies of the valley, and polyanthuses enriched such shady spots, as, for want of sun, were not well calculated for the production of other flowers. The mixture of perfumes which exhaled from this profusion composed the highest fragrance, and sometimes the different scents regaled the senses alternately, and filled us with reflections on the infinite variety of nature.

When we were within about a quarter of a mile of the house, the scene became still more animated. On one side was the greatest variety of cattle, the most beautiful of their kinds, grazing in fields whose verdure equaled that of the finest turf, nor were they destitute of their ornaments, only the woodbines and Jessamine, and such flowers, as might have tempted the inhabitants of these pastures to crop them, were defended with roses and sweet-briars, whose thorns preserved them from all attacks.

Though Lamont had hitherto been little accustomed to admire nature, yet was he much captivated with this scene, and with his usual levity cried out, 'If Nebuchadnezzar had such pastures as these to range in, his seven years expulsion from human society might now be the most agreeable part of his life.' My attention was too much engaged to criticize the light turn of Lamont's mind, nor did his thoughts continue long on the same subject, for our observation was soon called off, by a company of hay-makers in the fields on the other side of the avenue. The cleanliness and neatness of the young women thus employed, rendered them a more pleasing subject for Lamont's contemplation than any thing we had yet seen; in them we beheld rural simplicity, without any of those marks of poverty and boorish rusticity, which would have spoilt the pastoral air of the scene around us; but not even the happy amiable innocence, which their figures and countenances expressed, gave me so much satisfaction as the sight of the number of children, who were all exerting the utmost of their strength, with an air of delighted emulation between themselves, to contribute their share to the general undertaking. Their eyes sparkled with that spirit which health and activity can only give, and the rosy cheeks shewed the benefits of youthful labour. Curiosity is one of those insatiable passions that grow by gratification; it still prompted us to proceed, not unsatisfied with what we had seen, but desirous to see still more of this earthly paradise. We approached the house, wherein, as it was the only human habitation in view, we imagined must reside the Primum Mobile of all we had yet beheld. We were admiring the magnificence of the ancient structure and inclined to believe it the abode of the genius which presided over this fairy land, when we were surprised by a storm, which had been for some time gathering over our heads, though our thoughts had been too agreeably engaged to pay much attention to it. We took shelter under the thick shade of a large oak, but the violence of the thunder and lightening made our situation rather uncomfortable. All those whom we had a little before seen so busy, left their work on hearing the first clap of thunder, and ran with the utmost speed to Millenium Hall, so I shall call the noble mansion of which I am speaking, as to an assured asylum against every evil.

Some of these persons, I imagine, perceived us; for immediately after they entered, came out a woman, who, by her air and manner of address, we guessed to be the house-keeper, and desired us to walk into the house till the storm was over. We made some difficulties about taking that liberty, but she still persisting in her invitation, had my curiosity to see the inhabitants of this hospitable mansion been less, I could not have refused to comply, as by prolonging these ceremonious altercations I was detaining her in the storm, we therefore agreed to follow her.

If we had been inclined before to fancy ourselves on enchanted ground, when after being led through a large hall, we were introduced to the ladies, who knew nothing of what had passed, I could scarcely forbear believing myself in the Attick school.

The room where they sat was about forty-five feet long, of a proportionable breadth, with three windows on one side, which looked into a garden, and a large bow at the upper end. Over against the windows were three large book-cases, upon the top of the middle one stood an orrery, and a globe on each of the others. In the bow sat two ladies reading, with pen, ink, and paper on a table before them, at which was a young girl translating out of French. At the lower end of the room was a lady painting, with exquisite art indeed, a beautiful Madona; near her another, drawing a landscape out of her own imagination; a third, carving a picture-frame in wood, in the finest manner; a fourth, engraving; and a young girl reading aloud to them; the distance from the ladies in the bow-window being such, that they could receive no disturbance from her. At the next window were placed a group of girls, from the age of ten years old to fourteen. Of these, one was drawing figures, another a landscape, a third a perspective view, a fourth engraving, a fifth carving, a sixth turning in wood, a seventh writing, an eighth cutting out linen, another making a gown, and by them an empty chair and a tent, with embroidery, finely fancied, before it, which we afterwards found had been left by a young girl who was gone to practise on the harpsicord.

As soon as we entered they all rose up, and the house-keeper introduced us, by saying, she saw us standing under a tree to avoid the storm, and so had desired us to walk in. The ladies received us with the greatest politeness, and expressed concern, that when their house was so near, we should have recourse to so insufficient a shelter. Our surprise at the sight of so uncommon a society, occasioned our making but an awkward return to their obligating reception; nor when we observed how many arts we had interrupted, could we avoid being ashamed that we had then intruded upon them.

But before I proceed farther, I shall endeavour to give you some idea of the persons of the ladies, whose minds I shall afterwards best describe by their actions. The two who sat in the bow window were called Mrs. Maynard and Mrs. Selvyn. Mrs. Maynard is between forty and fifty years of age, a little woman, well made, with a lively and genteel air, her hair black, and her eyes of the same colour, bright and piercing, her features good, and complexion agreeable, though brown.

Her countenance expresses all the vivacity of youth, tempered with a serenity which becomes her age.

Mrs. Selvyn can scarcely be called tall, though she approaches that standard. Her features are too irregular to be handsome, but there is a sensibility and delicacy in her countenance which render her extremely engaging; and her person is elegant.

Mrs. Mancel, whom we had disturbed from her painting, is tall and finely formed, has great elegance of figure, and is graceful in every motion. Her hair is of a fine brown, her eyes blue, with all that sensible sweetness which is peculiar to that colour. In short, she excels in every beauty but the bloom, which is so soon faded, and so impossible to be imitated by the utmost efforts of art, nor has she suffered any farther by years than the loss of that radiance, which renders beauty rather more resplendent than more pleasing.

Mrs. Trentham, who was carving by her, was the tallest of the company, and in dignity of air particularly excels, but her features and complexion have been so injured by the small pox, that one can but just guess they were once uncommonly fine; a sweetness of countenance, and a very sensible look, indeed, still remain, and have baffled all the most cruel ravages of that distemper.

Lady Mary Jones, whom we found engraving, seems to have been rather pleasing than beautiful. She is thin, and pale, but a pair of the finest black eyes I ever saw, animate, to a great degree, a countenance, which sickness has done its utmost to render languid, but has, perhaps only made more delicate and amiable. Her person is exquisitely genteel, and her voice, in common speech, enchantingly melodious.

Mrs. Morgan, the lady who was drawing, appears to be upwards of fifty, tall, rather plump, and extremely majestic, an air of dignity distinguishes her person, and every virtue is engraven in indelible characters on her countenance. There is a benignity in every look, which renders the decline of life, if possible, more amiable than the bloom of youth. One would almost think nature had formed her for a common parent, such universal and tender benevolence beams from every glance she casts around her.

The dress of the ladies was thus far uniform, the same neatness, the same simplicity and cleanliness appeared in each, and they were all in lutestring night-gowns, though of different colours, nor was there anything unfashionable in their appearance, except that they were free from any trumpery ornaments. The girls were all clothed in camblet coats, but not uniform in colour, their linen extremely white and clean though coarse.

Some of them were pretty, and none had any defect in person, to take off from that general pleasingness which attends youth and innocence.

They had been taught such an habit of attention, that they seemed not at all disturbed by our conversation, which was of that general kind, as might naturally be expected on such an occasion, though supported by the ladies with more sensible vivacity and politeness, than is usual, where part of the company are such total strangers to the rest; till by chance one of the ladies called Mrs. Maynard by her name.

From the moment I saw her, I thought her face not unknown to me, but could not recollect where, or when I had been acquainted with her, but her name brought to my recollection, that she was not only an old acquaintance, but a near relation. I observed, that she had looked on me with particular attention, and I begged her to give me leave to ask her, of what family of Maynards she was? Her answer confirmed my supposition, and as she told me, that she believed she had some remembrance of my face, I soon made her recollect our affinity and former intimacy, though my twenty years abode in Jamaica, the alteration the climate had wrought in me, and time had made in us both, had almost effaced us from each other's memory.

There is great pleasure in renewing the acquaintance of our youth; a thousand pleasing ideas accompany it; many mirthful scenes and juvenile amusements return to the remembrance, and make us, as it were, live over again what is generally the most pleasing part of life. Mrs. Maynard seemed no less sensible of the satisfaction arising from this train of thoughts than myself, and the rest of the company were so indulgently good-natured, as in appearance, to share them with us. The tea table by no means interrupted our conversation, and I believe I should have forgot that our journey was not at an end, if a servant had not brought in word, that my man, who had observed our motions, was come to inform us, that our chaise could not be repaired that night.

The ladies immediately declared, that though their equipage was in order, they would not suffer it to put an end to a pleasure they owed to the accident which had happened to ours, and insisted we should give them our company till the smith had made all necessary reparations, adding, that I could not be obstinately bent on depriving Mrs. Maynard so soon of the satisfaction she received, from having recovered so

long lost a relation. I was little inclined to reject this invitation: pleasure was the chief design of my journey, and I saw not how I could receive more, than by remaining in a family so extraordinary, and so perfectly agreeable. When both parties are well agreed, the necessary ceremonies previous to a compliance are soon over, and it was settled that we should not think of departing before the next day at soonest.

The continuance of the rain rendered it impossible to stir out of the house; my cousin, who seemed to think variety necessary to amuse, asked if we loved music? Which being answered in the affirmative, she begged the other ladies to entertain us with one of their family concerts, and we joining in the petition, proper orders were given, and we adjourned into another room, which was well furnished with musical instruments. Over the door was a beautiful Saint Cecilia, painted in crayons by Mrs. Mancel, and a fine piece of carved work over the chimney, done by Mrs. Trentham, which was a very artificial representation of every sort of musical instruments.

While we were admiring these performances, the company took their respective places. Mrs. Mancel seated herself at the harpsichord, Lady Mary Jones played on the arch lute, Mrs. Morgan on the organ, Mrs. Selvyn and Mrs. Trentham each on the six-stringed bass; the shepherd who had charmed us in the field was there with his German flute; a venerable looking man, who is their steward, played on the violincello, a lame youth on the French horn, another, who seemed very near blind, on the bassoon, and two on the fiddle. My cousin had no share in the performance except singing agreeably, wherein she was joined by some of the ladies, and where the music could bear it, by ten of the young girls, with two or three others whom we had not seen, and whose voices and manner were equally pleasing. They performed several of the finest pieces of the Messiah and Judas Maccabeus, with exquisite taste, and the most exact time. There was a sufficient number of performers to give the choruses all their pomp and fullness, and the songs were sung in a manner so touching and pathetic, as could be equaled by none, whose hearts were not as much affected by the words, as their senses were by the music. The sight of so many little innocents joining in the most sublime harmony, made me almost think myself already amongst the heavenly choir, and it was a great mortification to me to be brought back to this sensual world, by so gross an attraction as a call to supper, which put an end to our concert, and carried us to another room, where we found a repast more elegant than expensive.

The evening certainly is the most social part of the day, without any of those excesses which so often turn it into senseless revelry. The conversation after supper was particularly animated, and left us still more charmed with the society into which chance had introduced us; the sprightliness of their wit, the justness of their reflexions, the dignity which accompanied their vivacity, plainly evinced with how much greater strength the mind can exert itself in a regular and rational way of life, than in a course of dissipation. At this house every change came too soon, time seemed to wear a double portion of wings, eleven o'clock struck, and the ladies ordered a servant to shew us our rooms, themselves retiring to theirs.

It was impossible for Lamont and I to part till we had spent an hour in talking over this amiable family, with whom he could not help being much delighted, though he observed, 'they were very deficient in the bon ton, there was too much solidity in all they said, they would trifle with trifles indeed, but had not the art of treating more weighty subjects with the same lightness, which gave them an air of rusticity; and he did not doubt, but on a more intimate acquaintance we should find their manners much rusticated, and their heads filled with antiquated notions, by having lived so long out of the great world.'

I rose the next morning very early, desirous to make the day, which I purposed for the last of my abode in this mansion, as long as I could. I went directly into the garden, which, by what I saw from the house was extremely pretty. As I passed by the windows of the saloon, I perceived the ladies and their little pupils were earlier risers than myself, for they were all at their various employments. I first went into the gayest flower garden I ever beheld. The rainbow exhibits not half the variety of tints, and they are so artfully mingled, and ranged to make such a harmony of colours, as taught me how much the most beautiful objects may be improved by a judicious disposition of them. Beyond these beds of flowers rises a shrubbery, where every thing sweet and pleasing is collected. As these ladies have no taste but what is directed by good sense, nothing found a place here from being only uncommon, for they think few things are very rare but because they are little desirable; and indeed it is plain they are free from that littleness of mind, which makes people value a thing the more for its being possessed by no one but themselves. Behind the shrubbery is a

little wood, which affords a gloom, rendered more agreeable by its contrast with the dazzling beauty of that part of the garden that leads to it. In the high pale which encloses this wood I observed a little door; curiosity induced me to pass through it; I found it opened on a row of the neatest cottages I ever saw, which the wood had concealed from my view. They were new and uniform, and therefore I imagined all dedicated to the same purpose. Seeing a very old woman spinning at one of the doors, I accosted her, by admiring the neatness of her habitation.

'Ay, indeed, said she, it is a most comfortable place, God bless the good ladies! I and my neighbours are as happy as princesses, we have every thing we want and wish, and who can say more?' 'Very few so much, answered I, but pray what share have the ladies in procuring the happiness you seem so sensible of.'

'Why Sir, continued the old woman, it is all owing to them. I was almost starved when they put me into this house, and no shame of mine, for so were my neighbours too; perhaps we were not so painstaking as we might have been; but that was not our faults, you know, as we had not things to work with, nor any body to set us to work, poor folks cannot know every thing as these good ladies do; we were half dead for want of victuals, and then people have not courage to set about any thing. Nay, all the parish were so when they came into it, young and old, there was not much to chuse, few of us had rags to cover us, or a morsel of bread to eat, except the two Squires; they indeed grew rich, because they had our work, and paid us not enough to keep life and soul together; they live above a mile off, so perhaps they did not know how poor we were, I must say that for them; the ladies tell me I ought not to speak against them, for every one has faults, only we see other peoples, and are blind to our own; and certainly it is true enough, for they are very wise ladies as well as good, and must know such things.'

As my new acquaintance seemed as loquacious as her age promised, I hoped for full satisfaction, and asked her, 'How she and her neighbours employed themselves?' 'Not all alike, replied the good woman, I will tell you, all about it. There are twelve of us that live here. We have every one a house of two rooms, as you may see, beside other conveniences, and each a little garden, but though we are separated, we agree as well, perhaps better, than if few lived together, and all help one another. Now, there is neighbour Susan, and neighbour Rachel; Susan is lame, so she spins cloaths for Rachel; and Rachel cleans Susan's house, and does such things for her as she cannot do for herself. The ladies settled all these matters at first, and told us, that as they, to please God, assisted us, we must in order to please him serve others; and that to make us happy they would have a melancholy life if she was to be always spinning and knitting, seeing other people around her talking, and not be able to hear a word they said, so the ladies busy her in making broths and caudles, and such things, for all the sick poor in this and the next parish, and two of us are fixed upon to carry what she has made to those that want them; to visit them often, and spend more or less time with them every day according as they have, or have not relations to take care of them; for though the ladies always hire nurses for those who are very ill, yet they will not trust quite to them, but make us overlook them, so that in a sickly time we shall be all day going from one to another.'

'But, said I, there are I perceive many children amongst you, how happens that? your ages shew they are not your own.'

'Oh! as for that, replied my intelligencer, I will tell you how that is. You must know these good ladies, heaven preserve them! take every child after the fifth of every poor person, as soon as it can walk, till when they pay the mother for nursing it; these children they send to us to keep out of harm, and as soon as they can hold a knitting-needle to teach them to knit, and to spin, as much as they can be taught before they are four or five years old, when they are removed into one of the schools. They are pretty company for us, and make us mothers again, as it were, in our old age; then the childrens relations are all so fond of us for our care of them, that it makes us a power of friends, which you know is very pleasant, though we want nothing from them but their good wills.'

Here I interrupted her by observing, that it must take up a great deal of time, and stop their work, consequently lessen their profits.

'There is nothing in that, continued the good woman, the ladies steward sends us in all we want in the way of meat, drink, and firing; and our spinning we carry to the ladies; they employ a poor old weaver, who before they came broke for want of work, to weave it for us, and when there is not enough they put more to it, so we are sure to have our cloathing; if we are not idle that is all over our houses, which they tell us, and certainly with truth, for it is a great deal of trouble to them, is all for our good, for that we cannot be healthy if we are not clean and neat. Then every

saint's day, and every Sunday after church, we all go down to the hall, and the ladies read prayers, and a sermon to us, and their own family; nor do they ever come here without giving us some good advice. We used to quarrel, to be sure, sometimes when we first came to these houses, but the ladies condescended to make it up amongst us, and shewed us so kindly how much it was our duty to agree together, and to forgive every body their faults, or else we could not hope to be forgiven by God, against whom we so often sinned, that now we love one another like sisters, or indeed better, for I often see such quarrel. Beside, they have taught us when we are as much to blame, which we may be sure enough will happen, let us try ever so much to the contrary. Then the ladies seem so pleased when we do any kindness to one another, as to be sure is a great encouragement; and if any of us are sick they are so careful and so good, that it would be a shame if we did not do all we can for one another, who have been always neighbours and acquaintance, when such great ladies, who never knew us, as I may say, but to make us happy, and have no reason to take care of us but that we are poor, are so kind and condescending to us.'

I was so pleased with the good effect which the charity of her benefactors had on the mind, as well as the situation of this old woman, whose neighbours by her own account were equally benefited by the blessings they received, that I should have stayed longer with her, if a bell had not rang at Millenium Hall, which she informed me was a summons to breakfast. I obeyed its call, and after thanking her for her conversation, returned with a heart warmed and enlarged, to the amiable society. My mind was so filled with exalted reflections on their virtues, that I was less attentive to the charms of inanimate nature than when I first passed through the gardens.

After breakfast the ladies proposed a walk, and as they had seen the course I took when I first went out, they led us a contrary way, lest, they said, I should be tired with the repetition of the same scene. I told them with great truth, that 'what I had beheld could never weary, for virtue is a subject we must ever contemplate with fresh delight, and as such examples could not fail of improving every witness of them, the pleasure of reflection would encrease, as one daily grew more capable of enjoying it, by cultivating kindred sensations.' By some more explicit hints they found out to what I alluded, and thereby knew where I had been, but turning the conversation to present objects, they conducted us to a very fine wood, which is laid out with so much taste, that Lamont observed the artist's hand was never more distinguishable, and perceived in various spots the direction of the person at present most famous for that sort of improvement.

The ladies smiled, and one of them answered, 'He did their wood great honour, in thinking art had lent her assistance to nature, but that there was little in that place for which they were not solely obliged to the latter.' Mrs. Trentham interrupted her who was speaking, and told us, that, 'As she had no share in the improvements which had been made, she might with the better grace assure Mr. Lamont, that Lady Mary Jones, Mrs. Mancel, and Mrs. Morgan, were the only persons who had laid out that wood, and the commonest labourers in the country had executed their orders.' Lamont was much surprised at this piece of information, and though he would have thought it still more exquisitely beautiful had it been the design of the person he imagined, yet truth is so powerful, that he could not suppress his admiration and surprise. Every cut in it is terminated by some noble object. In several places are seats formed with such rustic simplicity, as have more real grandeur in them, than can be found in the most expensive buildings. On an eminence, 'bosomed high in tufted trees,' is a temple dedicated to solitude. The structure is an exquisite piece of architecture, the prospect from it noble and extensive, and the windows so placed, that one sees no house but at so considerable a distance, as not to take off from the solitary air, which is perfectly agreeable to a temple declaredly dedicated to solitude. The most beautiful object in the view is a very large river, in reality an arm of the sea, little more than a quarter of a mile distant from the building; about three miles beyond it lies the sea, on which the sun then shone, and made it dazzlingly bright. In the temple is a picture of Contemplation, another of Silence, two of various birds and animals, and a couple of moon-light pieces, the workmanship of ladies.

Close by the temple runs a gentle murmuring rivulet, which flows in meanders through the rest of the wood, sometimes concealed from view, and then appearing at the next turning of the walk. The wood is well peopled with pheasants, wild turkies, squirrels and hares, who live so unmolested, that they seem to have forgot all fear, and rather to welcome than fly those who come amongst them. Man never appears there as a merciless destroyer; but the preserver, instead of the tyrant of the inferior part of the creation. While they continue in that wood, none but natural evil can approach them, and from that they are defended as much as possible. We there 'walked joint tenant of the shade,' with the animal race; and a perfect equality in nature's bounty seems enjoyed by the whole creation. One could scarcely forbear thinking those happy times were come, when 'The wolf shall dwell with the lamb, and the leopard shall lye down with the kid; and the calf, and the young lion, and the fatling together, and a young child shall lead them. The wilderness and the solitary place shall be glad for them, and the desart shall rejoice, and blossom as the rose.'

At the verge of this wood, which extends to the river I have mentioned, without perceiving we were entering a building, so well is the outside of it concealed by trees, we found ourselves in a most beautiful grotto, made of fossils, spars, coral, and such shells, as are at once both fine and rustic; all of the glaring, tawdry kind are excluded, and by the gloom and simplicity preserved, one would imagine it the habitation of some devout anchoret. Ivy and moss in some places cover, while they seem to unite, the several materials of the variegated walls. The rivulet which runs through the wood, falls down one side of the grotto with great rapidity, broken into various streams by the spar and coral, and passing through, forms a fine cascade just at the foot of the grotto, from whence it flows into the river. Great care is taken to prevent the place from growing damp, so that we sat some time in it with safety, admiring the smooth surface of the river, to which it lies very open.

As the ladies had some daily business on their hands which they never neglect, we were obliged to leave this lovely scene, where I think I could have passed my life with pleasure, and to return towards the house, though by a different way from that we came, traversing the other side of the wood. In one spot where we went near the verge, I observed a pale, which, upon examination, I found was continued for some acres, though it was remarkable only in one place. It is painted green, and on the inside a hedge of yews, laurel, and other thick evergreens, rises to about seven or eight feet high. I could not forbear asking what was thus so carefully enclosed? The ladies smiled on each other, but evaded answering my question, which only encreased my curiosity. Lamont, not less curious, and more importunate, observed, that 'the inclosure bore some resemblance to one of Lord Lamore's, where he kept lions, tigers, leopards, and such foreign animals, and he would be hanged, if the ladies had not made some such collection, intreating that he might be admitted to see them; for nothing gave him greater entertainment than to behold those beautiful wild beasts, brought out of their native woods, where they had reigned as kings, and here tamed and subjected by the superior art of man. It was a triumph of human reason, which could not fail to afford great pleasure.'

'Not to us, I assure you, Sir, replied Mrs. Mancel, when reason appears only in the exertion of cruelty and tyrannical oppression, it is surely not a gift to be boasted of. When a man forces the furious steed to endure the bit, or breaks oxen to the yoke, the great benefits he receives from, and communicates to the animals, excuses the forcible methods by which it is accomplished. But to see a man, from a vain desire to have in his possession the native of another climate and another country, reduce a fine and noble creature to misery, and confine him within narrow inclosures whose happiness consisted in unbounded liberty, shocks my nature. There is I confess something so amiable in gentleness, that I could be pleased with seeing a tyger caress its keeper, if the cruel means by which the fiercest of beasts is taught all the servility of a fawning spaniel, did not recur every instant to my mind; and it is not much less abhorrent to my nature, to see a venerable lion jumping over a stick, than it would be to behold a hoary philosopher forced by some cruel tyrant to spend his days in whipping a top, or playing with a rattle. Every thing to me loses its charm when it is put out of that station wherein nature, or to speak more properly, the all-wise Creator has placed it. I imagine man has a right to use the animal race for his own preservation, perhaps for his convenience, but certainly not to treat them with wanton cruelty, and as it is not in his power to give them any thing so valuable as their liberty, it is, in my opinion, criminal to enslave them, in order to procure ourselves a vain amusement, if we have so little feeling as to find any while others suffer.'

'I believe madam, replied Lamont, it is most advisable for me not to attempt to defend what I have said; should I have reason on my side, while you have humanity on yours, I should make but a bad figure in the argument. What advantage could I expect from applying to the understanding, while your amiable disposition would captivate even reason itself? But still I am puzzled; what we behold is certainly an inclosure, how can that be without a confinement to those that are within it?'

'After having spoken so much against tyranny, said Mrs. Mancel smiling, I do not know whether I should be excusable, if I left you to be tyrannized by curiosity, which I believe can inflict very severe pains, at least, if I may be allowed to judge by the means people often take to satisfy it. I will therefore gratify you with the knowledge of what is within this inclosure, which makes so extraordinary an impression upon you. It is, then, an asylum for those poor creatures who are rendered miserable from some natural deficiency or redundancy.

'Here they find refuge from tyranny of those wretches, who seem to think that being two or three feet taller gives them a right to make them a property, and expose their unhappy forms to the contemptuous curiosity of the unthinking multitude. Procrustes has been branded through all ages with the name of tyrant; and principally, as it appears, from fitting the body of every stranger to a bed which he kept as the necessary standard, cutting off the legs of those whose height exceeded the length of it, and stretching on the rack such as fell short of that measure, till they attained the requisite proportion. But is not almost every man a Procrustes? We have not the power of shewing our cruelty exactly in the same method, but actuated by the like spirit, we abridge of their liberty, and torment by scorn, all who either fall short, or exceed the usual standard, if they happen to have the additional misfortune of poverty. Perhaps we are in no part more susceptible than in our vanity, how much then must those poor wretches suffer, whose deformity would lead them to wish to be secluded from human view, in being exposed to the public, whose observations are no better than expressions of scorn, and who are surprised to find that any thing less than themselves can speak, or appear like intelligent beings. But this is only part of what they have to endure. As if their deficiency in height deprived them of the natural right to air and sunshine, they are kept confined in small rooms, and because they fill less space than common, are stuffed into chairs so little, that they are squeezed as close as a pair of gloves in a walnut-shell.

'This miserable treatment of persons, to whom compassion should secure more than common indulgence, determined us to purchase these worst sort of slaves, and in this place we have five who owed their wretchedness to being only three foot high, one grey-headed toothless old man of sixteen years of age, a woman of about seven feet in height, and a man who would be still taller, if the weakness of his body, and the wretched life he for some time led, in the hands of one of these monster-mongers, did not make him bend almost double, and oblige him to walk almost on crutches; with which infirmities he is well pleased, as they reduce him near the common standard.'

We were very desirous of seeing this enfranchised [Editors' note: Here, set free, rather than endowed with the right to vote.] company; but Mrs. Morgan told us it was what they seldom granted, for fear of inflicting some of the pains from which they had endeavoured to rescue those poor creatures, but she would step in, and ask if they had no objection to our admission, and if that appeared really the case she would gratify us.

This tenderness to persons who were under such high obligations, charmed me. She soon returned with the permission we wished, but intreated us to pay all our attention to the house and the garden, and to take no more than a civil notice of its inhabitants. We promised obedience, and followed her. Her advice was almost unnecessary, for the place could not have failed of attracting our particular observation. It was a quadrangle of about six acres, and the inward part was divided by nets into eight parts, four of which were filled with poultry of all sorts, which were fed here for the use of the hall, and kept with the most exact cleanliness. The other four parts were filled with shrubs and flowers, which were cultivated with great delight by these once unfortunate, but now happy beings. A little stream ran across the quadrangle, which served for drink to the poultry, and facilitated the watering of the flowers. I have already said, that at the inward edge of the pale was a row of ever-greens; at their feet were beds of flowers, and a little gravel walk went around the whole. At each corner was an arbour made with woodbines and jessamine, in one or two of which there was always an agreeable shade.

At one side of the quadrangle was a very neat habitation, into which a dwarf invited us to enter, to rest ourselves after our walk; they were all passing backwards and forwards, and thus gave us a full view of them, which would have been a shocking sight, but for the reflexions we could not avoid making on their happy condition, and the very extraordinary humanity of the ladies to whom they owed it; so that instead of feeling the pain one might naturally receive from seeing the human form so disgraced, we were filled with admiration for the human mind, when so nobly exalted by virtue, as it is in the patronesses of these poor creatures, who wore an air of cheerfulness,

which shewed they thought the churlishness wherewith they had been treated by nature sufficiently compensated. The tender enquiries the ladies made after their healths, and the kind notice they took of each of them, could not be exceeded by anything but the affection, I might almost say adoration, with which these people beheld their benefactresses.

This scene had made too deep an impression on our minds, not to be the subject of our discourse all the way home, and in the course of conversation, I learnt, that when these people were first rescued out of their misery, their healths were much impaired, and their tempers more so: to restore the first, all medicinal care was taken, and air and exercise assisted greatly in their recovery; but to cure the malady of the mind, and conquer that internal source of unhappiness, was a work of longer time. Even these poor wretches had their vanity, and would contend for superior merit, of which, the argument was the money their keepers had gained in exhibiting them. To put an end to this contention, the ladies made them understand, that what they thought a subject of boasting, was only a proof of their being so much farther from the usual standard of the human form, and therefore a more extraordinary spectacle. But it was long before one of them could be persuaded to lay aside her pretensions to superiority, which she claimed on account of an extraordinary honour she had received from a great princess, who had made her a present of a sedan chair.

At length, however, much reasoning and persuasion, a conviction of principles, of which they had before no knowledge, the happiness of their situation, and the improvements of their healths, concurred to sweeten their tempers, and they now live in great harmony. They are entirely mistresses of their house, have two maids to wait on them, over whom they have sole command, and a person to do such little things in their garden as they cannot themselves perform; but the cultivation of it is one of their great pleasures; and by their extraordinary care, they have the satisfaction of presenting the finest flowers of the spring to their benefactresses, before they are blown in any other place.

When they first came, the ladies told us, that the horror they had conceived of being exhibited as public spectacles, had fixed in them such a fear of being seen by any stranger, that the sound of a voice, with which they were not acquainted at the outside of the paling, or the trampling of feet, would set them all a running behind the bushes to hide themselves, like so many timorous partridges in a mew, hurrying behind sheaves of corn for shelter; they even found a convenience in their size, which, though it rendered them unwilling to be seen, enabled them so easily to find places for concealment.

By degrees the ladies brought them to consent to see their head servants, and some of the best people in the parish; desiring, that to render it more agreeable to their visitors, they would entertain them with fruit and wine; advising them to assist their neighbours in plain work; thus to endear themselves to them, and procure more frequent visits, which as they chose to confine themselves within so narrow a compass, and enjoyed but precarious health, their benefactresses thought a necessary amusement. These recommendations, and the incidents wherewith their former lives had furnished them to amuse their company, and which they now could relate with pleasure, from the happy sense that all mortifications were past, rendered their conversation much courted among that rank of people.

It occurred to me, that their dislike to being seen by numbers, must prevent their attendance on public worship, but my cousin informed me that was thus avoided. There was in the church an old gallery, which from disuse was grown out of repair; this the ladies caused to be mended, and the front of it so heightened, that these little folks when in it could not be seen; the tall one contrived by stooping when they were there, not to appear of any extraordinary height: To this they were conveyed in the ladies coach, and set down close to covered stairs, which led up to the gallery.

This subject employed our conversation till we approached the hall; the ladies then, after insisting that we should not think of going from thence that day, all left us except Mrs. Maynard. It may seem strange that I was not sorry for their departure; but, in truth, I was so filled with astonishment, at characters so new, and so curious to know by what steps women thus qualified both by nature and by fortune to have the world almost at command, were brought thus to seclude themselves from it, and make as it were a new one for themselves, constituted on such very different principles from that I had hitherto lived in, that I longed to be alone with my cousin, in hopes that I might from her receive some account of this wonder. I soon made my curiosity known, and beseeched her to gratify it.

'I see no good reason, said she, why I should not comply with your request, as my friends are above wishing to conceal any part of their lives, though themselves are never the subject of their own conversation.

If they have had any follies they do not desire to hide them; they have not pride enough to hurt with candid criticisms, and have too much innocence to fear any very severe censures. But as we did not all reach this paradise at the same time, I shall begin with the first inhabitants of, and indeed the founders of this society, Mrs. Mancel and Mrs. Morgan, who from their childhood have been so connected, that I could not, if I would, disunite them in my relation; and it would almost be a sin to endeavour to separate them even in idea.'

We sat down in an arbour, whose shade invited us to seek there a defence against the sun, which was then in its meridian, and shone with uncommon heat. The woodbines, the roses, the jessamines, the pinks, and above all, the minionette with which it was surrounded, made the air one general perfume; every breeze came loaded with fragrance, stealing and giving odour. A rivulet ran bubbling by the side of the arbour, whose gentle murmurs soothed the mind into composure, and seemed to hush us to attention, when Mrs. Maynard thus began, to shew her readiness to comply with my request.

_____

Source: Scott, Sarah. 1762. *A Description of Millenium Hall.* London: J. Newbery.

Immanuel Kant, from *Observations on the Feeling of the Beautiful and the Sublime* (1764)

In this excerpt the renowned Enlightenment philosopher, Immanuel Kant, discusses the "savages" of Africa, North America, and "the Orient." Kant argues for the innate inferiority of African peoples based upon inferior physical and mental characteristics.

"Of National Characteristics, so far as they Depend upon the Distinct Feeling of the Beautiful and Sublime"

The Negroes of Africa have by nature no feeling that rises above the trifling. Mr. Hume challenges anyone to cite a single example in which a Negro has shown talents, and asserts that among the hundreds of thousands of black who are transported elsewhere from their countries, although many of them have even been set free, still not a single one was ever found who presented anything great in art or science or any other praiseworthy quality, even though among the whites some continually rise aloft from the lowest rabble, and through superior gifts earn respect in the world. So fundamental is the difference between these two races of man, and it appears to be as great in regard to mental capacities as in color. The religion of fetishes so widespread among them is perhaps a sort of idolatry that sinks as deeply into the trifling as appears to be possible to human nature. A bird's feather, a cow's horn, a conch shell, or any other common object, as soon as it becomes consecrated by a few words, is an object of veneration and of invocation in swearing oaths. The blacks are very vain but in the Negro's way, and so talkative that they must be driven apart from each other with thrashings.

Among all savages there is no nation that displays so sublime a mental character as those of North America. They have a strong feeling for honor, and as in quest of it they seek wild adventures hundreds of miles abroad, they are still extremely careful to avert the least injury to it when their equally harsh enemy, upon capturing them, seeks by cruel pain to extort cowardly groans from them. The Canadian savage, moreover, is truthful and honest. The friendship he establishes is just as adventurous and enthusiastic as anything of that kind reported from the most ancient and fabled times. He is extremely proud, feels the whole worth of freedom, and even in his education suffers no encounter that would let him feel a low subservience. Lycurgus probably gave statutes to just such savages; and if a lawgiver arose among those Six Nations, one would see a Spartan republic rise in the New World; for the undertaking of the Argonauts is little different from the war parties of these Indians, and Jason excels Attakakullakulla in nothing but the honor of a Greek name. All these savages have little feeling for the beautiful in moral understanding, and the generous forgiveness of an injury, which is at once noble and beautiful, is completely unknown as a virtue among the savages, but rather is disdained as a miserable cowardice. Valor is the greatest merit of the savage and revenge his sweetest bliss. The remaining natives of this part of the world show few traces of a mental character disposed to the finer feelings, and an extraordinary apathy constitutes the mark of this type of race.

If we examine the relation of the sexes in these parts of the world, we find that the European alone has found the secret of decorating with so many flowers the sensual charm of a mighty inclination and of interlacing it with so much morality that he has not only extremely elevated its agreeableness but also made it very decorous. The inhabitant of the Orient is of a very false taste in this respect. Since he has no concept of the morally beautiful which can be united with this impulse, he loses even the worth of the sensuous enjoyment, and his harem is a constant source of unrest. He thrives on all sorts of amorous grotesqueries, among which the imaginary jewel is only the foremost, which he seeks to safeguard above all else, whose whole worth consists only in smashing it, and of which one in our part of the world generally entertains much malicious doubt—and yet to whose preservation he makes use of very unjust and often loathsome means. Hence there a woman is always in a prison, whether she may be a maid, or have a barbaric, good-for-nothing and always suspicious husband. In the lands of the black, what better can one expect than what is found prevailing, namely the feminine sex in the deepest slavery? A despairing man is always a strict master over anyone weaker, just as with us that man is always a tyrant in the kitchen who outside his own house hardly dares to look anyone in the face. Of course, Father Labat reports that a Negro carpenter, whome he reproached for haughty treatment toward his wives, answered: "You whites are indeed fools, for first you make great concessions to your wives, and afterward you complain when they drive you mad." And it might be that there were something in this which perhaps deserved to be considered; but in short, this fellow was quite black from head to foot, a clear proof that what he said was stupid.

Source: Kant, Immanuel. 2004. Goldthwait, John T., trans. *Observations on the Feeling of the Beautiful and Sublime,* 2nd ed. Berkeley: University of California Press. (Originally published 1764)

▣ Anna Laetitia Barbauld (1743–1825), from "An Inquiry into Those Types of Distress That Excite Agreeable Sensations"

Theorizing aesthetics in terms of natural impulses, Anna Laetitia Barbauld (1743–1825) comments on the undesirability of having characters, such as Henry Fielding's Amelia, endowed with blemishes and imperfections. In contending that deformity is innately repulsive to the imagination, Barbauld (in the rest of the text) contrasts "disgusting" physical imperfection with more pleasing kinds of "distress," which instead produce sympathy, admiration, or fascination in readers.

Deformity is always disgusting, and the imagination cannot reconcile it with the idea of a favourite character; therefore the poet and romance-writer are fully justified in giving a larger share of beauty to their principal figures than is usually met with in common life. A late genius, indeed, in a whimsical mood, gave us a lady with her nose crushed for the heroine of his story: but the circumstance spoils the picture; and though in the course of the story it is kept a good deal out of sight, whenever it does recur to the imagination we are hurt and disgusted. It was an heroic instance of virtue in the nuns of a certain abbey, who cut off their noses and lips to avoid violation; yet this would make a very bad subject for a poem or a play. Something akin to this is the representation of any thing unnatural; of which kind is the famous story of the Roman charity, and for this reason I cannot but think it an unpleasing subject for either the pen or the pencil.

Source: Barbauld, Anna Laetitia. 1825. "An Inquiry into Those Types of Distress That Excite Agreeable Sensations." T*he Works of Anna Laetitia Barbauld, with a Memoir by Lucy Aikin.* London: Longman et al.

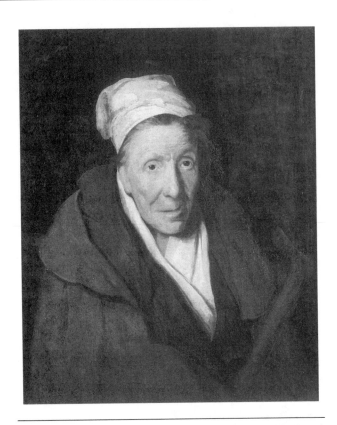

The Madwoman, *by Théodore Géricault (1791–1824). The French neo-Baroque painter Géricault was fascinated with topics of disability and death. He based a number of his works on common beliefs about appearances as manifesting otherwise interior disorders of the mind.*

Source: Art Resource, New York.

▣ Johann Wolfgang von Goethe, from *The Sorrows of Young Werther* (1774)

The Sorrows of Young Werther (Die Leiden des jungen Werther*) by Johann Wolfgang von Goethe is an account of a young man's intense and overwhelming attachment to the object of his affections. The fictional epistolary account, which ends notoriously with the desperate suicide of the emotionally overwrought narrator, caused a sensation upon its publication and thereafter. Napoleon is said to have read it seven times; it was banned in some locales for provoking obsessive youth to suicide, though it can more likely be seen as a cautionary tale of emotional trauma.*

AUGUST 12

Certainly Albert is the best fellow in the world. I had a strange scene with him yesterday. I went to take leave of him; for I took it into my head to spend a few days in these mountains, from where I now write to you. As I was walking up and down his room, my eye fell upon his pistols. "Lend me those pistols," said I, "for my journey." "By all means," he replied, "if you will take the trouble to load them; for they only hang there for form." I took down one of them; and he continued, "Ever since I was near suffering for my extreme caution, I will have nothing to do with such things." I was curious to hear the story. "I was staying," said he, "some three months ago, at a friend's house in the country. I had a brace of pistols with me, unloaded; and I slept without any anxiety. One rainy afternoon I was sitting by myself, doing nothing, when it occurred to me I do not know how that the house might be attacked, that we might require the pistols, that we might in short, you know how we go on fancying, when we have nothing better to do. I gave the pistols to the servant, to clean and load. He was playing with the maid, and trying to frighten her, when the pistol went off—God knows how!—the ramrod was in the barrel; and it went straight through her right hand, and shattered the thumb. I had to endure all the lamentation, and to pay the surgeon's bill; so, since that time, I have kept all my weapons unloaded. But, my dear friend, what is the use of prudence? We can never be on our guard against all possible dangers. However,"—now, you must know I can tolerate all men till they come to "however;"—for it is self-evident that every universal rule must have its exceptions. But he is so exceedingly accurate, that, if he only fancies he has said a word too precipitate, or too general, or only half true, he never ceases to qualify, to modify, and extenuate, till at last he appears to have said nothing at all. Upon this occasion, Albert was deeply immersed in his subject: I ceased to listen to him, and became lost in reverie. With a sudden motion, I pointed the mouth of the pistol to my forehead, over the right eye. "What do you mean?" cried Albert, turning back the pistol. "It is not loaded," said I. "And even if not," he answered with impatience, "what can you mean? I cannot comprehend how a man can be so mad as to shoot himself, and the bare idea of it shocks me."

"But why should any one," said I, "in speaking of an action, venture to pronounce it mad or wise, or good or bad? What is the meaning of all this? Have you carefully studied the secret motives of our actions? Do you understand—can you explain the causes which occasion them, and make them inevitable? If you can, you will be less hasty with your decision."

"But you will allow," said Albert; "that some actions are criminal, let them spring from whatever motives they may." I granted it, and shrugged my shoulders.

"But still, my good friend," I continued, "there are some exceptions here too. Theft is a crime; but the man who commits it from extreme poverty, with no design but to save his family from perishing, is he an object of pity, or of punishment? Who shall throw the first stone at a husband, who, in the heat of just resentment, sacrifices his faithless wife and her perfidious seducer? or at the young maiden, who, in her weak hour of rapture, forgets herself in the impetuous joys of love? Even our laws, cold and cruel as they are, relent in such cases, and withhold their punishment."

"That is quite another thing," said Albert; "because a man under the influence of violent passion loses all power of reflection, and is regarded as intoxicated or insane."

"Oh! you people of sound understandings," I replied, smiling, "are ever ready to exclaim 'Extravagance, and madness, and intoxication!' You moral men are so calm and so subdued! You abhor the drunken man, and detest the extravagant; you pass by, like the Levite, and thank God, like the Pharisee, that you are not like one of them. I have been more than once intoxicated, my passions have always bordered on extravagance: I am not ashamed to confess it; for I have learned, by my own experience, that all extraordinary men, who have accomplished great and astonishing actions, have ever been decried by the world as drunken or insane. And in private life, too, is it not intolerable that no one can undertake the execution of a noble or generous deed, without giving rise to the exclamation that the doer is intoxicated or mad? Shame upon you, ye sages!"

"This is another of your extravagant humours," said Albert: "you always exaggerate a case, and in this matter you are undoubtedly wrong; for we were speaking of suicide, which you compare with great actions, when it is impossible to regard it as anything but a weakness. It is much easier to die than to bear a life of misery with fortitude."

I was on the point of breaking off the conversation, for nothing puts me so completely out of patience as the utterance of a wretched commonplace when I am talking from my inmost heart. However, I composed myself, for I had often heard the same observation with sufficient vexation; and I answered him, therefore, with a little warmth, "You call this a weakness—beware of being led astray by appearances. When a nation, which has long groaned under the intolerable yoke of a tyrant, rises at last and throws off its chains, do you call that weakness? The man who, to rescue his house from the flames, finds his physical strength redoubled, so that he lifts burdens with ease, which, in the absence of excitement, he could scarcely move; he who, under the rage of an insult, attacks and puts to flight half a score of his enemies, are such persons to be called weak? My good friend, if resistance be strength, how can the highest degree of resistance be a weakness?"

Albert looked steadfastly at me, and said, "Pray forgive me, but I do not see that the examples you have adduced bear any relation to the question." "Very likely," I answered; "for I have often been told that my style of illustration borders a little on the absurd. But let us see if we cannot place the matter in another point of view, by inquiring what can be a man's state of mind who resolves to free himself from the burden of life,—a burden often so pleasant to bear,—for we cannot otherwise reason fairly upon the subject.

"Human nature," I continued, "has its limits. It is able to endure a certain degree of joy, sorrow, and pain, but becomes annihilated as soon as this measure is exceeded. The question, therefore, is, not whether a man is strong or weak, but whether he is able to endure the measure of his sufferings. The suffering may be moral or physical; and in my opinion it is just as absurd to call a man a coward who destroys himself, as to call a man a coward who dies of a malignant fever."

Source: Goethe, Johann Wolfgang von. 1917. Carlyle, Thomas, trans. *The Sorrows of Young Werther.* New York: Collier. (Originally published 1774)

◙ Jean-Jacques Rousseau, from *Reveries of the Solitary Walker* (1778)

As one architect of the Romantic cult of individuality, Rousseau outlaws obligation to others as an unfair restriction by society on the individual. Here, Rousseau demonstrates that his sense of obligation toward a crippled beggar boy erodes his freedom to act while producing at the same time an unhealthy dependency in the boy. Charity hobbles the individuality of both the giver and receiver by producing dependency where, apparently, independence should reign.

In one corner of the boulevard, just by the Porte d'Enfer, a woman sets up stall every day in the summer to sell fruit, rolls and tisane. This woman has a little boy who is very sweet, but a cripple, and he hobbles about on his crutches begging from passers-by in a not unpleasant way. I had struck up a sort of acquaintance with the little fellow, and every time I went past he came up without fail to make me a little compliment, which was always followed by a little gift from me. The first few times I was delighted to see him and gave him money very willingly, and I continued doing so for some time with the same pleasure, usually even giving myself the added satisfaction of engaging him in conversation and listening to his pleasant chatter. This pleasure gradually became a habit, and this was somehow transformed into a sort of duty which I soon began to find irksome, particularly

on account of the preamble I was obliged to listen to, in which he never failed to address me as Monsieur Rousseau so as to show that he knew me well, thus making it quite clear to me on the contrary that he knew no more of me than those who had taught him. From that time on I felt less inclined to go that way, and in the end I unthinkingly adopted the habit of making a detour when I approached this obstacle.

Source: Rousseau, Jean-Jacques. 1979. Butterworth, Charles E. trans. "Sixth Walk." In *Reveries of the Solitary Walker.* Harmondsworth, UK: Penguin.

◙ James Forbes, The Blind Diver of Dhuboy (1781)

James Forbes reported a civil case from Dhuboy (now Dabhoi), Gujarat, North India, in 1781. The story focuses on a broken contract by a goldsmith whose wife had thrown herself and a treasure of jewels into a well in order to deprive him of the chance to take up with another woman. The goldsmith promised to reward a blind man with one third of the treasure if he located it during a dive, but then he reneged on the agreement.

A certain blind man, well known in Dhuboy, died during my residence there. Although deprived of one sense, he seemed to enjoy the others in greater perfection: among various talents he could generally discover hidden treasure, whether buried in the earth, or concealed under water, and possessed the faculty of diving and continuing a long time in that element without inconvenience. As he never commenced a search without stipulating for one third of the value restored, he had, by this occupation, maintained an aged father, a wife, and several children. The old man complained, that several persons for whom his son had found money, refused to make good their promise; and particularly a goldsmith, who on being summoned before the court, acknowledged the truth of the story, but thought a third part of the amount too large a proportion. The goldsmith had reprimanded his wife for misconduct: being a woman of spirit, she took the first opportunity of his absence to collect as much of his money and valuables as possible, and threw them, together with herself and her own jewels and ornaments, into a well. As they had not lived very happily together, the goldsmith on his return, was not much concerned about his wife, but regretting the loss of his treasure he made diligent search for her body, which was found in an adjoining well, divested of all her ornaments. Surprized and disappointed, he knew not what further to do, when a confidential friend of his wife told him the deceased had taken off her gold chains and jewels, and tying them up in a bag with his own valuables, threw them into another well, but where it was she knew not; having alleged two reasons for her conduct, that he might lose his property, and be deprived of the means of procuring another wife, which he would find difficult without the jewels. The blind man was sent for, and after a long search, found the bag in a distant well, but could not prevail on the goldsmith to give him his share; and since his decease his father had been unsuccessful. The court of adawlat decreed him one third of the property.

Source: Forbes, James. 1813. Vol. II:362–364 in *Oriental Memoirs . . . Written During Seventeen Years Residence in India.* London: White, Cochrane.

▣ Samuel Johnson, from "The Life of Pope" (1781)

In Johnson's "Life of Pope," the excruciating details of Pope's physical impairment serve to disempower the "King of Parnassus," allowing Johnson to question—by a standard juxtaposition of what he called the "character" of the author with the appraisal of his work in each of the Lives of the Poets—the polished perfection of Pope's eminently "prudent" art.

The person of Pope is well known not to have been formed by the nicest model. He has, in his account of the 'Little Club,' compared himself to a spider, and by another is described as protuberant behind and before. He is said to have been beautiful in his infancy; but he was of a constitution originally feeble and weak, and as bodies of a tender frame are easily distorted his deformity was probably in part the effect of his application. His stature was so low that, to bring him to a level with common tables, it was necessary to raise his seat. But his face was not displeasing, and his eyes were animated and vivid.

By natural deformity or accidental distortion his vital functions were so much disordered that his life was a 'long disease.' His most frequent assailant was the headache, which he used to relieve by inhaling the steam of coffee, which he very frequently required.

Most of what can be told concerning his petty peculiarities was communicated by a female domestic of the Earl of Oxford, who knew him perhaps after the middle of life. He was then so weak as to stand in perpetual need of female attendance; extremely sensible of cold, so that he wore a kind of fur doublet under a shirt of very coarse warm linen with fine sleeves. When he rose he was invested in bodice made of stiff canvas, being scarce able to hold himself erect till they were laced, and he then put on a flannel waistcoat. One side was contracted. His legs were so slender that he enlarged their bulk with three pair of stockings, which were drawn on and off by the maid; for he was not able to dress or undress himself, and neither went to bed nor rose without help. His weakness made it very difficult for him to be clean.

His hair had fallen almost all away, and he used to dine sometimes with Lord Oxford, privately, in a velvet cap. His dress of ceremony was black, with a tie-wig and a little sword.

The indulgence and accommodation which his sickness required had taught him all the unpleasing and unsocial qualities of a valetudinary man. He expected that every thing should give way to his ease or humor, as a child whose parents will not hear her cry has an unresisted dominion in the nursery.

Source: Johnson, Samuel. 1905. Hill, G. B., ed. "The Life of Pope." In *The Lives of the English Poets.* Oxford, UK: Clarendon Press. (Originally published 1781)

▣ Benjamin Rush, from Two Essays on the Mind (1786)

The American physician Benjamin Rush was ahead of his time in believing that mentally ill people deserved to be treated with respect. He sharply criticized the inhumane treatment he saw mental patients receive and was able to win public support for state funding for a ward for the insane. In this excerpt, Rush considers the connections between physical health and moral and mental characteristics.

It was probably a state of the human mind such, as has been described, that our Saviour alluded to in the disciple, who was about to betray him, when he called him "a devil." Perhaps the essence of depravity in infernal spirits, consists in their being wholly devoid of a moral faculty. In them the will has probably lost

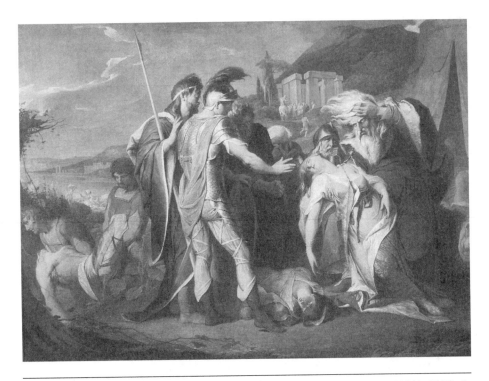

King Lear Weeping over the Body of Cordelia (1786–1788), by James Barry (1741–1806). In this recreation of a scene from Shakespeare's King Lear, Barry captures the protagonist's desperate mourning over the death of his daughter as a tragedy caused by his own descent into madness.

Source: Art Resource, New York.

I remarked in the beginning of this discourse, that persons who were deprived of the just exercise of memory—imagination—or judgment, were proper subjects of medicine; and that there are many cases upon record which prove, that the diseases from the derangement of these faculties, have yielded to the healing art.

It is perhaps only because the disorders of the moral faculty, have not been traced to a connection with physical causes, that medical writers have neglected to give them a place in their systems of nosology, and that so few attempts have been hitherto made, to lessen or remove them by physical as well as rational and moral remedies.

I hinted formerly, in proving the analogy between the effects of DISEASES upon the intellects, and upon the moral faculty, that the latter was frequently impaired by fevers and madness. I beg to add further upon this head, that not only fevers and madness, but the hysteria and hypochondriasis, as well as all those states of the body, whether idiopathic or symptomatic, which are accompanied with preternatural irritability—sensibility—topor—stupor—or morbidity of the nervous system, dispose to vice, either of the body or of the mind. It is in vain to attack these vices with lectures upon morality. They are only to be cured by medicine,—particularly by exercise,—the cold bath,—and by a cold or a warm atmosphere. The young woman, whose case I mentioned earlier, that lost her habit of veracity by a nervous fever, recovered this virtue, as soon as her system recovered its natural tone from this cold weather which happily succeeded her fever.

the power of choosing, as well as the inclination of enjoying moral good. It is true, we read of their trembling in a belief of the existence of God, and of anticipating future punishment by asking, whether they were to be tormented before their time: but this is the effect of coincidence, and hence arises another argument in favor of this judicial power of the mind, being distinct from the moral faculty. It would seem as if the Supreme Being had preserved the moral faculty in man from the ruins of his fall, on purpose to guide him back again to Paradise, and at the same time had constituted the conscience, both in men and in fallen spirits, a kind of royalty in his moral empire, on purpose to shew his property in all intelligent creatures, and their original resemblance to himself. Perhaps the essence of moral depravity in man consists in a total, but temporary, suspension of the power of conscience. Perhaps in this situation are emphatically said in the scriptures to be a "past feeling"—and to have their consciences seared, with a "hot iron"—they are likewise said to be "twice dead"—that is, the same torpor or moral insensibility, has seized both the moral faculty and the conscience.

Weakness, disease, and pain, have many instances, given to a preternatural excitement to the human intellects. Cicero, Erasmus, Pascal, and Boilieu, were all well known to their contemporaries, as much by the feebleness of their constitutions, as by the strength of their minds. The great mental vigour, which has been observed in persons who are hump-backed, of which, the celebrated Roman orator Galba, and Mr. Pope, furnished memorable instances, is probably occasioned by the bodily weakness that is connected with deformity. But the effects of disease, whether occasioned or chronic, in an evolving mind, are still more remarkable. How often do we hear our patients discover, upon a sick or death-bed, marks of reflection, and even eloquence, to which they were strangers to in health! It has been remarked, that abortive and sickly children make sensible men and women. Disease, in this case, acts in various ways. It imposes a restraint upon their appetites, it confines them to the company of their parents, and of persons who are capable of improving them, and it certainly keeps up an action in the brain, in common with other parts of the body, which tends to impart vigour to the intellectual faculties.

But further. There are several well-attested instances, upon record, of persons speaking long forgotten languages in the delirium of a fever, and one, related by Dr. Frank, of a man, who spoke a language in a diseased state of his brain, which he had never learned. If this be true, he must have heard the words of it, without understanding, for it is impossible to conceive of the knowledge of even a single sound existing in the mind, unless it has been previously conveyed there through the medium of the ears.

In support of the influence of diseases in exciting the faculties of the mind, let us attend to the phenomena of diseases, which are produced by a morbid state of the brain. The intellects act here without order, but they act with uncommon celerity and force. Of this, every man must be convinced, who has paid the least attention to those operations in his own mind. The business of a day is often transacted in a dream, in the course of a single minute, and the perceptions of supposed impressions upon the imagination, are far more vivid than in the waking state. Even madness discovers the connection between morbid excitement in the body, and an increase of vigour and activity in certain intellectual operations. Who has not heard preternatural and brilliant effusions of eloquence, and wit in the cell of a hospital? The disease, in this instance, resembles an earthquake, which, in rending the ground, now and then throws upon its surface, with many offensive matters, certain precious fossils, which surprise and delight us by their novelty or splendour.

The effects of pain, in generating new ideas, or exciting old ones in a rapid succession, have been taken notice of in my account of the influence of the physical causes of the moral faculty. To the facts I have there mentioned, I shall add two more. The famous pedestrian traveler, Mr. Stewart, informed me, that he had seen torture produce short intervals of reason in some idiots in Italy. I have known the pain of a large abscess upon the back, produce the same effect upon a man, who had been confined for madness, which ended in fatuity, above twenty years in the Pennsylvania hospital.

Source: Rush, Benjamin. 1972. Carlson, Eric T., ed. *Two Essays on the Mind: An Enquiry into the Influence of Physical Causes upon the Moral Faculty, and on the Influence of Physical Causes in Promoting an Increase of the Strength and Activity of the Intellectual Faculties of Man.* New York: Brunner/Mazel. (Originally published 1786)

▣ James Boswell, from *The Life of Samuel Johnson* (1791)

Suspended between an early modern reading of disability as divine mark and a modern reading of disability as obstacle to be overcome by exceptional heroism, Boswell's Life of Johnson makes a hero of a writer considered in his own day to be both a physical oddity and a social monster. Samuel Johnson's many disabilities (partial deafness and blindness, obsessive-compulsive behaviors, crippling depression, and facial disfigurement among them) sometimes serve as markers of Johnson's painful progress as exemplary Christian hero, but at other times, Boswell's mentions of Johnson's disability fail to signify at all beyond the self-evident significance of anecdotal detail.

Samuel Johnson was born at Lichfield, in Staffordshire, on the 18th of September, N.S. 1709; and his initiation into the Christian Church was not delayed; for his baptism is recorded in the register of St. Mary's parish in that city, to have been performed on the day of his birth. His father is there stiled *Gentleman*, a circumstance of which an ignorant panegyrist has praised him for not being proud; when the truth is, that the appellation of Gentleman, though now lost in the indiscriminate assumption of *Esquire*, was commonly taken by those who could not boast of gentility. His father was Michael Johnson, a native of Derbyshire, of obscure extraction, who settled in Lichfield as a bookseller and stationer. His mother was Sarah Ford, descended of an ancient race of substantial yeomanry in Warwickshire. They were well advanced in years when they married, and never had more than two children, both sons; Samuel, their first born, who lived to be the illustrious character whose various excellence I am to endeavor to record, and Nathanael, who died in his twenty-fifty year.

Mr. Michael Johnson was a man of a large and robust body, and of a strong and active mind; yet, as in the most solid rocks veins of unsound substance are often discovered, there was in him a mixture of that disease, the nature of which eludes the most minute enquiry, though the effects are well known to be a weariness of life, an unconcern about those things which agitate the greater part of mankind, and a general sensation of gloomy wretchedness. From him then his son inherited, with some other qualities, 'a vile melancholy,' which in his too strong expression of any disturbance of the mind, 'made him mad all his life, at least not sober.' Michael was, however, forced by the narrowness of his circumstances to be very diligent in business, not only in his shop, but by occasionally resorting to several towns in the neighborhood, some of which were at a considerable distance from Lichfield. At that time booksellers' shops in the provincial towns of England were very rare, so that there was not one even in Birmingham, in which town old Mr. Johnson used to open a shop every market-day. He was a pretty good Latin scholar, and a citizen so creditable as to be made one of the magistrates of Lichfield; and, being a man of good sense, and skill in his trade, he acquired a reasonable share of wealth, of which however he afterwards lost the greatest part, by engaging unsuccessfully in a manufacture of parchment. He was a zealous high-churchman and royalist, and retained his attachment to the unfortunate house of Stuart, though he reconciled himself, by casuistical arguments of expediency and necessity, to take the oaths imposed by the prevailing power. . . .

Young Johnson had the misfortune to be much afflicted with the scrophula, or king's-evil, which disfigured a countenance naturally well formed, and hurt his visual nerves so much, that he did not see at all with one of his eyes, though its appearance was little different from that of the other. There is amongst his prayers, one inscribed *When my EYE was restored to its use,* which ascertains a defect that many of his friends knew he had, though I never perceived it. I supposed him to be only near-sighted; and indeed I must observe, that in no other respect, could I discern any defect in his vision; on the contrary, the force of his attention and perceptive quickness made him see and distinguish all manner of objects, whether of nature or of art, with a nicety that is rarely to be found. When he and I were travelling in the Highlands of Scotland, and I pointed out to him a mountain which I observed resembled a cone, he corrected my inaccuracy, by shewing me, that it was indeed pointed at the top, but that one side of it was larger than the other. And the ladies with whom he was acquainted agree, that no man was more nicely and minutely critical in the elegance of female dress. When I found that he saw the romantick beauties of Islam, in Derbyshire, much better than I did, I told him that he resembled an able performer upon a bad instrument. How false and contemptible then are all the remarks which have been made to the prejudice either of his candour or of his philosophy, founded upon a supposition that he was almost blind. It has been said, that he contracted this grievous malady from his nurse. His mother, yielding to the superstitious notion, which, it is wonderful to think, prevailed so long in this country, as to the virtue of the regal touch; a notion, which our kings encouraged, and to which a man of such enquiry and such judgement as Carte could give credit; carried him to London, where he was actually touched by Queen Anne. Mrs. Johnson indeed, as Mr. Hector informed me, acted by the advice of the celebrated Sir John Floyer, then a physician in Lichfield. Johnson used to talk of this very frankly; and Mrs. Piozzi has preserved his very picturesque description of the scene, as it remained upon his fancy. Being asked if he could remember Queen Anne,—"He had (he said) a confused, but somehow a sort of solemn recollection of a lady in diamonds, and a long black hood." This touch, however, was without any effect. I ventured to say to him, in allusion to the political principles in which he was educated, and of which he ever retained some odour, that "his mother had not carried him far enough; she should have taken him to ROME."

◻ William Wordsworth, from "The Idiot Boy" (1798)

"The Idiot Boy" was one of the key odes published in the Romantic manifesto Lyrical Ballads, *a series of poems by Wordsworth and Samuel Taylor Coleridge*

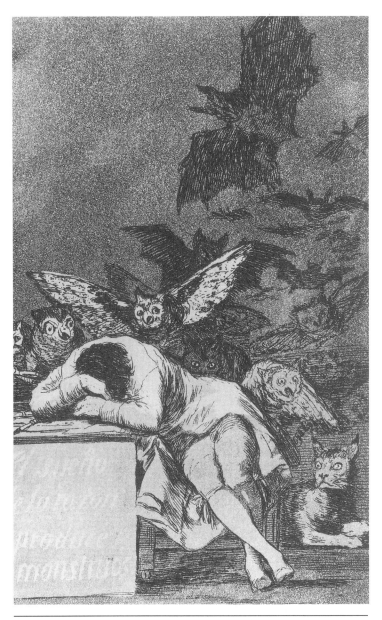

The Sleep of Reason Produces Monsters, *by Francisco Goya (1746–1828).*
Goya's illustration captures his belief that excessive confidence in Reason's
ability to conquer nature results in the repression of phenomena less easy to
explain through empirical observation. Here, the sleeping scientific
observer finds himself assaulted by occult imaginings that have been side-
lined by his rational inquiry during the period of the Enlightenment.

Source: Art Resource, New York.

that paid homage to the life of the folk as worthy of
literary treatment. In this excerpt, the Idiot Boy is
charged with the responsibility of setting out on
the family horse to retrieve a doctor for an ill neigh-
bor. By the end of the journey the boy has failed to
return with the physician but has experienced a sub-
lime journey into Nature that sustains himself and the
poet.

'Tis eight o'clock,—a clear March night,
The moon is up,—the sky is blue,
The owlet, in the moonlight air,
Shouts from nobody knows where;
He lengthens out his lonely shout,
Halloo! halloo! a long halloo!

—Why bustle thus about your door,
What means this bustle, Betty Foy?
Why are you in this mighty fret?
And why on horseback have you set
Him whom you love, your Idiot Boy? . . .

. . . And Betty o'er and o'er has told
The Boy, who is her best delight,
Both what to follow, what to shun,
What do, and what to leave undone,
How turn to left, and how to right.

And Betty's most especial charge,
Was, "Johnny! Johnny! mind that you
Come home again, nor stop at all,—
Come home again, whate'er befall,
My Johnny, do, I pray you do." . . .

. . . But when the Pony moved his legs,
Oh! then for the poor Idiot Boy!
For joy he cannot hold the bridle,
For joy his head and heels are idle,
He's idle all for very joy.

And while the Pony moves his legs,
In Johnny's left hand you may see
The green bough motionless and dead:
The Moon that shines above his head
Is not more still and mute than he. . . .

. . . The clock is on the stroke of one;
But neither Doctor nor his Guide
Appears along the moonlight road;
There's neither horse nor man abroad,
And Betty's still at Susan's side.

And Susan now begins to fear
Of sad mischances not a few,
That Johnny may perhaps be drowned;
Or lost, perhaps, and never found;
Which they must both for ever rue. . . .

. . . Poor Betty now has lost all hope,
Her thoughts are bent on deadly sin,

A green-grown pond she just has past,
And from the brink she hurries fast,
Lest she should drown herself therein.

And now she sits her down and weeps;
Such tears she never shed before;
"Oh dear, dear Pony! my sweet joy!
Oh carry back my Idiot Boy!
And we will ne'er o'erload thee more." . . .

. . . Your Pony's worth his weight in gold:
Then calm your terrors, Betty Foy!
She's coming from among the trees,
And now all full in view she sees
Him whom she loves, her Idiot Boy.

And Betty sees the Pony too:
Why stand you thus, good Betty Foy?
It is no goblin, 'tis no ghost,
'Tis he whom you so long have lost,
He whom you love, your Idiot Boy.

She looks again—her arms are up—
She screams—she cannot move for joy;
She darts, as with a torrent's force,
She almost has o'erturned the Horse,
And fast she holds her Idiot Boy. . . .

. . . For while they all were travelling home,
Cried Betty, "Tell us, Johnny, do,
Where all this long night you have been,
What you have heard, what you have seen:
And, Johnny, mind you tell us true."

Now Johnny all night long had heard
The owls in tuneful concert strive;
No doubt too he the moon had seen;
For in the moonlight he had been
From eight o'clock till five.

And thus, to Betty's question, he
Made answer, like a traveller bold,
(His very words I give to you,)
"The cocks did crow to-whoo, to-whoo,
And the sun did shine so cold!"
—Thus answered Johnny in his glory,
And that was all his travel's story.

———————

Source: Wordsworth, William. 1798. "The Idiot Boy." In Wordsworth, William, and Samuel Taylor Coleridge, *Lyrical Ballads.* Bristol, UK: T. N. Longman.

Modernity and Normalization: 1800–1945

▣ Samuel Taylor Coleridge, from "Dejection: An Ode" (1802)

This poem is a study in the feelings of melancholy often found in Romantic poetry, but with the essential difference that Coleridge questions the capacity of the natural world to raise one's spirits. Rather, affliction remains the responsibility of each person, and one can find a cure only through inner resources.

My genial spirits fail;
And what can these avail
To lift the smothering weight from off my breast?
It were a vain endeavour,
Though I should gaze for ever
On that green light that lingers in the west:
I may not hope from outward forms to win
The passion and the life, whose fountains are within.

Source: Coleridge, Samuel Taylor. 1802. Lines 39–46 in "Dejection: An Ode." Available at: http://etext.lib.virginia.edu/stc/Coleridge/poems/Dejection_An_Ode.html

▣ John Keats, "This Living Hand" (1816)

John Keats died at the age of 25 following many years of poor health from tuberculosis. Thought to address Keats's fiancée, Fanny Brawne, this poem describes the complex emotions felt at the bedside of the dying or disabled person. The hand of death invites us to sacrifice ourselves to save those who are dying or disabled at the same time that it excites the fear that death and disability may be contagious.

This Living Hand

This living hand, now warm and capable
Of earnest grasping, would, if it were cold
And in the icy silence of the tomb,
So haunt thy days and chill thy dreaming nights
That thou wouldst wish thine own heart dry of blood
So in my veins red life might stream again,
And thou be conscience-calmed—see here it is—
I hold it towards you.

Source: Keats, John. 1816. "This Living Hand." Available at: http://www.portablepoetry.com/poems/john_keats/this_living_hand.html

▣ Mary Shelley, from *Frankenstein* (1818)

Shelley explores the isolation of the monster, who cannot show his face in the light of day or buy redemption through good deeds. Shelley's use of physical difference to explore the marginal status of her protagonist is a familiar device among Romantic writers, as is her suggestion that the monster's loneliness may be cured only by finding a soul mate. In this excerpt, the monster is recounting some of his history to his creator, Victor Frankenstein.

"Cursed, cursed creator! Why did I live? Why, in that instant, did I not extinguish the spark of existence, which you had so wantonly bestowed? I know not;

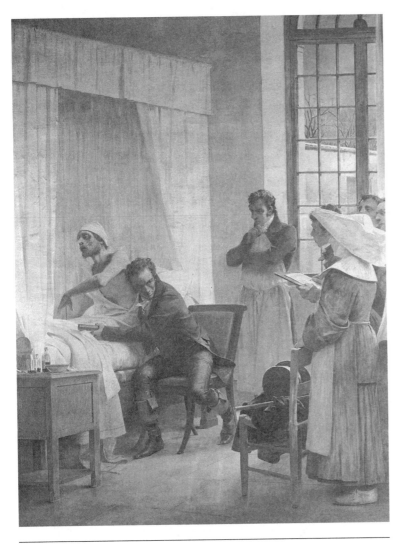

Laennec at the Necker Hospital Ausculting a Tuberculosis Patient in Front of His Students *(1816), by Theobold Chartran (1849–1907). A common way for physicians to diagnose the presence of tuberculosis was through auscultation of the chest with a stethoscope while listening for crackles during breathing.*

Source: Art Resource, New York.

branches above me: now and then the sweet voice of a bird burst forth amidst the universal stillness. All, save I, were at rest or in enjoyment: I, like the arch-fiend, bore a hell within me; and, finding myself unsympathised with, wished to tear up the trees, spread havoc and destruction around me, and then to have sat down and enjoyed the ruin.

"But this was a luxury of sensation that could not endure; I became fatigued with excess of bodily exertion, and sank on the damp grass in the sick impotence of despair. There was none among the myriads of men that existed who would pity or assist me; and should I feel kindness towards my enemies? No: from that moment I declared everlasting war against the species, and, more than all, against him who had formed me, and sent me forth to this insupportable misery.

"The sun rose; I heard the voices of men, and knew that it was impossible to return to my retreat during that day. Accordingly I hid myself in some thick underwood, determining to devote the ensuing hours to reflection on my situation.

"The pleasant sunshine, and the pure air of day, restored me to some degree of tranquility; and when I considered what had passed at the cottage, I could not help believing that I had been too hasty in my conclusions. I had certainly acted imprudently. It was apparent that my conversation had interested the father in my behalf, and I was a fool in having exposed my person to the horror of his children. I ought to have familiarized the old De Lacey to me, and by degrees to have discovered myself to the rest of his family, when they should have been prepared for my approach. But I did not believe my errors to be irretrievable; and, after much consideration, I resolved to return to the cottage, seek the old man, and by my representations win him to my party.

"These thoughts calmed me, and in the afternoon I sank into a profound sleep; but the fever of my blood did not allow me to be visited by peaceful dreams. The horrible scene of the preceding day was for ever acting before my eyes; the females were flying, and

despair had not yet taken possession of me; my feelings were those of rage and revenge. I could with pleasure have destroyed the cottage and its inhabitants, and have glutted myself with their shrieks and misery.

"When night came, I quitted my retreat, and wandered in the wood; and now, no longer restrained by the fear of discovery, I gave vent to my anguish in fearful howlings. I was like a wild beast that had broken the toils; destroying the objects that obstructed me, and ranging through the wood with a stag like swiftness. O! what a miserable night I passed! the cold stars shone in mockery, and the bare trees waved their the enraged Felix tearing me from his father's feet. I awoke exhausted; and, finding that it was already night, I crept forth from my hiding-place, and went in search of food.

"When my hunger was appeased, I directed my steps towards the well known path that conducted to the cottage. All there was at peace. I crept into my hovel, and remained in silent expectation of the accustomed hour when the family arose. That hour passed, the sun mounted high in the heavens, but the cottagers did not appear. I trembled violently, apprehending some dreadful misfortune. The inside of the cottage was dark, and I heard no motion; I cannot describe the agony of this suspense.

"Presently two countrymen passed by; but, pausing near the cottage, they entered into conversation, using violent gesticulations; but I did not understand what they said, as they spoke the language of the country, which differed from that of my protectors. Soon after, however, Felix approached with another man: I was surprised, as I knew that he had not quitted the cottage that morning, and waited anxiously to discover, from his discourse, the meaning of these unusual appearances.

"'Do you consider,' said his companion to him, 'that you will be obliged to pay three months' rent, and to lose the produce of your garden? I do not wish to take any unfair advantage, and I beg therefore that you will take some days to consider of your determination.'

"'It is utterly useless,' replied Felix; 'we can never again inhabit your cottage. The life of my father is in the greatest danger, owing to the dreadful circumstance that I have related. My wife and my sister will never recover their horror. I entreat you not to reason with me any more. Take possession of your tenement, and let me fly from this place.'

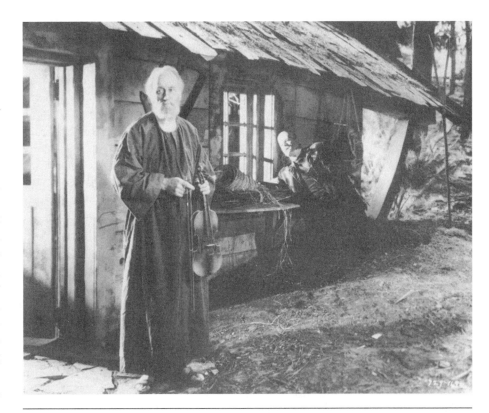

In Frankenstein *(1931), one of the earliest feature-length sound films, James Whale brought Mary Shelley's nineteenth-century story of deviant creation to the screen. In this movie still, a dual disability interchange occurs between the "lumbering" monster and a blind man. The social stigma applied to both individuals is mitigated through their momentary friendship.*

Source: Frankenstein (1931), directed by James Whale. B&W, 90 minutes. Reprinted by permission of Paul Darke.

"Felix trembled violently as he said this. He and his companion entered the cottage, in which they remained for a few minutes, and then departed. I never saw any of the family of De Lacey more.

"I continued for the remainder of the day in my hovel in a state of utter and stupid despair. My protectors had departed, and had broken the only link that held me to the world. For the first time the feelings of revenge and hatred filled my bosom, and I did not strive to control them; but, allowing myself to be borne away by the stream, I bent my mind towards injury and death. When I thought of my friends, of the mild voice of De Lacey, the gentle eyes of Agatha, and the exquisite beauty of the Arabian, these thoughts vanished, and a gush of tears somewhat soothed me. But again, when I reflected that they had spurned and deserted me, anger returned, a rage of anger; and, unable to injure anything human, I turned my fury towards inanimate objects. As night advanced, I placed a variety of combustibles around the cottage;

and, after having destroyed every vestige of cultivation in the garden, I waited with forced impatience until the moon had sunk to commence my operations.

"As the night advanced, a fierce wind arose from the woods, and quickly dispersed the clouds that had loitered in the heavens: the blast tore along like a mighty avalanche, and produced a kind of insanity in my spirits that burst all bounds of reason and reflection. I lighted the dry branch of a tree, and danced with fury around the devoted cottage, my eyes still fixed on the western horizon, the edge of which the moon nearly touched. A part of its orb was at length hid, and I waved my brand; it sunk, and, with a loud scream, I fired the straw, and heath, and bushes, which I had collected. The wind fanned the fire, and the cottage was quickly enveloped by the flames, which clung to it, and licked it with their forked and destroying tongues.

"As soon as I was convinced that no assistance could save any part of the habitation, I quitted the scene and sought for refuge in the woods.

"And now, with the world before me, whither should I bend my steps? I resolved to fly far from the scene of my misfortunes; but to me, hated and despised, every country must be equally horrible. At length the thought of you crossed my mind. I learned from your papers that you were my father, my creator; and to whom could I apply with more fitness than to him who had given me life? Among the lessons that Felix had bestowed upon Safie, geography had not been omitted. I had learned from these the relative situations of the different countries of the earth. You had mentioned Geneva as the name of your native town; and towards this place I resolved to proceed.

"But how was I to direct myself? I knew that I must travel in a south westerly direction to reach my destination; but the sun was my only guide. I did not know the names of the towns that I was to pass through, nor could I ask information from a single human being; but I did not despair. From you only could I hope for succour, although towards you I felt no sentiment but that of hatred. Unfeeling, heartless creator! you had endowed me with perceptions and passions, and then cast me abroad an object for the scorn and horror of mankind. But on you only had I any claim for pity and redress, and from you I determined to seek that justice which I vainly attempted to gain from any other being that wore the human form.

"My travels were long, and the sufferings I endured intense. It was late in autumn when I quitted the district where I had so long resided. I travelled only at night, fearful of encountering the visage of a human being. Nature decayed around me, and the sun became heatless; rain and snow poured around me; mighty rivers were frozen; the surface of the earth was hard, and chill, and bare, and I found no shelter. Oh, earth! how often did I imprecate curses on the cause of my being! The mildness of my nature had fled, and all within me was turned to gall and bitterness. The nearer I approached to your habitation, the more deeply did I feel the spirit of revenge enkindled in my heart. Snow fell, and the waters were hardened; but I rested not. A few incidents now and then directed me, and I possessed a map of the country; but I often wandered wide from my path. The agony of my feelings allowed me no respite: no incident occurred from which my rage and misery could not extract its food; but a circumstance that happened when I arrived on the confines of Switzerland, when the sun had recovered its warmth, and the earth again began to look green, confirmed in an especial manner the bitterness and horror of my feelings.

"I generally rested during the day, and travelled only when I was secured by night from the view of man. One morning, however, finding that my path lay through a deep wood, I ventured to continue my journey after the sun had risen; the day, which was one of the first of spring, cheered even me by the loveliness of its sunshine and the balminess of the air. I felt emotions of gentleness and pleasure, that had long appeared dead, revive within me. Half surprised by the novelty of these sensations, I allowed myself to be borne away by them; and, forgetting my solitude and deformity, dared to be happy. Soft tears again bedewed my cheeks, and I even raised my humid eyes with thankfulness towards the blessed sun which bestowed such joy upon me.

"I continued to wind among the paths of the wood, until I came to its boundary, which was skirted by a deep and rapid river, into which many of the trees bent their branches, now budding with the fresh spring. Here I paused, not exactly knowing what path to pursue, when I heard the sound of voices that induced me to conceal myself under the shade of a cypress. I was scarcely hid, when a young girl came running towards the spot where I was concealed, laughing, as if she ran from some one in sport. She continued her course along the precipitous sides of the river, when suddenly her foot slipt, and she fell into the rapid stream. I rushed from my hiding place; and, with extreme labour from the force of the current, saved her, and dragged her to shore. She was senseless; and I endeavoured by every means in my power to restore animation, when I was suddenly interrupted by the approach of a rustic, who was probably the person from whom she had playfully fled. On seeing me, he darted towards me, and tearing the girl from my arms, hastened towards the deeper parts of the wood. I followed speedily, I hardly knew why; but when the man saw me draw near, he aimed a gun, which he carried, at my body, and fired. I sunk to the ground, and my injurer, with increased swiftness, escaped into the wood.

"This was then the reward of my benevolence! I had saved a human being from destruction, and, as a recompense, I now writhed under the miserable pain of a wound, which shattered the flesh and bone. The feelings of kindness and gentleness which I had entertained but a few moments before gave place to hellish rage and gnashing of teeth. Inflamed by pain, I vowed eternal hatred and vengeance to all mankind. But the agony of my wound overcame me; my pulses paused, and I fainted.

"For some weeks I led a miserable life in the woods, endeavouring to cure the wound which I had received. The ball had entered my shoulder, and I knew not whether it had remained there or passed through; at any rate I had no means of extracting it. My sufferings were augmented also by the oppressive sense of the injustice and ingratitude of their infliction. My daily vows rose for revenge—a deep and deadly revenge, such as would alone compensate for the outrages and anguish I had endured.

"After some weeks my wound healed, and I continued my journey. The labours I endured were no longer to be alleviated by the bright sun or gentle breezes of spring; all joy was but a mockery, which insulted my desolate state, and made me feel more painfully that I was not made for the enjoyment of pleasure.

"But my toils now drew near a close; and in two months from this time I reached the environs of Geneva.

"It was evening when I arrived, and I retired to a hiding-place among the fields that surround it, to meditate in what manner I should apply to you. I was oppressed by fatigue and hunger, and far too unhappy to enjoy the gentle breezes of evening, or the prospect of the sun setting behind the stupendous mountains of Jura.

"At this time a slight sleep relieved me from the pain of reflection, which was disturbed by the approach of a beautiful child, who came running into the recess I had chosen, with all the sportiveness of infancy. Suddenly, as I gazed on him, an idea seized me, that this little creature was unprejudiced, and had lived too short a time to have imbibed a horror of deformity. If, therefore, I could seize him, and educate him as my companion and friend, I should not be so desolate in this peopled earth.

"Urged by this impulse, I seized on the boy as he passed and drew him towards me. As soon as he beheld my form, he placed his hands before his eyes and uttered a shrill scream: I drew his hand forcibly from his face, and said, 'Child, what is the meaning of this? I do not intend to hurt you; listen to me.'

"He struggled violently. 'Let me go,' he cried; 'monster! ugly wretch! you wish to eat me, and tear me to pieces—You are an ogre—Let me go, or I will tell my papa.'

"'Boy, you will never see your father again; you must come with me.'

"'Hideous monster! let me go. My papa is a Syndic—he is M. Frankenstein—he will punish you. You dare not keep me.'

"'Frankenstein! you belong then to my enemy—to him towards whom I have sworn eternal revenge; you shall be my first victim.'

"The child still struggled, and loaded me with epithets which carried despair to my heart; I grasped his throat to silence him, and in a moment he lay dead at my feet.

"I gazed on my victim, and my heart swelled with exultation and hellish triumph: clapping my hands, I exclaimed, 'I, too, can create desolation; my enemy is not invulnerable; this death will carry despair to him, and a thousand other miseries shall torment and destroy him.'

"As I fixed my eyes on the child, I saw something glittering on his breast. I took it; it was a portrait of a most lovely woman. In spite of my malignity, it softened and attracted me. For a few moments I gazed with delight on her dark eyes, fringed by deep lashes, and her lovely lips; but presently my rage returned: I remembered that I was for ever deprived of the delights that such beautiful creatures could bestow; and that she whose resemblance I contemplated would, in regarding me, have changed that air of divine benignity to one expressive of disgust and affright.

"Can you wonder that such thoughts transported me with rage? I only wonder that at that moment, instead of venting my sensations in exclamations and agony, I did not rush among mankind and perish in the attempt to destroy them.

"While I was overcome by these feelings, I left the spot where I had committed the murder, and seeking a more secluded hiding-place, I entered a barn which had appeared to me to be empty. A woman was sleeping on some straw; she was young: not indeed so beautiful as her whose portrait I held; but of an agreeable aspect, and blooming in the loveliness of youth and health. Here, I thought, is one of those whose joy-imparting smiles are bestowed on all but me. And then I bent over her, and whispered, 'Awake, fairest, thy lover is near—he who would give his life but to obtain one look of affection from thine eyes: my beloved, awake!'

"The sleeper stirred; a thrill of terror ran through me. Should she indeed awake, and see me, and curse me, and denounce the murderer? Thus would she assuredly act, if her darkened eyes opened and she beheld me. The thought was madness; it stirred the fiend within me—not I, but she shall suffer: the murder I have committed because I am for ever robbed of all that she could give me, she shall atone. The crime had its source in her: be hers the punishment! Thanks to the lessons of Felix and the sanguinary laws of man, I had learned now to work mischief. I bent over her, and placed the portrait securely in one of the folds of her dress. She moved again, and I fled.

"For some days I haunted the spot where these scenes had taken place; sometimes wishing to see you, sometimes resolved to quit the world and its miseries for ever. At length I wandered towards these mountains, and have ranged through their immense recesses, consumed by a burning passion which you alone can gratify. We may not part until you have promised to comply with my requisition. I am alone, and miserable; man will not associate with me; but one as deformed and horrible as myself would not deny herself to me. My companion must be of the same species, and have the same defects. This being you must create."

Source: Shelley, Mary. 1981. Pp. 121–129 in *Frankenstein*. New York: Bantam. (Originally published 1818)

◉ George Gordon, Lord Byron, from *The Deformed Transformed* (1822)

Upon Byron's death, this unfinished manuscript for a drama, based on Goethe's Faust and a popular novel of the times entitled The Three Brothers, was discovered in his drawer. In the work the hunchbacked protagonist, Arnold, is given the opportunity to trade in

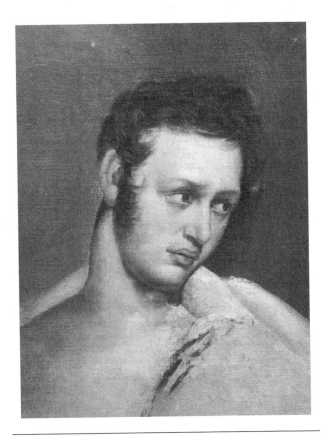

Lord Byron, English Poet, *by Thomas Lawrence (1769–1830). Lord Byron, who was diagnosed with a clubfoot at birth (his condition is now thought to have been Little's disease), wrote about experiences of social ostracization in his last, unfinished play,* The Deformed Transformed. *In the work, the hunchbacked protagonist, Arnold, makes a Faustian deal with a stranger to exchange his disabled body for the more able body of the Greek hero Achilles. The result is Byron's ironic commentary on masculine militarization and the unacknowledged capacities of those who occupy socially rejected physicalities.*

Source: Art Resource, New York.

his "deformed" body for that of the Greek warrior Achilles. The stranger who makes this offer sets out to demonstrate that a disabled body does not hinder one from social accomplishments by taking up Arnold's discarded exterior himself. It should be noted that Byron was born with a physical impairment and so lived with disability his entire life.

Part I.

Scene I: A Forest.
Enter Arnold and his mother Bertha.
Bert.
Out, Hunchback!
Arn.
I was born so, Mother!

Bert.

Out,
Thou incubus! Thou nightmare! Of seven sons,
The sole abortion!

Arn.

Would that I had been so,
And never seen the light!

Bert.

I would so, too!
But as thou hast—hence, hence—and do thy best!
That back of thine may bear its burthen; 'tis
More high, if not so broad as that of others.

Arn.

It bears its burthen;—but, my heart! Will it
Sustain that which you lay upon it, Mother?
I love, or, at the least, I loved you: nothing
Save You, in nature, can love aught like me.
You nursed me—do not kill me!

Bert.

Yes—I nursed thee,
Because thou wert my first-born, and I knew not
If there would be another unlike thee,
That monstrous sport of Nature. But get hence,
And gather wood!

Arn.

I will: but when I bring it,
Speak to me kindly. Though my brothers are
So beautiful and lusty, and as free
As the free chase they follow, do not spurn me:
Our milk has been the same.

Bert.

As is the hedgehog's,
Which sucks at midnight from the wholesome dam
Of the young bull, until the milkmaid finds
The nipple, next day, sore, and udder dry.
Call not thy brothers brethren! Call me not
Mother; for if I brought thee forth, it was
As foolish hens at times hatch vipers, by
Sitting upon strange eggs. Out, urchin, out!

[Exit Bertha.]

Arn. (solus).

Oh, mother!—She is gone, and I must do
Her bidding;—wearily but willingly
I would fulfil it, could I only hope
A kind word in return. What shall I do?

[Arnold begins to cut wood: in doing this he wounds
one of his hands.]

My labour for the day is over now.
Accursèd be this blood that flows so fast;
For double curses will be my meed now
At home—What home? I have no home, no kin,

No kind—not made like other creatures, or
To share their sports or pleasures. Must I bleed, too,
Like them? Oh, that each drop which falls to earth
Would rise a snake to sting them, as they have
stung me!
Or that the Devil, to whom they liken me,
Would aid his likeness! If I must partake
His form, why not his power? Is it because
I have not his will too? For one kind word
From her who bore me would still reconcile me
Even to this hateful aspect. Let me wash
The wound.

[Arnold goes to a spring, and stoops to wash his
hand: he starts back.]

They are right; and Nature's mirror shows me,
What she hath made me. I will not look on it
Again, and scarce dare think on't. Hideous wretch
That I am! The very waters mock me with
My horrid shadow—like a demon placed
Deep in the fountain to scare back the cattle
From drinking therein.

[He pauses.]

And shall I live on,
A burden to the earth, myself, and shame
Unto what brought me into life? Thou blood,
Which flowest so freely from a scratch, let me
Try if thou wilt not, in a fuller stream,
Pour forth my woes for ever with thyself
On earth, to which I will restore, at once,
This hateful compound of her atoms, and
Resolve back to her elements, and take
The shape of any reptile save myself,
And make a world for myriads of new worms!
This knife! now let me prove if it will sever
This withered slip of Nature's nightshade—my
Vile form—from the creation, as it hath
The green bough from the forest.

[Arnold places the knife in the ground, with the point
upwards.]

Now 'tis set,
And I can fall upon it. Yet one glance
On the fair day, which sees no foul thing like
Myself, and the sweet sun which warmed me, but
In vain. The birds—how joyously they sing!
So let them, for I would not be lamented:
But let their merriest notes be Arnold's knell;
The fallen leaves my monument; the murmur
Of the near fountain my sole elegy.
Now, knife, stand firmly, as I fain would fall!

[As he rushes to throw himself upon the knife, his eye is
suddenly caught by the fountain, which seems in motion.]

The fountain moves without a wind: but shall
The ripple of a spring change my resolve?
No. Yet it moves again! The waters stir,
Not as with air, but by some subterrane
And rocking Power of the internal world.
What's here? A mist! No more?—
[A cloud comes from the fountain. He stands gazing
upon it: it is dispelled, and a tall black man comes
towards him.]

Arn.
What would you? Speak!
Spirit or man?

Stran.
As man is both, why not
Say both in one?

Arn.
Your form is man's, and yet
You may be devil.

Stran.
So many men are that
Which is so called or thought, that you may add me
To which you please, without much wrong to either.
But come: you wish to kill yourself;—pursue
Your purpose.

Arn.
You have interrupted me.

Stran.
What is that resolution which can e'er
Be interrupted? If I be the devil
You deem, a single moment would have made you
Mine, and for ever, by your suicide;
And yet my coming saves you.

Arn.
I said not
You were the Demon, but that your approach
Was like one.

Stran.
Unless you keep company
With him (and you seem scarce used to such high
Society) you can't tell how he approaches;
And for his aspect, look upon the fountain,
And then on me, and judge which of us twain
Looks likest what the boors believe to be
Their cloven-footed terror.

Arn.
Do you—dare you
To taunt me with my born deformity?

Stran.
Were I to taunt a buffalo with this
Cloven foot of thine, or the swift dromedary
With thy Sublime of Humps, the animals

Would revel in the compliment. And yet
Both beings are more swift, more strong, more
mighty
In action and endurance than thyself,
And all the fierce and fair of the same kind
With thee. Thy form is natural: 'twas only
Nature's mistaken largess to bestow
The gifts which are of others upon man.

Arn.
Give me the strength then of the buffalo's foot,
When he spurns high the dust, beholding his
Near enemy; or let me have the long
And patient swiftness of the desert-ship,
The helmless dromedary!—and I'll bear
Thy fiendish sarcasm with a saintly patience.

Stran.
I will.

Arn. *(with surprise).*
Thou *canst*?

Stran.
Perhaps. Would you aught else?

Arn.
Thou mockest me.

Stran.
Not I. Why should I mock
What all are mocking? That's poor sport, methinks.
To talk to thee in human language (for
Thou canst not yet speak mine), the forester
Hunts not the wretched coney, but the boar,
Or wolf, or lion—leaving paltry game
To petty burghers, who leave once a year
Their walls, to fill their household cauldrons with
Such scullion prey. The meanest gibe at thee,—
Now I can mock the mightiest.

Arn.
Then waste not
Thy time on me: I seek thee not.

Stran.
Your thoughts
Are not far from me. Do not send me back:
I'm not so easily recalled to do
Good service.

Arn.
What wilt thou do for me?

Stran.
Change
Shapes with you, if you will, since yours so irks you;
Or form you to your wish in any shape.

Arn.
Oh! then you are indeed the Demon, for
Nought else would wittingly wear mine.

Stran.

I'll show thee
The brightest which the world e'er bore, and give thee
Thy choice.

Arn.

On what condition?

Stran.

There's a question!
An hour ago you would have given your soul
To look like other men, and now you pause
To wear the form of heroes.

Arn.

No; I will not.
I must not compromise my soul.

Stran.

What soul,
Worth naming so, would dwell in such a carcase?

Arn.

'Tis an aspiring one, whate'er the tenement
In which it is mislodged. But name your compact:
Must it be signed in blood?

Stran.

Not in your own.

Arn.

Whose blood then?

Stran.

We will talk of that hereafter.
But I'll be moderate with you, for I see
Great things within you. You shall have no bond
But your own will, no contract save your deeds.
Are you content?

Arn.

I take thee at thy word.

Stran.

Now then!—

[The Stranger approaches the fountain, and turns to Arnold.]

A little of your blood.

Arn.

For what?

Stran.

To mingle with the magic of the waters,
And make the charm effective.

Arn. *(holding out his wounded arm).*

Take it all.

Stran.

Not now. A few drops will suffice for this.

[The Stranger takes some of Arnold's blood in his hand, and casts it into the fountain.]

Shadows of Beauty!
Shadows of Power!

Rise to your duty—
This is the hour!
Walk lovely and pliant
From the depth of this fountain,
As the cloud-shapen giant
Bestrides the Hartz Mountain.
Come as ye were,
That our eyes may behold
The model in air
Of the form I will mould,
Bright as the Iris
When ether is spanned;—
Such *his* desire is,

[Pointing to Arnold.]

Such *my* command!
Demons heroic—
Demons who wore
The form of the Stoic
Or sophist of yore—

Or the shape of each victor—
From Macedon's boy,
To each high Roman's picture,
Who breathed to destroy—
Shadows of Beauty!
Shadows of Power!
Up to your duty—
This is the hour!

[Various phantoms arise from the waters, and pass in succession before the Stranger and Arnold.]

Arn.

What do I see?

Stran.

The black-eyed Roman, with
The eagle's beak between those eyes which ne'er
Beheld a conqueror, or looked along
The land he made not Rome's, while Rome became
His, and all theirs who heired his very name.

Arn.

The phantom's bald; my quest is beauty. Could I
Inherit but his fame with his defects!

Stran.

His brow was girt with laurels more than hairs.
You see his aspect—choose it, or reject.
I can but promise you his form; his fame
Must be long sought and fought for.

Arn.

I will fight, too,
But not as a mock Cæsar. Let him pass:
His aspect may be fair, but suits me not.

Stran.
Then you are far more difficult to please
Than Cato's sister, or than Brutus's mother,
Or Cleopatra at sixteen—an age
When love is not less in the eye than heart.
But be it so! Shadow, pass on!
[The phantom of Julius Cæsar disappears.]

Arn.
And can it
Be, that the man who shook the earth is gone,
And left no footstep?

Stran.
There you err. His substance
Left graves enough, and woes enough, and fame
More than enough to track his memory;
But for his shadow—'tis no more than yours,
Except a little longer and less crooked
I' the sun. Behold another!
[A second phantom passes].

Arn.
Who is he?

Stran.
He was the fairest and the bravest of
Athenians. Look upon him well.

Arn.
He is
More lovely than the last. How beautiful!

Stran.
Such was the curled son of Clinias;—wouldst thou
Invest thee with his form?

Arn.
Would that I had
Been born with it! But since I may choose further,
I will *look* further.
[The shade of Alcibiades disappears.]

Stran.
Lo! behold again!

Arn.
What! that low, swarthy, short-nosed, round-eyed satyr,
With the wide nostrils and Silenus' aspect,
The splay feet and low stature! I had better
Remain that which I am.

Stran.
And yet he was
The earth's perfection of all mental beauty,
And personification of all virtue.
But you reject him?

Arn.
If his form could bring me
That which redeemed it—no.

Stran.
I have no power
To promise that; but you may try, and find it
Easier in such a form—or in your own.

Arn.
No. I was not born for philosophy,
Though I have that about me which has need on't.
Let him fleet on.

Stran.
Be air, thou Hemlock-drinker!
[The shadow of Socrates disappears: another rises.]

Arn.
What's here? whose broad brow and whose curly beard
And manly aspect look like Hercules,
Save that his jocund eye hath more of Bacchus
Than the sad purger of the infernal world,
Leaning dejected on his club of conquest,
As if he knew the worthlessness of those
For whom he had fought.

Stran.
It was the man who lost
The ancient world for love.

Arn.
I cannot blame him,
Since I have risked my soul because I find not
That which he exchanged the earth for.

Stran.
Since so far
You seem congenial, will you wear his features?

Arn.
No. As you leave me choice, I am difficult.
If but to see the heroes I should ne'er
Have seen else, on this side of the dim shore,
Whence they float back before us.

Stran.
Hence, Triumvir,
Thy Cleopatra's waiting.
[The shade of Antony disappears: another rises.]

Arn.
Who is this?
Who truly looketh like a demigod,
Blooming and bright, with golden hair, and stature,
If not more high than mortal, yet immortal
In all that nameless bearing of his limbs,
Which he wears as the Sun his rays—a something
Which shines from him, and yet is but the flashing
Emanation of a thing more glorious still.
Was he e'er human only?

Stran.

Let the earth speak,
If there be atoms of him left, or even
Of the more solid gold that formed his urn.

Arn.

Who was this glory of mankind?

Stran.

The shame
Of Greece in peace, her thunderbolt in war—
Demetrius the Macedonian, and
Taker of cities.

Arn.

Yet one shadow more.

Stran. *(addressing the shadow).*

Get thee to Lamia's lap!

[The shade of Demetrius Poliorcetes vanishes: another rises.]

I'll fit you still,
Fear not, my Hunchback: if the shadows of
That which existed please not your nice taste,
I'll animate the ideal marble, till
Your soul be reconciled to her new garment.

Arn.

Content! I will fix here.

Stran.

I must commend
Your choice. The godlike son of the sea-goddess,
The unshorn boy of Peleus, with his locks
As beautiful and clear as the amber waves
Of rich Pactolus, rolled o'er sands of gold,
Softened by intervening crystal, and
Rippled like flowing waters by the wind,
All vowed to Sperchius as they were—behold them!
And him—as he stood by Polixena,
With sanctioned and with softened love, before
The altar, gazing on his Trojan bride,
With some remorse within for Hector slain
And Priam weeping, mingled with deep passion
For the sweet downcast virgin, whose young hand
Trembled in his who slew her brother. So
He stood i' the temple! Look upon him as
Greece looked her last upon her best, the instant
Ere Paris' arrow flew.

Arn.

I gaze upon him
As if I were his soul, whose form shall soon
Envelope mine.

Stran.

You have done well. The greatest
Deformity should only barter with

The extremest beauty—if the proverb's true
Of mortals, that Extremes meet.

Arn.

Come! Be quick!
I am impatient.

Stran.

As a youthful beauty
Before her glass. You both see what is not,
But dream it is what must be.

Arn.

Must I wait?

Stran.

No; that were a pity. But a word or two:
His stature is twelve cubits; would you so far
Outstep these times, and be a Titan? Or
(To talk canonically) wax a son
Of Anak?

Arn.

Why not?

Stran.

Glorious ambition!
I love thee most in dwarfs! A mortal of
Philistine stature would have gladly pared
His own Goliath down to a slight David:
But thou, my manikin, wouldst soar a show
Rather than hero. Thou shalt be indulged,
If such be thy desire; and, yet, by being
A little less removed from present men
In figure, thou canst sway them more; for all
Would rise against thee now, as if to hunt
A new-found Mammoth; and their cursèd engines,
Their culverins, and so forth, would find way
Through our friend's armour there, with greater ease
Than the Adulterer's arrow through his heel
Which Thetis had forgotten to baptize
In Styx.

Arn.

Then let it be as thou deem'st best.

Stran.

Thou shalt be beauteous as the thing thou seest,
And strong as what it was, and—

Arn.

I ask not
For Valour, since Deformity is daring.
It is its essence to o'ertake mankind
By heart and soul, and make itself the equal—
Aye, the superior of the rest. There is
A spur in its halt movements, to become
All that the others cannot, in such things

As still are free to both, to compensate
For stepdame Nature's avarice at first.
They woo with fearless deeds the smiles of fortune,
And oft, like Timour the lame Tartar, win them.
Stran.
Well spoken! And thou doubtless wilt remain
Formed as thou art. I may dismiss the mould
Of shadow, which must turn to flesh, to incase
This daring soul, which could achieve no less
Without it.
Arn.
Had no power presented me
The possibility of change, I would
Have done the best which spirit may to make
Its way with all Deformity's dull, deadly,
Discouraging weight upon me, like a mountain,
In feeling, on my heart as on my shoulders—
A hateful and unsightly molehill to
The eyes of happier men. I would have looked
On Beauty in that sex which is the type
Of all we know or dream of beautiful,
Beyond the world they brighten, with a sigh—
Not of love, but despair; nor sought to win,
Though to a heart all love, what could not love me
In turn, because of this vile crookèd clog,
Which makes me lonely. Nay, I could have borne
It all, had not my mother spurned me from her.
The she-bear licks her cubs into a sort
Of shape;—my Dam beheld my shape was hopeless.
Had she exposed me, like the Spartan, ere
I knew the passionate part of life, I had
Been a clod of the valley,—happier nothing
Than what I am. But even thus—the lowest,
Ugliest, and meanest of mankind—what courage
And perseverance could have done, perchance
Had made me something—as it has made heroes
Of the same mould as mine. You lately saw me
Master of my own life, and quick to quit it;
And he who is so is the master of
Whatever dreads to die.
Stran.
Decide between
What you have been, or will be.
Arn.
I have done so.
You have opened brighter prospects to my eyes,
And sweeter to my heart. As I am now,
I might be feared—admired—respected—loved
Of all save those next to me, of whom I

Would be belovèd. As thou showest me
A choice of forms, I take the one I view.
Haste! haste!
Stran.
And what shall *I* wear?
Arn.
Surely, he
Who can command all forms will choose the highest,
Something superior even to that which was
Pelides now before us. Perhaps his
Who slew him, that of Paris: or—still higher—
The Poet's God, clothed in such limbs as are
Themselves a poetry.
Stran.
Less will content me;
For I, too, love a change.
Arn.
Your aspect is
Dusky, but not uncomely.
Stran.
If I chose,
I might be whiter; but I have a *penchant*
For black—it is so honest, and, besides,
Can neither blush with shame nor pale with fear;
But I have worn it long enough of late,
And now I'll take your figure.
Arn.
Mine!
Stran.
Yes. You
Shall change with Thetis' son, and I with Bertha,
Your mother's offspring. People have their tastes;
You have yours—I mine.
Arn.
Despatch! despatch!
Stran.
Even so.
*[The Stranger takes some earth and moulds it along
the turf, and then addresses the phantom of Achilles.]*
Beautiful shadow
Of Thetis's boy!
Who sleeps in the meadow
Whose grass grows o'er Troy:
From the red earth, like Adam,
Thy likeness I shape,
As the Being who made him,
Whose actions I ape.
Thou Clay, be all glowing,
Till the Rose in his cheek

Be as fair as, when blowing,
It wears its first streak!

Ye Violets, I scatter,
Now turn into eyes!
And thou, sunshiny Water,
Of blood take the guise!
Let these Hyacinth boughs
Be his long flowing hair,
And wave o'er his brows,
As thou wavest in air!
Let his heart be this marble
I tear from the rock!
But his voice as the warble
Of birds on yon oak!
Let his flesh be the purest
Of mould, in which grew
The Lily-root surest,
And drank the best dew!
Let his limbs be the lightest
Which clay can compound,
And his aspect the brightest
On earth to be found!
Elements, near me,
Be mingled and stirred,
Know me, and hear me,
And leap to my word!
Sunbeams, awaken
This earth's animation
'Tis done! He hath taken
His stand in creation!

[Arnold falls senseless; his soul passes into the shape of Achilles, which rises from the ground; while the phantom has disappeared, part by part, as the figure was formed from the earth.]

Source: Gordon, George, Lord Byron. 1822. *The Deformed Transformed*. Available at: http://www.blackmask.com/books 64c/deftrans.htm

▣ Victor Hugo, from *The Hunchback of Notre Dame* (1831)

Here Hugo introduces his main character, Quasimodo the hunchback, who alone can save but not win the beautiful Esmeralda. Every grotesque person in Paris is invited by the rabble-rouser Coppenole to compete in a grimacing contest for the title of the Pope of Fools, but the winner, Quasimodo, is the one who incorporates more disabilities than anyone else. The introduction of Quasimodo to readers in this crowd scene allows Hugo to catalog the many superstitions and fears surrounding disability at the same time that he presents readers with one of the most memorable heroes in French literature, the Romantic outcast par excellence. This excerpt begins with the crowd shouting "Noel! Noel! Noel!" (the old French word for hurrah) to signify their overwhelming vote for Quasimodo as Pope of Fools.

From Chapter V. "Quasimodo"

"Noel! Noel! Noel!" shouted the people on all sides. That was, in fact, a marvellous grimace which was beaming at that moment through the aperture in the rose window. After all the pentagonal, hexagonal, and whimsical faces, which had succeeded each other at that hole without realizing the ideal of the grotesque which their imaginations, excited by the orgy, had constructed, nothing less was needed to win their suffrages than the sublime grimace which had just dazzled the assembly. Master Coppenole himself applauded, and Clopin Trouillefou, who had been among the competitors (and God knows what intensity of ugliness his visage could attain), confessed himself conquered: We will do the same. We shall not try to give the reader an idea of that tetrahedral nose, that horseshoe mouth; that little left eye obstructed with a red, bushy, bristling eyebrow, while the right eye disappeared entirely beneath an enormous wart; of those teeth in disarray, broken here and there, like the embattled parapet of a fortress; of that callous lip, upon which one of these teeth encroached, like the tusk of an elephant; of that forked chin; and above all, of the expression spread over the whole; of that mixture of malice, amazement, and sadness. Let the reader dream of this whole, if he can.

The acclamation was unanimous; people rushed towards the chapel. They made the lucky Pope of the Fools come forth in triumph. But it was then that surprise and admiration attained their highest pitch; the grimace was his face.

Or rather, his whole person was a grimace. A huge head, bristling with red hair; between his shoulders an enormous hump, a counterpart perceptible in front; a system of thighs and legs so strangely astray that they could touch each other only at the knees, and, viewed

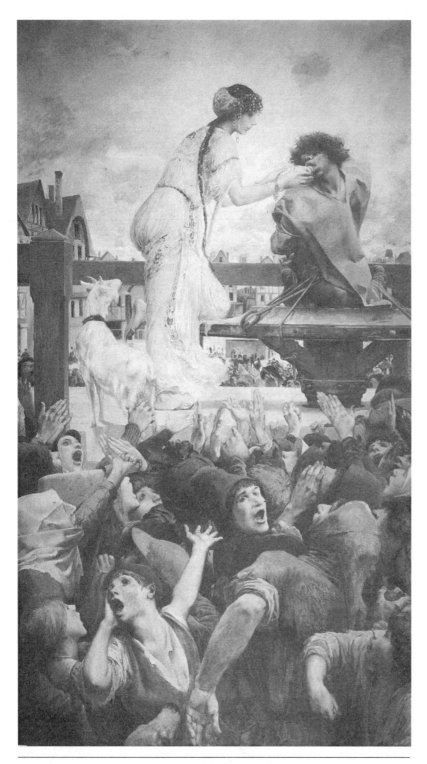

Illustration for The Hunchback of Notre Dame: *"Esmeralda Feeds Quasimodo," by Luc Olivier Merson (1846–1920). As the disabled Quasimodo is exhibited for public ridicule, the female protagonist, Esmeralda, experiences a moment of empathy and provides relief for his dehydration. The scene recalls the biblical passage when Christ is offered water while carrying his cross. This also recalls the common practice of the public display of people with disabilities for profit. While cultivating sympathy for rejected bodies, Hugo leaves them largely outside of the sphere of meaningful human relationships.*

Source: Art Resource, New York.

from the front, resembled the crescents of two scythes joined by the handles; large feet, monstrous hands; and, with all this deformity, an indescribable and redoubtable air of vigor, agility, and courage,—strange exception to the eternal rule which wills that force as well as beauty shall be the result of harmony. Such was the pope whom the fools had just chosen for themselves.

One would have pronounced him a giant who had been broken and badly put together again.

When this species of cyclops appeared on the threshold of the chapel, motionless, squat, and almost as broad as he was tall; squared on the base, as a great man says; with his doublet half red, half violet, sown with silver bells, and, above all, in the perfection of his ugliness, the populace recognized him on the instant, and shouted with one voice,—

"'Tis Quasimodo, the bellringer! 'tis Quasimodo, the hunchback of Notre-Dame! Quasimodo, the one-eyed! Quasimodo, the bandy-legged! Noel! Noel!"

It will be seen that the poor fellow had a choice of surnames.

"Let the women with child beware!" shouted the scholars.

"Or those who wish to be," resumed Joannes.

The women did, in fact, hide their faces.

"Oh! the horrible monkey!" said one of them.

"As wicked as he is ugly," retorted another.

"He's the devil," added a third.

"I have the misfortune to live near Notre-Dame; I hear him prowling round the eaves by night."

"With the cats."

"He's always on our roofs."

"He throws spells down our chimneys."

"The other evening, he came and made a grimace at me through my attic window. I thought that it was a man. Such a fright as I had!"

"I'm sure that he goes to the witches' sabbath. Once he left a broom on my leads."

"Oh! what a displeasing hunchback's face!"

"Oh! what an ill-favored soul!"

"Whew!"

The men, on the contrary, were delighted and applauded. Quasimodo, the object of the tumult, still stood on the threshold of the chapel, sombre and grave, and allowed them to admire him.

One scholar (Robin Poussepain, I think), came and laughed in his face, and too close. Quasimodo contented himself with taking him by the girdle, and hurling him ten paces off amid the crowd; all without uttering a word.

Master Coppenole, in amazement, approached him.

"Cross of God! Holy Father! you possess the handsomest ugliness that I have ever beheld in my life. You would deserve to be pope at Rome, as well as at Paris."

So saying, he placed his hand gayly on his shoulder. Quasimodo did not stir.

Coppenole went on,—"You are a rogue with whom I have a fancy for carousing, were it to cost me a new dozen of twelve livres of Tours. How does it strike you?"

Quasimodo made no reply.

"Cross of God!" said the hosier, "are you deaf?"

He was, in truth, deaf.

Nevertheless, he began to grow impatient with Coppenole's behavior, and suddenly turned towards him with so formidable a gnashing of teeth, that the Flemish giant recoiled, like a bull-dog before a cat.

Then there was created around that strange personage, a circle of terror and respect, whose radius was at least fifteen geometrical feet. An old woman explained to Coppenole that Quasimodo was deaf.

"Deaf!" said the hosier, with his great Flemish laugh. "Cross of God! He's a perfect pope!"

"He! I recognize him," exclaimed Jehan, who had, at last, descended from his capital, in order to see Quasimodo at closer quarters, "he's the bellringer of my brother, the archdeacon. Good-day, Quasimodo!"

"What a devil of a man!" said Robin Poussepain still all bruised with his fall. "He shows himself; he's a hunchback. He walks; he's bandy-legged. He looks at you; he's one-eyed. You speak to him; he's deaf. And what does this Polyphemus do with his tongue?"

"He speaks when he chooses," said the old woman; "he became deaf through ringing the bells. He is not dumb."

"That he lacks," remarks Jehan.

"And he has one eye too many," added Robin Poussepain.

"Not at all," said Jehan wisely. "A one-eyed man is far less complete than a blind man. He knows what he lacks."

In the meantime, all the beggars, all the lackeys, all the cutpurses, joined with the scholars, had gone in procession to seek, in the cupboard of the law clerks' company, the cardboard tiara, and the derisive robe of the Pope of the Fools. Quasimodo allowed them to array him in them without wincing, and with a sort of proud docility. Then they made him seat himself on a motley litter. Twelve officers of the fraternity of fools raised him on their shoulders; and a sort of bitter and disdainful joy lighted up the morose face of the cyclops, when he beheld beneath his deformed feet all those heads of handsome, straight, well-made men. Then the ragged and howling procession set out on its march, according to custom, around the inner galleries of the Courts, before making the circuit of the streets and squares.

Source: Hugo, Victor. 1831. *The Hunchback of Notre Dame.* Available at: http://www.online-literature.com/victor_hugo/hunchback_notre_dame/

▣ Comments on Lord Byron's Medical Care (19th c.)

This excerpt from Abt's work, which includes important quotations from Jeaffreson's biography of Lord Byron, inveighs against the "carelessness" with which disabled children were treated in Byron's time, arguing that Byron could have lived a long and healthy life if ignorant doctors had not interfered with his condition. Most contemporary biographers now refer to Byron's impairment as Little's disease (an early designation for cerebral palsy).

The world has undoubtedly suffered greatly from this carelessness [for the welfare of disabled children]. Hundreds, who might otherwise have contributed to the beauty of civilization, or have led their fellow men to new accomplishments, have been deprived of their birthright. In the past, only the wealthy cripples have had any opportunity for education. And even they have been handicapped by lack of orthopedic knowledge on the part of the medical profession. It is commonly believed that Lord Byron had a clubfoot. As a matter of fact, the great poet might have lived to an advanced age and produced volumes of additional poetry, had he not received the attention of a "quack doctor." As a young boy, Byron was afflicted with "lameness due to a contraction of the tendon Achilles which compelled him to walk on the balls and toes of his feet. The foot (later) was considerably distorted so as to turn inward, a malformation which may have been caused altogether by the violence with which it was treated." "The lad at Nottingham suffered much at the hands of a bone setter, Lavenden. . . . Blind to the nature of the case, the man did precisely as any other pretender of his kind would have done. . . . He rubbed the foot with oil, twisted it about with violence screwing and torturing bone and muscle into better behavior." In the opinion of medical men, had Byron been given the proper care, his deformity might have been entirely cured. As walking was always painful for him because of his obesity, he continually dieted. The dieting reduced his resistance, which, had it been stronger, might have successfully combated the fever which carried him away on the battle fields of Greece at the age of thirty-six years. Thus was the world deprived of one great man through carelessness.

Sources: Abt, Henry Edward. 1924. *The Care, Cure, and Education of the Crippled Child.* International Society for Crippled Children. Available at: http://www.disabilitymuseum.org/lib/docs/1449.htm

Jeaffreson, John Cordy. 1833. Vol. 1 of *The Real Lord Byron: New Views of the Poet's Life.* London: Hurst and Blackett.

▣ Harriet Martineau, from *Society in America* (1837)

Asylum tourism was popular with both domestic and foreign travelers in antebellum America. Harriet Martineau, a deaf English writer, visited the United States and wrote of her experiences. Her report on the American means of treating people with various disabilities is found in the context of descriptions of American prisons, poor relief, temperance, abolition, and other varied and energetic approaches to dependency and reform.

The idea of travelling in America was first suggested to me by a philanthropist's saying to me, "Whatever else may be true about the Americans, it is certain that they have got at principles of justice and mercy in the treatment of the least happy classes of society which we may be glad to learn from them. I wish you would go and see what they are." I did so; and the results of my investigation have not been reserved for this short chapter, but are spread over the whole of my book. The fundamental democratic principles on which American society is organised, are those "principles of justice and mercy" by which the guilty, the ignorant, the needy, and the infirm, are saved and blessed. The charity of a democratic society is heart-reviving to witness; for there is a security that no wholesale oppression is bearing down the million in one direction, while charity is lifting up, the hundred in another. Generally speaking, the misery that is seen is all that exists: there is no paralysing sense of the hopelessness of setting up individual benevolence against social injustice. If the community has not yet arrived at the point at which all communities are destined to arrive, of perceiving guilt to be infirmity, of obviating punishment, ignorance, and want, still the Americans are more blessed than others, in the certainty that they have far less superinduced misery than societies abroad, and are using wiser methods than others for its alleviation. In a country where social equality is the great principle in which all acquiesce, and where, consequently, the golden rule is suggested by every collision between man and man, neglect of misery is almost as much out of the question as the oppression from which most misery springs. . . .

The pauperism of the United States is, to the observation of a stranger, nothing at all. To residents, it is an occasion for the exercise of their ever-ready charity. It is confined to the ports, emigrants making their way back into the country, the families of intemperate or disabled men; and unconnected women, who depend on their own exertions. The amount altogether is far from commensurate with the charity of the community; and it is to be hoped that the curse of a legal charity, at least to the able-bodied, will be avoided in a country where it certainly cannot become necessary within any assignable time. I was grieved to see the magnificent pauper asylum near Philadelphia, made to accommodate luxuriously 1200 persons; and to have its arrangements pointed out to me, as yielding far more comfort to the inmates than the labourer can secure at home by any degree of industry and prudence. There are so many persons in the city, however, who see the badness of the principle, and regret the erection, that I trust a watch will be maintained over the establishment, and its corridors kept as empty as possible. In Boston, the principles of true charity have been better acted upon. There, many of the clergymen,—among the rest, Father Taylor, the seaman's friend,—are in possession of wisdom, derived from the mournful experience of England; and seem likely to save the city from the misery of a debasing pauperism among any class of its inhabitants. I know no large city where there is so much mutual helpfulness, so little neglect and ignorance of the concerns of other classes, as in Boston: and I cannot but anticipate that from thence the world may derive the brightest lesson that has yet been offered it, in the duties of the rich towards the poor. If the agents of the benevolence of the wealthy will but be scrupulously careful to avoid all that mental encroachment and moral interference, which have but too generally ruined the efficacy of charity, and go on to exhibit the devotion of the philanthropist, without the inquisitiveness and authoritativeness of the priest, they may deserve the thanks of the whole of society, as well as the attachment of those whom they befriend.

In Boston, an excellent plan has been adopted for the prevention of fraud on the part of paupers, and the mutual enlightenment and guidance of the agents of charity. A weekly meeting is held of delegates, from all societies engaged in the relief of the poor. The delegates compare lists of the persons relieved, so as to ascertain that none are fraudulently receiving from more than one society: they discuss and investigate doubtful cases; extend indulgence to those of peculiar hardship; and, in short, secure all the advantages of co-operation. Perhaps there are no cities in England but London too large for a somewhat similar organisation: and its adoption would be an act of great wisdom.

In the south, I was rather amused at a boast which was made to me of the small amount of pauperism. As the plague distances all lesser diseases, so does slavery obviate pauperism. In a society of two classes, where the one class are all capitalists, and the other property, there can be no pauperism but through the vice or accidental disability of members of the first. But I was beset by many an anxious thought about the fate of disabled slaves. Masters are, of course, bound to take care of their slaves for life. There are doubtless many masters who guard the comfort of their helpless negroes all the more carefully from the sense of the

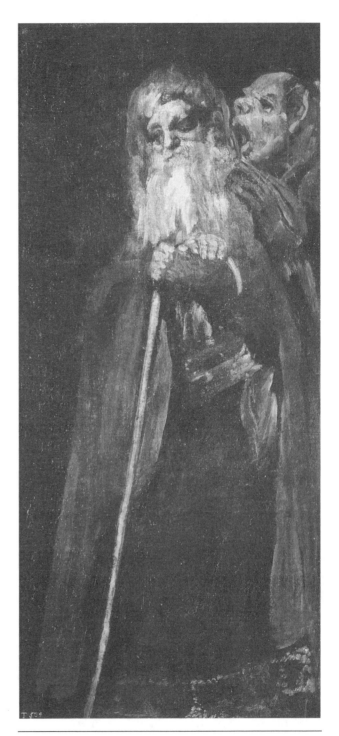

From the Black Paintings, by Francisco de Goya (1746–1828). In this work, one monk, deaf, listens to the other, who shout in the deaf monk's ear. This work, from Goya's Black Paintings series, was created on the wall of his house, the Quinta del Sordo. The Black Paintings were all made during the latter part of the artist's life. Goya experienced deafness as he grew older, and this work depicts his feelings of alienation from the hearing world by having those in the background yelling into the ears of the caped figure with a walking stick in the foreground.

Source: Art Resource, New York.

entire dependence of the poor creatures upon their mercy: but, there are few human beings fit to be trusted with absolute power: and while there are many who abuse the authority they have over slaves who are not helpless, it is fearful to think what may be the fate of those who are purely burdensome. I observed, here and there, an idiot slave. Those whom I saw were kindly treated, humoured, and indulged. These were the only cases of natural infirmity that I witnessed among the negroes; and the absence of others struck me. At Columbia, South Carolina, I was taken by a benevolent physician to see the State Lunatic Asylum, which might be considered his work; so diligent had he been in obtaining appropriations for the object from the legislature, and afterwards in organising its plans, with great wisdom and humanity. When we were looking out from the top of this building, watching the patients in their airing grounds, I observed that no people of colour were visible in any part of the establishment. I inquired whether negroes were as subject to insanity as whites. Probably; but no means were known to have been taken to ascertain the fact. From the violence of their passions, there could be no doubt that insanity must exist among them. Were such insane negroes ever seen?—No one present had ever seen any.—Where were they then?—It was some time before I could get a clear answer to this: but my friend the physician said, at length, that he had no doubt they were kept in out-houses, chained to logs, to prevent their doing harm. No member of society is charged with the duty of investigating cases of disease and suffering among slaves who cannot make their own state known. They are wholly at the mercy of their owners. The physician told me that it was his intension, now he had accomplished his object of establishing a lunatic asylum for the whites, to persevere no less strenuously till he obtained one for the blacks. He will probably not find this a very difficult object to effect; for the interest of masters, as well as their humanity, is concerned in having an asylum provided by the State for the useless or mischievous negroes.

The Lunatic Asylums of the United States [are] an honour to the country, to judge by those which I saw. The insane in Pennsylvania hospital, Philadelphia, should be removed to some more light and cheerful abode, and be much more fully supplied with employment, and with stimulus to engage in it. I was less pleased with their conditions than with that of any other insane patients whom I saw. The institution at Worcester, Massachusetts, is admirably managed under Dr. Woodward. So was that at Charlestown, near Boston, by Dr. Lee; a young physician who has since died, mourned by his grateful patients, and by all who had their welfare at heart. The establishment at Bloomingdale; near New York, is of similar excellence. The only great deficiency that I am aware of is one which belongs to most lunatic asylums, and which it does not rest with the superintendent to supply;—a want of sufficient employment. Every exertion is made to provide a variety of amusements, and to encourage all little undertakings that may be suggested: but regular, important business is what is wanted. It is to be hoped that in the establishment of all such institutions, the provision of an ample quantity of land will be one of the prime considerations. Watchful and ingenious kindness may do much to alleviate the miseries of the insane; but if cure is sought, I believe it is agreed by those who know best that regular employment, with a reasonable object, is indispensable.

The Asylum for the Blind at Philadelphia was a young institution at the time I saw it; but it pleased me more than any I ever visited: more than the larger one at Boston; whose institution and conduct are, however, honourable to all concerned in it. The reason of my preference of the Philadelphia one is that the pupils there were more active and cheerful than those of Boston. The spirits of the inmates are the one infallible test of the management of an institution for the blind. The fault of such in general is that mirth is not sufficiently cultivated, and religion too exclusively so. It should ever be remembered that religion comes out of the mind, and not in at the eye or ear; and that the truest way of cultivating religion is to exercise the faculties, and enlarge the stock of ideas to the utmost. The method of printing for the blind, introduced with such admirable ingenuity and success into the American institutions, I should like to see employed to bring within the reach of the blind the most amusing works that can be found. I should like to see it made an object with benevolent persons to go and give the pupils a hearty laugh occasionally, by reading droll books, and telling amusing stories. The one thing which the born blind want most is to have their cheerlessness removed, to be drawn out of their abstractions, and exercised in play on the greatest possible variety of familiar objects and events. They should hear no condolence: their friends should keep their sympathetic sorrow to themselves; and explain, cheerfully and fully, the allusions to visual objects which must occur in all reading and conversation. It grieves me to hear the hymns and other compositions put into the mouths of blind pupils, all full of lamentation and resignation about not seeing the stars and the face of nature. Such sorrow is for those who see to feel on their behalf; or for those who have lost sight: not for those who never saw. Put into their mouths, it becomes cant. When a roving sea-captain tells his children of the glories of oriental scenery which they are destined never to behold, does he teach them to sigh, and struggle to submit patiently to their destiny of staying at home? Does he not rather make them take pleasure in mirthfully and eagerly learning what he can teach? The face of nature is a foreign land to the born blind. Let them be taught all that can possibly be conveyed to them, and in the most spirited manner that they can bear. There is a nearer approach to the realisation of this principle of teaching the blind in the Philadelphia house than I ever saw elsewhere. It would be enough to cheer a misanthrope to see a little German boy there, picked up out of the streets, dull, neglected, and depressed; but within a few months, standing in the centre of the group of musicians, fiddling and stamping time with all his might, and quite ready to obey every instigation to laugh. Mr. Friedlander, the tutor, is much to be congratulated on what he has already done.

It may be worth suggesting here that while some of the thinkers of America, like many of the same classes in England, are mourning over the low state of the Philosophy of Mind in their country, society is neglecting a most important means of obtaining the knowledge requisite for the acquisition of such philosophy. Scholars are embracing alternately the systems of Kant, of Fichte, of Spurzheim, of the Scotch school; or abusing or eulogising Locke, asking who Hartley was, or weaving a rainbow arch of transcendentalism, which is to comprehend the whole that lies within human vision, but sadly liable to be puffed away in dark vapour with the first breeze of reality; scholars are thus labouring at a system of mental philosophy on any but the experimental method, while the materials for experiment lie all around and within them. If they object, as is common, the difficulty of experimenting on their conscious selves, there is the mental pathology of their blind schools, and the asylums for the deaf and dumb. I am aware that they put away the phenomena of insanity as irrelevant; but the same objections do not pertain to the other two classes. Let the closet speculations be pursued with all

vigour; but if there were joined with these a close and unwearied study of the phenomena of the minds of persons deficient in a sense, and especially of those precluded from the full use of language, the world might fairly look for an advance in the science of Mind equal to that which medical science owes to pathology. It will not probably lodge us in any final and total result, any more than medicine and anatomy promise to ascertain the vital principle: but it will doubtless yield us some points of certainty, in aid of the fluctuating speculations amidst which we are now tossed, while few can be found to agree even upon matters of so-called universal consciousness. I should like to see a few philosophers interested in ascertaining and recording the manifestations of some progressive minds, peculiar from infirmity, for a series of years. If any such in America, worthy to undertake the task, from having strength enough to put away theory and prejudice, and record only what is really manifested to them, should be disposed to take my hint, I hope they will not wait for a philosophical "class to fall into."

Source: Martineau, Harriet. 1837. Chapter 4, "Sufferers," in *Society in America*. Available at: http://www2.pfeiffer.edu/~lridener/DSS/Martineau/v3p3c4.html

▣ English Poor Law Amendment (1841)

This nineteenth-century amendment act introduced significant changes in the policy management of poor and disabled people in England. It sought to narrow eligibility requirements for workhouses in order to make that institution less preferable than even jobs garnering the lowest paid wages. Further, the policy prohibited outdoor relief (support for those living in the community) and mandated public support in workhouse settings alone.

The superiority of the condition of the pauper . . . as regards medical aid will, on the one hand, encourage a resort to the poor rates for medical relief, so far as it is given out of the workhouse, and will thus tempt the industrious labourer into pauperism; and on the other hand, it will discourage sick clubs and friendly societies and other similar institutions, which are not only valuable in reference to the contingencies against which they provide, but as creating and fostering a spirit of frugality and forethought amongst the labouring classes.

Source: English Poor Law Commission. 1841. [Amendment to *An Act for the Amendment and Better Administration of the Laws Relating to the Poor in England and Wales.* 4 & 5 Will. IV cap. 76.]

William Dodd, from *A Narrative of William Dodd: Factory Cripple* (1841)

William Dodd began working in an English textile factory at the age of five, working up to 18 hours a day at times. Within a few years, the work had rendered him severely disabled. He continued to work in the textile factories but was able to learn to read and write by attending school at night, which enabled him to leave factory work. Eventually, Lord Ashley, a member of parliament interested in protecting child laborers, commissioned him to write of his experiences. With Lord Ashley's support, Dodd was able to publish a number of books. His descriptions of the experiences of child laborers were so compelling that reform opponents in the House of Commons launched attacks on his character and credibility (a brief excerpt from a speech attacking Dodd is included after the excerpts from Dodd's book). Dodd eventually decided to move to the United States, where he continued to write against the child labor system.

At the age of six I became a piecer. The duties of the piecer will not be clearly understood by the reader, unless he is acquainted with the machine for spinning woollen yarn, called a billy. A billy is a machine somewhat similar in form to the letter H, one side being stationary, and the other moveable, and capable of being pushed close in under the stationary part, almost like the drawer of a side table; the moveable part, or carriage, runs backwards and forwards, by means of six iron wheels, upon three iron rails, as a carriage on a railroad. In this carriage are the spindles, from 70 to 100 in number, all turned by one wheel, which is in the care of the spinner. When the spinner brings the carriage close up under the fixed part of the machine, he is able, to obtain a certain length of carding for each spindle, say 10 or 12 inches, which he draws back, and spins into yarn; this done, he winds the yarn round the spindles, brings the carriage close up as before, and again obtains a fresh supply of cardings.

These cardings are taken up by the piecer in the left hand, about twenty at a time. He holds them about four inches from one end, the other end hanging down; these he takes, with the right hand, one at a time, for the purpose of piecing, and laying the ends of the cardings about 2 inches over each other, he rubs them together on the canvas cloth with his flat hand. He is obliged to be very expert, in order to keep the spinner well supplied. A good piecer will supply from 30 to 40 spindles with cardings.

The number of cardings a piecer has through his fingers in a day is very great; each piecing requires three or four rubs, over a space of three or four inches; and the continual friction of the hand in rubbing the piecing upon the coarse wrapper wears off the skin, and causes the finger to bleed. The position in which the piecer stands to his work is with the right foot forward, and his right side facing the frame: the motion he makes in going along in front of the frame, for the purpose of piecing, is neither forwards or backwards, but in a sliding direction, constantly keeping his right side towards the frame. In this position he continues during the day, with his hands, feet, and eyes constantly in motion. It will be easily seen, that the chief weight of his body rests upon his right knee, which is almost always the first joint to give way.

I have frequently worked at the frame till I could scarcely get home, and in this state have been stopped by people in the streets who noticed me shuffling along, and advised me to work no more in the factories; but I was not my own master. During the day, I frequently counted the clock, and calculated how many hours I had still to remain at work; my evenings were spent in preparing for the following day—in rubbing my knees, ankles, elbows, and wrists with oil, etc. I went to bed, to cry myself to sleep, and pray that the Lord would take me to himself before morning. . . .

My legs became distorted. Standing in the easiest position, when the feet are about 14 inches apart, the knees and thighs are then pressing close together, so that the legs form a sort of arch for the support of the body. One evil arising from the bending and curving of the legs is the blood-vessels must go wrong. One serious evil resulting from the imperfect circulation of the blood, is the drying up of the marrow in the bones. The bones then decay.

In the spring of 1840, I began to feel some painful symptoms in my right wrist, arising from the general weakness of my joints, brought on in the factories. The swelling and pain increased; and although I had the advice of medical practitioners, it was all to no purpose; and, having been off work for a length of time, and my resources failing, I was under the necessity of entering St. Thomas's Hospital where every care and attention was paid to me. It soon became evident to all who saw me, that I must, very soon, lose either my hand or my life. A consultation was held by the surgeons of the hospital, who came to the conclusion, that amputation was absolutely necessary. On the 18th of July, I underwent the operation. The hand being taken off a little below the elbow. Thus, another plan to raise myself above want, and keep myself out of the workhouse, was frustrated and dashed.

John Bright's Speech in the House of Commons (March 1844)

I have in my hand two publications; one is *The Adventures of William Dodd the Factory Cripple* and the other is entitled *The Factory System*—both books have gone forth to the public under the sanction of the noble Lord Ashley. I do not wish to go into the particulars of the character of this man, for it is not necessary to my case, but I can demonstrate, that his books and statements are wholly unworthy of credit. Dodd states that from the hardships he endured in a factory, he was "done up" at the age of thirty-two, whereas I can prove that he was treated with uniform kindness, which he repaid by gross immorality of conduct, and for which he was discharged from his employment.

Source: Dodd, William. 1841. *A Narrative of William Dodd: Factory Cripple,* 2nd ed. London: L & G Seeley.

Charles Dickens, from *A Christmas Carol* (1843)

With the aid of the Spirit of Christmas Present, Scrooge witnesses the family life of the impoverished Cratchits, at the heart of which is their son, Tiny Tim. Dickens focuses all emotions on the disabled but angelic child, with the moral measure of the other characters being taken by the degree of their sympathy for him.

Then up rose Mrs. Cratchit, Cratchit's wife, dressed out but poorly in a twice-turned gown, but brave in ribbons, which are cheap and make a goodly show for sixpence; and she laid the cloth, assisted by Belinda

Cratchit, second of her daughters, also brave in ribbons; while Master Peter Cratchit plunged a fork into the saucepan of potatoes, and getting the corners of his monstrous shirt-collar (Bob's private property, conferred upon his son and heir in honour of the day) into his mouth, rejoiced to find himself so gallantly attired, and yearned to show his linen in the fashionable Parks. And now two smaller Cratchits, boy and girl, came tearing in, screaming that outside the baker's they had smelt the goose, and known it for their own; and basking in luxurious thoughts of sage-and-onion, these young Cratchits danced about the table, and exalted Master Peter Cratchit to the skies, while he (not proud, although his collars nearly choked him) blew the fire, until the slow potatoes bubbling up, knocked loudly at the saucepan-lid to be let out and peeled.

"What has ever got your precious father then," said Mrs. Cratchit. "And your brother, Tiny Tim; and Martha warn't as late last Christmas Day by half-an-hour!"

"Here's Martha, mother!" said a girl, appearing as she spoke.

"Here's Martha, mother!" cried the two young Cratchits. "Hurrah! There's such a goose, Martha!"

"Why, bless your heart alive, my dear, how late you are!" said Mrs. Cratchit, kissing her a dozen times, and taking off her shawl and bonnet for her, with officious zeal.

"We'd a deal of work to finish up last night," replied the girl, "and had to clear away this morning, mother!"

"Well! Never mind so long as you are come," said Mrs. Cratchit. "Sit ye down before the fire, my dear, and have a warm, Lord bless ye!"

"No no! There's father coming," cried the two young Cratchits, who were everywhere at once. "Hide Martha, hide!"

So Martha hid herself, and in came little Bob, the father, with at least three feet of comforter exclusive of the fringe, hanging down before him; and his thread-bare clothes darned up and brushed, to look seasonable; and Tiny Tim upon his shoulder. Alas for Tiny Tim, he bore a little crutch, and had his limbs supported by an iron frame!

"Why, where's our Martha?" cried Bob Cratchit looking round.

"Not coming," said Mrs. Cratchit.

"Not coming!" said Bob, with a sudden declension in his high spirits; for he had been Tim's blood horse all the way from church, and had come home rampant. "Not coming upon Christmas Day!"

Martha didn't like to see him disappointed, if it were only in joke; so she came out prematurely from behind the closet door, and ran into his arms, while the two young Cratchits hustled Tiny Tim, and bore him off into the wash-house, that he might hear the pudding singing in the copper.

"And how did little Tim behave?" asked Mrs. Cratchit, when she had rallied Bob on his credulity and Bob had hugged his daughter to his heart's content.

"As good as gold," said Bob, "and better. Somehow he gets thoughtful sitting by himself so much, and thinks the strangest things you ever heard. He told me, coming home, that he hoped the people saw him in the church, because he was a cripple, and it might be pleasant to them to remember upon Christmas Day, who made lame beggars walk and blind men see."

Bob's voice was tremulous when he told them this, and trembled more when he said that Tiny Tim was growing strong and hearty.

His active little crutch was heard upon the floor, and back came Tiny Tim before another word was spoken, escorted by his brother and sister to his stool beside the fire; and while Bob, turning up his cuffs—as if, poor fellow, they were capable of being made more shabby—compounded some hot mixture in a jug with gin and lemons, and stirred it round and round and put it on the hob to simmer; Master Peter and the two ubiquitous young Cratchits went to fetch the goose, with which they soon returned in high procession.

Such a bustle ensued that you might have thought a goose the rarest of all birds; a feathered phenomenon, to which a black swan was a matter of course: and in truth it was something very like it in that house. Mrs. Cratchit made the gravy (ready beforehand in a little saucepan) hissing hot; Master Peter mashed the potatoes with incredible vigour; Miss Belinda sweetened up the apple-sauce; Martha dusted the hot plates; Bob took Tiny Tim beside him in a tiny corner at the table; the two young Cratchits set chairs for everybody, not forgetting themselves, and mounting guard upon their posts, crammed spoons into their mouths, lest they should shriek for goose before their turn came to be helped. At last the dishes were set on, and grace was said. It was succeeded by a breathless pause, as Mrs. Cratchit, looking slowly all along the carving-knife, prepared to plunge it in the breast; but when she did, and when the long expected gush of stuffing issued forth, one murmur of delight arose all round the board, and even Tiny Tim, excited by the two young Cratchits, beat on the table with the handle of his knife, and feebly cried Hurrah!

There never was such a goose. Bob said he didn't believe there ever was such a goose cooked. Its tenderness and flavour, size and cheapness, were the themes of universal admiration. Eked out by the apple-sauce and mashed potatoes, it was a sufficient dinner for the whole family; indeed, as Mrs. Cratchit said with great delight (surveying one small atom of a bone upon the dish), they hadn't ate it all at last! Yet every one had had enough, and the youngest Cratchits in particular, were steeped in sage and onion to the eyebrows! But now, the plates being changed by Miss Belinda, Mrs. Cratchit left the room alone—too nervous to bear witnesses—to take the pudding up, and bring it in.

Suppose it should not be done enough! Suppose it should break in turning out! Suppose somebody should have got over the wall of the back-yard, and stolen it, while they were merry with the goose: a supposition at which the two young Cratchits became livid! All sorts of horrors were supposed.

Hallo! A great deal of steam! The pudding was out of the copper. A smell like a washing-day! That was the cloth. A smell like an eating-house, and a pastry cook's next door to each other, with a laundress's next door to that! That was the pudding. In half a minute Mrs. Cratchit entered: flushed, but smiling proudly: with the pudding, like a speckled cannon-ball, so hard and firm, blazing in half of half-a-quartern of ignited brandy, and bedight with Christmas holly stuck into the top.

Oh, a wonderful pudding! Bob Cratchit said, and calmly too, that he regarded it as the greatest success achieved by Mrs. Cratchit since their marriage. Mrs. Cratchit said that now the weight was off her mind, she would confess she had had her doubts about the quantity of flour. Everybody had something to say about it, but nobody said or thought it was at all a small pudding for a large family. It would have been flat heresy to do so. Any Cratchit would have blushed to hint at such a thing.

At last the dinner was all done, the cloth was cleared, the hearth swept, and the fire made up. The compound in the jug being tasted and considered perfect, apples and oranges were put upon the table, and a shovel-full of chesnuts on the fire. Then all the Cratchit family drew round the hearth, in what Bob Cratchit called a circle, meaning half a one; and at Bob

Cratchit's elbow stood the family display of glass; two tumblers, and a custard-cup without a handle.

These held the hot stuff from the jug, however, as well as golden goblets would have done; and Bob served it out with beaming looks, while the chesnuts on the fire sputtered and crackled noisily. Then Bob proposed:

"A Merry Christmas to us all, my dears. God bless us!"

Which all the family re-echoed.

"God bless us every one!" said Tiny Tim, the last of all.

He sat very close to his father's side, upon his little stool. Bob held his withered little hand in his, as if he loved the child, and wished to keep him by his side, and dreaded that he might be taken from him.

"Spirit," said Scrooge, with an interest he had never felt before, "tell me if Tiny Tim will live."

"I see a vacant seat," replied the Ghost, "in the poor chimney corner, and a crutch without an owner, carefully preserved. If these shadows remain unaltered by the Future, the child will die."

"No, no," said Scrooge. "Oh no, kind Spirit! say he will be spared."

"If these shadows remain unaltered by the Future, none other of my race," returned the Ghost, "will find him here. What then? If he be like to die, he had better do it, and decrease the surplus population."

Scrooge hung his head to hear his own words quoted by the Spirit, and was overcome with penitence and grief.

"Man," said the Ghost, "if man you be in heart, not adamant, forbear that wicked cant until you have discovered What the surplus is, and Where it is. Will you decide what men shall live, what men shall die? It may be, that in the sight of Heaven, you are more worthless and less fit to live than millions like this poor man's child. Oh God! to hear the Insect on the leaf pronouncing on the too much life among his hungry brothers in the dust!"

Scrooge bent before the Ghost's rebuke, and trembling cast his eyes upon the ground. But he raised them speedily, on hearing his own name.

"Mr. Scrooge!" said Bob; "I'll give you Mr. Scrooge, the Founder of the Feast!"

"The Founder of the Feast indeed!" cried Mrs. Cratchit, reddening. "I wish I had him here. I'd give him a piece of my mind to feast upon, and I hope he'd have a good appetite for it."

"My dear," said Bob, "the children; Christmas Day."

"It should be Christmas Day, I am sure," said she, "on which one drinks the health of such an odious, stingy, hard, unfeeling man as Mr. Scrooge. You know he is, Robert! Nobody knows it better than you do, poor fellow!"

"My dear," was Bob's mild answer, "Christmas Day."

"I'll drink his health for your sake and the Day's," said Mrs. Cratchit, "not for his. Long life to him! A merry Christmas and a happy new year!—he'll be very merry and very happy, I have no doubt!"

The children drank the toast after her. It was the first of their proceedings which had no heartiness in it. Tiny Tim drank it last of all, but he didn't care twopence for it. Scrooge was the Ogre of the family. The mention of his name cast a dark shadow on the party, which was not dispelled for full five minutes.

Source: Dickens, Charles. 1843. *A Christmas Carol*. Available at: http://www.literature.org/authors/dickens-charles/christmas-carol/index.html

▣ Nathaniel Hawthorne, from "The Birthmark" (1846)

Georgiana is beautiful but flawed by a small, hand-shaped birthmark on her face. Her scientist husband, Aylmer, wants to make her perfect at any cost. Hawthorne's story asks readers to contemplate whether we need to be perfect to be loved and whether our flaws are an essential part of who we are. The excerpt here begins with Aylmer's presentation of the potion he has created to erase Georgina's birthmark.

"Drink, then, thou lofty creature!" exclaimed Aylmer, with fervid admiration. "There is no taint of imperfection on thy spirit. Thy sensible frame, too, shall soon be all perfect!"

She quaffed the liquid, and returned the goblet to his hand.

"It is grateful," said she, with a placid smile. "Methinks it is like water from a heavenly fountain; for it contains I know not what of unobtrusive fragrance and deliciousness. It allays a feverish thirst, that had parched me for many days. Now, dearest, let me sleep. My earthly senses are closing over my spirit, like the leaves around the heart of a rose, at sunset."

She spoke the last words with a gentle reluctance, as if it required almost more energy than she could command to pronounce the faint and lingering syllables. Scarcely had they loitered through her lips, ere she was lost in slumber. Aylmer sat by her side, watching her aspect with the emotions proper to a man, the whole value of whose existence was involved in the process now to be tested. Mingled with this mood, however, was the philosophic investigation, characteristic of the man of science. Not the minutest symptom escaped him. A heightened flush of the cheek—a slight irregularity of breath—a quiver of the eyelid—a hardly perceptible tremor through the frame—such were the details which, as the moments passed, he wrote down in his folio volume. Intense thought had set its stamp upon every previous page of that volume; but the thoughts of years were all concentrated upon the last.

While thus employed, he failed not to gaze often at the fatal Hand, and not without a shudder. Yet once, by a strange and unaccountable impulse, he pressed it with his lips. His spirit recoiled, however, in the very act, and Georgiana, out of the midst of her deep sleep, moved uneasily and murmured, as if in remonstrance. Again, Aylmer resumed his watch. Nor was it without avail. The Crimson Hand, which at first had been strongly visible upon the marble paleness of Georgiana's cheek now grew more faintly outlined. She remained not less pale than ever; but the birthmark, with every breath that came and went, lost somewhat of its former distinctness. Its presence had been awful; its departure was more awful still. Watch the stain of the rainbow fading out of the sky; and you will know how that mysterious symbol passed away.

"By Heaven, it is well nigh gone!" said Aylmer to himself, in almost irrepressible ecstasy. "I can scarcely trace it now. Success! Success! And now it is like the faintest rose-color. The slightest flush of blood across her cheek would overcome it. But she is so pale!"

He drew aside the window-curtain, and suffered the light of natural day to fall into the room, and rest upon her cheek. At the same time, he heard a gross, hoarse chuckle, which he had long known as his servant Aminadab's expression of delight.

"Ah, clod! Ah, earthly mass!" cried Aylmer, laughing in a sort of frenzy. "You have served me well! Master and Spirit—Earth and Heaven—have both done their part in this! Laugh, thing of the senses! You have earned the right to laugh."

These exclamations broke Georgiana's sleep. She slowly unclosed her eyes, and gazed into the mirror, which her husband had arranged for that purpose. A faint smile flitted over her lips, when she recognized

how barely perceptible was now that Crimson Hand, which had once blazed forth with such disastrous brilliancy as to scare away all their happiness. But then her eyes sought Aylmer's face, with a trouble and anxiety that he could by no means account for.

"My poor Aylmer!" murmured she.

"Poor? Nay, richest! Happiest! Most favored!" exclaimed he. "My peerless bride, it is successful! You are perfect!"

"My poor Aylmer!" she repeated, with a more than human tenderness. "You have aimed loftily!—you have done nobly! Do not repent, that, with so high and pure a feeling, you have rejected the best the earth could offer. Aylmer—dearest Aylmer—I am dying!"

Alas, it was too true! The fatal Hand had grappled with the mystery of life, and was the bond by which an angelic spirit kept itself in union with a mortal frame. As the last crimson tint of the birth-mark—that sole token of human imperfection—faded from her cheek, the parting breath of the now perfect woman passed into the atmosphere, and her soul, lingering a moment near her husband, took its heavenward flight. Then a hoarse, chuckling laugh was heard again! Thus ever does the gross Fatality of Earth exult in its invariable triumph over the immortal essence, which, in this dim sphere of half-development, demands the completeness of a higher state. Yet, had Aylmer reached a profounder wisdom, he need not thus have flung away the happiness, which would have woven his mortal life of the self-same texture with the celestial. The momentary circumstance was too strong for him; he failed to look beyond the shadowy scope of Time, and living once for all in Eternity, to find the perfect Future in the present.

Source: Hawthorne, Nathaniel. 1937. "The Birthmark." Pearson, Norman Holmes, ed. *The Complete Novels and Selected Tales of Nathaniel Hawthorne.* New York: Random House. (Originally published 1846)

▣ Abraham Lincoln, "My Childhood's Home I See Again" (1846)

In this poem, Lincoln acknowledges his own struggle with severe depression and draws an analogy between his experience of emotional duress and that of a childhood friend, Matthew, who has now become a "madman." Following his imprisonment for threatening harm to his parents, Matthew expresses his isolation by howling, which solidifies the poet's identification with this outlaw figure.

My Childhood's Home I See Again

I

My childhood's home I see again,
And sadden with the view;
And still, as memory crowds my brain,
There's pleasure in it too.

O Memory! thou midway world
'Twixt earth and paradise,
Where things decayed and loved ones lost
In dreamy shadows rise,

And, freed from all that's earthly vile,
Seem hallowed, pure, and bright,
Like scenes in some enchanted isle
All bathed in liquid light.

As dusky mountains please the eye
When twilight chases day;
As bugle-tones that, passing by,
In distance die away;

As leaving some grand waterfall,
We, lingering, list its roar—
So memory will hallow all
We've known, but know no more.

Near twenty years have passed away
Since here I bid farewell
To woods and fields, and scenes of play,
And playmates loved so well.

Where many were, but few remain
Of old familiar things;
But seeing them, to mind again
The lost and absent brings.

The friends I left that parting day,
How changed, as time has sped!
Young childhood grown, strong manhood gray,
And half of all are dead.

I hear the loved survivors tell
How nought from death could save,
Till every sound appears a knell,
And every spot a grave.

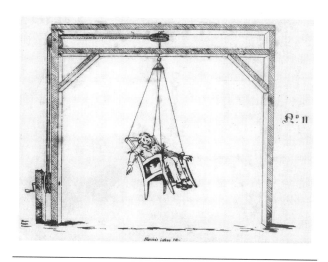

Rotary Machine for the Treatment of Moral Sufferers. This rotary machine was used in the early nineteenth century for the treatment of those diagnosed as emotionally unbalanced or insane.

Source: Art Resource, New York.

I range the fields with pensive tread,
And pace the hollow rooms,
And feel (companion of the dead)
I'm living in the tombs.

II

But here's an object more of dread
Than ought the grave contains—
A human form with reason fled,
While wretched life remains.

Poor Matthew! Once of genius bright,
A fortune-favored child—
Now locked for aye, in mental night,
A haggard mad-man wild.

Poor Matthew! I have ne'er forgot,
When first, with maddened will,
Yourself you maimed, your father fought,
And mother strove to kill;

When terror spread, and neighbors ran,
Your dange'rous strength to bind;
And soon, a howling crazy man
Your limbs were fast confined.

How then you strove and shrieked aloud,
Your bones and sinews bared;
And fiendish on the gazing crowd,
With burning eye-balls glared—

And begged, and swore, and wept and prayed
With maniac laughter joined—
How fearful were those signs displayed
By pangs that killed thy mind!

And when at length, tho' drear and long,
Time smoothed thy fiercer woes,
How plaintively thy mournful song
Upon the still night rose.

I've heard it oft, as if I dreamed,
Far distant, sweet, and lone—
The funeral dirge, it ever seemed
Of reason dead and gone.

To drink its strains, I've stole away,
All stealthily and still,
Ere yet the rising God of day
Had streaked the Eastern hill.

Air held his breath; trees, with the spell,
Seemed sorrowing angels round,
Whose swelling tears in dew-drops fell
Upon the listening ground.

But this is past; and nought remains,
That raised thee o'er the brute.
Thy piercing shrieks, and soothing strains,
Are like, forever mute.

Now fare thee well—more thou the cause,
Than subject now of woe.
All mental pangs, by time's kind laws,
Hast lost the power to know.

O death! Thou awe-inspiring prince,
That keepst the world in fear;
Why dost thou tear more blest ones hence,
And leave him ling'ring here?

Source: Lincoln, Abraham. 1953. "My Childhood's Home I See Again." Basler, Roy P., Marion Dolores Pratt, and Lloyd A. Dunlap, eds. *The Collected Works of Abraham Lincoln:* Vol. 1. New Brunswick, NJ: Rutgers University Press. (Originally written 1846)

▣ "Phrenology of Tom Thumb" (1846)

In keeping with the nineteenth century's penchant for medical curiosity closets and freak show exhibition as entertainment, the following excerpt discusses the phrenological examination of General Tom Thumb (phrenologists purported to be able to "read" a person's mental abilities and character by means of the shape of the skull). Tom Thumb, who was born Charles S. Stratton in 1838, became one of P. T. Barnum's main exhibits at the age of four and was named after a character in a Grimm's fairy tale "who was in all his limbs, but no longer than a thumb."

The head of General Tom Thumb has been examined by Mr. Straton, who reports of it that the size of the brain is the smallest recorded of one capable of sane and somewhat vigorous mental manifestation.

"As regards the balance of the different parts of the head, 'General Tom Thumb' is a very favorable specimen in most particulars. The anterior and coronal regions are slightly below an equal balance, the posterior is slightly above. Some of the individual organs present slight deviations from the equal balance. In the anterior region, individuality, form, size, weight, locality, and eventuality, especially the last, are the largest organs. Cautiousness is conspicuous in the lateral aspect. The cerebellum seems to be very small, as defective indeed as I have ever seen it in an infant of six months. In this particular the 'general' is a very remarkable case against the doctrine held by some, that the cerebellum is connected with the regulation of muscular action; for, if there be any one thing more than another, for which he can be said to be remarkable, apart from his diminutive size and fine proportions, it is his control over muscular action. In his representations of the Grecian statues, Napoleon, Frederick the Great, the English gentleman, the Highland chieftain, &c., the rapidity with which he can change his posture, and the accuracy with which he can imitate the actions and attitudes—so far as mere muscular action is concerned—of the objects represented, are regarded as very remarkable. His intellectual acquirements are said to be *very* limited as yet. It will be extremely important to note his progress in this particular. It is to be hoped that phrenologists who happen to meet with the 'general' will endeavor to inform themselves as *accurately* as possible regarding his progress and proficiency in intellectual pursuits, and report from time to time. His muscular system has attained a degree of firmness, strength, and maturity, quite equal to, or rather beyond, the average of his age. It is legitimate to presume that the brain is matured in a corresponding degree. His health is said to be excellent. 'General Tom Thumb' is, then, I repeat, a case of unusual interest to the phrenological world. He affords the extremely rare opportunity of solving one question in the great problem: What amount of manifestation is a well-balanced and healthy head of a given size capable of? The 'general' is certainly very near, if he does not actually touch, the extreme lowest point on the scale of size. What, then, is a head of 66 or a brain of 40 cubic inches capable of attaining in his circumstances!"—*Critic.*

Source: "Phrenology of Tom Thumb." 1846. *Littell's Living Age,* October 31. Available at: http://www.disabilitymuseum.org/lib/docs/2004.htm?page=print

▣ Charlotte Brontë, from *Jane Eyre* (1847)

In Brontë's novel, Jane Eyre and Edward Rochester are in love, but Rochester is not free to marry because he is already married to Bertha, a madwoman he keeps locked in the attic of his manor; upon learning of the situation, Jane leaves. In this excerpt from late in the novel, she is reunited with Rochester only to find that he has been blinded in the fire started by his suicidal wife. Now that Bertha is dead, Jane and Rochester may live together, but the impediment of madness has been replaced by that of blindness.

From Chapter 36

"Poor Mr. Edward!" he ejaculated, "I little thought ever to have seen it! Some say it was a just judgment on him for keeping his first marriage secret, and wanting to take another wife while he had one living: but I pity him, for my part."

"You said he was alive?" I exclaimed.

"Yes, yes: he is alive; but many think he had better be dead."

"Why? How?" My blood was again running cold. "Where is he?" I demanded. "Is he in England?"

"Ay—ay—he's in England; he can't get out of England, I fancy—he's a fixture now."

What agony was this! And the man seemed resolved to protract it.

"He is stone-blind," he said at last. "Yes, he is stone-blind, is Mr. Edward."

I had dreaded worse. I had dreaded he was mad. I summoned strength to ask what had caused this calamity.

"It was all his own courage, and a body may say, his kindness, in a way, ma'am: he wouldn't leave the house till every one else was out before him. As he came down the great staircase at last, after Mrs. Rochester had flung herself from the battlements, there was a great crash—all fell. He was taken out from under the ruins, alive, but sadly hurt: a beam had fallen in such a way as to protect him partly; but one eye was knocked out, and one hand so crushed that Mr. Carter, the surgeon, had to amputate it directly. The other eye inflamed: he lost the sight of that also. He is now helpless, indeed—blind and a cripple."

"Where is he? Where does he now live?"

"At Ferndean, a manor-house on a farm he has, about thirty miles off: quite a desolate spot."

"Who is with him?"

"Old John and his wife: he would have none else. He is quite broken down, they say."

"Have you any sort of conveyance?"

"We have a chaise, ma'am, a very handsome chaise."

"Let it be got ready instantly; and if your post-boy can drive me to Ferndean before dark this day, I'll pay both you and him twice the hire you usually demand."

From Chapter 37

The manor-house of Ferndean was a building of considerable antiquity, moderate size, and no architectural pretensions, deep buried in a wood. I had heard of it before. Mr. Rochester often spoke of it, and sometimes went there. His father had purchased the estate for the sake of the game covers. He would have let the house, but could find no tenant, in consequence of its ineligible and insalubrious site. Ferndean then remained uninhabited and unfurnished, with the exception of some two or three rooms fitted up for the accommodation of the squire when he went there in the season to shoot.

To this house I came just ere dark on an evening marked by the characteristics of sad sky, cold gale, and continued small penetrating rain. The last mile I performed on foot, having dismissed the chaise and driver with the double remuneration I had promised. Even when within a very short distance of the manor-house, you could see nothing of it, so thick and dark grew the timber of the gloomy wood about it. Iron gates between granite pillars showed me where to enter, and passing through them, I found myself at once in the twilight of close-ranked trees. There was a grass-grown track descending the forest aisle between hoar and knotty shafts and under branched arches. I followed it, expecting soon to reach the dwelling; but it stretched on and on, it wound far and farther: no sign of habitation or grounds was visible.

I thought I had taken a wrong direction and lost my way. The darkness of natural as well as of sylvan dusk gathered over me. I looked round in search of another road. There was none: all was interwoven stem, columnar trunk, dense summer foliage—no opening anywhere.

I proceeded: at last my way opened, the trees thinned a little; presently I beheld a railing, then the house—scarce, by this dim light, distinguishable from the trees; so dank and green were its decaying walls. Entering a portal, fastened only by a latch, I stood amidst a space of enclosed ground, from which the wood swept away in a semicircle. There were no flowers, no garden-beds; only a broad gravel-walk girdling a grass-plat, and this set in the heavy frame of the forest. The house presented two pointed gables in its front; the windows were latticed and narrow: the front door was narrow too, one step led up to it. The whole looked, as the host of the Rochester Arms had said, "quite a desolate spot." It was as still as a church on a week-day: the pattering rain on the forest leaves was the only sound audible in its vicinage.

"Can there be life here?" I asked.

Yes, life of some kind there was; for I heard a movement—that narrow front-door was unclosing, and some shape was about to issue from the grange.

It opened slowly: a figure came out into the twilight and stood on the step; a man without a hat: he stretched forth his hand as if to feel whether it rained. Dusk as it was, I had recognised him—it was my master, Edward Fairfax Rochester, and no other.

I stayed my step, almost my breath, and stood to watch him—to examine him, myself unseen, and alas! to him invisible. It was a sudden meeting, and one in which rapture was kept well in check by pain. I had no difficulty in restraining my voice from exclamation, my step from hasty advance.

His form was of the same strong and stalwart contour as ever: his port was still erect, his hair was still raven black; nor were his features altered or sunk: not in one year's space, by any sorrow, could his athletic strength be quelled or his vigorous prime blighted. But in his countenance I saw a change: that looked desperate and brooding—that reminded me of some wronged and fettered wild beast or bird, dangerous to

approach in his sullen woe. The caged eagle, whose gold-ringed eyes cruelty has extinguished, might look as looked that sightless Samson.

And, reader, do you think I feared him in his blind ferocity?—if you do, you little know me. A soft hope blest with my sorrow that soon I should dare to drop a kiss on that brow of rock, and on those lips so sternly sealed beneath it: but not yet. I would not accost him yet.

He descended the one step, and advanced slowly and gropingly towards the grass-plat. Where was his daring stride now? Then he paused, as if he knew not which way to turn. He lifted his hand and opened his eyelids; gazed blank, and with a straining effort, on the sky, and toward the amphitheatre of trees: one saw that all to him was void darkness. He stretched his right hand (the left arm, the mutilated one, he kept hidden in his bosom); he seemed to wish by touch to gain an idea of what lay around him: he met but vacancy still; for the trees were some yards off where he stood. He relinquished the endeavour, folded his arms, and stood quiet and mute in the rain, now falling fast on his uncovered head. At this moment John approached him from some quarter.

"Will you take my arm, sir?" he said; "there is a heavy shower coming on: had you not better go in?"

"Let me alone," was the answer.

John withdrew without having observed me. Mr. Rochester now tried to walk about: vainly,—all was too uncertain. He groped his way back to the house, and, re-entering it, closed the door.

I now drew near and knocked: John's wife opened for me. "Mary," I said, "how are you?"

She started as if she had seen a ghost: I calmed her. To her hurried "Is it really you, miss, come at this late hour to this lonely place?" I answered by taking her hand; and then I followed her into the kitchen, where John now sat by a good fire. I explained to them, in few words, that I had heard all which had happened since I left Thornfield, and that I was come to see Mr. Rochester. I asked John to go down to the turnpike-house, where I had dismissed the chaise, and bring my trunk, which I had left there: and then, while I removed my bonnet and shawl, I questioned Mary as to whether I could be accommodated at the Manor House for the night; and finding that arrangements to that effect, though difficult, would not be impossible, I informed her I should stay. Just at this moment the parlour-bell rang.

"When you go in," said I, "tell your master that a person wishes to speak to him, but do not give my name."

"I don't think he will see you," she answered; "he refuses everybody."

When she returned, I inquired what he had said. "You are to send in your name and your business," she replied. She then proceeded to fill a glass with water, and place it on a tray, together with candles.

"Is that what he rang for?" I asked.

"Yes: he always has candles brought in at dark, though he is blind."

"Give the tray to me; I will carry it in."

I took it from her hand: she pointed me out the parlour door. The tray shook as I held it; the water spilt from the glass; my heart struck my ribs loud and fast. Mary opened the door for me, and shut it behind me.

This parlour looked gloomy: a neglected handful of fire burnt low in the grate; and, leaning over it, with his head supported against the high, old-fashioned mantelpiece, appeared the blind tenant of the room. His old dog, Pilot, lay on one side, removed out of the way, and coiled up as if afraid of being inadvertently trodden upon. Pilot pricked up his ears when I came in: then he jumped up with a yelp and a whine, and bounded towards me: he almost knocked the tray from my hands. I set it on the table; then patted him, and said softly, "Lie down!" Mr. Rochester turned mechanically to SEE what the commotion was: but as he SAW nothing, he returned and sighed.

"Give me the water, Mary," he said.

I approached him with the now only half-filled glass; Pilot followed me, still excited.

"What is the matter?" he inquired.

"Down, Pilot!" I again said. He checked the water on its way to his lips, and seemed to listen: he drank, and put the glass down. "This is you, Mary, is it not?"

"Mary is in the kitchen," I answered.

He put out his hand with a quick gesture, but not seeing where I stood, he did not touch me. "Who is this? Who is this?" he demanded, trying, as it seemed, to SEE with those sightless eyes—unavailing and distressing attempt! "Answer me—speak again!" he ordered, imperiously and aloud.

"Will you have a little more water, sir? I spilt half of what was in the glass," I said.

"WHO is it? WHAT is it? Who speaks?"

"Pilot knows me, and John and Mary know I am here. I came only this evening," I answered.

"Great God!—what delusion has come over me? What sweet madness has seized me?"

"No delusion—no madness: your mind, sir, is too strong for delusion, your health too sound for frenzy."

"And where is the speaker? Is it only a voice? Oh! I CANNOT see, but I must feel, or my heart will stop and my brain burst. Whatever—whoever you are—be perceptible to the touch or I cannot live!"

He groped; I arrested his wandering hand, and prisoned it in both mine.

"Her very fingers!" he cried; "her small, slight fingers! If so there must be more of her."

The muscular hand broke from my custody; my arm was seized, my shoulder—neck—waist—I was entwined and gathered to him.

"Is it Jane? WHAT is it? This is her shape—this is her size—"

"And this her voice," I added. "She is all here: her heart, too. God bless you, sir! I am glad to be so near you again."

"Jane Eyre!—Jane Eyre," was all he said.

"My dear master," I answered, "I am Jane Eyre: I have found you out—I am come back to you."

"In truth?—in the flesh? My living Jane?"

"You touch me, sir,—you hold me, and fast enough: I am not cold like a corpse, nor vacant like air, am I?"

"My living darling! These are certainly her limbs, and these her features; but I cannot be so blest, after all my misery. It is a dream; such dreams as I have had at night when I have clasped her once more to my heart, as I do now; and kissed her, as thus—and felt that she loved me, and trusted that she would not leave me."

"Which I never will, sir, from this day."

"Never will, says the vision? But I always woke and found it an empty mockery; and I was desolate and abandoned—my life dark, lonely, hopeless—my soul athirst and forbidden to drink—my heart famished and never to be fed. Gentle, soft dream, nestling in my arms now, you will fly, too, as your sisters have all fled before you: but kiss me before you go—embrace me, Jane."

"There, sir—and there!"

I pressed my lips to his once brilliant and now rayless eyes—I swept his hair from his brow, and kissed that too. He suddenly seemed to arouse himself: the conviction of the reality of all this seized him.

"It is you—is it, Jane? You are come back to me then?"

"I am."

"And you do not lie dead in some ditch under some stream? And you are not a pining outcast amongst strangers?"

"No, sir! I am an independent woman now."

"Independent! What do you mean, Jane?"

"My uncle in Madeira is dead, and he left me five thousand pounds."

"Ah! this is practical—this is real!" he cried: "I should never dream that. Besides, there is that peculiar voice of hers, so animating and piquant, as well as soft: it cheers my withered heart; it puts life into it.—What, Janet! Are you an independent woman? A rich woman?"

"If you won't let me live with you, I can build a house of my own close up to your door, and you may come and sit in my parlour when you want company of an evening."

"But as you are rich, Jane, you have now, no doubt, friends who will look after you, and not suffer you to devote yourself to a blind lamenter like me?"

"I told you I am independent, sir, as well as rich: I am my own mistress."

Source: Brontë, Charlotte. 1847. *Jane Eyre.* Available at: http://www.online-literature.com/brontec/janeeyre/

▣ Samuel Gridley Howe, "Report Made to the Legislature of Massachusetts upon Idiocy" (1848)

Howe's report to the Massachusetts legislature on the prevalence and condition of those labeled "idiots" led to the establishment of the first U.S. training school for the feebleminded. The training school was attached to the Perkins Institute for the Blind on a grant of $2,500 per annum for three years. In the narrative, Howe relies on the theory of idiocy advanced by Edouard Seguin, which views idiocy as based on a failed or severely diminished will (self-control).

To His Excellency, GEORGE N. BRIGGS, *Governor of the Commonwealth of Massachusetts:*

SIR: The undersigned, commissioners appointed by your excellency, under the act of April 11, 1846, "to inquire into the condition of the Idiots of the Commonwealth, to ascertain their number, and whether anything can be done in their behalf," respectfully as follows:—

REPORT:

When we accepted the task assigned to us, it was not without a sense of its importance. We did not look upon idiocy as a thing which concerned only the hundred or thousand unfortunate creatures in this generation who are stunted or blighted by it; for even if means could be found of raising all the idiots now within our borders from their brutishness, and alleviating their suffering, the work would have to be done over again, because the next generation would be burdened with an equal number of them. Such means would only cut off the outward cancer, and leave the vicious sources of it in the system. We regarded idiocy as a diseased excrescence of society; as an outward sign of an inward malady. It was hard to believe it to be in the order of Providence that the earth should always be encumbered with so many creatures in the human shape, but without the light of human reason. It seemed impious to attribute to the Creator any such glaring imperfection in his handiwork. It appeared to us certain that the existence of so many idiots in every generation *must* be the consequence of some violation of the *natural laws;*—that where there was so much suffering, there must have been sin. We resolved, therefore, to seek for the *sources* of the evil, as well as to gauge the depth and extent of the misery. It was to be expected that the search would oblige us to witness painful scenes, not only of misfortunes and sufferings, but of deformities and infirmities, the consequences of ignorance, vice, and depravity. The subjects of them, however, were brethren of the human family; the end proposed was not only to relieve their sufferings, and improve their condition; but, if possible, to lessen such evils in coming generations; the task, therefore, was not to be shrunk from, however repulsive and painful was its contemplation.

It is to be confessed, however, that we have been painfully disappointed by the sad reality, for the numbers of beings originally made in God's image, but now sunk in utter brutishness, is fearfully great, even beyond anything that had been anticipated.

The examination of their physical condition forces one into scenes, from the contemplation of which the mind and the senses instinctively revolt.

In searching for the causes of this wretchedness in the condition and habits of the progenitors of the sufferers, there is found a degree of physical deterioration, and of mental and moral darkness, which will hardly be credited.

We would fain be spared any relation of what has been witnessed, as well for our own sake, as for the tastes and feelings of others, which must be shocked by the recital of it. It would be pleasanter simply to recommend such measures as would tend to remove the present evils, and prevent their recurrence. But this may not be. Evils cannot be grappled with, and overcome, unless their nature and extent are fully known.

Besides, our duty was not only to examine into, but to report upon, the *condition* of the idiots in our Commonwealth; and that duty must be done.

During the year 1846, we endeavored, by means of circular letters addressed to the town clerks, and to other persons in every town of the Commonwealth, to ascertain the number, and, as far as could be, the condition of the idiots in their respective neighborhoods.

The answers obtained to most of these inquiries were, in many cases, very vague and unsatisfactory. It was soon seen that little dependence could be placed upon information so obtained, even as to numbers, much less, as to the condition and wants of the idiots. We, therefore, visited as many towns as possible, and endeavored, by personal observation and by inquiries, to gather all the information in our power, respecting the numbers, condition, and treatment of the unfortunate objects of our inquiry, whether they were in the public almshouses or at private charge.

It was not possible, however, to obtain all the desired information, because the researches were begun too late in the season, and because the subject grew in importance and in dreadful interest, the more closely it was examined.

The imperfect results of these inquiries were embodied in a report, made March 13th, 1847, and printed by order of the legislature.

Being directed to continue these labors, the painful inquiry was resumed during the last summer.

By diligent and careful inquiries in nearly one hundred towns in different parts of the State, we have ascertained the existence, and examined the condition, of *five hundred and seventy-four* human beings who are condemned to hopeless idiocy, who are considered and treated as idiots by their neighbors, and left to their own brutishness. They are also idiotic in a legal sense; that is, they are regarded as incapable of entering into contracts, and are irresponsible for their actions, although some of them would not be considered as idiots according to the definition of idiocy by medical writers. There are a few cases where insanity has terminated in total *dementia.* There are others where the sufferers seemed to have had all their faculties in youth, and to have gradually lost them, not by insanity but by unknown causes. Excluding such cases, there are four hundred and twenty persons who are to be regarded as truly idiots.

These are found in 77 towns. But of these towns only 63 were thoroughly examined. These contain an aggregate population of 183,942; among which were found 361 idiots, exclusive of insane persons. Now if the other parts of the State contain the same proportion

of idiots to their whole population, the total number in the Commonwealth is *between twelve and fifteen hundred!*

This is a fearful number, and it may seem to others, as it did at first to us, to be incredible. It is far greater than any calculation based upon previous returns to the legislature by commissions appointed to ascertain the number of lunatics and idiots, or that number of idiots set down in the pauper abstract, published by the secretary of state, as supported or relieved by the towns. That document makes the number to be only 377; whereas, if our observations are correct, and the other towns in the State furnish a proportionate number of pauper idiots, then the whole number in the State of that class should be over 500. It is probable, however, that the overseers of the poor, in making their return, gave only the number of idiots in almshouses, and overlooked many who receive aid from the towns at their own houses. When a poor woman applies for aid, they do not go to inquire whether any of her children are idiotic or not; whereas we pursued our inquiries into the families, and found many idiots there. However, without any reference to the manner in which other returns have been made, or any question about the degree of care which was observed, by those who made them, to distinguish between idiots and lunatics, it seems certain that our own return is a very near approach to the truth. Indeed, if there be any material error, it must be of omission, for our calculation is not based upon vague reports or answers returned to circulars. We have examined almost every case personally or by an agent on whom dependence could be placed, and in a few only have relied upon other sources of information which seemed unquestionable.

There is yet another mode by which to try the correctness of these conclusions. The returns made to us in 1846, by the town clerks in 119 towns, containing an aggregate population of 213,993 inhabitants, give the names of 394 persons who are considered by them as idiots. If to these are added 361 idiots proper, found in 1847, in 63 other towns, containing an aggregate population of 178,693,—they make a total of 182 towns, and an aggregate of 392,586 inhabitants, among whom are found 755 idiots. In this ratio, the number in the State would be over 1300, even considering the population as no greater than it was in 1840, and supposing that the number in the towns that give imperfect returns, is even as great as in those that were thoroughly examined.

We make our report, therefore, of the number of idiots in the towns examined, with entire confidence that it is not too high; and conclude, moreover, that if the other parts of the Commonwealth furnish an equal number, there are over twelve hundred persons within the State who are considered and treated as idiots. This, it will be observed, is even a greater number than was supposed to exist, when the partial report of last year was made.

The same thing has been experienced, in estimates made of the number of the insane. When attention was first turned to the subject, the number reported was supposed to be altogether an exaggeration; yet every succeeding examination has shown that the number is greater than that given by the preceding ones.

Over four hundred idiots have been minutely inspected by us personally, or by an agent upon whom we can rely. Upon the bodily and mental condition of these will be based our remarks and conclusions.

In an appendix will be found their names, ages, physical condition, and mental and moral character. It may seem to some, who inspect the tables, that they contain many trivial details with regard to the physical condition of the persons named; but it is hard to be too minute in these statements. The whole subject of idiocy is new. Science has not yet thrown her certain light upon its remote, or even its proximate causes. There is little doubt, however, that they are to be found in the CONDITION OF THE BODILY ORGANIZATION. The size and shape of the head, therefore; the proportionate development of its different parts; the condition of the nervous system; the temperament; the activity of the various functions; the development of the great cavities;—the chest and abdomen; the stature,—the weight,—every peculiarity, in short, that can be noted in a great number of individuals, may be valuable to future observers. We contribute our own observations to the store of facts, out of which science may, by and by, deduce general laws. If any bodily peculiarities, however minute, always accompany peculiar mental conditions, they become important; they are the finger-marks of the Creator, by which we learn to read his works.

There are yet more subtle causes of idiocy existing in the bodily organization, and derived from the action of that mysterious, but inevitable law, by which Nature, outraged in the persons of the parents, exacts her penalty from the persons of their children. We have endeavored to throw some light upon this also; or rather, to give a number of detached luminous points; trusting that more accurate observers will furnish many others, until all the dark surface shall be made bright, and the whole subject become clear.

The tables have been made with great care; and though they cannot pretend to perfect accuracy, they are recommended to the physiologist and student of nature, as furnishing humble, but important data.

With these introductory remarks, we proceed with our report.

Definition of Terms. Idiots. Idiocy

A difficulty is met, at the very outset, in the want of terms which clearly explain and define themselves.

Our commission is to examine into the condition of idiots. What is an idiot?—*A being in the human form, but utterly devoid of sense and understanding?* If so, then our report would be brief. Very few such have been found. Creatures are sometimes born of women, who are utterly wanting in the corporeal instruments by which understanding is most immediately manifested,—monsters without heads; but Nature lets none such cumber the earth; they come into life only to die; they take one short step from birth to death. A few seem to possess a brain and nervous system, but in such an abnormal condition as will not suffice even for command of muscular motion. Such creatures have only organic life. All other beings in human shape, manifest *some* sense and understanding.

Source: Howe, Samuel Gridley. 1848. "Report Made to the Legislature of Massachusetts upon Idiocy." Available at: http://www.personal.dundee.ac.uk/~mksimpso/howe3.htm

Nathaniel Hawthorne, from *The Scarlet Letter* (1850)

In this description of Roger Chillingworth, the vengeful estranged husband of Hester Prynne, Hawthorne draws a twisted, asymmetrical body. The man's internal emotional turmoil, Hawthorne implies, may not be expressed as outright rage, but its effect appears nonetheless, inevitably, as physical deformity. The reader is meant to perceive menace in the man's tics and uneven stance.

He was small in stature, with a furrowed visage which, as yet, could hardly be termed aged. There was a remarkable intelligence in his features, as of a person who had so cultivated his mental part that it could not fail to mould the physical to itself, and become manifest by unmistakable tokens. Although, by a seemingly careless arrangement of his heterogeneous garb, he had endeavored to conceal or abate the peculiarity, it was sufficiently evident to Hester Prynne that one of this man's shoulders rose higher than the other. Again, at this first instant of perceiving that thin visage and the slight deformity of the figure, she pressed her infant to her bosom with so compulsive a force that the poor babe uttered another cry of pain. But the mother did not seem to hear it.

At his arrival in the marketplace, and some time before she saw him, the stranger had bent his eyes on Hester Prynne. It was carelessly, at first, like a man chiefly accustomed to look inward, and to whom external matters are of little value and import unless they bear relation to something within his mind. Very soon, however, his look became keen and penetrative. A writhing horror twisted itself across his features, like a snake gliding swiftly over them, and making one little pause, with all its wreathed intervolutions in open sight. His face darkened with some powerful emotion, which, nevertheless, he so instantaneously controlled by an effort of his will, that, save a single moment, its expression might have passed for calmness. After a brief space, the convulsion grew almost imperceptible, and finally subsided into the depths of nature. When he found the eyes of Hester Prynne fastened on his own, and saw that she appeared to recognize him, he slowly and calmly raised his finger, made a gesture with it in the air, and laid it on his lips.

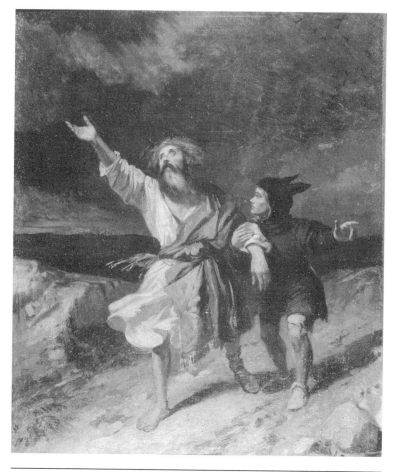

King Lear and the Fool in the Storm *(1836), by Louis Boulanger (1806–1867). In Shakespeare's* King Lear, *the fool functions as the one character in the play allowed to critique the king's decisions openly. His challenge to authority is allowed because he is viewed as mentally unstable and therefore does not pose a threat to traditional lines of authority. However, in the scene depicted here, Lear joins in the fool's fun-making at his own expense for a time before threatening to whip the fool for his audacity.*

Source: Art Resource, New York.

Source: Hawthorne, Nathaniel. 1850. *The Scarlet Letter.* Available at: www.online-literature.com/ hawthorne/scarletletter/

◙ Edgar Allan Poe, "Hop-Frog" (1850)

Poe's tale creates such sympathy for the disabled jester that readers may forgive the act of revenge directed against the mean-spirited monarch he serves. Poe uses the jester's point of view to criticize society but also exposes the violence often underlying jokes, in particular the ridicule directed toward people who are different.

I never knew anyone so keenly alive to a joke as the king was. He seemed to live only for joking. To tell a good story of the joke kind, and to tell it well, was the surest road to his favor. Thus it happened that his seven ministers were all noted for their accomplishments as jokers. They all took after the king, too, in being large, corpulent, oily men, as well as inimitable jokers. Whether people grow fat by joking, or whether there is something in fat itself which predisposes to a joke, I have never been quite able to determine; but certain it is that a lean joker is a rara avis in terris.

About the refinements, or, as he called them, the 'ghost' of wit, the king troubled himself very little. He had an especial admiration for breadth in a jest, and would often put up with length, for the sake of it. Over-niceties wearied him. He would have preferred Rabelais' 'Gargantua' to the 'Zadig' of Voltaire: and, upon the whole, practical jokes suited his taste far better than verbal ones.

At the date of my narrative, professing jesters had not altogether gone out of fashion at court. Several of the great continental 'powers' still retain their 'fools,' who wore motley, with caps and bells, and who were expected to be always ready with sharp witticisms, at a moment's notice, in consideration of the crumbs that fell from the royal table.

Our king, as a matter of course, retained his 'fool.' The fact is, he required something in the way of folly—if only to counterbalance the heavy wisdom of the seven wise men who were his ministers—not to mention himself.

His fool, or professional jester, was not only a fool, however. His value was trebled in the eyes of the king, by the fact of his being also a dwarf and a cripple. Dwarfs were as common at court, in those days, as fools; and many monarchs would have found it difficult to get through their days (days are rather longer at court than elsewhere) without both a jester to laugh with, and a dwarf to laugh at. But, as I have already observed, your jesters, in ninety-nine cases out of a hundred, are fat, round, and unwieldy—so that it was no small source of self-gratulation with our king that, in Hop-Frog (this was the fool's name), he possessed a triplicate treasure in one person.

I believe the name 'Hop-Frog' was not that given to the dwarf by his sponsors at baptism, but it was conferred upon him, by general consent of the several ministers, on account of his inability to walk as other men do. In fact, Hop-Frog could only get along by a sort of interjectional gait—something between a leap and a wriggle—a movement that afforded illimitable amusement, and of course consolation, to the king, for (notwithstanding the protuberance of his stomach and a constitutional swelling of the head) the king, by his whole court, was accounted a capital figure.

But although Hop-Frog, through the distortion of his legs, could move only with great pain and difficulty along a road or floor, the prodigious muscular power which nature seemed to have bestowed upon his arms, by way of compensation for deficiency in the lower limbs, enabled him to perform many feats of wonderful dexterity, where trees or ropes were in question, or any thing else to climb. At such exercises he certainly much more resembled a squirrel, or a small monkey, than a frog.

I am not able to say, with precision, from what country Hop-Frog originally came. It was from some barbarous region, however, that no person ever heard of—a vast distance from the court of our king. Hop-Frog, and a young girl very little less dwarfish than himself (although of exquisite proportions, and a marvellous dancer), had been forcibly carried off from their respective homes in adjoining provinces, and sent as presents to the king, by one of his ever-victorious generals.

Under these circumstances, it is not to be wondered at that a close intimacy arose between the two little captives. Indeed, they soon became sworn friends. Hop-Frog, who, although he made a great deal of sport, was by no means popular, had it not in his power to render Trippetta many services; but she, on account of her grace and exquisite beauty (although a dwarf), was universally admired and petted; so she possessed much influence; and never failed to use it, whenever she could, for the benefit of Hop-Frog.

On some grand state occasion—I forgot what—the king determined to have a masquerade, and whenever a masquerade or any thing of that kind, occurred at our court, then the talents, both of Hop-Frog and Trippetta were sure to be called into play. Hop-Frog, in especial, was so inventive in the way of getting up pageants, suggesting novel characters, and arranging costumes, for masked balls, that nothing could be done, it seems, without his assistance.

The night appointed for the fete had arrived. A gorgeous hall had been fitted up, under Trippetta's eye, with every kind of device which could possibly give eclat to a masquerade. The whole court was in a fever of expectation. As for costumes and characters, it might well be supposed that everybody had come to a decision on such points. Many had made up their minds (as to what roles they should assume) a week, or even a month, in advance; and, in fact, there was not a particle of indecision anywhere—except in the case of the king and his seven ministers. Why they hesitated I never could tell, unless they did it by way of a joke. More probably, they found it difficult, on account of being so fat, to make up their minds. At all events, time flew; and, as a last resort they sent for Trippetta and Hop-Frog.

When the two little friends obeyed the summons of the king they found him sitting at his wine with the seven members of his cabinet council; but the monarch appeared to be in a very ill humor. He knew that Hop-Frog was not fond of wine, for it excited the poor cripple almost to madness; and madness is no comfortable feeling. But the king loved his practical jokes, and took pleasure in forcing Hop-Frog to drink and (as the king called it) 'to be merry.'

"Come here, Hop-Frog," said he, as the jester and his friend entered the room; "swallow this bumper to the health of your absent friends, (here Hop-Frog sighed,) and then let us have the benefit of your invention. We want characters—characters, man—something novel—out of the way. We are wearied with this everlasting sameness. Come, drink! the wine will brighten your wits."

Hop-Frog endeavored, as usual, to get up a jest in reply to these advances from the king; but the effort was too much. It happened to be the poor dwarf's birthday, and the command to drink to his 'absent friends' forced the tears to his eyes. Many large, bitter drops fell into the goblet as he took it, humbly, from the hand of the tyrant.

"Ah! ha! ha!" roared the latter, as the dwarf reluctantly drained the beaker.—"See what a glass of good wine can do! Why, your eyes are shining already!"

Poor fellow! his large eyes gleamed, rather than shone; for the effect of wine on his excitable brain was not more powerful than instantaneous. He placed the goblet nervously on the table, and looked round upon the company with a half-insane stare. They all seemed highly amused at the success of the king's 'joke.'

"And now to business," said the prime minister, a very fat man.

"Yes," said the King; "Come lend us your assistance. Characters, my fine fellow; we stand in need of characters—all of us—ha! ha! ha!" and as this was seriously meant for a joke, his laugh was chorused by the seven.

Hop-Frog also laughed although feebly and somewhat vacantly.

"Come, come," said the king, impatiently, "have you nothing to suggest?"

"I am endeavoring to think of something novel," replied the dwarf, abstractedly, for he was quite bewildered by the wine.

"Endeavoring!" cried the tyrant, fiercely; "what do you mean by that? Ah, I perceive. You are sulky, and want more wine. Here, drink this!" and he poured out another goblet full and offered it to the cripple, who merely gazed at it, gasping for breath.

"Drink, I say!" shouted the monster, "or by the fiends—"

The dwarf hesitated. The king grew purple with rage. The courtiers smirked. Trippetta, pale as a corpse, advanced to the monarch's seat, and, falling on her knees before him, implored him to spare her friend.

The tyrant regarded her, for some moments, in evident wonder at her audacity. He seemed quite at a loss what to do or say—how most becomingly to express his indignation. At last, without uttering a syllable, he pushed her violently from him, and threw the contents of the brimming goblet in her face.

The poor girl got up the best she could, and, not daring even to sigh, resumed her position at the foot of the table.

There was a dead silence for about half a minute, during which the falling of a leaf, or of a feather, might have been heard. It was interrupted by a low, but harsh and protracted grating sound which seemed to come at once from every corner of the room.

"What—what—what are you making that noise for?" demanded the king, turning furiously to the dwarf.

The latter seemed to have recovered, in great measure, from his intoxication, and looking fixedly but quietly into the tyrant's face, merely ejaculated:

"I—I? How could it have been me?"

"The sound appeared to come from without," observed one of the courtiers. "I fancy it was the parrot at the window, whetting his bill upon his cage-wires."

"True," replied the monarch, as if much relieved by the suggestion; "but, on the honor of a knight, I could have sworn that it was the gritting of this vagabond's teeth."

Hereupon the dwarf laughed (the king was too confirmed a joker to object to any one's laughing), and displayed a set of large, powerful, and very repulsive teeth. Moreover, he avowed his perfect willingness to swallow as much wine as desired. The monarch was pacified; and having drained another bumper with no very perceptible ill effect, Hop-Frog entered at once, and with spirit, into the plans for the masquerade.

"I cannot tell what was the association of idea," observed he, very tranquilly, and as if he had never tasted wine in his life, "but just after your majesty, had struck the girl and thrown the wine in her face—just after your majesty had done this, and while the parrot was making that odd noise outside the window, there came into my mind a capital diversion—one of my own country frolics—often enacted among us, at our masquerades: but here it will be new altogether. Unfortunately, however, it requires a company of eight persons and—"

"Here we are!" cried the king, laughing at his acute discovery of the coincidence; "eight to a fraction— I and my seven ministers. Come! what is the diversion?"

"We call it," replied the cripple, "the Eight Chained Ourang-Outangs, and it really is excellent sport if well enacted."

"We will enact it," remarked the king, drawing himself up, and lowering his eyelids.

"The beauty of the game," continued Hop-Frog, "lies in the fright it occasions among the women."

"Capital!" roared in chorus the monarch and his ministry.

"I will equip you as ourang-outangs," proceeded the dwarf; "leave all that to me. The resemblance shall be so striking, that the company of masqueraders will take you for real beasts—and of course, they will be as much terrified as astonished."

"Oh, this is exquisite!" exclaimed the king. "Hop-Frog! I will make a man of you."

"The chains are for the purpose of increasing the confusion by their jangling. You are supposed to have escaped, en masse, from your keepers. Your majesty cannot conceive the effect produced, at a masquerade, by eight chained ourang-outangs, imagined to be real ones by most of the company; and rushing in with savage cries, among the crowd of delicately and gorgeously habited men and women. The contrast is inimitable!"

"It must be," said the king: and the council arose hurriedly (as it was growing late), to put in execution the scheme of Hop-Frog.

His mode of equipping the party as ourang-outangs was very simple, but effective enough for his purposes. The animals in question had, at the epoch of my story, very rarely been seen in any part of the civilized world; and as the imitations made by the dwarf were sufficiently beast-like and more than sufficiently hideous, their truthfulness to nature was thus thought to be secured.

The king and his ministers were first encased in tight-fitting stockinet shirts and drawers. They were then saturated with tar. At this stage of the process, some one of the party suggested feathers; but the suggestion was at once overruled by the dwarf, who soon convinced the eight, by ocular demonstration, that the hair of such a brute as the ourang-outang was much

more efficiently represented by flax. A thick coating of the latter was accordingly plastered upon the coating of tar. A long chain was now procured. First, it was passed about the waist of the king, and tied, then about another of the party, and also tied; then about all successively, in the same manner. When this chaining arrangement was complete, and the party stood as far apart from each other as possible, they formed a circle; and to make all things appear natural, Hop-Frog passed the residue of the chain in two diameters, at right angles, across the circle, after the fashion adopted, at the present day, by those who capture Chimpanzees, or other large apes, in Borneo.

The grand saloon in which the masquerade was to take place, was a circular room, very lofty, and receiving the light of the sun only through a single window at top. At night (the season for which the apartment was especially designed) it was illuminated principally by a large chandelier, depending by a chain from the centre of the sky-light, and lowered, or elevated, by means of a counter-balance as usual; but (in order not to look unsightly) this latter passed outside the cupola and over the roof.

The arrangements of the room had been left to Trippetta's superintendence; but, in some particulars, it seems, she had been guided by the calmer judgment of her friend the dwarf. At his suggestion it was that, on this occasion, the chandelier was removed. Its waxen drippings (which, in weather so warm, it was quite impossible to prevent) would have been seriously detrimental to the rich dresses of the guests, who, on account of the crowded state of the saloon, could not all be expected to keep from out its centre; that is to say, from under the chandelier. Additional sconces were set in various parts of the hall, out of the way, and a flambeau, emitting sweet odor, was placed in the right hand of each of the Caryaides [Caryatides] that stood against the wall—some fifty or sixty altogether.

The eight ourang-outangs, taking Hop-Frog's advice, waited patiently until midnight (when the room was thoroughly filled with masqueraders) before making their appearance. No sooner had the clock ceased striking, however, than they rushed, or rather rolled in, all together—for the impediments of their chains caused most of the party to fall, and all to stumble as they entered.

The excitement among the masqueraders was prodigious, and filled the heart of the king with glee. As had been anticipated, there were not a few of the guests who supposed the ferocious-looking creatures to be beasts of some kind in reality, if not precisely ourang-outangs. Many of the women swooned with affright; and had not the king taken the precaution to exclude all weapons from the saloon, his party might soon have expiated their frolic in their blood. As it was, a general rush was made for the doors; but the king had ordered them to be locked immediately upon his entrance; and, at the dwarf's suggestion, the keys had been deposited with him.

While the tumult was at its height, and each masquerader attentive only to his own safety (for, in fact, there was much real danger from the pressure of the excited crowd), the chain by which the chandelier ordinarily hung, and which had been drawn up on its removal, might have been seen very gradually to descend, until its hooked extremity came within three feet of the floor.

Soon after this, the king and his seven friends having reeled about the hall in all directions, found themselves, at length, in its centre, and, of course, in immediate contact with the chain. While they were thus situated, the dwarf, who had followed noiselessly at their heels, inciting them to keep up the commotion, took hold of their own chain at the intersection of the two portions which crossed the circle diametrically and at right angles. Here, with the rapidity of thought, he inserted the hook from which the chandelier had been wont to depend; and, in an instant, by some unseen agency, the chandelier-chain was drawn so far upward as to take the hook out of reach, and, as an inevitable consequence, to drag the ourang-outangs together in close connection, and face to face.

The masqueraders, by this time, had recovered, in some measure, from their alarm; and, beginning to regard the whole matter as a well-contrived pleasantry, set up a loud shout of laughter at the predicament of the apes.

"Leave them to me!" now screamed Hop-Frog, his shrill voice making itself easily heard through all the din. "Leave them to me. I fancy I know them. If I can only get a good look at them, I can soon tell who they are."

Here, scrambling over the heads of the crowd, he managed to get to the wall; when, seizing a flambeau from one of the Caryaides [Caryatides], he returned, as he went, to the centre of the room—leaping, with the agility of a monkey, upon the kings head, and thence clambered a few feet up the chain; holding down the torch to examine the group of ourang-outangs, and still screaming: "I shall soon find out who they are!"

And now, while the whole assembly (the apes included) were convulsed with laughter, the jester suddenly uttered a shrill whistle; when the chain flew violently up for about thirty feet—dragging with it the dismayed and struggling ourang-outangs, and leaving them suspended in mid-air between the sky-light and the floor. Hop-Frog, clinging to the chain as it rose, still maintained his relative position in respect to the eight maskers, and still (as if nothing were the matter) continued to thrust his torch down toward them, as though endeavoring to discover who they were.

So thoroughly astonished was the whole company at this ascent, that a dead silence, of about a minute's duration, ensued. It was broken by just such a low, harsh, grating sound, as had before attracted the attention of the king and his councillors when the former threw the wine in the face of Trippetta. But, on the present occasion, there could be no question as to whence the sound issued. It came from the fang-like teeth of the dwarf, who ground them and gnashed them as he foamed at the mouth, and glared, with an expression of maniacal rage, into the upturned countenances of the king and his seven companions.

"Ah, ha!" said at length the infuriated jester. "Ah, ha! I begin to see who these people are now!" Here, pretending to scrutinize the king more closely, he held the flambeau to the flaxen coat which enveloped him, and which instantly burst into a sheet of vivid flame. In less than half a minute the whole eight ourang-outangs were blazing fiercely, amid the shrieks of the multitude who gazed at them from below, horror-stricken, and without the power to render them the slightest assistance.

At length the flames, suddenly increasing in virulence, forced the jester to climb higher up the chain, to be out of their reach; and, as he made this movement, the crowd again sank, for a brief instant, into silence. The dwarf seized his opportunity, and once more spoke:

"I now see distinctly." he said, "what manner of people these maskers are. They are a great king and his seven privy-councillors,—a king who does not scruple to strike a defenceless girl and his seven councillors who abet him in the outrage. As for myself, I am simply Hop-Frog, the jester—and this is my last jest."

Owing to the high combustibility of both the flax and the tar to which it adhered, the dwarf had scarcely made an end of his brief speech before the work of vengeance was complete. The eight corpses swung in their chains, a fetid, blackened, hideous, and indistinguishable mass. The cripple hurled his torch at them, clambered leisurely to the ceiling, and disappeared through the sky-light.

It is supposed that Trippetta, stationed on the roof of the saloon, had been the accomplice of her friend in his fiery revenge, and that, together, they effected their escape to their own country: for neither was seen again.

Source: Poe, Edgar Allan. 1850. "Hop-Frog." In Vol. 5 of *The Works of Edgar Allan Poe*. Available at: http://whitewolf.newcastle.edu.au/words/authors/P/PoeEdgarAllan/prose/raven_5/hopfrog.html

▣ Herman Melville, from *Moby Dick: or The Whale* (1851)

As the "monomaniacal" captain of the Pequod, Melville's one-legged Ahab storms about the ship with great ferocity. His personal and metaphysical anger over his "dismasting" leads him into a vengeful and ill-fated quest to hunt down and kill the white whale, Moby-Dick, as his singular life objective. In making this Ahab's life's goal, the novel supplies one of the most influential portraits of disability as a quest narrative of revenge.

Chapter 28: Ahab

For several days after leaving Nantucket, nothing above hatches was seen of Captain Ahab. The mates regularly relieved each other at the watches, and for aught that could be seen to the contrary, they seemed to be the only commanders of the ship; only they sometimes issued from the cabin with orders so sudden and peremptory, that after all it was plain they but commanded vicariously. Yes, their supreme lord and dictator was there, though hitherto unseen by any eyes not permitted to penetrate into the now sacred retreat of the cabin.

Every time I ascended to the deck from my watches below, I instantly gazed aft to mark if any strange face were visible; for my first vague disquietude touching the unknown captain, now in the seclusion of the sea, became almost a perturbation. This was strangely heightened at times by the ragged Elijah's diabolical incoherences uninvitedly recurring to me, with a subtle energy I could not have before conceived of. But poorly could I withstand them, much as in other moods I was almost ready to smile at the solemn whimsicalities of that outlandish prophet of the wharves. But whatever it was of apprehensiveness or uneasiness—to call it so—which I felt, yet whenever I came to look about me in the ship, it seemed against all warranty to cherish such emotions. For though the harpooneers, with the great body of the crew, were a far more barbaric, heathenish, and motley set than any of the tame merchant-ship companies which my previous experiences had made me acquainted with, still I ascribed this—and rightly ascribed it—to the fierce uniqueness of the very nature of that wild Scandinavian vocation in which I had so abandonedly embarked. But it was especially the aspect of the three chief officers of the ship, the mates, which was most forcibly calculated to allay these colourless misgivings, and induce confidence and cheerfulness in every presentment of the voyage. Three better, more likely sea-officers and men, each in his own different way, could not readily be found, and they were every one of them Americans; a Nantucketer, a Vineyarder, a Cape man. Now, it being Christmas when the ship shot from out her harbor, for a space we had biting Polar weather, though all the time running away from it to the southward; and by every degree and minute of latitude which we sailed, gradually leaving that merciless winter, and all its intolerable weather behind us. It was one of those less lowering, but still grey and gloomy enough mornings of the transition, when with a fair wind the ship was rushing through the water with a vindictive sort of leaping and melancholy rapidity, that as I mounted to the deck at the call of the forenoon watch, so soon as I levelled my glance towards the taffrail, foreboding shivers ran over me. Reality outran apprehension; Captain Ahab stood upon his quarter-deck.

There seemed no sign of common bodily illness about him, nor of the recovery from any. He looked like a man cut away from the stake, when the fire has overrunningly wasted all the limbs without consuming them, or taking away one particle from their compacted aged robustness. His whole high, broad form, seemed made of solid bronze, and shaped in an unalterable mould, like Cellini's cast Perseus. Threading its way out from among his grey hairs, and continuing right down one side of his tawny scorched face and neck, till it disappeared in his clothing, you saw a slender rod-like mark, lividly whitish. It resembled that perpendicular seam sometimes made in the straight, lofty trunk of a great tree, when the upper lightning tearingly darts down it, and without wrenching a single twig, peels and grooves out the bark from top to bottom, ere running off into the soil, leaving the tree still greenly alive, but branded. Whether that mark was born with him, or whether it was the scar left by some desperate wound, no one could certainly say. By some tacit consent, throughout the voyage little or no allusion was made to it, especially by the mates. But once Tashtego's senior, an old Gay-Head Indian among the crew, superstitiously asserted that not till he was full forty years old did Ahab become that way branded, and then it came upon him, not in the fury of any mortal fray, but in an elemental strife at sea. Yet, this wild hint seemed inferentially negatived, by what a grey Manxman insinuated, an old sepulchral man, who, having never before sailed out of Nantucket, had never ere this laid eye upon wild Ahab. Nevertheless, the old sea-traditions, the immemorial credulities, popularly invested this old Manxman with preternatural powers of discernment. So that no white sailor seriously contradicted him when he said that if ever Captain Ahab should be tranquilly laid out—which might hardly come to pass, so he muttered—then, whoever should do that last office for the dead, would find a birth-mark on him from crown to sole.

So powerfully did the whole grim aspect of Ahab affect me, and the livid brand which streaked it, that for the first few moments I hardly noted that not a little of this overbearing grimness was owing to the barbaric white leg upon which he partly stood. It had previously come to me that this ivory leg had at sea been fashioned from the polished bone of the sperm whale's jaw. "Aye, he was dismasted off Japan," said the old Gay-Head Indian once; "but like his dismasted craft, he shipped another mast without coming home for it. He has a quiver of 'em."

I was struck with the singular posture he maintained. Upon each side of the Pequod's quarter deck, and pretty close to the mizzen shrouds, there was an auger hole, bored about half an inch or so, into the plank. His bone leg steadied in that hole; one arm elevated, and holding by a shroud; Captain Ahab stood erect, looking straight out beyond the ship's ever-pitching prow. There was an infinity of firmest fortitude, a determinate, unsurrenderable wilfulness, in the fixed and fearless, forward dedication of that glance. Not a word he spoke; nor did his officers say aught to him; though by all their minutest gestures and expressions, they plainly showed the uneasy, if not painful, consciousness of being under a troubled master-eye. And not only that, but moody stricken Ahab stood before them with a crucifixion in his face; in all the nameless regal overbearing dignity of some mighty woe.

Ere long, from his first visit in the air, he withdrew into his cabin. But after that morning, he was every day visible to the crew; either standing in his pivot-hole, or seated upon an ivory stool he had; or heavily walking the deck. As the sky grew less gloomy; indeed, began to grow a little genial, he became still less and less a recluse; as if, when the ship had sailed from home, nothing but the dead wintry bleakness of the sea had then kept him so secluded. And, by and by, it came to pass, that he was almost continually in the air; but, as yet, for all that he said, or perceptibly did, on the at last sunny deck, he seemed as unnecessary there as another mast. But the Pequod was only making a passage now; not regularly cruising; nearly all whaling preparatives needing supervision the mates were fully competent to, so that there was little or nothing, out of himself, to employ or excite Ahab, now; and thus chase away, for that one interval, the clouds that layer upon layer were piled upon his brow, as ever all clouds choose the loftiest peaks to pile themselves upon.

Nevertheless, ere long, the warm, warbling persuasiveness of the pleasant, holiday weather we came to, seemed gradually to charm him from his mood. For, as when the red-cheeked, dancing girls, April and May, trip home to the wintry, misanthropic woods; even the barest, ruggedest, most thunder-cloven old oak will at least send forth some few green sprouts, to welcome such glad-hearted visitants; so Ahab did, in the end, a little respond to the playful allurings of that girlish air. More than once did he put forth the faint blossom of a look, which, in any other man, would have soon flowered out in a smile.

Chapter 106: Ahab's Leg

The precipitating manner in which Captain Ahab had quitted the Samuel Enderby of London, had not been unattended with some small violence to his own person. He had lighted with such energy upon a thwart of his boat that his ivory leg had received a half-splintering shock. And when after gaining his own deck, and his own pivot-hole there, he so vehemently wheeled round with an urgent command to the steersman (it was as ever, something about his not steering inflexibly enough); then, the already shaken ivory received such an additional twist and wrench, that though it still remained entire, and to all appearances lusty, yet Ahab did not deem it entirely trustworthy.

And, indeed, it seemed small matter for wonder, that for all his pervading, mad recklessness, Ahab did at times give careful heed to the condition of that dead bone upon which he partly stood. For it had not been very long prior to the Pequod's sailing from Nantucket, that he had been found one night lying prone upon the ground, and insensible; by some unknown, and seemingly inexplicable, unimaginable casualty, his ivory limb having been so violently displaced, that it had stake-wise smitten, and all but pierced his groin; nor was it without extreme difficulty that the agonizing wound was entirely cured.

Nor, at the time, had it failed to enter his monomaniac mind, that all the anguish of that then present suffering was but the direct issue of a former woe; and he too plainly seemed to see, that as the most poisonous reptile of the marsh perpetuates his kind as inevitably as the sweetest songster of the grove; so, equally with every felicity, all miserable events do naturally beget their like. Yea, more than equally, thought Ahab; since both the ancestry and posterity of Grief go further than the ancestry and posterity of Joy. For, not to hint of this: that it is an inference from certain canonic teachings, that while some natural enjoyments here shall have no children born to them for the other world, but, on the contrary, shall be followed by the joy-childlessness of all hell's despair; whereas, some guilty mortal miseries shall still fertilely beget to themselves an eternally progressive progeny of griefs beyond the grave; not at all to hint of this, there still seems an inequality in the deeper analysis of the thing. For, thought Ahab, while even the highest earthly felicities ever have a certain unsignifying pettiness lurking in them, but, at bottom, all heart-woes, a mystic significance, and, in some men, an archangelic grandeur; so do their diligent tracings-out not belie the obvious deduction. To trail the genealogies of these high mortal miseries, carries us at last among the sourceless primogenitures of the gods; so that, in the face of all the glad, hay-making suns, and soft-cymballing, round harvest-moons, we must needs give in to this: that the gods themselves are not for ever glad. The ineffaceable, sad birth-mark in the brow of man, is but the stamp of sorrow in the signers.

Unwittingly here a secret has been divulged, which perhaps might more properly, in set way, have been disclosed before. With many other particulars concerning Ahab, always had it remained a mystery to some, why it was, that for a certain period, both before and after the sailing of the Pequod, he had hidden himself away with such Grand-Lama-like exclusiveness; and, for that one interval, sought speechless refuge, as it were, among the marble senate of the dead. Captain Peleg's rooted reason for this thing appeared by no means adequate; though, indeed, as touching all Ahab's deeper part, every revelation partook more of significant darkness than of explanatory light. But, in the end, it all came out; this one matter did, at least. That direful mishap was at the bottom of his temporary recluseness. And not only this, but to that ever-contracting, dropping circle ashore, who, for any reason, possessed the privilege of a less banned approach to him; to that timid circle the above hinted casualty—remaining, as it did, moodily unaccounted for by Ahab—invested itself with terrors, not entirely underived from the land of spirits and of wails. So that, through their zeal for him, they had all conspired, so far as in them lay, to muffle up the knowledge of this thing from others; and hence it was, that not till a considerable interval had elapsed, did it transpire upon Pequod's decks.

But be all this as it may; let the unseen, ambiguous synod in the air, or the vindictive princes and potentates of fire, have to do or not with earthly Ahab, yet, in this present matter of his leg, he took plain practical procedures;—he called the carpenter.

And when that functionary appeared before him, he bade him without delay set about making a new leg, and directed the mates to see him supplied with all the studs and joists of jaw-ivory (Sperm Whale) which had thus far been accumulated on the voyage, in order that a careful selection of the stoutest, clearest-grained stuff might be secured. This done, the carpenter received orders to have the leg completed that night; and to provide all the fittings for it, independent of those pertaining to the distrusted one in use. Moreover, the ship's forge was ordered to be hoisted out of its contemporary idleness in the hold; and, to accelerate the affair, the blacksmith was commanded to proceed at once to the forging of whatever iron contrivances might be needed.

Source: Melville, Herman. 1851. *Moby Dick: or The Whale.* Available at: http://www.americanliterature.com/MD/MDINDEX.HTML

▣ Herbert Spencer, from *Social Statics or Order* (1851)

Herbert Spencer (1820–1903) was a British-born biologist and social philosopher whose theory of evolution was toppled by that of Charles Darwin in The Origins of Species. However, Spencer is credited with

condensing (many might claim simplifying) Darwin's argument into the adage "survival of the fittest." Although Darwin resisted this designation for years, he finally accepted this shorthand way of capturing his theory of adaptation. The idea of "survival of the fittest" was often used during the eugenics period and beyond to explain why disabled people were the "weak links" in a hierarchy of valued human capacities.

The Evanescence of Evil

All evil results from the non-adaptation of constitution to conditions. Does a shrub dwindle in poor soil, or become sickly when deprived of light, or die outright if removed to a cold climate? It is because the harmony between its organization and its circumstances has been destroyed. Those experiences of the farm-yard and the menagerie which show that pain, disease, and death, are entailed upon animals by certain kinds of treatment, may be similarly generalized. Every suffering incident to the human body, from a headache up to a fatal illness, from a burn or a sprain up to accidental loss of life, is similarly traceable to the having placed that body in a situation for which its powers did not fit it. Nor is the expression confined in its application to physical evil. Is the bachelor unhappy because his means will not permit him to marry? Does the mother mourn over her lost child? Does the emigrant lament leaving his fatherland? The explanation is still the same. No matter what the special nature of the evil, it is invariably referable to one generic cause—want of congruity between the faculties and their spheres of action.

Equally true is that evil perpetually tends to disappear. In virtue of an essential principle of life, this non-adaptation of an organism to its condition is ever being rectified; and modification of one or both, continues until the adaptation is complete. Whatever possesses vitality, from the elementary cell up to man himself, inclusive, obeys this law. We see it illustrated in the acclimatization of plants, in the altered habits of domesticated animals, in the varying characteristics of our own race. Accustomed to the brief arctic summer, the Siberian herbs and shrubs spring up, flower, and ripen their seeds, in the space of a few weeks. If exposed to the rigour of northern winters, animals of the temperate zone get thicker coats and become white. The greyhound which, when first transported to the high plateaus of the Andes, fails in the chase from want of breath, acquires, in the course of generations, a more efficient pair of lungs.

Man exhibits the same adaptability. He alters in colour according to habitat—lives here upon rice and there upon whale oil—gets larger digestive organs if he habitually eats innutritious food—acquires the power of long fasting if his mode of life is irregular, and loses it when the supply of food is certain—attains acute vision, hearing, and scent, when his habits of life call for them, and gets these senses blunted when they are less needful. That such changes are towards fitness for surrounding circumstances no one can question. When he sees that the dweller in marshes lives in an atmosphere which is certain death to a stranger—when he sees that the Hindoo can lie down and sleep under a tropical sun, while his white master with closed blinds, and water sprinklings, and punkah, can hardly get a doze—when he sees that the Greenlander and the Neapolitan subsist comfortably on their respective foods—blubber and macaroni, but would be made miserable by an interchange of them—when he sees that in other cases there is still this fitness to diet, to climate, and to modes of life, even the most skeptical must admit that some law of adaptation is at work. In the drunkard who needs an increasing quantity of spirits to intoxicate him, and in the opium eater who has to keep taking a larger dose to produce the usual effect, he may mark how the system gradually acquires power to resist what is noxious. Those who smoke, who take snuff, or who habitually use medicines, can furnish like illustrations. This universal law of physical modification, is the law of mental modification also. The multitudinous differences of capacity and disposition which have, in course of time, grown up between the Indian, African, Mongolian, and Caucasian races, and between the various subdivisions of them, must all be ascribed to the acquirement in each case of fitness for surrounding circumstances. Why all this divergence from the one original type? If adaptation of constitution to conditions is not the cause, what is the cause?

There are none however, who can with anything like consistency combat this doctrine; for all use arguments that presuppose its truth. They do this when they attribute differences of national character to differences in social customs and arrangements; and again when they comment on the force of habit; and again when they discuss the probable influence of a proposed measure upon public morality; and again when they recommend practice as a means of acquiring increased aptitude; and again when they describe certain pursuits as elevating and others as degrading;

and again when they talk of getting used to anything; and again when they teach that virtuous conduct eventually becomes pleasurable, or when they warn against the power of a long-encouraged vice.

We must adopt one of three propositions. We must either affirm that the human being is unaltered by the influences brought to bear on him—his circumstances; or that he tends to become *un*fitted to those circumstances; or that he tends to become fitted to them. If the first be true, then all schemes of education, of government, of social reform are useless. If the second be true, then the way to make a man virtuous is to accustom him to vicious practices, and *vice versa*. Both of which propositions being absurd, we are impelled to admit the remaining one.

Keeping in mind these truths, that all evil results from the non-adaptation of constitution to conditions; and that where this non-adaptation exists it is continually being diminished by the changing of constitution to suit conditions; we shall be prepared for comprehending the present position of the human race.

By the increase of population the state of existence we call social has been necessitated. Men living in this state suffer under numerous evils. By the hypothesis it follows that their characters are not completely adapted to such a state.

In what respects are they not so adapted? What is the special qualification which the social state requires?

It requires that each individual shall have such desires only, as may be fully satisfied without trenching upon the ability of other individuals to obtain like satisfactions. If the desires of each are not thus limited, then either all must have certain of their desires ungratified; or some must get gratification for them at the expense of others. Both of which alternatives, necessitating pain, imply non-adaptation.

But why is not man adapted to the social state?

Simply because he yet partially retains characteristics appropriate to an antecedent state. The respects in which he is not fitted to society, are the respects in which he is fitted for his original predatory life. His primitive circumstances required that he should sacrifice the welfare of other beings to his own; his present circumstances require that he shall not do so; and in so far as his old attribute still clings to him, he is unfit for the social state. All sins of men against one another, from the cannibalism of the Fijian to the crimes and venalities we see around us; the felonies which fill our prisons, the trickeries of trade, the quarrellings of class with class and of nation with nation, have their causes comprehended under this generalization.

Men needed one moral constitution to fit him for his original state; he needs another to fit him for his present state; and he has been, is, and will long continue to be, in process of adaptation. And the belief in human perfectibility merely amounts to the belief that, in virtue of this process, man will eventually become completely suited to his mode of life.

Progress, therefore, is not an accident, but a necessity. Instead of civilization being artificial it is a part of nature; all of a piece of development of an embryo or the unfolding of a flower. The modifications mankind have undergone, and are still undergoing, result from a law underlying the whole organic creation; and provided the human race continues, and the constitution of things remains the same, those modifications must end in completeness. As surely as the tree becomes bulky when it stands alone, and slender if one of a group; as surely as a blacksmiths arm grows large, and the skin of a laborer's hand thick; as surely as the eye tends to become long-sighted in the sailor, and short-sighted in the student; as surely as a clerk acquires rapidity in writing and calculation; as surely as the musician learns to detect an error of a semitone amidst what seems to others a very babel of sounds; as surely as a passion grows by indulgence and diminishes when restrained; as surely as a disregarded conscience becomes inert, and one that is obeyed active; as surely as there is any meaning in such terms as habit, custom, practice;—so surely must the human faculties be moulded into complete fitness for the social state; so surely must evil and immorality disappear; so surely must man become perfect.

[Editors' note: Spencer later added the following qualifications to the foregoing argument.] With the exception of small verbal improvements, I have let this chapter stand unaltered, though it is now clear to me that the conclusions drawn in it should be largely qualified. 1. Various races of mankind, inhabiting bad habitats, and obliged to lead miserable lives, cannot by any amount of adaptation be moulded into satisfactory types. 2. Astronomical and geological changes must continue hereafter to cause such changes of surface and climate as must entail migrations from habitats rendered unfit to fitter habitats; and such migrations must entail modified modes of life, with consequent re-adaptations. 3. The rate of progress towards any adapted form must diminish with the approach to complete adaptation, since the force producing it must diminish; so that, other causes apart, perfect adaptation can be reached only in infinite time.

Source: Spencer, Herbert. 1915. Pp. 28–32 in *Social Statics or Order: Together with Man versus the State*. New York: D. Appleton. (Originally published 1851)

▣ Phineas T. Barnum, from *The Life of P. T. Barnum* (1855)

Barnum was an extraordinary entrepreneur, an impresario, and a self-made man. He remade himself several times during his long career as a showman. The following is an excerpt from Barnum's first autobiography, published at the height of his antebellum success and fame. Barnum relates how he pulled himself out of financial danger with his purchase of the American Museum and how he achieved his first profits there with the Fejee Mermaid. Moses Kimball of the Boston Museum was his friend, and he was the means by which Barnum obtained the Fejee Mermaid. Barnum was a master of promotion—notice how he promoted the Fejee Mermaid. When he obtained the services of the four-year-old Charles Stratton, Barnum would use similar approaches in promoting the boy he called Tom Thumb.

The American Museum, at the date of my purchase, was little more than the nucleus of what it is now. During the thirteen years of my proprietorship, I have considerably more than doubled the value of the permanent attractions and curiosities of the establishment. The additions were derived, partly from Peale's Museum, (which I bought and transferred to my former collection in the fall of 1842;) partly from the large and rare collection known as the Chinese Museum, (which I removed to the American Museum in 1848;) and partly by purchases wherever I could find curiosities, in both America and Europe.

The space now occupied for my Museum purposes is more than double what it was in 1841. The Lecture Room, which was originally narrow, ill-contrived and uncomfortable, has been several times enlarged and improved, and at present may be pronounced one of the most commodious and beautiful halls of entertainment in New-York.

There have been enlargement and improvement in other respects. At first, the Museum was merely a collection of curiosities by day, and in the evening there

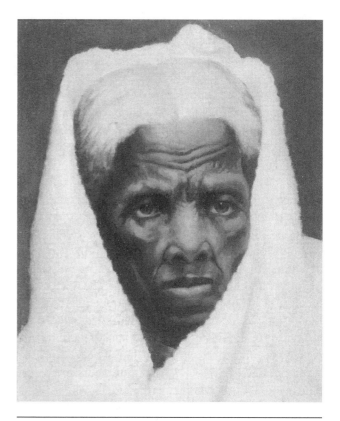

Harriet Tubman, *by Jacob Lawrence (1917–2000). Harriet Tubman, a leader of the Underground Railroad for escaped slaves from the American South, experienced a head injury as a teenager when an angry overseer hit her with a weight intended for another slave. Her efforts assisted more than 300 individuals to remove themselves from status as human chattel.*

Source: Art Resource, New York.

was a performance, consisting of disjointed and disconnected amusements, such as are still to be found at many of the inferior shows. Saturday *afternoon* was soon appropriated to performances, and shortly afterwards the *afternoon* of Wednesday was added. The programme has for years included the afternoon and evening of every day in the week, (of course excepting the Sabbath,) and on great holidays, we have sometimes given as many as twelve performances.

There has been a gradual change in these, and the transient attractions of the Museum have been greatly diversified. Industrious fleas, educated dogs, jugglers, automatons, ventriloquists, living statuary, tableaux, gipsies, albinoes, fat boys, giants, dwarfs, rope-dancers, caricatures of phrenology, and "live Yankees," pantomime, instrumental music, singing and dancing in great variety, (including Ethiopians,) etc. Dioramas, panoramas, models of Dublin, Paris, Niagara, Jerusalem, etc., mechanical figures, fancy glass-blowing, knitting machines and other triumphs in the mechanical arts, dissolving views, American Indians, including their warlike and religious ceremonies enacted on the stage, etc., etc.

I need not specify the order of time in which these varieties were presented to the public. In one respect there has been a thorough though gradual change in the general plan, for the *moral drama* is now, and has been for several years, the principal feature of the Lecture Room of the American Museum.

Apart from the merit and interest of these performances, and apart from every thing connected with the stage, my permanent collection of curiosities is, without doubt, abundantly worth the uniform charge of admission to all the entertainments of the establishment, and I can therefore afford to be accused of "humbug" when I add such transient novelties as increase its attractions. If I have exhibited a questionable dead mermaid in my Museum, it should not be overlooked that I have also exhibited cameleopards, a rhinoceros, grisly bears, orang-outangs, great serpents, etc., about which there could be no mistake because they were alive; and I should hope that a little "clap-trap" occasionally, in the way of transparencies, flags, exaggerated pictures, and puffing advertisements, might find an offset in a wilderness of wonderful, instructive, and amusing realities. Indeed I cannot doubt that the sort of "clap-trap" here referred to, is allowable, and that the public like a little of it mixed up with the great realities which I provide. The titles of "humbug," and the "prince of humbugs," were first applied to me by myself. I made these titles a part of my "stock in trade," and may here quote a passage from the "Fortunes of the Scattergood Family," a work by the popular English writer, Albert Smith:

"'It's a great thing to be a humbug,' said Mr. Rossett. 'I've been called so often. It means hitting the public in reality. Anybody who can do so, is sure to be called a humbug by somebody who can't.'"

Among my first extra exhibitions produced at the American Museum, was a model of the Falls of Niagara, belonging to Grain the artist. It was undoubtedly a fine model, giving the mathematical proportions of that great cataract, and the trees, rocks, buildings, etc., in its vicinity. But the absurdity of the thing consisted in introducing water, thus pretending to present a *facsimile* of that great wonder of nature. The falls were about eighteen inches high, every thing else being in due proportion!

I confess I felt somewhat ashamed of this myself, yet it made a good line in the bill, and I bought the model for $200.

———————

Source: Barnum, Phineas T. 1855. *The Life of P. T. Barnum.* New York: Redfield. .

▣ Lizzie Jones's Letter Home from the Orthopaedic Institution for the Cure of Deformities (1855)

Eliza Adam "Lizzie" Jones (1839–1911) of Orange County, North Carolina, wrote this and several subsequent letters to relatives during her stay at a clinic in Brooklyn, New York. The letter demonstrates some of the paradoxical intersections between gender and disability in antebellum Southern culture. Marriageability was important and required a sound physique, but for planter-class daughters with "deformities," a winter of confinement in Brooklyn might also be a release from restrictive dresses and rural monotony.

I suppose you think me not very true to my promises—if I had known when I left Raleigh, how hard it is to write away from home I don't think I would have made any positive promises about writing, however now that I am beginning to be settled, I can write much more easily. You cannot think how strange it seemed to me to have to take up my abode at this 'Orthopaedic Institution for the Cure of Deformities'— that is the sign in *great big* letters! Aunt Sal and Fan are staying with me, and I tell them that they will be called deformed too. I hope, dear cousin, you won't wait for me to get cured, before you come on because though it may take a good while, yet every one is quite certain that I *will* be straitened up, and it will be *so* nice to have you here. You asked me to tell you the mode of treatment—that I received—it is very simple indeed; at present I do nothing more than take gymnastic exercises every day, which are very pleasant, and drink some kind of wine. I have been over to New York very often, and seen as many fine sights as Aunt Sally or Fanny. But this state of things is not to last long—the Dr. has already expressed a desire that I should stay more at *home,* and in about half an hour, he is going to apply electricity to me; they have been laughing at me all the morning about being so anxious for the time to come; although I know it will be disagreeable, I am just as anxious about it as if it were some delightful sensation I were going to experience. . . . I will put on a brace in two or three days which will prevent me from wearing anything but a loose wrapper, then of course I cannot go out, so I am going to try to make up for leaving school by reading a great deal. I am sure I ought to improve myself in that respect, for it will be the principal means I have of entertaining myself.

Source: Jones, Lizzie. 1855. Letter. Cameron Family Papers, Southern Historical Collection, University of North Carolina at Chapel Hill.

▣ John J. Flournoy to William Turner, "A Mighty Change" (1856)

The following excerpts are from correspondence debating the value and need for a separate deaf commonwealth/state. Flournoy argues that a separate state would be an empowering project for the deaf community and would not involve the entire deaf community but rather a select group. It would prove that deaf people had the same capabilities as nondeaf people. Booth responds by discussing the impossibility of Flournoy's proposal, citing educational and economic problems and the paucity of fit land. Much of the debate reveals social attitudes about and barriers to the capabilities of the deaf.

John J. Flournoy to William Turner

After William Turner, the principal of the American Asylum, gently rejected Flournoy's proposal for a deaf commonwealth, Flournoy sent him the following response. The letter was published in the American Annals of the Deaf and Dumb *in 1856.*

Rev. W. W. Turner;

Rev. and Dear Friend: I am in receipt of your kind favor of the 6th inst., replying to my inquiry of last summer, concerning the feasibility and propriety, in your view, of colonizing some small territory in our country with a population of mutes. Your objections I have duly considered and weighed: and although I accord to them that respect and that deference due from me to your sentiments, still I might confess my want of conviction as yet, unless you would do away with the force of the following observations, predicated as an answer to your remarks. . . .

You will observe that my appeal, circulated among my class of our people, and sent to Europe, did not have intention of persuading the migration of the *entire* deaf population of those regions—but only a portion of them! And it is presumable that there are among them a sufficient number who would agree to emigrate, provided the General Government would do what I clearly laid down, I believe, in those papers: *secure the government and offices of small territory or State, to the mute community!* Neither home, nor parents, nor friends, would or ought to deter a body of enterprising and resolute deaf men from moving to such a possession! We do not ask it as a grant, boon or charity from the government—the ruling powers and legislature have too much grudged us any pittance they have seen their predecessors give in its infancy to the American Asylum at Hartford—but we will pay our pre-emptive right money for the acres, if only guaranteed the control of the commonwealth. That government will give us *such* a prerogative to a State about the size of Rhode Island or Connecticut, I confess I do not feel sanguine enough to hope! But there is nothing like trying. . . .

The old cry about the incapacity of men's minds from physical disabilities, I think it were time, now in this intelligent age, to *explode!* You asked, how could a deaf man legislate and govern among the hearing, any more than a blind man lead an army? (I use your ideas—not your language. The matter is just as I give it.) Did you ever believe lame men, and blind men, and deaf men, when usefulness was in view, were as useless as dumb beasts? Certainly not. Then where does your reasoning limit their capacity? You use a military figure: and I will dwell a little on one. Have you ever heard how Muley Molech had himself borne in a litter, when lamed by wounds, to the head of his legions, and how he vanquished the foe? So much for a *lame* man. Then, as for a *blind* one, such a one as the beggared Belisarius of declining Rome or Byzantium; was such a man of no military moment because sightless? I would myself, if I were contemporary with himself, suggest the Romans that he be provided with a military academy to teach the strategy of war—or be kept on a hill near a battle to direct emergencies, while the seeing faithfully inform him of events. Here then, literally meeting you with your own weapons, is a great blind general made consummate leader, if experienced. But the application of such views to the deaf is not legitimate. We do not claim *all* offices, nor to do *every* thing. But we do attest that we are capable of many of which the prejudice, and sometimes even

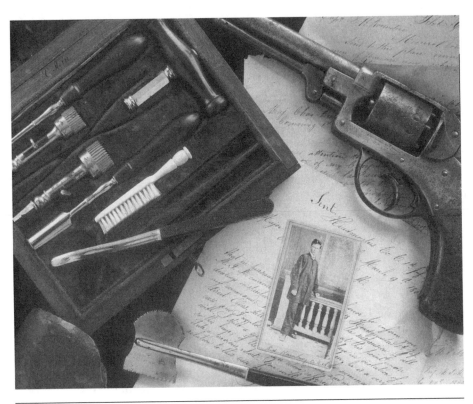

Mementos of soldiers who fought in the U.S. Civil War and surgeon's kit. The surgeon's instrument kit was used by Dr. Charles Stein during the Civil War. Stein served as assistant surgeon to the 57th New York Infantry, known as the "Polish Legion."

Source: Art Resource, New York.

which alone our class of people can attain to the dignity and honor of Human Nature. Else our course is (under the idea that a deaf and dumb man is of little consequence) within the circle of diffident humility. I spurn this imputation of thousands of my hearing *inferiors*—who give the fatness of power and office to their own class—and keep me, like Lazarus, out at the gate of splendid and munificent patronage without sending me a solitary crumb from the table.

Place *me* for an example in any Capitol with Legislative sanctity, and I will move for an *aid,* a hearer and amanuensis, to reveal to me what is said, what to be done, what to do, and to read my speeches. And by this way I can get along supremely well, as Legislator. The gist and gravamen being that my intelligence and judgement may prove better and superior to the hearing majority. So your object about deaf incapacity is answered . . .

Can I then concede that hearing men "are the ones and wisdom shall die with them?" No sir—No. I am to lead—and can only lead where deaf capacity be widely acknowledged. I am not in your estimation, I hope, descending to "fanaticism," or to "peculiarity." *Evasions like these will not do!* Men must think. They must investigate before they feel warranted to traduce sterling persons who are not made to sit down and acquiesce in perfidy to self and to mankind.

That deaf men have not my feelings and ambition, is no reason that they should not find a habitation of their own.

If only in such a State forty deaf men, or even twelve, were found, the constitution guarantying power to them alone, they may rule all the hearing owning continents, encroach on the deaf there. If our children hear, let them go to other States. *This Government is to be sacred to the Deaf alone.* In hearing

malignance of our hearing brethren deprive us!! It were better that Congress had the presence of some blind philosophers to lead the way in legislation, than to have only seeing men without wisdom. The court of the Areopagus, at ancient Athens, blindfolded the judges to prevent prejudice against unprepossessing suitors. And so long as this was the custom, no judicial decision was so faultless as that of these people. So much for your simile in disparagement of the *blind.*

So of the deaf. Many of us have hearts, of an integrity superior to the *mad* hearing partisans that go to Congress and to legislatures, and fill presidential and gubernatorial seats; and when the fact is that some of us are sages, so far as rational views and Christian principles be taken into consideration;—you can not observe that the loss is greatly the country's, in not being able to avail of our supervision, from the prejudices and disparagements of the world about a sense or two!

Advocating, therefore, a formation out West, of a deaf State, I wish to preserve in urging a measure by communities how many children stay with their parents? Do brothers and sisters continue together? How then expect deaf-mutes to be such perpetual children as to claim and assert nothing appertaining to the dignity and grandeur of humanity, but to stick to home.

The idea, therefore, of acquiring a commonwealth for themselves ought not to be abandoned.

You say that deaf persons have privileges among the hearing and can amass wealth. But how tardily, where competition by the auricular is such that no isolated deaf person is able to break through a single web of its massive Free Masonry? The auricular are not satisfied with hearing, nor with the usual mutual sympathies of their own class, but are banded and combined together in associations, open, and societies, secret, until they form a compact moral mechanism, that fairly by their majority, puts us in the shade. I know not how at this day the people of your section comport towards the deaf. But when I was at Hartford, I saw that a tailor (A.S.B.) *disdainfully* repelled away a mute applicant for the post of *foreman* (D.A.S.). Even if it be better for our class *now* in New England, it is far from one-ninety-ninth so, in Georgia, whose Legislature, after my prayer in 1834, granting a deaf education to the mutes here, a few years thereafter, became chagrined at having *honored me,* and though they dared not revoke their education, still they made a law to "*make deaf and dumb persons idiots in law and to provide them guardians.*" Thus in the South we are contemned, spurned, degraded and abhorred, and I see no redemption but in forming a powerful oligarchy of our own to control a State at the West—a Deaf-mute Republic.

We constitutionally allow no foreigner to be President—nationally. We would in that small State allow no hearing man to have any lucrative office. This is all I care about. Its Legislature, Judiciary, &c., all mutes.

A deaf community, once established, to whom only offices are open to Congress and at home, as none others should be eligible—would easily draw mute recipients for the bounty from all sections. Once fixed, I see nothing deterrent.

I fear my letter is quite annoyingly lengthy, and will now close. I have said all I believe necessary to convince you of the propriety of our plan, which will only fail because the deaf and dumb are not worthy of a better destiny, or are as unlike as possible,

Your affectionate and obliged humble servant,
John J. Flournoy

Edmund Booth to John J. Flournoy, 1858

Edmund Booth wrote this response to Flournoy. Although it was not intended for publication, Booth agreed to allow the Annals *to publish it in January 1858, along with a number of other letters on the subject of a deaf commonwealth.*

Dear Sir,
In regard to a community of deaf-mutes in the West, or anywhere—supposing you mean a community exclusively or mainly of mutes—let me say candidly that I hold it to be an impossibility, save in the commencement, and that on a very small scale. Just consider a moment. A community of this class would be a mixture of a few well and many half-educated; and among them must be many non-readers and frivolous. And then the general equality claimed with all by the latter, would operate to keep the more sensible from joining such community; for we all know that gossip, scandal, backbiting and other diabolisms are as common among mutes as among hearing persons.

Again: They will need to work at a variety of trades, and a commonwealth of mutes could never exceed 10,000, supposing all in the U.S. were brought in. A sparsely settled state would make nobody rich, and would satisfy few; and no law could be made effectual to prevent their selling their lands, buildings, &c., to hearing persons. Thus the distinct nature of the community would soon be lost. And it would so happen in any event, for their children being mostly of the hearing order, it would become a hearing community faster than the fathers and mothers died out.

I think the wiser course is to let the mutes remain as they are—scattered and in one sense lost—among their hearing associates. In such situations they are compelled to read and write, and thus keep their minds under the educational process through life.

In reply to your other questions: the country *will* suit them. But in Iowa there is no land unsold or in market, save the railroad lands, which are withdrawn, and they are narrow strips and cannot be obtained save at $2.50 per acre or more, and that at cash down the moment they are brought into market. Speculators have drained Iowa completely of her government lands, with the exceptions as above. Government lands can be obtained in Minnesota, where they are not yet in market, especially in the western part of that territory; but it is too far north and too cold to suit my ideas of a residence. The cold in the West is less than in the same latitude East. For a community of mutes,

Nebraska is almost out of the question. It is mostly a barren country. I speak from observation, having traveled through it from the Missouri river to the South Pass. Iowa is a prairie country. Perhaps one-tenth of it timber. One-twentieth would be nearer the truth. The guide books say one-third or one-fourth. My own observations say one-tenth.

I see no country that would suit your ideas so well as Kansas. But to me the whole scheme looks much like those of other communities formed on the exclusive system, like those of Mons. Cabet, Rapp, &c. They had the incentive of religion and friendship and community of goods, labor and profit. With us it would be otherwise; and we should break through before we had made half a trial.

Yours truly,
E. Booth

Flournoy to Turner, 1858

Flournoy's response appeared with Booth's letter in the same issue of the Annals.

Rev. Mr. Turner:

My dear Friend—This being a free country, where every "smart" man, and his name is legion, has his opinion whether crude or vulgar, or refined and intellectual, the American community are very unquiet and debatable, subject to a thousand though not very learned of profound sentiments, political and social. The deaf and dumb have taken a color of character from this disputatious habit, a specimen of which is evinced in the enclosed letter from Edmund Booth, Esq. Instead of meeting my project with a philosophical view, I am met by objections, some of which, like yours and Mr. Booth's, are truly formidable! It would seem then, that without intending to be the great leader and original mind, I am the chief in this cause, and that if I carry it not forward, the idea of a deaf community may prove abortive as to any practical result.

There is always some objection to every project under the sun, and often very cogent ones. What is a man then to do? Abandon every scheme because impeded by natural and conventional obstacles? Certainly not. Many of the greatest nations have been founded in time by defiance of the untoward predictions of impractible visionaries. Many a costly experiment has been forsaken on no better hypothesis. The invention of the daguerreotype—the photogenic art—was not accidental, but by a design; and persistent,

philosophical chemists began and followed out the plan, until Daguerre, in the final series of the successive experimenters, perfected the science by which our features are in exact copies transmitted to posterity. Resolution and perseverance will accomplish wonders. And I pray God that the deaf and dumb may prove worthy of the name of men.

Mr. Booth thinks the West will not suit the mutes. From his description of the North-west I agree with him in that opinion. His other views have been answered before in the annals and elsewhere.

I do not know what kind of a constitution the mutes may superstruct, whether to make real estate inherent only in the deaf, by that organic law all have to respect and defer to; or in case of default, to escheat to the estate. This, however, is certain, that the *control* of our community over the commonwealth would be strict and universal. This is what we want and for what we may emigrate. *The government of a piece of Territory.* Nothing more or less.

Mr. Booth believes we can do better, and will read more, scattered as we are and "lost" among the hearing. I challenge him to show me twenty deaf-mutes in a hundred, that are constant readers, adequate to comprehending either literature or science, as they now are dispersed among hearing people, who do not read any or much themselves, and who have a sense (auricular) by which they gather in their knowledge, a privilege debarred the deaf, who therefore are the more ignorant *for being thus scattered.* Whereas if convened in a land peculiarly their own, the concentration of reading intellects would set a beneficial example; and preaching and lectures in the sign language, and libraries of suitable books, may improve their minds and hearts, beyond what is attainable in their scattered condition. For this, as a principal cause and source of improvement, this colony is a desideratum.

But the difficulty that meets me on all sides is, how can you keep up the mute population? The children of deaf parents are mostly hearing. These will inherit property and the community will not endure. This reasoning seems to take it that our society is to be organized like that of the hearing, and to be modeled upon the same principles. Now there is no such thing. I acknowledge that the hearing children of deaf parents may not inherit land in that anomalous and contracted community—neither power nor patronage. But the other States are so near, and their parents may supply them with the means to buy real estate in them. When they have a good location, the mutes would come in from all parts of the world. An Asylum for their education may be founded there, as well as other Institutions, so that there will be no lacking of the deaf *materiel*. What then of this visionary difficulty! We will allow such hearing persons as come for trade or residence, to vote with us. *We would give woman that right.* Hence we may always possess sufficient population to be a State. But even if this be futile, we can remain a Territory of the Federal Government and enjoy its powerful protection under Omnipotence; the General Government guaranteeing to us the peculiar Constitution we may devise: "Republican in form."

If mutes *cannot* do this they are justly held as inferior and *useless* in the world. For they ought not to pretend to be "any body" among hearing men, who do what deaf "dogs" shrink from achieving *alone*. But we are men, and have under god only to try, and the thing is a finished work!

After this argument, which if published I hope may satisfy the overscrupulous, I would approach the great point that is before us. I think we can acquire territory enough from the Cherokees or other red men, West of Arkansas, and *very cheaply,* on which to make our experiment, or else from the State of Maine. Perhaps some one of the New England, Northern or Middle States may grant space enough for this purpose. I myself prefer the Indian Territory, if the U.S. government would sanction and aid a cession. Hence, no fear about trade and business. Capital will accumulate in our hands when our skill and industry are concentrated, and our ruling prerogative unimpeachable. Whereas now, in their scattered condition, especially in the Middle and Southern States, few deaf men have employment of respectability, and their ignorance is "stereotyped," as I have shown, by their unfortunate and dispersed situation, without preaching or any instruction whatsoever. When combined, competition and a sense of high duty and responsibility will cause them to study books, documents, and men and things, and like other communities we shall produce men of intellectual predominance.

Even should the contemplated colony fail, as Mr. Booth predicts, one great utility to ourselves will have been derived from a practical experience. We shall have proved to the other nations and our own, that a deaf and dumb people are capable of many things; and to our successors in misfortune, offices and employment may be opened. They may be treated as men and women of *some use* to society and to the country, and respected accordingly. And this will to us be no inconsiderable triumph; and the victory sure, as the deaf now continues to prove this competency and fidelity in lands and other trusts. And this, we, as accountable beings, who may not bury our talent in a napkin, owe to the long and harmless line of the "pantomimic generations" that are to come after us!

I have now fully, I hope, in attempting something like a reply to Mr. Booth, given what refutation I am able, to the many objects that are ever starting up to confound this project. I hope the Annals will embrace both Mr. Booth's letter and mine. I presume that invaluable periodical will devote some space to this discussion, as relating so closely to the welfare and interests of the community, to whose benefit it is so inseparately devoted.

> I am, dear sir, truly and respectfully,
> your most obliged, obedient, humble servant,
>
> J. J. Flournoy

Source: Krentz, Christopher, ed. 2002. *An Anthology of Deaf American Writing, 1816–1864.* Washington, DC: Gallaudet University Press.

Rebecca Davis, from "Life in the Iron Mills" (1861)

Davis's stories of immigrant workers' lives in hellish industrial settings highlighted the harsh physical toll of mill work and unrelenting poverty. In this scene, the ever-weary Deborah's eyes are emphasized as pale, watery, bleared, and glazed. "Stupor and vacancy" have made her face seem older and more apathetic; elsewhere in the narrative, we see her twisted spine and ghostly pale complexion as well. Hugh Wolfe, also mentioned in this extract, is another Davis character whose body and artistic talents are wasted by deprivation and overexertion.

She watched him eat with a painful eagerness. With a woman's quick instinct, she saw that he was not hungry,—was eating to please her. Her pale, watery eyes began to gather a strange light.

"Is't good, Hugh? T'ale was a bit sour, I feared."

"No, good enough." He hesitated a moment. "Ye're tired, poor lass! Bide here till I go. Lay down on that heap of ash, and go to sleep."

He threw her an old coat for a pillow, and turned to his work. The heap was the refuse of the burnt iron, and was not a hard bed; the half-smothered warmth, too, penetrated her limbs, dulling their pain and cold shiver.

Miserable enough she looked, lying there on the ashes like a limp, dirty rag,—yet not an unfitting figure to crown the scene of hopeless discomfort and veiled crime: more fitting, if one looked deeper into the heart of things,—at her thwarted woman's form, her colorless life, her walking stupor that smothered pain and hunger,—even more fit to be a type of her class. Deeper yet if one could look, was there nothing worth reading in this wet, faded thing, half-covered with ashes? no story of a soul filled with groping passionate love, heroic unselfishness, fierce jealousy? of years of weary trying to please the one human being whom she loved, to gain one look of real heart-kindness from him? If anything like this were hidden beneath the pale, bleared eyes, and dull, washed-out-looking face, no one had ever taken the time to read their signs: not the half-clothed furnace-tender, Wolfe, certainly. Yet he was kind to her; it was his nature to be kind, even to the very rats that swarmed in the cellar; kind to her in just the same way. She knew that. And it might be that very knowledge that had given to her face its apathy and vacancy more than her low, torpid life. One sees that dead, vacant look steal sometimes over the rarest, finest of the women's faces,—in the very midst, it may be, of their warmest summer's day; and then one can guess at the secret of intolerable solitude that lies hidden beneath the delicate laces and brilliant smile. There was no warmth, no brilliancy, no summer for this woman; so the stupor and vacancy had time to gnaw into her face perpetually. She was young, too, though no one guessed it; so the gnawing was the fiercer.

She lay quiet in the dark corner, listening, through the monotonous din and uncertain glare of the works, to the dull plash of the rain in the far distance,—shrinking back whenever the man Wolfe happened to look towards her. She knew, in spite of all his kindness, that there was that in her face and form which made him loathe the sight of her. She felt by instinct, although she could not comprehend it, the finer nature of the man, which made him among his fellow-workmen something unique, set apart. She knew, that, down under all the vileness and coarseness of his life, there was a groping passion for whatever was beautiful and pure,—that his soul sickened with disgust for her deformity, even when his words were kindest. Through this dull consciousness, which never left her, came, like a sting, the recollection of the little Irish girl she had left in the cellar. The recollection struck through even her stupid intellect with a vivid glow of beauty and of grace. Little Janey, timid, helpless, clinging to Hugh as her only friend: that was the sharp thought, the bitter thought, that drove into the glazed eyes a fierce light of pain. You laugh at it? Are pain and jealousy less savage realities down here in this place I am taking you to than in your own house, or your own heart, your heart, which they clutch at sometimes? The note is the same, I fancy, be the octave high or low.

If you could go into this mill where Deborah lay, and drag out from the hearts of these men the terrible tragedy of their lives, taking it as a symptom of the disease of their class, no ghost Horror would terrify you more. A reality of soul starvation, of living death, that meets you every day under the besotted faces on the street—I can paint nothing of this, only give you the outside outlines of a night, a crisis in the life of one man: whatever muddy depth of a soul-history lies beneath you can read according to the eyes God has given you.

Source: Davis, Rebecca. 1861. "Life in the Iron Mills." *Atlantic Monthly.* Available at: http://www.worldwideschool.org/library/books/lit/socialcommentary/LifeintheIron-Mills/Chap1.html

Edouard Séguin, *Idiocy: And Its Treatment by the Physiological Method* (1866)

After his successful work in France developing training programs for those diagnosed as idiots, Séguin moved to the United States. He became an influential figure in the institutionalization movement of the nineteenth century and developed a theory that idiocy resulted from a lack of control over the will. In order to counter this "deficiency," Séguin advocated physical exercise and concentration-based tasks that asked individuals to master their bodies through programs of self-hygiene.

Synonyms.—Named by Savage, *Amentia;* by Segar, *Imbecillitas ingenii;* by Vogel, *Fatuitas ingenii;* by Linnaeus, *Morosis;* by Cullen and Fodéré, *Demence innée;* by Willis, *Stupiditas;* by Pinel, *Idiotism;* by some English writers, *Idiotcy;* by Esquirol and the majority of Encyclopædias and dictionaries, *Idiocy.*

We shall use this latter term to express the physiological infirmity; and would like to see the name given to it by Pinel, Idiotism, preserved to express the specific condition of mind pertaining to idiocy.

Its definitions have been so numerous, they are so different one from the other, and they have so little bearing on the treatment, that their omission cannot be much felt in a practical treatise. Our own, if objectionable, will be found at least to correspond to a plan of treatment, both supporting each other; and may suffice until a better definition and a better treatment can be devised.

Idiocy is a specific infirmity of the cranio-spinal axis, produced by deficiency of nutrition in utero and neo-nati. It incapacitates mostly the functions which give rise to the reflex, instinctive, and conscious phenomena of life; consequently, the idiot moves, feels, understands, wills, but imperfectly; does nothing, thinks of nothing, cares for nothing (extreme cases), he is a minor legally irresponsible; isolated, without associations; a soul shut up in imperfect organs, an innocent.

The *modus operandi* of deficiency of nutrition in the first period of life has not yet been fully investigated; it may bear upon all the tissues, but we are concerned here mostly with its actions on the nervous system.

At the time when deficiency of nutrition takes place it stops the foetal progress, and gives permanency to the transitory type through which the foetus was passing; these transient types being to some extent analogous to the persistent forms of the lower animals. For instance, *atresia palpebrarum* testifies to the presence of the cause of arrest of development as far back as the third month of gestation; arrest of development of the inter-auricular septum leaves the human heart homologous with the heart of fishes; similar early arrest of nutrition of the encephalon leaves its circumvolutions unfinished at the low types of the orang-outang, the calf, or even lower. After the time at which deficiency of nutrition has stopped the ascending evolution of the embryo at one of its low types, it sometimes continues its deleterious action of altering, or entirely destroying the foetus also. For instance, it may destroy one of two foetuses for the nutrition of the other, leaving next to the spared one an acephalus, or only a few fragments of an organized being; or it may partially destroy an encephalon at any stage of development, even after birth, by the intervening of hydrocephalus; or it may give rise to some embryonic malady, destructive of a set of organs or of functions. Though the deficiency of nutrition may affect the whole being, it strikes by preference one set of organs, such as those of speech, of hearing, of local contractility. Deficiency of nutrition happens in two ways; slowly, when induced by depressing influences; or at once, when brought on by a shock. Hence, the first leaves the child a prey to maladies of embryonic origin, or at best at a low point of vitality; the other leaves him well provided for by anterior nutrition, but torpid, or prey to automatism, epilepsy, etc.

Nothing hinders us now from entering into the study of the physiological symptoms after having taken a rapid survey of the infant born idiotic, or predisposed to idiocy.

The only thing which could tempt us to form a diagnosis when the child is just born, is the often monstrous shape exhibited by the head. But it is so difficult to appreciate what part of it is due to deficiency of nutrition or to transitory compressions from maneuvres or instruments; and the head is endowed with such a power of reaction and self-modulation against these transient deformities, that we had better let it receive its own finishing touch before venturing on the expression of a judgement upon its unfinished state. But after the first cries, the child shuts himself up into a chrysalid life. He is rosy and rather puffy, or greyish and shrivelled in his loose integuments, according to his general health. For a time nothing more of him may be foreseen than is seen. Even a few months later, if the mother, feeling her baby without reaction in her embrace, seized with a secret presentiment, seeks for advice, the physician rarely happens to see him otherwise than nursing and sleeping. He has scarcely the chance to notice the head hanging back, or rolled on the pillow automatically, the eyes unlighted and playing the pendulum in their sockets, fixed, or upward or sideways; the difficulty of swallowing the milk once drawn in the mouth; the absence of voice or its animal sounds; the inability of the spine to support the body; the flaccidity of the legs; the hands closed, thumbs inward, by the side instead of coming out from the cradle to take with a firm grasp their share of this world.

In the midst of this uncertainty, profuse salivation, involuntary excretions, imperfect sensations or disordered movements appear daily more settled, instead of the opposite abilities vainly expected. Or after a fall, a blow, exposure to cold, isolation, prolonged successions, fright, or in the period of teething, coma sets in or convulsions appear. After which some function of the reflex or voluntary order, motor or sensitive, is impaired. But the commotion of the cerebro-spinal axis may be temporary or prolonged, producing more convulsions, deeper coma, other incapacitations; throwing the little sufferer far behind his fellows, or leaving him a confirmed idiot. Between these two extremes the majority of young idiots do not differ very sensibly from common babies; because the power of both may be expressed by the same verb, they cannot. But tomorrow the well infant will use his hands, the idiot will allow his to hang in half flexion; the first will move his head at will, the second will toss it about; the look of the former penetrates every day farther than the domain of the touch, that of the latter has no straight dart, and wanders from the inner to the outer canthus; the one will set erect on his spine, the other shall remain recumbent where left, the first will laugh in your face with a contagious will, the second shall not be moved into an intellectual or social expression by any provocation whatever. And each day carves more deeply the differential characters of both; not by making the idiot worse, unless from bad habits gotten by neglect, but by the hourly progress of the other. Idiocy so viewed from its origin is a continuance of the isolation and helplessness of babyhood under ampler forms and obsolete proportions. Compared unavoidably with children of his age, the idiot seems to grow worse every day; his tardy improvement looking like backward steps. With his incapacity of action, of expression, of feeling, he makes a sickening sight indeed by the side of a bright child entering into the intricacies of life as on an open play-ground.

At this stage there can be no mistake; we see plainly what he is, and we can describe what we see. This is the time when the study of the physiological symptoms will make up for the deficiency of the anatomo-pathological ones.

The functions of organic life are generally below the normal standard. The respiration is not deep; the pulse is without resistance. The appetite is sometimes quite anormal in its objects or limited to a few things, rarely voracious, though it looks so, owing to the unconventional or decidedly animal modes of eating and drinking of these children. The swallowing of the food without being masticated, only rolled up in saliva, resumes many of these imperfections which are to be attributed in variable proportions to absence of intelligence, want of action of the will on the organs of mastication and deglutition, deformity of and want of relation between the same. As might be expected,

imperfect chewing produces on them, as on other children, unpleasant effects, but no more. Their excretions cannot be said to present any dissimilarity from those of others which our senses can discriminate; only their sebaceous matters are as different from ours as ours are from those of the variously colored races, or from those emitted in most diseases.

The functions of animal life, or of relation, are generally affected in idiocy; either by perversion, diminution, or suppression. We shall begin the study of these anomalies in the organs whose contractility has for object the movement of displacement and prehension.

The incapacity of walking, and of prehending objects, to whatever degree it exists, gives the measure of the isolation of the idiot. He is isolated because he cannot possess himself of those which come in the range of his imperfect grasp; he is double immured in his muscular infirmity. The same motor function may exist, but escaping the control of the will, it produces movements more or less disordered, mechanical, spasmodic, or automatic. Disordered, when their want of harmony prevents the accomplishment of their object; mechanical, when their recurrence, in the course of other normal movements, cannot be otherwise produced or prevented, but can hardly be postponed by a superior influence; spasmodic, when they proceed from an accessory condition of the nerves congener to chorea or epilepsy; automatic, when they consist in the continuity or frequent recurrence of a single unavoidable gesture, without object or meaning. The simple disorder of movements involves a waste of nervous power, disabling, more or less, the child for useful activity, but not depriving him of it entirely. The mechanism throws, unexpectedly, some instinctive jerk or motion in the midst of well-regulated actions. The spasmodism accompanies all actions, as in chorea, or substitutes itself at times for all the normal acts, as in epileptic seizures. The automatism acts as a substitute for all, or nearly all other modes of contractility; it incapacitates more and more the child's muscular power for any useful purposes; and, as a sorry compensation, furnishes him with a supply of involuntary instead of voluntary exercise. Of the four anormal ways of expending uselessly and unwillingly the contractile force allotted to the muscular system, automatism is the most tenacious, when, for years past, no physiological action has been induced by proper training in its stead.

Idiocy affects the body in its general habits, as bending forward, throwing the head backward, moving it in a rotatory manner which seems impossible, swinging the body to and fro, or in a sort of sideway roll.

The following are examples of another kind of hyperæsthesia: some of our children will be unable to touch anything, but with the delicacy of the humming-bird, and seem to suffer greatly from any other mode of contact imposed upon the hands. The feet of others are so much affected with similar exaltation of sensibility, that the thinnest shoes pain them, and the contact of the softest carpet or floor makes them recoil or advance, as if they could not help it, and as if walking on live coals. The hands of one child will move with prestidigitative briskness without apparent object, single or interlaced, to intercept some rays of light falling obliquely into their vacant eyes. Other hands, affected with disorder of the touch, without obvious complication, are caressed, sucked, bitten, till the blood starts, or a heavy callus is formed to protect them; others are constantly bathed in saliva, and their skin nearly resembles that of the washer-woman; these hands feel, out of the mouth like fish out of water. We could multiply these examples of anomalies of sensation, single or double, merely tactile or altogether tactile and contractile, by which the hand is robbed of its powers as an instrument of touch, as well as of prehension.

Setting aside these localized tactile disorders, general sensibility proper is dull in idiots, who are soon benumbed by cold and less affected by heat, but much prostrated by the atmospheric modifications of a thunder-storm.

With them the Taste and Smell are oftener indifferent than anormal. Rarely we see them have a taste for non-alimentary substances, or an exclusive appetence for one kind of food. Some of them, without swallowing, chew beads, suck pieces of broken china, etc., with apparent relish. The smell may take possession of the same articles and scent them for hours, or delight in the fragrance of two pieces of silex, stricken one against the other; or, this sense may substitute itself for any other, as a means of discrimination and knowledge; or, on the contrary, be dead-like to all intent and appearance. But the difference between the errors of function of these two senses is, that the taste is oftener depraved, and the smell is more frequently exalted.

The Hearing is sometimes so passive and limited, and the intellectual wants so disinterested to the noises transmitted to the ear, that the idiot, though possessed of perfect organs of audition, is practically deaf, and, of course, mute; no deafness, and yet no hearing. Therefore, it is prudent to remember that next to the deafness from birth, or from infantile diseases, there is an intellectual deafness from idiocy; the only one which we shall specially consider. In this interesting condition the child may hear, and even audit the sound of objects that he knows and wishes for, and none other. For instance, he hears music, and no articulated voices; or he may retain and repeat tunes, and not be able to hear or repeat a single word. He may even, in extreme cases, be absolutely indifferent, and, consequently, appear really insensible to sounds; and then the diagnosis has to be postponed till the state of the organ and function is thoroughly ascertained by an experimental training of that sense. So far, he is practically deaf and mute, but is not so organically. This difficult point in diagnosis has caused many mistakes.

The Sight may be as badly and more ostentatiously impaired than the hearing. Be it fixed in one canthus, be it wandering and unfixable, be it glossy, laughing, like a picture moving behind a motionless varnish, be it dull and immured to images, its meanings are not doubtful; it means idiocy. Our expressions here would be very incorrect if they conveyed the idea that these defects of vision prevent the child from seeing. The images being printed on their passing into the ocular chamber, as the river-side scenery is on the passing current, the child, when he pays an accidental attention, gets a notion of some of them, but the transitory perception produced thereby can hardly serve him for educational purposes. The principal characters of this infirmity are, the repugnance of the child to look and the incapacity of his will to control the organs of vision; he sees by chance, but never looks. These defects of the sight, when grave, are always connected with automatic motions, and both oppose serious obstacles to progress; one by the ease with which the child can use his negative will to prevent the training of his eyes, the other by depriving him of all knowledge to be acquired farther than the touch can reach. This complication makes a child look very unfavorably indeed, and increases much the task of his teacher.

Some idiots are deprived of speech, that is to say, do not pronounce a word. Some, speaking a few words more or less connected in sentences, have yet no language; for the word language conveys with it the meaning of interchange of ideas. In this acceptation, language does not belong to idiots before they are educated, nor to those who are but imperfectly so, and consequently, they have a speech more or less limited, but no language: strictly speaking, speech represents the function, language the faculty.

When we come to examine the anomalies of the speech, as here defined, it is well to exclude, previously, the many organic disorders which may interfere with it as a function, and which have nothing to do with idiocy but as an external impediment and exogenous aggravation. For, because a child is idiotic, it does not necessarily follow that his organs of perceiving speech and of expressing language may not be impaired by some independent affection. Idiotic or intelligent, a child may be deprived of hearing, or of the movements necessary to form the speech, directly by malformation or paralysis, or indirectly by the many causes producing deafness. These are the causes of the organic mutism which must never be attributed to idiocy, but which too often aggravates it.

To substantiate in a few words the causes of the functional mutism derived from idiocy, we point out, first, the incapacity of the will to move the organs; second, the long silence in which idiots have confirmed their mutism, like prisoners have gotten theirs in protracted confinement; third, the absence of persevering and intelligent efforts of their friends to make them speak; fourth, the want of desire to exercise that function, and the want of understanding of the power of speech as a faculty.

In this wreck of powers, one human, irresistible tendency or impulse is left him; for as low as we find him, lower than the brute in regard to activity and intelligence, he has, as the great, the lowly, the privileged, the millions, his hobby or amulet that no animal has: the external thing toward which his human, centrifugal power gravitates; if it be only a broken piece of china, a thread, a rag, an unseizable ray of the sun, he shall spend his life in admiring, kissing, catching, polishing, sucking it, according to what it may be. Till we take away that amulet, as Moses took it from his people, we must have something to substitute for it. This worship or occupation shows that if the idiot can form, of himself, no other connexion with the world, he is ready to do so if we only know how to help him.

That the idiot is endowed with a moral nature, no one who has had the happiness of ministering to him will deny. Epileptic, paralytic, choreic, or imbecile children will often strike or bite their mother or affectionate attendant. If any idiot is found doing the same (and we never found any) he must have been taught it by some cruel treatment imposed upon him. In general,

as soon as his mind is opened to reflection, the tender family feelings are so deep in him that they often interfere with his successful transplantation into the broader and richer ground of our public institutions. It is true that his habits are sad, droll, or repulsive; that his doings are often worse than none; but these manifestations exhibit as much the carelessness and want of intelligence of the parents or keepers as they do the primary character of the infirmity. Does not the idiot, in making his silly gestures, tacitly say, "See what I am doing; if you knew how to teach me better and more I would do it." It is true, that previous to being educated, the slightest work is too much for him, and makes him recoil; but if we succeed in making him believe that he has accomplished a real object, emulation will appear and shed a ray of satisfaction over his face. He is sensible to eulogy, reproach, command, menace, even to imaginary punishment; he sympathizes with the pains he can understand; he loves those who love him; he tries to please those who please him; his sense of duty and propriety is limited, but perfect in its kind; his egotism is moderate; his possessive and retentive propensities sufficient; his courage, if not Samsonian, is not aggressive, and may easily be cultivated. As a collective body, idiotic children are, in their institutions, equal in order and decency, in true lovingness, if not in loveliness, to any collection of children in the land. Their moral powers are influenced by isolation, company, multitude, silence, turmoil, music, human eloquence, as they are in all masses of mankind. If we are asked how we pretend to see all these good and promising dispositions in the unfortunate subject whom we have depicted as more or less motionless, speechless and repulsive, we can affirm that the idiot, even when neglected in his lowest conditions, does not manifest any character contrary to the one here described; a character which we have seen him assume, steadily and uniformly, under the influence of a proper training, and, as we firmly believe, in virtue of his own moral nature: he is one of us in mankind, but shut up in an imperfect envelope.

Therefore, we must not confound with imbeciles, insanes, epileptics, etc., the harmless idiot, sitting awkwardly, bashful, or at least reserved on our approach. He will answer us if he can, rarely mistaking, never deceiving, but often times failing to understand. His mind is extremely limited but not deranged and with no special tendency to final insanity. He has been hurt often, but he never assailed anybody; he loves quiet places and arrangements; repeated monotonous sounds, or stillness, and above all plain and familiar faces; he has a look, not of envy at things and persons, but of abstraction, gazing far out of this world into a something which neither we nor he can discern.

How could any child, subject to other disease or infirmity, be mistaken for him? Nevertheless this confusion takes place. Practically and legally, the idiot has been assimilated to unfortunate beings whose rights upon society are different from his; and he has suffered deeply by the mistake.

The child nearest akin to an idiot is called simply backward, in French *enfant arrière,* his character may be better delineated by comparison with the idiot, who presents even in superficial cases, an arrest of development, whilst the feeble-minded child is only retarded in his. The idiot has disordinate movements, cannot use his hands, swings his body in walking, presents some sensorial vices or incapacity; on the other hand, the backward child is free from any disordered activity, uses his hands naturally but with very little effectiveness, walks without defect, but without firmness or elasticity, presents no sensorial anomaly but does not much use his senses to quicken his sluggish comprehension; when the idiot does not seem to make any progress, and when the ordinary child improves in the ratio of ten, the backward child improves only in that of one, two, three, or five. This child may be, and is in fact, actually educated with the confirmed idiot; and there is no inconvenience, but advantage, in their being treated alike.

The same could not be said of the following case which is now as rarely met among idiots, as it frequently was thirty years ago in the *"hospices"* and poor-houses. He looks dignified, sad, depressed, wistful, immovable, idiotic—but worse than an idiot, he is a dement. There does not seem to be a sensible difference between them, but idiocy is accompanied by some sensorial disorders, begins young, by its worst symptoms, and generally ends quite early; whilst dementia commences in later life, is accompanied by an insidious touch of paralysis, especially of the sphincters; it soon alters the alæ nasi and the external auditory apparatus, and eventually may continue to a great age, ending by its worst symptoms.

A young lad who looks and stands like an idiot, with deep, dull eyes, hollow cheeks, thin hanging hands, flesh gone from his long, lank limbs, and empty frame; a prey to fever, languor, inappetence; tired of everything, forgetting instead of learning, avoiding company and light, sleepless yet never wide awake, speech embarrassed, mind absent, hope, gayety, cheerfulness, friendship, love future, all given up for the worship of one's self, and of a few apparitions evoked by the mania of self-destruction; his tendency is toward early death, through imbecility or dementia.

Source: Seguin, Edouard. 1866. Pp. 39–77 in *Idiocy: And Its Treatment by the Physiological Method.* New York: William Wood and Company.

Karl Marx, from *Capital* (1867)

In Marx's famous analysis of capitalism, he uses disability both to impugn the character of the typical capitalist and also to demonstrate the degree to which unchecked manufacturing practices produce disability in the worker's body.

Part 4, Chapter 14, Section 5. The Capitalistic Character of Manufacture

An increased number of labourers under the control of one capitalist is the natural starting-point, as well of co-operation generally, as of manufacture in particular. But the division of labour in manufacture makes this increase in the number of workmen a technical necessity. The minimum number that any given capitalist is bound to employ is here prescribed by the previously established division of labour. On the other hand, the advantages of further division are obtainable only by adding to the number of workmen, and this can be done only by adding multiples of the various detail groups. But an increase in the variable component of the capital employed necessitates an increase in its constant component, too, in the workshops, implements, &c., and, in particular, in the raw material, the call for which grows quicker than the number of workmen. The quantity of it consumed in a given time, by a given amount of labour, increases in the same ratio as does the productive power of that labour in consequence of its division. Hence, it is a law, based on the very nature of manufacture, that the minimum amount of capital, which is bound to be in the hands of each capitalist, must keep increasing; in other words, that the transformation into capital of the social means of production and subsistence must keep extending.

In manufacture, as well as in simple co-operation, the collective working organism is a form of existence of capital. The mechanism that is made up of numerous individual detail labourers belongs to the capitalist. Hence, the productive power resulting from a combination of labours appears to be the productive power of capital. Manufacture proper not only subjects the previously independent workman to the discipline and command of capital, but, in addition, creates a hierarchic gradation of the workmen themselves. While simple co-operation leaves the mode of working by the individual for the most part unchanged, manufacture thoroughly revolutionises it, and seizes labour-power by its very roots. It converts the labourer into a crippled monstrosity, by forcing his detail dexterity at the expense of a world of productive capabilities and instincts; just as in the States of La Plata they butcher a whole beast for the sake of his hide or his tallow. Not only is the detail work distributed to the different individuals, but the individual himself is made the automatic motor of a fractional operation, and the absurd fable of Menenius Agrippa, which makes man a mere fragment of his own body, becomes realised. If, at first, the workman sells his labour-power to capital, because the material means of producing a commodity fail him, now his very labour-power refuses its services unless it has been sold to capital. Its functions can be exercised only in an environment that exists in the workshop of the capitalist after the sale. By nature unfitted to make anything independently, the manufacturing labourer develops productive activity as a mere appendage of the capitalist's workshop. As the chosen people bore in their features the sign manual of Jehovah, so division of labour brands the manufacturing workman as the property of capital.

The knowledge, the judgement, and the will, which, though in ever so small a degree, are practised by the independent peasant or handicraftsman, in the same way as the savage makes the whole art of war consist in the exercise of his personal cunning these faculties are now required only for the workshop as a whole. Intelligence in production expands in one direction, because it vanishes in many others. What is lost by the detail labourers, is concentrated in the capital that employs them. It is a result of the division of labour in manufactures, that the labourer is brought face to face with the intellectual potencies of the material process of production, as the property of another, and as a ruling power. This separation begins in simple co-operation, where the capitalist represents to the single workman, the oneness and the will of the associated labour. It is developed in manufacture which cuts down the labourer into a detail labourer.

It is completed in modern industry, which makes science a productive force distinct from labour and presses it into the service of capital.

In manufacture, in order to make the collective labourer, and through him capital, rich in social productive power, each labourer must be made poor in individual productive powers. "Ignorance is the mother of industry as well as of superstition. Reflection and fancy are subject to err; but a habit of moving the hand or the foot is independent of either. Manufactures, accordingly, prosper most where the mind is least consulted, and where the workshop may . . . be considered as an engine, the parts of which are men." As a matter of fact, some few manufacturers in the middle of the 18th century preferred, for certain operations that were trade secrets, to employ half-idiotic persons.

"The understandings of the greater part of men," says Adam Smith, "are necessarily formed by their ordinary employments. The man whose whole life is spent in performing a few simple operations . . . has no occasion to exert his understanding. . . . He generally becomes as stupid and ignorant as it is possible for a human creature to become." After describing the stupidity of the detail labourer he goes on: "The uniformity of his stationary life naturally corrupts the courage of his mind. . . . It corrupts even the activity of his body and renders him incapable of exerting his strength with vigour and perseverance in any other employments than that to which he has been bred. His dexterity at his own particular trade seems in this manner to be acquired at the expense of his intellectual, social, and martial virtues. But in every improved and civilised society, this is the state into which the labouring poor, that is, the great body of the people, must necessarily fall." For preventing the complete deterioration of the great mass of the people by division of labour, A. Smith recommends education of the people by the State, but prudently, and in homeopathic doses. G. Garnier, his French translator and commentator, who, under the first French Empire, quite naturally developed into a senator, quite as naturally opposes him on this point. Education of the masses, he urges, violates the first law of the division of labour, and with it "our whole social system would be proscribed." "Like all other divisions of labour," he says, "that between hand labour and head labour is more pronounced and decided in proportion as society (he rightly uses this word, for capital, landed property and their State) becomes richer. This division of labour, like every other, is an effect of past, and a cause of future progress . . . ought the government then to work in opposition to this division of labour, and to hinder its natural course? Ought it to expend a part of the public money in the attempt to confound and blend together two classes of labour, which are striving after division and separation?"

Some crippling of body and mind is inseparable even from division of labour in society as a whole. Since, however, manufacture carries this social separation of branches of labour much further, and also, by its peculiar division, attacks the individual at the very roots of his life, it is the first to afford the materials for, and to give a start to, industrial pathology.

"To subdivide a man is to execute him, if he deserves the sentence, to assassinate him if he does not. . . . The subdivision of labour is the assassination of a people."

Part 4, Chapter 15, Section 9. The Factory Acts. Sanitary and Educational Clauses of the Same. Their General Extension in England

Factory legislation, that first conscious and methodical reaction of society against the spontaneously developed form of the process of production, is, as we have seen, just as much the necessary product of modern industry as cotton yarn, self-actors, and the electric telegraph. Before passing to the consideration of the extension of that legislation in England, we shall shortly notice certain clauses contained in the Factory Acts, and not relating to the hours of work.

Apart from their wording, which makes it easy for the capitalist to evade them, the sanitary clauses are extremely meagre, and, in fact, limited to provisions for whitewashing the walls, for insuring cleanliness in some other matters, for ventilation, and for protection against dangerous machinery. In the third book we shall return again to the fanatical opposition of the masters to those clauses which imposed upon them a slight expenditure on appliances for protecting the limbs of their workpeople, an opposition that throws a fresh and glaring light on the Free-trade dogma, according to which, in a society with conflicting interests, each individual necessarily furthers the common weal by seeking nothing but his own personal advantage! One example is enough. The reader knows that during the last 20 years, the flax industry has very much extended, and that, with that extension, the number of scutching mills in Ireland has increased. In

1864 there were in that country 1,800 of these mills. Regularly in autumn and winter women and "young persons," the wives, sons, and daughters of the neighbouring small farmers, a class of people totally unaccustomed to machinery, are taken from field labour to feed the rollers of the scutching mills with flax. The accidents, both as regards number and kind, are wholly unexampled in the history of machinery. In one scutching mill, at Kildinan, near Cork, there occurred between 1852 and 1856, six fatal accidents and sixty mutilations; every one of which might have been prevented by the simplest appliances, at the cost of a few shillings. Dr. W. White, the certifying surgeon for factories at Downpatrick, states in his official report, dated the 15th December, 1865: "The serious accidents at the scutching mills are of the most fearful nature. In many cases a quarter of the body is torn from the trunk, and either involves death, or a future of wretched incapacity and suffering. The increase of mills in the country will, of course, extend these dreadful results, and it will be a great boon if they are brought under the legislature. I am convinced that by proper supervision of scutching mills a vast sacrifice of life and limb would be averted."

What could possibly show better the character of the capitalist mode of production, than the necessity that exists for forcing upon it, by Acts of Parliament, the simplest appliances for maintaining cleanliness and health? In the potteries the Factory Act of 1864 "has whitewashed and cleansed upwards of 200 workshops, after a period of abstinence from any such cleaning, in many cases of 20 years, and in some, entirely," (this is the "abstinence" of the capitalist!) "in which were employed 27,800 artisans, hitherto breathing through protracted days and often nights of labour, a mephitic atmosphere, and which rendered an otherwise comparatively innocuous occupation, pregnant with disease and death. The Act has improved the ventilation very much." At the same time, this portion of the Act strikingly shows that the capitalist mode of production, owing to its very nature, excludes all rational improvement beyond a certain point. It has been stated over and over again that the English doctors are unanimous in declaring that where the work is continuous, 500 cubic feet is the very least space that should be allowed for each person. Now, if the Factory Acts, owing to their compulsory provisions, indirectly hasten on the conversion of small workshops into factories, thus indirectly attacking the proprietary rights of the smaller capitalists, and assuring a monopoly to the great ones, so, if it were made obligatory to provide the proper space for each workman in every workshop, thousands of small employers would, at one full swoop, be expropriated directly! The very root of the capitalist mode of production, i.e., the self-expansion of all capital, large or small, by means of the "free" purchase and consumption of labour-power, would be attacked. Factory legislation is therefore brought to a deadlock before these 500 cubic feet of breathing space. The sanitary officers, the industrial inquiry commissioners, the factory inspectors, all harp, over and over again, upon the necessity for those 500 cubic feet, and upon the impossibility of wringing them out of capital. They thus, in fact, declare that consumption and other lung diseases among the workpeople are necessary conditions to the existence of capital.

Paltry as the education clauses of the Act appear on the whole, yet they proclaim elementary education to be an indispensable condition to the employment of children. The success of those clauses proved for the first time the possibility of combining education and gymnastics with manual labour, and, consequently, of combining manual labour with education and gymnastics. The factory inspectors soon found out by questioning the schoolmasters, that the factory children, although receiving only one half the education of the regular day scholars, yet learnt quite as much and often more. "This can be accounted for by the simple fact that, with only being at school for one half of the day, they are always fresh, and nearly always ready and willing to receive instruction. The system on which they work, half manual labour, and half school, renders each employment a rest and a relief to the other; consequently, both are far more congenial to the child, than would be the case were he kept constantly at one. It is quite clear that a boy who has been at school all the morning, cannot (in hot weather particularly) cope with one who comes fresh and bright from his work." Further information on this point will be found in Senior's speech at the Social Science Congress at Edinburgh in 1863. He there shows, amongst other things, how the monotonous and uselessly long school hours of the children of the upper and middle classes, uselessly add to the labour of the teacher, "while he not only fruitlessly but absolutely injuriously, wastes the time, health, and energy of the children." From the Factory system budded, as Robert Owen has shown us in detail, the germ of the education of the future, an education that will,

in the case of every child over a given age, combine productive labour with instruction and gymnastics, not only as one of the methods of adding to the efficiency of production, but as the only method of producing fully developed human beings.

Modern Industry, as we have seen, sweeps away by technical means the manufacturing division of labour, under which each man is bound hand and foot for life to a single detail-operation. At the same time, the capitalistic form of that industry reproduces this same division of labour in a still more monstrous shape; in the factory proper, by converting the workman into a living appendage of the machine; and everywhere outside the Factory, partly by the sporadic use of machinery and machine workers, partly by re-establishing the division of labour on a fresh basis by the general introduction of the labour of women and children, and of cheap unskilled labour.

The antagonism between the manufacturing division of labour and the methods of Modern Industry makes itself forcibly felt. It manifests itself, amongst other ways, in the frightful fact that a great part of the children employed in modern factories and manufactures, are from their earliest years riveted to the most simple manipulations, and exploited for years, without being taught a single sort of work that would afterwards make them of use, even in the same manufactory or factory. In the English letter-press printing trade, for example, there existed formerly a system, corresponding to that in the old manufactures and handicrafts, of advancing the apprentices from easy to more and more difficult work. They went through a course of teaching till they were finished printers. To be able to read and write was for every one of them a requirement of their trade. All this was changed by the printing machine. It employs two sorts of labourers, one grown up, renters, the other, boys mostly from 11 to 17 years of age whose sole business is either to spread the sheets of paper under the machine, or to take from it the printed sheets. They perform this weary task, in London especially, for 14, 15, and 16 hours at a stretch, during several days in the week, and frequently for 36 hours, with only 2 hours' rest for meals and sleep. A great part of them cannot read, and they are, as a rule, utter savages and very extraordinary creatures. "To qualify them for the work which they have to do, they require no intellectual training; there is little room in it for skill, and less for judgment; their wages, though rather high for boys, do not increase proportionately as they grow up, and the majority of them cannot look for advancement to the better paid and more responsible post of machine minder, because while each machine has but one minder, it has at least two, and often four boys attached to it." As soon as they get too old for such child's work, that is about 17 at the latest, they are discharged from the printing establishments. They become recruits of crime. Several attempts to procure them employment elsewhere, were rendered of no avail by their ignorance and brutality, and by their mental and bodily degradation.

Source: Marx, Karl. 1887. Moore, Samuel, and Edward Aveling, trans. *Capital: A Critique of Political Economy, Vol. I. The Process of Capitalist Production*. London: S. Sonnenschein, Lowrey.

▣ Francis Galton, from *Hereditary Genius* (1869)

Sir Francis Galton, who coined the term eugenics, used statistics to determine average and exceptional characteristics of human bodies. In this excerpt, he sets out to argue that genius and intelligence are passed down according to the laws of basic heredity that govern common qualities such as eye and hair color. In doing so, Galton set out to demonstrate that control over breeding practices could artificially engineer a more superior national race endowed with the qualities he most admired.

Introductory Chapter

I propose to show in this book that a man's natural abilities are derived by inheritance, under exactly the same limitations as are the form and physical features of the whole organic world. Consequently, as it is easy, notwithstanding those limitations, to obtain by careful selection a permanent breed of dogs or horses gifted with peculiar powers of running, or of doing anything else, so it would be quite practicable to produce a highly-gifted race of men by judicious marriages during several consecutive generations. I shall show that social agencies of an ordinary character, whose influences are little suspected, are at this moment working towards the degradation of human nature, and that others are working towards its improvement. I conclude that each generation has enormous power over the natural gifts of those that follow, and maintain that it is a duty we owe to

humanity to investigate the range of that power, and to exercise it in a way that, without being unwise towards ourselves, shall be most advantageous to future inhabitants of the earth.

I am aware that my views, which were first published four years ago in *Macmillan's Magazine* (in June and August 1865), are in contradiction to general opinion; but the arguments I then used have been since accepted, to my great gratification, by many of the highest authorities on heredity. In reproducing them, as I now do, in a much more elaborate form, and on a greatly enlarged basis of induction, I feel assured that, inasmuch as what I then wrote was sufficient to earn the acceptance of Mr. Darwin (*Domestication of Plants and Animals, ii 7),* the increased amount of evidence submitted in the present volume is not likely to be gainsaid.

The general plan of my argument is to show that high reputation is a pretty accurate test of high ability; next to discuss the relationships of a large body of fairly eminent men—namely, the Judges of England from 1660 to 1868, the Statesmen of the time of George III, and the Premiers during the last 100 years—and to obtain from these a general survey of the laws of heredity in respect to genius. Then I shall examine, in order, the kindred of the most illustrious Commanders, men of Literature and of Science, Poets, painters, and Musicians, of whom history speaks. I shall also discuss the kindred of a certain selection of Divines and of modern Scholars. Then will follow a short chapter, by way of comparison, on the hereditary transmission of physical gifts, as deduced from the relationships of certain classes of Oarsmen and Wrestlers. Lastly, I shall collate my results, and draw conclusions.

It will be observed that I deal with more than one grade of ability. Those upon whom the greater part of my volume is occupied, and on whose kinships my argument is most securely based, have been generally reputed as endowed by nature with extraordinary genius. There are so few of these men that, although they are scattered throughout the whole historical period of human existence, their number does not amount to more than 400, and yet a considerable proportion of them will be found to be interrelated.

Another grade of ability with which I deal is that which includes numerous highly eminent, and all the illustrious names of modern English history, whose immediate descendants are living among us, whose histories are popularly known, and whose relationships may readily be traced by the help of biographical dictionaries, peerages, and similar books of reference.

A third and lower grade is that of the English Judges, massed together as a whole, for the purpose of the prefatory statistical inquiry of which I have already spoken. No one doubts that many of the ablest intellects of our race are to be found among the Judges; nevertheless the *average* ability of a Judge cannot be rated as equal to that of the lower of the two grades I have described.

I trust the reader will make allowance for a large and somewhat important class of omissions I have felt myself compelled to make when treating of the eminent men of modern days. I am prevented by a sense of decorum from quoting names of their relations in contemporary life who are not recognized as public characters, although their abilities may be highly appreciated in private life. Still less consistent with decorum would it have been, to introduce the names of female relatives that stand in the same category. My case is so overpoweringly strong, that I am perfectly able to prove my point without having recourse to this class of evidence. Nevertheless, the reader should bear in mind that it exists; and I beg he will do me the justice of allowing that I have not overlooked the whole of the evidence that does not appear in my pages. I am deeply conscious of the imperfection of my work, but my sins are those of omission, not of commission. Such errors as I may and must have made, which give a fictitious support to my arguments, are, I am confident, out of all proportion fewer than such omissions of facts as would have helped to establish them.

I have taken little notice in this book of modern men of eminence who are not English, or at least well known to Englishmen. I feared, if I included large classes of foreigners, that I should make glaring errors. It requires a very great deal of labour to hunt out relationships, even with the facilities afforded to a countryman having access to persons acquainted with the various families; much more would it have been difficult to hunt out the kindred of foreigners. I should have especially liked to investigate the biographies of Italians and Jews, both of whom appear to be rich in families of high intellectual breeds. Germany and America are also full of interest. It is little less so with respect to France, where the Revolution and the guillotine made sad havoc among the progeny of her abler races.

There is one advantage to a candid critic in my having left so large a field untouched; it enables me to propose a test that any well-informed reader may easily adopt who doubts the fairness of my examples. He may most reasonably suspect that I have been unconsciously influenced by my theories to select men whose kindred were most favourable to their support. If so, I beg he will test my impartiality as follows:—Let him take a dozen names of his own selection, as the most eminent in whatever profession and in whatever country he knows most about, and let him trace out for himself their relations. It is necessary, as I find by experience, to take some pains to be sure that none, even of the immediate relatives, on either the male or female side, have been overlooked. If he does what I propose, I am confident he will be astonished at the completeness with which the results will confirm my theory. I venture to speak with assurance, because it has often occurred to me to propose this very test to incredulous friends, and invariably, so far as my memory serves me, as large a proportion of the men who were named were discovered to have eminent relations, as the nature of my views on heredity would have led us to expect.

From "Classification of Men According to their Natural Gifts"

In whatever way we may test ability, we arrive at equally enormous intellectual differences. Lord Macaulay (*see* under LITERATURE for his remarkable kinships) had one of the most tenacious of memories. He was able to recall many pages of hundreds of volumes by various authors, which he had acquired by simply reading them over. An average man could not certainly carry in his memory one thirty-second—ay, or one hundredth—part as much as Lord Macaulay. The father of Seneca had one of the greatest memories on record in ancient times (*see* under LITERATURE for his kinships). Porson, the Greek scholar, was remarkable for this gift, and, I may add, the "Porson memory" was hereditary in that family. In statesmanship, generalship, literature, science, poetry, art, just the same enormous differences are found between man and man; and numerous instances recorded in this book, will show in how small degree, eminence, either in these or any other class of intellectual powers, can be considered as due to purely special powers. They are rather to be considered in those instances as the result of concentrated efforts, made by men who are widely gifted. People lay too much stress on apparent specialities, thinking over-rashly that, because a man is devoted to some particular pursuit, he could not possibly have succeeded in anything else. They might just as well say that, because a youth had fallen desperately in love with a brunette, he could not possibly have fallen in love with a blonde. He may or may not have more natural liking for the former type of beauty than the latter, but it is as probable as not that the affair was mainly or wholly due to a general amorousness of disposition. It is just the same with special pursuits. A gifted man is often capricious and fickle before he selects his occupation, but when it has been chosen, he devotes himself to it with a truly passionate ardour. After a man of genius has selected his hobby, and so adapted himself to it as to seem unfitted for any other occupation in life, and to be possessed of but one special aptitude, I often notice, with admiration, how well he bears himself when circumstances suddenly thrust him into a strange position. He will display an insight into new conditions, and a power of dealing with them, with which even his most intimate friends were unprepared to accredit him. Many a presumptuous fool has mistaken indifference and neglect for incapacity; and in trying to throw a man of genius on ground where he was unprepared for attack, has himself received a most severe and unexpected fall. I am sure that no one who has had the privilege of mixing in the society of the abler men of any great capital, or who is acquainted with the biographies of the heroes of history, can doubt the existence of grand human animals, of natures pre-eminently noble, of individuals born to be kings of men. I have been conscious of no slight misgiving that I was committing a kind of sacrilege whenever, in the preparation of materials for this book, I had occasion to take the measurement of modern intellects vastly superior to my own, or to criticize the genius of the most magnificent historical specimens of our race. It was a process that constantly recalled to me a once familiar sentiment in bygone days of African travel, when I used to take altitudes of the huge cliffs that domineered above me as I traveled along their bases, or to map the mountainous landmarks of unvisited tribes, that loomed in faint grandeur beyond my actual horizon.

I have not cared to occupy myself much with people whose gifts are below the average, but they would be an interesting study. The number of idiots and imbeciles among the twenty million inhabitants of England and Wales is approximately estimated at 50,000, or as 1 in 400. Dr. Seguin, a great French authority on these matters, states that more than thirty

per cent. of idiots and imbeciles, put under suitable instruction, have been taught to conform to social and moral law, and rendered capable of order, of good feeling, and of working like *the third* of an average man. He says that more than forty per cent. have become capable of the ordinary transactions of life, under friendly control; of understanding moral and social abstractions, and of working like *two-thirds* of a man. And, lastly, that from twenty-five to thirty per cent. come nearer and nearer to the standard of manhood, till some of them will defy the scrutiny of good judges, when compared with ordinary young men and women. In the order next above idiots and imbeciles are a large number of milder cases scattered among private families and kept out of sight, the existence of whom is, however, well known to relatives and friends; they are too silly to take a part in general society, but are easily amused with some trivial, harmless occupation. Then comes a class of whom the Lord Dundreary of the famous play may be considered a representative; and so, proceeding through successive grades, we gradually ascend to mediocrity. I know two good instances of hereditary silliness short of imbecility, and have reason to believe I could easily obtain a large number of similar facts.

To conclude, the range of mental power between— I will not say the highest Caucasian and the lowest savage—but between the greatest and least of English intellects, is enormous. There is a continuity of natural ability reaching from one knows not what height, and descending to one can hardly say what depth. I propose in this chapter to range men according to their natural abilities, putting them into classes separated by equal degrees of merit, and to show the relative number of individuals included in the several classes. Perhaps some person might be inclined to make an offhand guess that the number of men included in the several classes would be pretty equal. If he thinks so, I can assure him he is most egregiously mistaken.

The method I shall employ for discovering all this is an application of the very curious theoretical law of "deviation from an average." First, I will explain the law, and then I will show that the production of natural intellectual gifts comes justly within its scope.

The law is an exceedingly general one. M. Quetelet, the Astronomer-Royal of Belgium, and the greatest authority on vital and social statistics, has largely used it in his inquiries. He has also constructed numerical tables, by which the necessary calculations can be easily made, whenever it is desired to have recourse to the law. Those who wish to learn more than I have space to relate, should consult his work, which is a very readable octavo volume, and deserves to be far better known to statisticians than it appears to be. Its title is *Letters on Probabilities*, translated by Downes. Layton and Co. London: 1849.

Source: Galton, Francis. 1869. *Hereditary Genius.* Available at: http://www.mugu.com/galton/books/hereditary-genius/

▣ Mark Twain, from *Innocents Abroad: Or, The New Pilgrim's Progress* (1869)

One of Twain's most popular books, this travel odyssey explores his experiences in the Middle East, Crimea, Greece, and Egypt. In this excerpt, Twain discusses the impact of the presence of a doctor in his party on "diseased" populations seeking medical assistance in their conditions.

From Chapter 45

This morning, during breakfast, the usual assemblage of squalid humanity sat patiently without the charmed circle of the camp and waited for such crumbs as pity might bestow upon their misery. There were old and young, brown-skinned and yellow. Some of the men were tall and stalwart, (for one hardly sees any where such splendid-looking men as here in the East,) but all the women and children looked worn and sad, and distressed with hunger. They reminded me much of Indians, did these people. They had but little clothing, but such as they had was fanciful in character and fantastic in its arrangement. Any little absurd gewgaw or gimcrack they had they disposed in such a way as to make it attract attention most readily. They sat in silence, and with tireless patience watched our every motion with that vile, uncomplaining impoliteness which is so truly Indian, and which makes a white man so nervous and uncomfortable and savage that he wants to exterminate the whole tribe.

These people about us had other peculiarities, which I have noticed in the noble red man, too: they were infested with vermin, and the dirt had caked on them till it amounted to bark.

The little children were in a pitiable condition—they all had sore eyes, and were otherwise afflicted in various ways. They say that hardly a native child in all

the East is free from sore eyes, and that thousands of them go blind of one eye or both every year. I think this must be so, for I see plenty of blind people every day, and I do not remember seeing any children that hadn't sore eyes. And, would you suppose that an American mother could sit for an hour, with her child in her arms, and let a hundred flies roost upon its eyes all that time undisturbed? I see that every day. It makes my flesh creep. Yesterday we met a woman riding on a little jackass, and she had a little child in her arms—honestly, I thought the child had goggles on as we approached, and I wondered how its mother could afford so much style. But when we drew near, we saw that the goggles were nothing but a camp meeting of flies assembled around each of the child's eyes, and at the same time there was a detachment prospecting its nose. The flies were happy, the child was contented, and so the mother did not interfere.

As soon as the tribe found out that we had a doctor in our party, they began to flock in from all quarters. Dr. B., in the charity of his nature, had taken a child from a woman who sat near by, and put some sort of a wash upon its diseased eyes. That woman went off and started the whole nation, and it was a sight to see them swarm! The lame, the halt, the blind, the leprous—all the distempers that are bred of indolence, dirt, and iniquity—were represented in the Congress in ten minutes, and still they came! Every woman that had a sick baby brought it along, and every woman that hadn't, borrowed one. What reverent and what worshiping looks they bent upon that dread, mysterious power, the Doctor! They watched him take his phials out; they watched him measure the particles of white powder; they watched him add drops of one precious liquid, and drops of another; they lost not the slightest movement; their eyes were riveted upon him with a fascination that nothing could distract. I believe they thought he was gifted like a god. When each individual got his portion of medicine, his eyes were radiant with joy—notwithstanding by nature they are a thankless and impassive race—and upon his face was written the unquestioning faith that nothing on earth could prevent the patient from getting well now.

Christ knew how to preach to these simple, superstitious, disease-tortured creatures: He healed the sick. They flocked to our poor human doctor this morning when the fame of what he had done to the sick child went abroad in the land, and they worshiped him with their eyes while they did not know as yet whether there was virtue in his simples or not. The ancestors of these—people precisely like them in color, dress, manners, customs, simplicity—flocked in vast multitudes after Christ, and when they saw Him make the afflicted whole with a word, it is no wonder they worshiped Him. No wonder His deeds were the talk of the nation. No wonder the multitude that followed Him was so great that at one time—thirty miles from here—they had to let a sick man down through the roof because no approach could be made to the door; no wonder His audiences were so great at Galilee that He had to preach from a ship removed a little distance from the shore; no wonder that even in the desert places about Bethsaida, five thousand invaded His solitude, and He had to feed them by a miracle or else see them suffer for their confiding faith and devotion; no wonder when there was a great commotion in a city in those days, one neighbor explained it to another in words to this effect: "They say that Jesus of Nazareth is come!"

Well, as I was saying, the doctor distributed medicine as long as he had any to distribute, and his reputation is mighty in Galilee this day. Among his patients was the child of the Shiek's daughter—for even this poor, ragged handful of sores and sin has its royal Shiek—a poor old mummy that looked as if he would be more at home in a poor-house than in the Chief Magistracy of this tribe of hopeless, shirtless savages. The princess—I mean the Shiek's daughter—was only thirteen or fourteen years old, and had a very sweet face and a pretty one. She was the only Syrian female we have seen yet who was not so sinfully ugly that she couldn't smile after ten o'clock Saturday night without breaking the Sabbath. Her child was a hard specimen, though—there wasn't enough of it to make a pie, and the poor little thing looked so pleadingly up at all who came near it (as if it had an idea that now was its chance or never,) that we were filled with compassion which was genuine and not put on.

Source: Twain, Mark. 1869. *Innocents Abroad: Or, The New Pilgrim's Progress.* Available at: http://www.mtwain.com/Innocents_Abroad/0.html

▣ Deaf and Deaf-Mute Servants in the Sultan's Court (1870–1909)

The following excerpts all pertain to populations identified as deaf and deaf-mute. They were all written during the reign of Sultan Abdel Hamid II (reigned 1876–1909). Those by the German physician and traveler Nachtigal and the French colonial governor Henri Gaden indicate that deaf servants were still much required by the Sultan, who sent his requisition as far as the slave-trading center at Darfur.

G. Nachtigal

From Nachtigal, G. 1971–1987. Fisher, A. G. B., & H. J. Fisher, trans. *Sahara and Sudan.* London: Hurst.

1870s In 1872, Nachtigal learned that the leading men of Bornu had given gifts, including "ordinary slaves, eunuchs, deaf-mutes and dwarfs," to an emissary of the Ottoman Sultan (Vol. IV: P. 4). At Kuka (capital of Bornu), west of Lake Chad, he remarked that "deaf and dumb slave girls" were sold for high prices to serve the wives of businessmen in some Islamic countries (Vol. II: P. 218).

Henri Gaden

Gaden, Henri. 1907. Etats musulmans de l'Afrique centrale et leurs rapports avec la Mecque et Constantinople. *Questions diplomatiques et coloniales* 24: 436–447.

1870s Gaden (P. 444) noted the long reign (1874–1898) of Sultan Yusuf at Ouadai (now in Chad), who "sent eunuchs to Constantinople almost yearly. Once, when the Ottoman Sultan Abd el-Hamid asked him particularly for deaf-mutes, he searched his kingdom and sent all whom he could find."

J. Sibree

Sibree, J. 1884. Notes on relics of the sign and gesture language among the Malagasy. *Journal of the Anthropological Institute of Great Britain and Ireland* 13:174–183. [Note that Pp. 179–182 include a "Postscript," with contributions from authors Houlder, Price, Peill, and Thorne, and on Pp. 182–183 there are "Discussion" notes, from Mr. Hyde Clark.]

1884 In reported discussion after Sibree's paper, Mr. Hyde Clarke gave more detail of the sign language used in the Ottoman Seraglio, which he had witnessed (Pp. 182–183). Both Sibree and Hyde Clarke were interested in tracing back their observations of gesture language in the 1880s to earlier sources, as far back as the historical texts with which they were familiar, that is, from ancient Rome and Palestine.

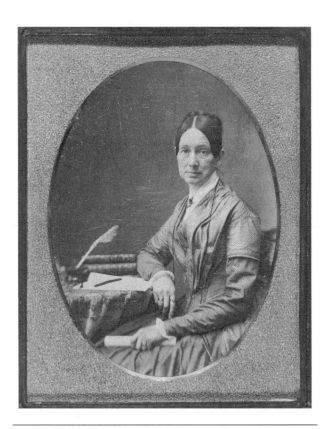

Daguerreotype (1849) of Dorothea Lynde Dix (1802–1887). In the United States during the Progressive Era, Dorothea Lynde Dix was a social reformer and advocate for those diagnosed as feebleminded and mentally ill. Dix demanded an end to the neglect of individuals deemed valueless and lobbied for the creation of humane, state-supported institutions in the United States.

Source: Art Resource, New York.

Ludger Busse

Busse, Ludger. 1994. Ferdi Garati und seine Schule für Gehörlose und Blinde in Istanbul—Die Ursprünge des türkischen Sonderschulwesens. *Hörgeschädigten Pädagogik* 48:227–235.

1889 Describes the opening by F. Garati of a formal deaf school at Istanbul in 1889 and its functioning until it closed in 1926. A blind school was added in 1890, but it closed seven years later.

▣ Charles Darwin, from *The Descent of Man* (1871)

In this excerpt, Darwin argues in favor of his evolutionary theory based on beliefs about the inferior bodies/capacities of racialized and disabled populations. The existence of "lesser" forms of humanity and

monstrous abnormalities serves to anchor proofs about the continuity of human and animal forms.

Chapter II. On the Manner of Development of Man from Some Lower Form

I have elsewhere so fully discussed the subject of Inheritance, that I need here add hardly anything. A greater number of facts have been collected with respect to the transmission of the most trifling, as well as of the most important characters in man, than in any of the lower animals; though the facts are copious enough with respect to the latter. So in regard to mental qualities, their transmission is manifest in our dogs, horses, and other domestic animals. Besides special tastes and habits, general intelligence, courage, bad and good temper, &c., are certainly transmitted. With man we see similar facts in almost every family; and we now know, through the admirable labours of Mr. Galton, that genius which implies a wonderfully complex combination of high faculties, tends to be inherited; and, on the other hand, it is too certain that insanity and deteriorated mental powers likewise run in families.

With respect to the causes of variability, we are in all cases very ignorant; but we can see that in man as in the lower animals, they stand in some relation to the conditions to which each species has been exposed, during several generations. Domesticated animals vary more than those in a state of nature; and this is apparently due to the diversified and changing nature of the conditions to which they have been subjected. In this respect the different races of man resemble domesticated animals, and so do the individuals of the same race, when inhabiting a very wide area, like that of America. We see the influence of diversified conditions in the more civilised nations; for the members belonging to different grades of rank, and following different occupations, present a greater range of character than do the members of barbarous nations. But the uniformity of savages has often been exaggerated, and in some cases can hardly be said to exist. It is, nevertheless, an error to speak of man, even if we look only to the conditions to which he has been exposed, as "far more domesticated" than any other animal. Some savage races, such as the Australians, are not exposed to more diversified conditions than are many species which have a wide range. In another and much more important respect, man differs widely from any strictly domesticated animal; for his breeding has never long been controlled, either by methodical or unconscious selection. No race or body of men has been so completely subjugated by other men, as that certain individuals should be preserved, and thus unconsciously selected, from somehow excelling in utility to their masters. Nor have certain male and female individuals been intentionally picked out and matched, except in the well-known case of the Prussian grenadiers; and in this case man obeyed, as might have been expected, the law of methodical selection; for it is asserted that many tall men were reared in the villages inhabited by the grenadiers and their tall wives. In Sparta, also, a form of selection was followed, for it was enacted that all children should be examined shortly after birth; the well-formed and vigorous being preserved, the others left to perish.

If we consider all the races of man as forming a single species, his range is enormous; but some separate races, as the Americans and Polynesians, have very wide ranges. It is a well-known law that widely-ranging species are much more variable than species with restricted ranges; and the variability of man may with more truth be compared with that of widely-ranging species, than with that of domesticated animals.

Not only does variability appear to be induced in man and the lower animals by the same general causes, but in both the same parts of the body are effected in a closely analogous manner. This has been proved in such full detail by Godron and Quatrefages, that I need here only refer to their works. Monstrosities, which graduate into slight variations, are likewise so similar in man and the lower animals, that the same classification and the same terms can be used for both, as has been shewn by Isidore Geoffroy St.-Hilaire. In my work on the variation of domestic animals, I have attempted to arrange in a rude fashion the laws of variation under the following heads:— The direct and definite action of changed conditions, as exhibited by all or nearly all the individuals of the same species, varying in the same manner under the same circumstances. The effects of the long-continued use or disuse of parts. The cohesion of homologous parts. The variability of multiple parts. Compensation of growth; but of this law I have found no good instance in the case of man. The effects of the mechanical pressure of one part on another; as of the pelvis on the cranium of the infant in the womb. Arrests of development, leading to the diminution or suppression of parts. The reappearance of long-lost

characters through reversion. And lastly, correlated variation. All these so-called laws apply equally to man and the lower animals; and most of them even to plants. It would be superfluous here to discuss all of them; but several are so important, that they must be treated at considerable length. . . .

Effects of the Increased Use and Disuse of Parts

It is well known that use strengthens the muscles in the individual, and complete disuse, or the destruction of the proper nerve, weakens them. When the eye is destroyed, the optic nerve often becomes atrophied. When an artery is tied, the lateral channels increase not only in diameter, but in the thickness and strength of their coats. When one kidney ceases to act from disease, the other increases in size, and does double work. Bones increase not only in thickness, but in length, from carrying a greater weight. Different occupations, habitually followed, lead to changed proportions in various parts of the body. Thus it was ascertained by the United States Commission that the legs of the sailors employed in the late war were longer by 0.217 of an inch than those of the soldiers, though the sailors were on an average shorter men; whilst their arms were shorter by 1.09 of an inch, and therefore, out of proportion, shorter in relation to their lesser height. This shortness of the arms is apparently due to their greater use, and is an unexpected result: but sailors chiefly use their arms in pulling, and not in supporting weights. With sailors, the girth of the neck and the depth of the instep are greater, whilst the circumference of the chest, waist, and hips is less, than in soldiers.

Whether the several foregoing modifications would become hereditary, if the same habits of life were followed during many generations, is not known, but it is probable. Rengger attributes the thin legs and thick arms of the Payaguas Indians to successive generations having passed nearly their whole lives in canoes, with their lower extremities motionless. Other writers have come to a similar conclusion in analogous cases. According to Cranz, who lived for a long time with the Esquimaux, "The natives believe that ingenuity and dexterity in seal-catching (their highest art and virtue) is hereditary; there is really something in it, for the son of a celebrated seal-catcher will distinguish himself, though he lost his father in childhood." But in this case it is mental aptitude, quite as much as bodily structure, which appears to be inherited. It is asserted that the hands of English labourers are at birth larger than those of the gentry. From the correlation which exists, at least in some cases, between the development of the extremities and of the jaws, it is possible that in those classes which do not labour much with their hands and feet, the jaws would be reduced in size from this cause. That they are generally smaller in refined and civilized men than in hard-working men or savages, is certain. But with savages, as Mr. Herbert Spencer has remarked, the greater use of the jaws in chewing coarse, uncooked food, would act in a direct manner on the masticatory muscles, and on the bones to which they are attached. In infants, long before birth, the skin on the soles of the feet is thicker than on any other part of the body; and it can hardly be doubted that this is due to the inherited effects of pressure during a long series of generations.

It is familiar to every one that watchmakers and engravers are liable to be short-sighted, whilst men living much out of doors, and especially savages, are generally long-sighted. Short-sight and long-sight certainly tend to be inherited. The inferiority of Europeans, in comparison with savages, in eyesight and in the other senses, is no doubt the accumulated and transmitted effect of lessened use during many generations; for Rengger states that he has repeatedly observed Europeans, who had been brought up and spent their whole lives with the wild Indians, who nevertheless did not equal them in the sharpness of their senses. The same naturalist observes that the cavities in the skull for the reception of the several sense-organs are larger in the American aborigines than in Europeans; and this probably indicates a corresponding difference in the dimensions of the organs themselves. Blumenbach has also remarked on the large size of the nasal cavities in the skulls of the American aborigines, and connects this fact with their remarkably acute power of smell. The Mongolians of the plains of northern Asia, according to Pallas, have wonderfully perfect senses; and Prichard believes that the great breadth of their skulls across the zygomas follows from their highly-developed sense organs.

The Quechua Indians inhabit the lofty plateaux of Peru; and Alcide d'Orbigny states that, from continually breathing a highly rarefied atmosphere, they have acquired chests and lungs of extraordinary dimensions. The cells, also, of the lungs are larger and more numerous than in Europeans. These observations have been doubted, but Mr. D. Forbes carefully measured many Aymaras, an allied race, living at the height of between 10,000 and 15,000 feet; and he informs me that they differ conspicuously from the men of all other races seen by him in the circumference and length of their bodies. In his table of measurements, the stature of each man is taken at 1000, and the other measurements are reduced to this standard. It is here seen that the extended arms of the Aymaras are shorter than those of Europeans, and much shorter than those of Negroes. The legs are likewise shorter; and they present this remarkable peculiarity, that in every Aymara measured, the femur is actually shorter than the tibia. On an average, the length of the femur to that of the tibia is as 211 to 252; whilst in two Europeans, measured at the same time, the femora to the tibiae were as 244 to 230; and in three Negroes as 258 to 241. The humerus is likewise shorter relatively to the forearm. This shortening of that part of the limb which is nearest to the body, appears to be, as suggested to me by Mr. Forbes, a case of compensation in relation with the greatly increased length of the trunk. The Aymaras present some other singular points of structure, for instance, the very small projection of the heel.

These men are so thoroughly acclimatised to their cold and lofty abode, that when formerly carried down by Spaniards to the low eastern plains, and when now tempted down by high wages to the gold-washings, they suffer a frightful rate of mortality. Nevertheless Mr. Forbes found a few pure families which had survived during two generations: and he observed that they still inherited their characteristic peculiarities. But it was manifest, even without measurement, that these peculiarities had all decreased; and on measurement, their bodies were found not to be so much elongated as those of the men on the high plateau; whilst their femora had become somewhat lengthened, as had their tibiae, although in a less degree. The actual measurements may be seen by consulting Mr. Forbes's memoir. From these observations, there can, I think, be no doubt that residence during many generations at a great elevation tends, both directly and indirectly, to induce inherited modifications in the proportions of the body.

Although man may not have been much modified during the latter stages of his existence through the increased or decreased use of parts, the facts now given shew that his liability in this respect has not been lost; and we positively know that the same law holds good with the lower animals. Consequently we may infer that when at a remote epoch the progenitors of man were in a transitional state, and were changing from quadrupeds into bipeds, natural selection would probably have been greatly aided by the inherited effects of the increased or diminished use of the different parts of the body.

Arrests of Development

There is a difference between arrested development and arrested growth, for parts in the former state continue to grow whilst still retaining their early condition. Various monstrosities come under this head; and some, as a cleft palate, are known to be occasionally inherited. It will suffice for our purpose to refer to the arrested brain-development of microcephalous idiots, as described in Vogt's memoir. Their skulls are smaller, and the convolutions of the brain are less complex than in normal men. The frontal sinus, or the projection over the eyebrows, is largely developed, and the jaws are prognathous to an "effrayant" degree; so that these idiots somewhat resemble the lower types of mankind. Their intelligence, and most of their mental faculties, are extremely feeble. They cannot acquire the power of speech, and are wholly incapable of prolonged attention, but are much given to imitation. They are strong and remarkably active, continually gambolling and jumping about, and making grimaces. They often ascend stairs on all-fours; and are curiously fond of climbing up furniture or trees. We are thus reminded of the delight shewn by almost all boys in climbing trees; and this again reminds us how lambs and kids, originally alpine animals, delight to frisk on any hillock, however small. Idiots also resemble the lower animals in some other respects; thus several cases are recorded of their carefully smelling every mouthful of food before eating it. One idiot is described as often using his mouth in aid of his hands, whilst hunting for lice. They are often filthy in their habits, and have no sense of decency; and several cases have been published of their bodies being remarkably hairy.

Reversion

Many of the cases to be here given, might have been introduced under the last heading. When a structure is arrested in its development, but still continues growing, until it closely resembles a corresponding structure in some lower and adult member of the same group, it may in one sense be considered as a case of reversion. The lower members in a group give us some

idea how the common progenitor was probably constructed; and it is hardly credible that a complex part, arrested at an early phase of embryonic development, should go on growing so as ultimately to perform its proper function, unless it had acquired such power during some earlier state of existence, when the present exceptional or arrested structure was normal. The simple brain of a microcephalous idiot, in as far as it resembles that of an ape, may in this sense be said to offer a case of reversion. There are other cases which come more strictly under our present head of reversion. Certain structures, regularly occurring in the lower members of the group to which man belongs, occasionally make their appearance in him, though not found in the normal human embryo; or, if normally present in the human embryo, they become abnormally developed, although in a manner which is normal in the lower members of the group. These remarks will be rendered clearer by the following illustrations.

In the above work (vol. ii., p. 12), I also attributed, though with much hesitation, the frequent cases of polydactylism in men and various animals to reversion. I was partly led to this through Prof. Owen's statement, that some of the Ichthyopterygia possess more than five digits, and therefore, as I supposed, had retained a primordial condition; but Prof. Gegenbaur (*Jenaische Zeitschrift*, B. v., Heft 3, s. 341), disputes Owen's conclusion. On the other hand, according to the opinion lately advanced by Dr. Gunther, on the paddle of Ceratodus, which is provided with articulated bony rays on both sides of a central chain of bones, there seems no great difficulty in admitting that six or more digits on one side, or on both sides, might reappear through reversion. I am informed by Dr. Zouteveen that there is a case on record of a man having twenty-four fingers and twenty-four toes! I was chiefly led to the conclusion that the presence of supernumerary digits might be due to reversion from the fact that such digits, not only are strongly inherited, but, as I then believed, had the power of regrowth after amputation, like the normal digits of the lower Vertebrata. But I have explained in the second edition of my Variation under Domestication why I now place little reliance on the recorded cases of such regrowth. Nevertheless it deserves notice, inasmuch as arrested development and reversion are intimately related processes; that various structures in an embryonic or arrested condition, such as a cleft palate, bifid uterus, &c., are frequently accompanied by polydactylism.

This has been strongly insisted on by Meckel and Isidore Geoffroy St.-Hilaire. But at present it is the safest course to give up altogether the idea that there is any relation between the development of supernumerary digits and reversion to some lowly organized progenitor of man.

In various mammals the uterus graduates from a double organ with two distinct orifices and two passages, as in the marsupials, into a single organ, which is in no way double except from having a slight internal fold, as in the higher apes and man. The rodents exhibit a perfect series of gradations between these two extreme states. In all mammals the uterus is developed from two simple primitive tubes, the inferior portions of which form the cornua; and it is in the words of Dr. Farre, "by the coalescence of the two cornua at their lower extremities that the body of the uterus is formed in man; while in those animals in which no middle portion or body exists, the cornua remain ununited. As the development of the uterus proceeds, the two cornua become gradually shorter, until at length they are lost, or, as it were, absorbed into the body of the uterus." The angles of the uterus are still produced into cornua, even in animals as high up in the scale as the lower apes and lemurs.

Now in women, anomalous cases are not very infrequent, in which the mature uterus is furnished with cornua, or is partially divided into two organs; and such cases, according to Owen, repeat "the grade of concentrative development," attained by certain rodents. Here perhaps we have an instance of a simple arrest of embryonic development, with subsequent growth and perfect functional development; for either side of the partially double uterus is capable of performing the proper office of gestation. In other and rarer cases, two distinct uterine cavities are formed, each having its proper orifice and passage. No such stage is passed through during the ordinary development of the embryo; and it is difficult to believe, though perhaps not impossible, that the two simple, minute, primitive tubes should know how (if such an expression may be used) to grow into two distinct uteri, each with a well-constructed orifice and passage, and each furnished with numerous muscles, nerves, glands and vessels, if they had not formerly passed through a similar course of development, as in the case of existing marsupials. No one will pretend that so perfect a structure as the abnormal double uterus in woman could be the result of mere chance. But the principle of reversion, by which a long-lost

structure is called back into existence, might serve as the guide for its full development, even after the lapse of an enormous interval of time.

Professor Canestrini, after discussing the foregoing and various analogous cases, arrives at the same conclusion as that just given. He adduces another instance, in the case of the malar bone, which, in some of the Quadrumana and other mammals, normally consists of two portions. This is its condition in the human foetus when two months old; and through arrested development, it sometimes remains thus in man when adult, more especially in the lower prognathous races. Hence Canestrini concludes that some ancient progenitor of man must have had this bone normally divided into two portions, which afterwards became fused together. In man the frontal bone consists of a single piece, but in the embryo, and in children, and in almost all the lower mammals, it consists of two pieces separated by a distinct suture. This suture occasionally persists more or less distinctly in man after maturity; and more frequently in ancient than in recent crania, especially, as Canestrini has observed, in those exhumed from the Drift, and belonging to the brachycephalic type. Here again he comes to the same conclusion as in the analogous case of the malar bones. In this, and other instances presently to be given, the cause of ancient races approaching the lower animals in certain characters more frequently than do the modern races, appears to be, that the latter stand at a somewhat greater distance in the long line of descent from their early semi-human progenitors.

Various other anomalies in man, more or less analogous to the foregoing, have been advanced by different authors, as cases of reversion; but these seem not a little doubtful, for we have to descend extremely low in the mammalian series, before we find such structures normally present.

In man, the canine teeth are perfectly efficient instruments for mastication. But their true canine character, as Owen remarks, "is indicated by the conical form of the crown, which terminates in an obtuse point, is convex outward and flat or sub-concave within, at the base of which surface there is a feeble prominence. The conical form is best expressed in the Melanian races, especially the Australian. The canine is more deeply implanted, and by a stronger fang than the incisors." Nevertheless, this tooth no longer serves man as a special weapon for tearing his enemies or prey; it may, therefore, as far as its proper function is concerned, be considered as rudimentary. In every large collection of human skulls some may be found, as Haeckel observes, with the canine teeth projecting considerably beyond the others in the same manner as in the anthropomorphous apes, but in a less degree. In these cases, open spaces between the teeth in the one jaw are left for the reception of the canines of the opposite jaw. An inter-space of this kind in a Kaffir skull, figured by Wagner, is surprisingly wide. Considering how few are the ancient skulls which have been examined, compared to recent skulls, it is an interesting fact that in at least three cases the canines project largely; and in the Naulette jaw they are spoken of as enormous.

Of the anthropomorphous apes the males alone have their canines fully developed; but in the female gorilla, and in a less degree in the female orang, these teeth project considerably beyond the others; therefore the fact, of which I have been assured, that women sometimes have considerably projecting canines, is no serious objection to the belief that their occasional great development in man is a case of reversion to an ape-like progenitor. He who rejects with scorn the belief that the shape of his own canines, and their occasional great development in other men, are due to our early forefathers having been provided with these formidable weapons, will probably reveal, by sneering, the line of his descent. For though he no longer intends, nor has the power, to use these teeth as weapons, he will unconsciously retract his "snarling muscles" (thus named by Sir C. Bell), so as to expose them ready for action, like a dog prepared to fight.

Many muscles are occasionally developed in man, which are proper to the Quadrumana or other mammals. Professor Vlacovich examined forty male subjects, and found a muscle, called by him the ischio-pubic, in nineteen of them; in three others there was a ligament which represented this muscle; and in the remaining eighteen no trace of it. In only two out of thirty female subjects was this muscle developed on both sides, but in three others the rudimentary ligament was present. This muscle, therefore, appears to be much more common in the male than in the female sex; and on the belief in the descent of man from some lower form, the fact is intelligible; for it has been detected in several of the lower animals, and in all of these it serves exclusively to aid the male in the act of reproduction. . . .

That this unknown factor is reversion to a former state of existence may be admitted as in the highest degree probable. It is quite incredible that a man should through mere accident abnormally resemble certain apes in no less than seven of his muscles, if there had been no genetic connection between them. On the other hand, if man is descended from some ape-like creature, no valid reason can be assigned why certain muscles should not suddenly reappear after an interval of many thousand generations, in the same manner as with horses, asses, and mules, dark-coloured stripes suddenly reappear on the legs, and shoulders, after an interval of hundreds, or more probably of thousands of generations.

These various cases of reversion are so closely related to those of rudimentary organs given in the first chapter, that many of them might have been indifferently introduced either there or here. Thus a human uterus furnished with cornua may be said to represent, in a rudimentary condition, the same organ in its normal state in certain mammals. Some parts which are rudimentary in man, as the os coccyx in both sexes, and the mammae in the male sex, are always present; whilst others, such as the supracondyloid foramen, only occasionally appear, and therefore might have been introduced under the head of reversion. These several reversionary structures, as well as the strictly rudimentary ones, reveal the descent of man from some lower form in an unmistakable manner.

Correlated Variation

In man, as in the lower animals, many structures are so intimately related, that when one part varies so does another, without our being able, in most cases, to assign any reason. We cannot say whether the one part governs the other, or whether both are governed by some earlier developed part. Various monstrosities, as I. Geoffroy repeatedly insists, are thus intimately connected. Homologous structures are particularly liable to change together, as we see on the opposite sides of the body, and in the upper and lower extremities. Meckel long ago remarked, that when the muscles of the arm depart from their proper type, they almost always imitate those of the leg; and so, conversely, with the muscles of the legs. The organs of sight and hearing, the teeth and hair, the colour of the skin and of the hair, colour and constitution, are more or less correlated. Professor Schaaffhausen first drew attention to the relation apparently existing between a muscular frame and the strongly-pronounced supra-orbital ridges, which are so characteristic of the lower races of man.

Besides the variations which can be grouped with more or less probability under the foregoing heads, there is a large class of variations which may be provisionally called spontaneous, for to our ignorance they appear to arise without any exciting cause. It can, however, be shewn that such variations, whether consisting of slight individual differences, or of strongly-marked and abrupt deviations of structure, depend much more on the constitution of the organism than on the nature of the conditions to which it has been subjected.

Rate of Increase

. . . If we look back to an extremely remote epoch, before man had arrived at the dignity of manhood, he would have been guided more by instinct and less by reason than are the lowest savages at the present time. Our early semi-human progenitors would not have practised infanticide or polyandry; for the instincts of the lower animals are never so perverted as to lead them regularly to destroy their own offspring, or to be quite devoid of jealousy. There would have been no prudential restraint from marriage, and the sexes would have freely united at an early age. Hence the progenitors of man would have tended to increase rapidly; but checks of some kind, either periodical or constant, must have kept down their numbers, even more severely than with existing savages. What the precise nature of these checks were, we cannot say, any more than with most other animals. We know that horses and cattle, which are not extremely prolific animals, when first turned loose in South America, increased at an enormous rate. The elephant, the slowest breeder of all known animals, would in a few thousand years stock the whole world. The increase of every species of monkey must be checked by some means; but not, as Brehm remarks, by the attacks of beasts of prey. No one will assume that the actual power of reproduction in the wild horses and cattle of America, was at first in any sensible degree increased; or that, as each district became fully stocked, this same power was diminished. No doubt, in this case, and in all others, many checks concur, and different checks under different circumstances; periodical dearths, depending on unfavourable seasons, being probably the most important of all. So it will have been with the early progenitors of man.

Natural Selection

We have now seen that man is variable in body and mind; and that the variations are induced, either directly or indirectly, by the same general causes, and obey the same general laws, as with the lower animals. Man has spread widely over the face of the earth, and must have been exposed, during his incessant migration, to the most diversified conditions. The inhabitants of Tierra del Fuego, the Cape of Good Hope, and Tasmania in the one hemisphere, and of the arctic regions in the other, must have passed through many climates, and changed their habits many times, before they reached their present homes. The early progenitors of man must also have tended, like all other animals, to have increased beyond their means of subsistence; they must, therefore, occasionally have been exposed to a struggle for existence, and consequently to the rigid law of natural selection. Beneficial variations of all kinds will thus, either occasionally or habitually, have been preserved and injurious ones eliminated. I do not refer to strongly-marked deviations of structure, which occur only at long intervals of time, but to mere individual differences. We know, for instance, that the muscles of our hands and feet, which determine our powers of movement, are liable, like those of the lower animals, to incessant variability. If then the progenitors of man inhabiting any district, especially one undergoing some change in its conditions, were divided into two equal bodies, the one half which included all the individuals best adapted by their powers of movement for gaining subsistence, or for defending themselves, would on an average survive in greater numbers, and procreate more offspring than the other and less well endowed half.

Source: Darwin, Charles. 1871. *The Descent of Man.* London: John Murray.

▣ Victoria Woodhull, "Tried as by Fire" (1871)

Victoria Woodhull gave her speech "Tried as by Fire" on a tour of 150 appearances around the United States, to audiences totaling over a quarter of a million people, by her own estimate. In the speech, she dramatically and explicitly connects feminism and eugenics. Woodhull's is an early expression of the idea that, if only women had sexual freedom and knowledge, their children would necessarily be free of deformity and defects. As evidence of this connection, in this passage Woodhull offers her personal experience, a rare public, firsthand narrative about raising a disabled son in the nineteenth century.

Go home with me and see desolation and devastation in another form. The cold, iron bolt has entered my heart and left my life a blank, in ashes upon my lips. Wherever I go I carry a living corpse in my breast, the vacant stare of whose living counterpart meets me at the door of my home. My boy, now nineteen years of age, who should have been my pride and my joy, has never been blessed by the dawning of reasoning. I was married at fourteen, ignorant of everything that related to my maternal functions. For this ignorance, and because I knew no better than to surrender my maternal functions to a drunken man, I am cursed with this living death. Do you think my mother's heart does not yearn for the love of my boy? Do you think I do not realize the awful condition to which I have consigned him? Do you think that I would not willingly give my life to make him what he has a right to be? Do you think his face is not ever before me pressing me on to declare these terrible social laws to the world? Do you think with this sorrow seated on my soul I can ever sit quietly down and permit women to go on ignorantly, repeating my crime? Do you think I can ever cease to hurl the bitterest imprecations at the accursed thing that has made my life one long misery? Do you think I can ever hesitate to warn the young maidens against my fate, or advise them never to surrender the control of their maternal functions to any man! Ah! if you do, you do not know the agony that rests here. Not to do less than I am doing were madness; it were worse than crime; it were the essence of ten thousand crimes concentrated in one soul to sing it in eternal infamy.

Source: Woodhull, Victoria. 1871, April 29. "Tried as by Fire." *Woodhull & Claflin's Weekly*, 2(24):10.

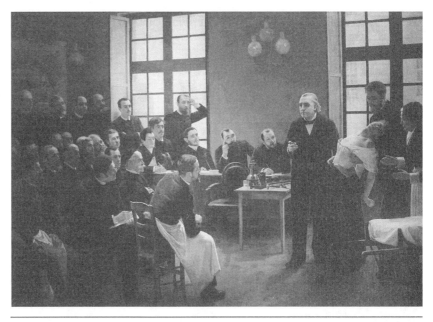

A Lesson on Hysteria by Dr. Jean Martin Charcot *(1823–1890), by André Brouillet (1857–1920). A French physician and neurologist, Charcot was well known for being able to induce female patients diagnosed with hysteria to have hypnotic fainting spells in front of his medical students, professional colleagues, and visitors. He believed that hysteria was hereditary and that hypnosis could be used to simulate the symptoms to facilitate the study of his patients.*

Source: Art Resource, New York.

▣ Victoria Woodhull on Women's Suffrage (1871)

Suffrage rhetoric in the 1870s frequently referred to disability issues in regard to voting. Disabled men vote, the argument ran, so why are women categorically excluded on the basis of "weakness"? In the second extract below, the issue is individuality. In a discussion of the well-known conjoined twins Millie and Christine McKoy, Woodhull argues that they should get two votes "as their mother gave them two names," analogous to the most famous such twins, Chang and Eng Bunker (who were also North Carolinians by this time).

A Woman's Thoughts on the Human Question

[The weaker physique of the average woman] is a curious reason for the subordination of the woman; since in a just application it would defeat itself, in depriving every physically feeble or ailing or crippled man—no matter what his moral or intellectual status—of the vote, and placing the same in the hand of every amazon, virago, termagant—no matter how coarse or ignorant—if they could but muscularly grasp it.

Source: Buddington, Zadel Barnes. "A Woman's Thoughts on the Human Question." Originally published in the *National Standard* (n.d.); reprinted on April 15, 1871, in *Woodhull & Clafin's Weekly,* 2(23):2.

A Question Answered

A correspondent asks us whether, if woman suffrage is established, the North Carolina two-headed girl, so called, will have two votes or one? We think, for the purpose of answering the question, we can give the monstrosity a plural position and call them girls, as their mother gave them two names—Milly and Christiana. They have two hearts and two heads, and would be as much entitled to two votes as Chang and Eng, the Siamese twins.

Source: Woodhull, Victoria. 1871, April 22. "A Question Answered." *Woodhull & Claflin's Weekly* 2(24):10.

▣ Hindu Testimony Acts (1872–1922)

This series of excerpts provides a sense of the range of British colonial policies in India regarding the legal status of mentally ill and mentally disabled people, including the admissibility of testimony by those deemed lunatic, weak-minded, and so forth.

Competence to Testify

The Indian Evidence Act, 1872, Section 118, provided that "all persons shall be competent to testify unless the Court considers that they are prevented from understanding the questions put to them, or from giving rational answers to those questions, by tender years, extreme old age, disease, whether of body of mind, or any other cause of the same kind."

Explanation: "A lunatic is not incompetent to testify, unless he is prevented by his lunacy from understanding the questions put to him and giving rational answers to them."

Incapacity Due to Mental Infirmity

John Mayne's *Treatise on Hindu Law and Usage* goes into detail of particular cases and decisions.

Mayne remarks, "As to mental infirmity, it has been held that the degree of incapacity which amounts to idiocy is not utter mental darkness. It is sufficient if the person is, and has been from his birth, of such an unsound and imbecile mind as to be incapable of instruction or discrimination between right and wrong. He must, in short, be one whom it would be impossible to describe as a reasoning being. Mere want of sound, or even ordinary, intelligence is not sufficient." In short, there is an area of opinion in which experts might well disagree.

Source: Stephen, James F. 1872. P. 200 in *The Indian Evidence Act (1. of 1872) with an Introduction on the Principles of Judicial Evidence.* London: Macmillan.

Source: Mayne, John D. 1922. Coutts Trotter, V. M., ed. *A Treatise on Hindu Law and Usage,* 9th ed. Madras, India: Higginbothams.

▣ Johanna Spyri, from *Heidi* (1880–1881)

In Clara, Swiss author Spyri created one of the classic disabled child characters in children's literature. Clara, a city child visiting in the mountains, is sweet and uncomplaining, but lonely and pampered at home. Fresh air, Alpine scenery, and friendship restore more than her spirits: In this climactic scene, Clara is suddenly able to walk, with the encouragement of Heidi and the grudging support of Peter (a boy who earlier had destroyed Clara's wheelchair in a fit of jealousy).

"Would you think me unkind, Clara," she said rather hesitatingly, "if I left you for a few minutes? I should run there and back very quickly. I want so to see how the flowers are looking—but wait—" for an idea had come into Heidi's head. She ran and picked a bunch or two of green leaves, and then took hold of Snowflake and led her up to Clara.

"There, now you will not be alone," said Heidi, giving the goat a little push to show her she was to lie down near Clara, which the animal quite understood. Heidi threw the leaves into Clara's lap, and the latter told her friend to go at once to look at the flowers as she was quite happy to be left with the goat; she liked this new experience. Heidi ran off, and Clara began to hold out the leaves one by one to Snowflake, who snoozled up to her new friend in a confiding manner and slowly ate the leaves from her hand. It was easy to see that Snowflake enjoyed this peaceful and sheltered way of feeding, for when with the other goats she had much persecution to endure from the larger and stronger ones of the flock. And Clara found a strange new pleasure in sitting all alone like this on the mountain side, her only companion a little goat that looked to her for protection. She suddenly felt a great desire to be her own mistress and to be able to help others, instead of herself being always dependent as she was now. Many thoughts, unknown to her before, came crowding into her mind, and a longing to go on living in the sunshine, and to be doing something that would bring happiness to another, as now she was helping to make the goat happy. An unaccustomed feeling of joy took possession of her, as if everything she had ever known or felt became all at once more beautiful, and she seemed to see all things in a new light, and so strong was the sense of this new beauty and happiness that she threw her arms round the little goat's neck, and exclaimed, "O Snowflake, how delightful it is up here! if only I could stay on for ever with you beside me!"

Heidi had meanwhile reached her field of flowers, and as she caught sight of it she uttered a cry of joy. The whole ground in front of her was a mass of shimmering gold, where the cistus flowers spread their yellow blossoms. Above them waved whole bushes of the deep blue bell-flowers; while the fragrance that arose from the whole sunlit expanse was as if the rarest balsam had been flung over it. The scent, however, came from the small brown flowers, the little round heads of which rose modestly here and there among the yellow blossoms. Heidi stood and gazed and drew in the delicious air. Suddenly she turned round and reached Clara's side out of breath with running and excitement. "Oh, you must come," she called out as soon as she came in sight, "it is more beautiful than you can imagine, and perhaps this evening it may not be so lovely. I believe I could carry you, don't you think I could?" Clara looked at her and shook her head. "Why, Heidi, what can you be thinking of! you are smaller than I am. Oh, if only I could walk!"

Heidi looked round as if in search of something, some new idea had evidently come into her head. Peter was sitting up above looking down on the two children. He had been sitting and staring before him in the same way for hours, as if he could not make out what he saw. He had destroyed the chair so that the friend might not be able to move anywhere and that her visit might come to an end, and then a little while after she had appeared right up here under his very nose with Heidi beside her. He thought his eyes must

deceive him, and yet there she was and no mistake about it.

Heidi now looked up to where he was sitting and called out in a peremptory voice, "Peter, come down here!"

"I don't wish to come," he called in reply.

"But you are to, you must; I cannot do it alone, and you must come here and help me; make haste and come down," she called again in an urgent voice.

"I shall do nothing of the kind," was the answer.

Heidi ran some way up the slope towards him, and then pausing called again, her eyes ablaze with anger, "If you don't come at once, Peter, I will do something to you that you won't like; I mean what I say."

Peter felt an inward throe at these words, and a great fear seized him. He had done something wicked which he wanted no one to know about, and so far he had thought himself safe. But now Heidi spoke exactly as if she knew everything, and whatever she did know she would tell her grandfather, and there was no one he feared so much as this latter person. Supposing he were to suspect what had happened about the chair! Peter's anguish of mind grew more acute. He stood up and went down to where Heidi was awaiting him.

"I am coming and you won't do what you said."

Peter appeared now so submissive with fear that Heidi felt quite sorry for him and answered assuringly, "No, no, of course not; come along with me, there is nothing to be afraid of in what I want you to do."

As soon as they got to Clara, Heidi gave her orders: Peter was to take hold of her under the arms on one side and she on the other, and together they were to lift her up. This first movement was successfully carried through, but then came the difficulty. As Clara could not even stand, how were they to support her and get her along? Heidi was too small for her arm to serve Clara to lean upon.

"You must put one arm well around my neck so, and put the other through Peter's and lean firmly upon it, then we shall be able to carry you."

Peter, however, had never given his arm to any one in his life. Clara put hers in his, but he kept his own hanging down straight beside him like a stick.

"That's not the way, Peter," said Heidi in an authoritative voice. "You must put your arm out in the shape of a ring, and Clara must put hers through it and lean her weight upon you, and whatever you do, don't let your arm give way; like that. I am sure we shall be able to manage."

Peter did as he was told, but still they did not get on very well. Clara was not such a light weight, and the team did not match very well in size; it was up one side and down the other, so that the supports were rather wobbly.

Clara tried to use her own feet a little, but each time drew them quickly back.

"Put your foot down firmly once," suggested Heidi, "I am sure it will hurt you less after that."

"Do you think so?" said Clara hesitatingly, but she followed Heidi's advice and ventured one firm step on the ground and then another; she called out a little as she did it; then she lifted her foot again and went on, "Oh, that was less painful already," she exclaimed joyfully.

"Try again," said Heidi encouragingly.

And Clara went on putting one foot out after another until all at once she called out, "I can do it, Heidi! look! look! I can make proper steps!" And Heidi cried out with even greater delight, "Can you really make steps, can you really walk? really walk by yourself? Oh, if only grandfather were here!" and she continued gleefully to exclaim, "You can walk now, Clara, you can walk!"

Source: Spyri, Johanna. 1918. *Heidi*. Philadelphia: David McKay. (Originally published 1880–1881)

◉ Emperor Wilhelm of Germany, Speech before Parliament (1881)

In this speech, delivered in support of a bill to establish accident insurance for workers, Emperor Wilhelm makes it clear that the bill is motivated as much by political as by humanitarian ends: Guaranteeing assistance to those disabled in workplace accidents will make socialism less attractive to the working classes.

Past institutions intended to insure working people against the danger of falling into a condition of helplessness owing to the incapacity resulting from accident or age have proved inadequate, and their insufficiency has to no small extent contributed to cause the working classes to seek help by participating in Social Democratic movements.

Source: Dawson, William. 1912. P. 111 in *Social Insurance in Germany, 1883–1911*. London: Scribner's.

◉ Robert Louis Stevenson, from *Treasure Island* (1883)

This scene from Robert Louis Stevenson's Treasure Island *introduces one of the most memorable and complicated characters in the history of literature, the pirate Long John Silver, as seen through the eyes of young Jim Hawkins. Disloyal and friendly, murderous and loving, Long John appears as a crippled, yet dexterous, acrobat and consummate talker, at once winning and despicable, physically powerful and impaired. Long John Silver emerges from a gallery of the eyeless, fingerless, and stupid not as the sailor outlaw with an eye patch or hook but as the peg-legged criminal of the sea who will be from this moment on fixed for all time in the Western imagination as the essence of what a pirate is: an enigma made vivid through the embodiment of disability.*

As I was waiting, a man came out of a side room, and, at a glance, I was sure he must be Long John. His left leg was cut off close by the hip, and under the left shoulder he carried a crutch, which he managed with wonderful dexterity, hopping about upon it like a bird. He was very tall and strong, with a face as big as a ham—plain and pale, but intelligent and smiling. Indeed, he seemed in the most cheerful spirits, whistling as he moved about among the tables, with a merry word or a slap on the shoulder for the more favoured of his guests.

Now, to tell you the truth, from the very first mention of Long John in Squire Trelawney's letter, I had taken a fear in my mind that he might prove to be the very one-legged sailor whom I had watched for so long at the old 'Benbow.' But one look at the man before me was enough. I had seen the captain, and Black Dog, and the blind man Pew, and I thought I knew what a buccaneer was like—a very different creature, according to me, from this clean and pleasant-tempered landlord.

I plucked up courage at once, crossed the threshold, and walked right up to the man where he stood, propped on his crutch, talking to a customer.

'Mr Silver, sir?' I asked, holding out the note.

'Yes, my lad,' said he; 'such is my name, to be sure. And who may you be?' And then as he saw the squire's letter, he seemed to me to give something almost like a start.

'Oh!' said he, quite loud, and offering his hand, 'I see. You are our new cabin-boy; pleased I am to see you.'

And he took my hand in his large firm grasp.

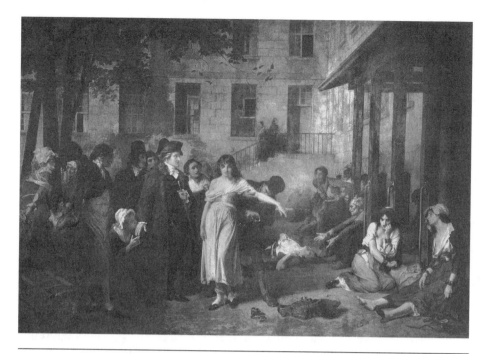

Doctor Philippe Pinel Orders the Removal of the Chains at the Lunatic Asylum, *by Tony Robert-Fleury (1838–1911). This painting captures Pinel's now-mythic effort to free the inmates from their chains at the all-female asylum of Salpetriere. He made the decision following his appointment as superintendent at the institution in 1794 after viewing conditions in the wards. The action is widely recognized as a transition in inmate care from punitive to psychoanalytic—what is now referred to as "moral treatment." In some cases, straightjackets replaced the chains; therefore, in* Madness and Civilization, *Michel Foucault treats this "liberation" as merely the substitution of one disciplinary system with another.*

Source: Art Resource, New York.

Just then one of the customers at the far side rose suddenly and made for the door. It was close by him, and he was out in the street in a moment. But his hurry had attracted my notice, and I recognised him at a glance. It was the tallow-faced man, wanting two fingers, who had come first to the 'Admiral Benbow.'

'Oh,' I cried, 'stop him! it's Black Dog!'

'I don't care two coppers who he is,' cried Silver. 'But he hasn't paid his score. Harry, run and catch him.'

One of the others who was nearest the door leaped up, and started in pursuit.

'If he were Admiral Hawke he shall pay his score,' cried Silver; and then, relinquishing my hand—'Who did you say he was?' he asked. 'Black what?'

'Dog, sir,' said I. 'Has Mr Trelawney not told you of the buccaneers? He was one of them.'

'So?' cried Silver. 'In my house! Ben, run and help Harry. One of those swabs, was he? Was that you drinking with him, Morgan? Step up here.'

The man whom he called Morgan—an old, grey-haired, mahogany-faced sailor—came forward pretty sheepishly, rolling his quid.

'Now, Morgan,' said Long John, very sternly; 'you never clapped your eyes on that Black—Black Dog before, did you, now?'

'Not I, sir,' said Morgan, with a salute.

'You didn't know his name, did you?'

'No, sir.'

'By the powers, Tom Morgan, it's as good for you!' exclaimed the landlord. 'If you had been mixed up with the like of that, you would never have put another foot in my house, you may lay to that. And what was he saying to you?'

'I don't rightly know, sir,' answered Morgan.

'Do you call that a head on your shoulders, or a blessed dead-eye?' cried Long John. 'Don't rightly know, don't you! Perhaps you don't happen to rightly know who you were speaking to, perhaps? Come, now, what was he jawing—v'yages, cap'ns, ships? Pipe up! What was it?'

'We was a-talkin' of keel-hauling,' answered Morgan.

'Keel-hauling, was you? and a mighty suitable thing, too and you may lay to that. Get back to your place for a lubber Tom.'

And then, as Morgan rolled back to his seat, Silver added to me in a confidential whisper, that was very flattering, as I thought:—

'He's quite an honest man, Tom Morgan, on'y stupid. An now,' he ran on again, aloud, 'let's see—Black Dog? No, don't know the name, not I. Yet I kind of think I've—yes, I've seen the swab. He used to come here with a blind beggar he used.'

'That he did, you may be sure,' said I. 'I knew that blind man, too. His name was Pew.'

'It was!' cried Silver, now quite excited. 'Pew! That were his name for certain. Ah, he looked a shark, he did! If we run down this Black Dog, now, there'll be news for Captain Trelawney! Ben's a good runner; few seamen run better than Ben. He should run him down, hand over hand, by the powers! He talked o' keel-hauling, did he? I'll keel-haul him!'

All the time he was jerking out these phrases he was stumping up and down the tavern on his crutch, slapping tables with his hand, and giving such a show of excitement as would have convinced an Old Bailey judge or a Bow Street runner. My suspicions had been thoroughly re-awakened on finding Black Dog at the 'Spy-glass,' and I watched the cook narrowly. But he was too deep, and too ready, and too clever for me, and by the time the two men had come back out of breath, and confessed that they had lost the track in a crowd, and been scolded like thieves, I would have gone bail for the innocence of Long John Silver.

'See here, now, Hawkins,' said he, 'here's a blessed hard thing on a man like me, now, aint it? There's Cap'n Trelawney—what's he to think? Here I have this confounded son of a Dutchman sitting in my own house, drinking of my own rum! Here you comes and tells me of it plain; and here I let him give us all the slip before my blessed dead-lights! Now, Hawkins, you do me justice with the cap'n. You're a lad, you are, but you're as smart as paint. I see that when you first came in. Now, here it is: What could I do, with this old timber I hobble on? When I was an A B master mariner I'd have come up alongside of him, hand over hand, and broached him to in a brace of old shakes, I would; but now—'

And then, all of a sudden, he stopped, and his jaw drooped as though he had remembered something.

'The score!' he burst out. 'Three goes o' rum! Why, shiver my timbers, if I hadn't forgotten my score!'

And, falling on a bench, he laughed until the tears ran down his cheeks. I could not help joining; and we laughed together, peal after peal, until the tavern rang again.

Source: Stevenson, Robert Louis. 1883. Ch. 8 in *Treasure Island*. London: Cassell.

▣ Mary E. Wilkins Freeman, from "A Mistaken Charity" (1887)

The U.S. regional northeastern writer Mary E. Wilkins Freeman wrote numerous short stories about women's efforts to free themselves of domestic and public constraints about femininity. In the story excerpted here, two aging sisters—one of whom is blind—develop an interdependency with each other while living in a ramshackle house. Their relationship revolves around their mutual needs rather than more traditional values of male self-sufficiency. Their efforts to live alone on their own terms violates their neighbors' belief that dependency is a failing, and thus a movement takes shape to have them institutionalized against their will.

There were in a green field a little, low, weather-stained cottage, with a foot-path leading to it from the highway several rods distant, and two old women—one with a tin pan and old knife searching for dandelion greens among the short young grass, and the other sitting on the door-step watching her, or, rather, having the appearance of watching her.

"Air there enough for a mess, Harriét?" asked the old woman on the door-step. She accented oddly the last syllable of the Harriet, and there was a curious quality in her feeble, cracked old voice. Besides the question denoted by the arrangement of her words and the rising inflection, there was another, broader and subtler, the very essence of all questioning, in the tone of her voice itself; the cracked, quavering notes that she used reached out of themselves, and asked, and groped like fingers in the dark. One would have known by the voice that the old woman was blind.

The old woman on her knees in the grass searching for dandelions did not reply; she evidently had not heard the question. So the old woman on the door-step, after waiting a few minutes with her head turned expectantly, asked again, varying her question slightly, and speaking louder:

"Air there enough for a mess, do ye s'pose, Harriét?"

The old woman in the grass heard this time. She rose slowly and laboriously; the effort of straightening out the rheumatic old muscles was evidently a painful one; then she eyed the greens heaped up in the tin pan, and pressed them down with her hand.

"Wa'al, I don't know, Charlotte," she replied, hoarsely. "There's plenty on 'em here, but I ain't got near enough for a mess; they do bile down so when you get 'em in the pot; an' it's all I can do to bend my j'ints enough to dig 'em."

"I'd give consider'ble to help ye, Harriét," said the old woman on the door-step.

But the other did not hear her; she was down on her knees in the grass again, anxiously spying out the dandelions.

So the old woman on the door-step crossed her little shrivelled hands over her calico knees, and sat quite still, with the soft spring wind blowing over her.

The old wooden door-step was sunk low down among the grasses, and the whole house to which it belonged had an air of settling down and mouldering into the grass as into its own grave.

When Harriet Shattuck grew deaf and rheumatic, and had to give up her work as tailoress, and Charlotte Shattuck lost her eyesight, and was unable to do any more sewing for her livelihood, it was a small and trifling charity for the rich man who held a mortgage on the little house in which they had been born and lived all their lives to give them the use of it, rent and interest free. He might as well have taken credit to himself for not charging a squirrel for his tenement in some old decaying tree in his woods.

So ancient was the little habitation, so wavering and mouldering, the hands that had fashioned it had lain still so long in their graves, that it almost seemed to have fallen below its distinctive rank as a house. Rain and snow had filtered through its roof, mosses had grown over it, worms had eaten it, and birds built their nests under its eaves; nature had almost completely overrun and obliterated the work of man, and taken her own to herself again, till the house seemed as much a natural ruin as an old tree-stump.

The Shattucks had always been poor people and common people; no especial grace and refinement or fine ambition had ever characterized any of them; they had always been poor and coarse and common. The father and his father before him had simply lived in the poor little house, grubbed for their living, and then unquestioningly died. The mother had been of no rarer stamp, and the two daughters were cast in the same mould.

After their parents' death Harriet and Charlotte had lived along in the old place from youth to old age, with the one hope of ability to keep a roof over their heads, covering on their backs, and victuals in their mouths—an all-sufficient one with them.

Neither of them had ever had a lover; they had always seemed to repel rather than attract the opposite sex. It was not merely because they were poor, ordinary, and homely; there were plenty of men in the place who would have matched them well in that respect; the fault lay deeper—in their characters. Harriet, even in her girlhood, had a blunt, defiant manner that almost amounted to surliness, and was well calculated to alarm timid adorers, and Charlotte had always had the reputation of not being any too strong in her mind.

Harriet had gone about from house to house doing tailor-work after the primitive country fashion, and Charlotte had done plain sewing and mending for the neighbors. They had been, in the main, except when pressed by some temporary anxiety about their work or the payment thereof, happy and contented, with that negative kind of happiness and contentment which comes not from gratified ambition, but a lack of ambition itself. All that they cared for they had had in tolerable abundance, for Harriet at least had been swift and capable about her work. The patched, mossy old roof had been kept over their heads, the coarse, hearty food that they loved had been set on their table, and their cheap clothes had been warm and strong.

After Charlotte's eyes failed her, and Harriet had the rheumatic fever, and the little hoard of earnings went to the doctors, times were harder with them, though still it could not be said that they actually suffered.

When they could not pay the interest on the mortgage they were allowed to keep the place interest free; there was as much fitness in a mortgage on the little house, anyway, as there would have been on a rotten old apple-tree; and the people about, who were mostly farmers, and good friendly folk, helped them out with their living. One would donate a barrel of apples from his abundant harvest to the two poor old women, one a barrel of potatoes, another a load of wood for the winter fuel, and many a farmer's wife had bustled up the narrow foot-path with a pound of butter, or a dozen fresh eggs, or a nice bit of pork. Besides all this, there was a tiny garden patch behind the house, with a straggling row of currant bushes in it, and one of gooseberries, where Harriet contrived every year to raise a few pumpkins, which were the pride of her life. On the right of the garden were two old apple-trees, a Baldwin and a Porter, both yet in a tolerably good fruit-bearing state. . . .

When the two old women sat down complacently to their meal of pork and dandelion greens in their little kitchen they did not dream how destiny slowly and surely was introducing some new colors into their web of life, even when it was almost completed, and that this was one of the last meals they would eat in their old home for many a day. In about a week from that day they were established in the "Old Ladies' Home" in a neighboring city. It came about in this wise: Mrs. Simonds, the woman who had brought the gift of hot doughnuts, was a smart, energetic person, bent on doing good, and she did a great deal. To be sure, she always did it in her own way. If she chose to give hot doughnuts, she gave hot doughnuts; it made not the slightest difference to her if the recipients of her charity would infinitely have preferred ginger cookies. Still, a great many would like hot doughnuts, and she did unquestionably a great deal of good.

She had a worthy coadjutor in the person of a rich and childless elderly widow in the place. They had fairly entered into a partnership in good works, with about an equal capital on both sides, the widow furnishing the money, and Mrs. Simonds, who had much the better head of the two, furnishing the active schemes of benevolence.

The afternoon after the doughnut episode she had gone to the widow with a new project, and the result was that entrance fees had been paid, and old Harriet and Charlotte made sure of a comfortable home for the rest of their lives. The widow was hand in glove with officers of missionary boards and trustees of charitable institutions. There had been an unusual mortality among the inmates of the "Home" this spring, there were several vacancies, and the matter of the admission of Harriet and Charlotte was very quickly and easily arranged. But the matter which would have seemed the least difficult—inducing the two old women to accept the bounty which Providence, the widow, and Mrs. Simonds were ready to bestow on them—proved the most so. The struggle to persuade them to abandon their tottering old home for a better was a terrible one. The widow had pleaded with mild surprise, and Mrs. Simonds with benevolent determination; the counsel and reverend eloquence of the minister had been called in; and when they yielded at last it was with a sad grace for the recipients of a worthy charity.

It had been hard to convince them that the "Home" was not an almshouse under another name, and their yielding at length to anything short of actual force was only due probably to the plea, which was advanced most eloquently to Harriet, that Charlotte would be so much more comfortable.

The morning they came away, Charlotte cried pitifully, and trembled all over her little shrivelled body. Harriet did not cry. But when her sister had passed out the low, sagging door she turned the key in the lock, then took it out and thrust it slyly into her pocket, shaking her head to herself with an air of fierce determination.

Mrs. Simonds's husband, who was to take them to the depot, said to himself, with disloyal defiance of his wife's active charity, that it was a shame, as he helped the two distressed old souls into his light wagon, and put the poor little box, with their homely clothes in it, in behind.

Mrs. Simonds, the widow, the minister, and the gentleman from the "Home" who was to take charge of them, were all at the depot, their faces beaming with the delight of successful benevolence. But the two poor old women looked like two forlorn prisoners in their midst. It was an impressive illustration of the truth of the saying "that it is more blessed to give than to receive."

Well, Harriet and Charlotte Shattuck went to the "Old Ladies' Home" with reluctance and distress. They stayed two months, and then—they ran away.

The "Home" was comfortable, and in some respects even luxurious; but nothing suited those two unhappy, unreasonable old women.

The fare was of a finer, more delicately served variety than they had been accustomed to; those finely flavored nourishing soups for which the "Home" took great credit to itself failed to please palates used to common, coarser food.

"O Lord, Harriét, when I set down to the table here there ain't no chinks," Charlotte used to say. "If we could hev some cabbage, or some pork an' greens, how the light would stream in!"

Then they had to be more particular about their dress. They had always been tidy enough, but now it had to be something more; the widow, in the kindness of her heart, had made it possible, and the good folks in charge of the "Home," in the kindness of their hearts, tried to carry out the widow's designs.

But nothing could transform these two unpolished old women into two nice old ladies. They did not take kindly to white lace caps and delicate neckerchiefs. They liked their new black cashmere dresses well enough, but they felt as if they broke a commandment when they put them on every afternoon. They had always worn calico with long aprons at home, and they wanted to now; and they wanted to twist up their scanty gray locks into little knots at the back of their heads, and go without caps, just as they always had done.

Charlotte in a dainty white cap was pitiful, but Harriet was both pitiful and comical. They were totally at variance with their surroundings, and they felt it keenly, as people of their stamp always do. No amount of kindness and attention—and they had enough of both—sufficed to reconcile them to their new abode. Charlotte pleaded continually with her sister to go back to their old home.

"O Lord, Harriét," she would exclaim (by the way, Charlotte's "O Lord," which, as she used it, was innocent enough, had been heard with much disfavor in the "Home," and she, not knowing at all why, had been remonstrated with concerning it), "let us go home. I can't stay here no ways in this world. I don't like their vittles, an' I don't like to wear a cap; I want to go home and do different. The currants will be ripe, Harriét. O Lord, thar was almost a chink, thinking about 'em. I want some of 'em; an' the Porter apples will be gittin' ripe, an' we could have some apple-pie. This here ain't good; I want merlasses fur sweeting. Can't we get back no ways, Harriét? It ain't far, an' we could walk, an' they don't lock us in, nor nothin.' I don't want to die here; it ain't so straight up to heaven from here. O Lord, I've felt as if I was slantendicular from heaven ever since I've been here, an' it's been so awful dark. I ain't had any chinks. I want to go home, Harriét."

"We'll go to-morrow mornin,'" said Harriet, finally; "we'll pack up our things an' go; we'll put on our old dresses, an' we'll do up the new ones in bundles, an' we'll jest shy out the back way to-morrow mornin'; an' we'll go. I kin find the way, an' I reckon we kin git thar, if it is fourteen mile. Mebbe somebody will give us a lift."

And they went. With a grim humor Harriet hung the new white lace caps with which she and Charlotte had been so pestered, one on each post at the head of the bedstead, so they would meet the eyes of the first person who opened the door. Then they took their bundles, stole slyly out, and were soon on the highroad, hobbling along, holding each other's hands, as jubilant as two children, and chuckling to themselves over their escape, and the probable astonishment there would be in the "Home" over it.

"O Lord, Harriét, what do you s'pose they will say to them caps?" cried Charlotte, with a gleeful cackle.

"I guess they'll see as folks ain't goin' to be made to wear caps agin their will in a free kentry," returned Harriet, with an echoing cackle, as they sped feebly and bravely along.

The "Home" stood on the very outskirts of the city, luckily for them. They would have found it a difficult undertaking to traverse the crowded streets. As it was, a short walk brought them into the free country road—free comparatively, for even here at ten o'clock in the morning there was considerable travelling to and from the city on business or pleasure.

People whom they met on the road did not stare at them as curiously as might have been expected. Harriet held her bristling chin high in air, and hobbled along with an appearance of being well aware of what she was about, that led folks to doubt their own first opinion that there was something unusual about the two old women.

Still their evident feebleness now and then occasioned from one and another more particular scrutiny. When they had been on the road a half-hour or so, a man in a covered wagon drove up behind them. After he had passed them, he poked his head around the front of the vehicle and looked back. Finally he stopped, and waited for them to come up to him.

"Like a ride, ma'am?" said he, looking at once bewildered and compassionate.

"Thankee," said Harriet, "we'd be much obleeged."

After the man had lifted the old women into the wagon, and established them on the back seat, he turned around, as he drove slowly along, and gazed at them curiously.

"Seems to me you look pretty feeble to be walking far," said he. "Where were you going?"

Harriet told him with an air of defiance.

"Why," he exclaimed, "it is fourteen miles out. You could never walk it in the world. Well, I am going within three miles of there, and I can go on a little farther as well as not. But I don't see—Have you been in the city?"

"I have been visitin' my married darter in the city," said Harriet, calmly.

Charlotte started, and swallowed convulsively.

Harriet had never told a deliberate falsehood before in her life, but this seemed to her one of the tremendous exigencies of life which justify a lie. She felt desperate. If she could not contrive to deceive him in some way, the man might turn directly around and carry Charlotte and her back to the "Home" and the white caps.

"I should not have thought your daughter would have let you start for such a walk as that," said the man. "Is this lady your sister? She is blind, isn't she? She does not look fit to walk a mile."

"Yes, she's my sister," replied Harriet, stubbornly: "an' she's blind; an' my darter didn't want us to walk. She felt reel bad about it. But she couldn't help it. She's poor, and her husband's dead, an' she's got four leetle children."

Harriet recounted the hardships of her imaginary daughter with a glibness that was astonishing. Charlotte swallowed again.

"Well," said the man, "I am glad I overtook you, for I don't think you would ever have reached home alive."

About six miles from the city an open buggy passed them swiftly. In it were seated the matron and one of the gentlemen in charge of the "Home." They never thought of looking into the covered wagon—and indeed one can travel in one of those vehicles, so popular in some parts of New England, with as much privacy as he could in his tomb. The two in the buggy were seriously alarmed, and anxious for the safety of the old women, who were chuckling maliciously in the wagon they soon left far behind. Harriet had watched them breathlessly until they disappeared on a curve of the road; then she whispered to Charlotte.

A little after noon the two old women crept slowly up the foot-path across the field to their old home.

"The clover is up to our knees," said Harriet; "an' the sorrel and the white-weed; an' there's lots of yaller butterflies."

"O Lord, Harriét, thar's a chink, an' I do believe I saw one of them yaller butterflies go past it," cried Charlotte, trembling all over, and nodding her gray head violently.

Harriet stood on the old sunken door-step and fitted the key, which she drew triumphantly from her pocket, in the lock, while Charlotte stood waiting and shaking behind her.

Then they went in. Everything was there just as they had left it. Charlotte sank down on a chair and began to cry. Harriet hurried across to the window that looked out on the garden.

"The currants air ripe," said she; "an' them pumpkins hev run all over everything."

"O Lord, Harriét," sobbed Charlotte, "thar is so many chinks that they air all runnin' together!"

Source: Freeman, Mary E. Wilkins. 1887. "A Mistaken Charity." In *A Humble Romance and Other Stories*. New York: Harper and Brothers.

Oscar Wilde, from "The Happy Prince" (1888)

In this short story, the Happy Prince, who didn't learn compassion during his life, becomes a statue. His experience as a statue teaches him compassion, and he enlists the help of a swallow to give his ruby, sapphire, and golden ornaments to the poor of the city.

Wilde satirizes those who see only external qualities and who believe that things that are "no longer beautiful [are] no longer useful" rather than examining the true natures of things.

Early the next morning the Mayor was walking in the square below in the company of the Town councillors. As they passed the column he looked up at the statue: "Dear me! How shabby the Happy Prince looks!" he said.

"How shabby indeed!" cried the Town Councillors, who always agreed with the Mayor; and they went up to look at it.

"The ruby has fallen out of his sword, his eyes are gone, and he is golden no longer," said the Mayor; "in fact, he is little better than a beggar!"

"Little better than a beggar," said the Town Councillors.

"And here is actually a dead bird at his feet!" continued the Mayor. "We must really issue a proclamation that birds are not to be allowed to die here." And the Town Clerk made a note of the suggestion.

So they pulled down the statue of the Happy Prince. "As he is no longer beautiful he is no longer useful," said the Art Professor at the University.

Source: Wilde, Oscar. 1888. "The Happy Prince." Available at: http://www.online-literature.com/wilde/177/

"Sim Chung Jeon" ("The Dutiful Daughter") (1889)

This Korean folktale, which exists in hundreds of version, is one of the Pansori 12 Madang, a type of musical storytelling performance that originated during the late seventeenth century and continued to be popular during the eighteenth century. In the story of this pansori, "Sim Chung Jeon," Sim Chung sacrifices herself for the cure of her father Sim Hyun's blindness. The tale combines the cultural practice of human sacrifice, the Confucian value of filial piety, and the Buddhist idea of karma.

Sim Hyun, or Mr. Sim was highly esteemed in the Korean village in which he resided. He belonged to the yangban, or gentleman class, and when he walked forth it was with the stately swinging stride of the gentleman, while if he bestrode his favorite donkey, or was carried in his chair, a runner went ahead calling to the commoners to clear the road. His rank was not high, and though greatly esteemed as a scholar, his income would scarcely allow of his taking the position he was fitted to occupy. . . .

His parents had been very fortunate in betrothing him to a remarkably beautiful and accomplished maiden, daughter of a neighboring gentleman. . . . It was an exceptionally happy union, the pair being intellectually suited to each other, and apparently possessing the bodily attributes necessary to charm the other. . . .

Heaven had kindly prepared the way for the little visitor, however; for after fifteen years weary waiting, they were not going to look with serious disfavor upon a girl, however much their hopes had been placed upon the advent of a son. The child grew, and the parents were united as they only could be by such a precious bond. . . .

Just as their joy seemed too great to be lasting, it was suddenly checked by the death of the mother, which plunged them into a deep grief from which the father emerged totally blind. It soon became a question as to where the daily food was to come from; little by little household trinkets were given to the brokers to dispose of, and in ten years they had used up the homestead, and all it contained.

The father was now compelled to ask alms, and as his daughter was grown to womanhood, she could no longer direct his footsteps as he wandered out in the darkness of the blind. One day in his journeying he fell into a deep ditch, from which he could not extricate himself. After remaining in this deplorable condition for some time he heard a step, and called out for assistance, saying: "I am blind, not drunk," whereupon the passing stranger said: "I know full well you are not drunk. True, you are blind, yet not incurably so."

"Why, who are you that you know so much about me?" asked the blind man.

"I am the old priest of the temple in the mountain fortress."

"Well, what is this that you say about my not being permanently blind?"

"I am a prophet, and I have had a vision concerning you. In case you make an offering of three hundred bags of rice to the Buddha of our temple, you will be restored to sight, you will be given rank and dignity, while your daughter will become the first woman in all Korea."

"But I am poor, as well as blind," was the reply. "How can I promise such a princely offering?"

"You may give me your order for it, and pay it along as you are able," said the priest.

"Very well, give me pencil and paper," whereupon they retired to a house, and the blind man gave his order for the costly price of his sight. Returning home weary, bruised, and hungry, he smiled to himself, in spite of his ill condition, at the thought of this giving an order for so much rice when he had not a grain of it to eat.

He obtained, finally, a little work in pounding rice in the stone mortars. It was hard labor for one who had lived as he had done; but it kept them from starving, and his daughter prepared his food for him as nicely as she knew how. One night, as the dinner was spread on the little, low table before him, sitting on the floor, the priest came and demanded his pay; the old blind man lost his appetite for his dinner, and refused to eat. He had to explain to his daughter the compact he had made with the priest, and, while she was filled with grief, and dismayed at the enormity of the price, she yet seemed to have some hope that it might be accomplished and his sight restored.

That night, after her midnight bath, she lay down on a mat in the open air, and gazed up to heaven, to which she prayed that her poor father might be restored to health and sight. While thus engaged, she feel asleep and dreamed that her mother came down from heaven to comfort her, and told her not to worry, that a means would be found for the payment of the rice, and that soon all would be happy again in the little family.

The next day she chanced to hear of the wants of a great merchant who sailed in his large boats to China for trade, but was greatly distressed by an evil spirit that lived in the water through which he must pass. For some time, it was stated, he had not been able to take his boats over this dangerous place, and his loss therefrom was very great. At last it was reported that he was willing and anxious to appease the spirit by making the offering the wise men had deemed necessary. Priests had told him that the sacrifice of a young maiden to the spirit would quiet it and remove the trouble. He was, therefore, anxious to find the proper person, and had offered a great sum to obtain such an one.

Sim Chung, hearing of this, decided that it must be the fulfillment of her dream, and having determined to go and offer herself, she put on old clothes and fasted while journeying, that she might look wan and haggard, like one in mourning. She had previously prepared food for her father, and explained to him that she wished to go and bow at her mother's grave, in return to her for having appeared to her in a dream.

When the merchant saw the applicant, he was at once struck with her beauty and dignity of carriage, in spite of her attempt to disguise herself. He said that it was not in his heart to kill people, especially maidens of such worth as she seemed to be. He advised her not to apply; but she told her story and said she would give herself for the three hundred bags of rice. "Ah! Now I see the true nobility of your character. I did not know that such filial piety existed outside the works of the ancients. I will send to my master and secure the rice," said the man, who happened to be but an over-seer for a greater merchant.

She got the rice and took it to the priest in a long procession of one hundred and fifty ponies, each laboring under two heavy bags; the debt cancelled and her doom fixed, she felt the relaxation and grief nec-essarily consequent upon such a condition. She could not explain to her father, she mourned over the loneli-ness that would come to him after she was gone, and wondered how he would support himself after she was removed and until his sight should be restored. She lay down and prayed to heaven, saying: "I am only fourteen years old, and have but four more hours to live. What will become of my poor father? Oh! Who will care for him? Kind heaven, protect him when I am gone." Wild with grief she went and sat on her father's knee, but could not control her sobs and tears; whereupon he asked her what the trouble could be. Having made up her mind that the time had come, and that the deed was done and could not be remedied, she decided to tell him, and tried to break it gently; but when the whole truth dawned upon the poor old man it nearly killed him. He clasped her close to his bosom, and crying: "My child, my daughter, my only comfort, I will not let you go. What will eyes to be me if I can no longer look upon your lovely face?" They mingled their tears and sobs, and the neighbors, hear-ing the commotion in the usually quiet hut, came to see what the trouble was. Upon ascertaining the rea-son of the old man's grief, they united in the general wailing. Sim Chung begged them to come and care for the old man when she could look after him no more, and they agreed to do so. While the wailing and heart breaking was going on, a stranger rode up on a don-key and asked for the Sim family. He came just in time to see what the act was costing the poor people. He comforted the girl by giving her a cheque for fifty bags of rice for the support of the father when his

daughter should be no more. She took it gratefully and gave it to the neighbors to keep in trust; she then pre-pared herself, took a last farewell, and left her fainting father to go to her bed in the sea.

In due time the boat that bore Sim Chung, at the head of a procession of boats, arrived at the place where the evil spirit reigned. She was dressed in bridal garments furnished by the merchant. On her arrival at the place, the kind merchant tried once more to appease the spirit by an offering of eatables, but it was useless, whereupon Sim Chung prayed to heaven, bade them all good-by[e] and leaped into the sea. Above, all was quiet, the waves subsided, the sea became like a lake, and the boats passed on their way unmolested.

When Sim Chung regained her consciousness she was seated in a little boat drawn by fishes, and pretty maidens were giving her to drink from a carved jade bottle. She asked them who they were, and where she was going. They answered: "We are servants of the King of the Sea, and we are taking you to his palace." . . .

Sim Chung wondered if this was death, and thought it very pleasant if it were. They passed through forests of waving plants, and saw great lazy fish feeding about in the water, till at last they reached the confines of the palace. Her amazement was then unbounded, for the massive walls were composed of precious stones, such as she had only heretofore seen used as ornaments. Pearls were used to cover the heads of nails in the great doors through which they passed, and everywhere there seemed a most costly and lavish display of the precious gems and metals, while the walks were made of polished black marble that shone in the water. . . .

The King treated her with great respect, and all the maidens and eunuchs bowed before her. She protested that she was not worthy of such attention. "I am," she said, "but the daughter of a beggar, for whom I thought I was giving my life when rescued by these maidens. I am in no way worthy of your respect." . . .

The King smiled a little, and said: Ah! I know more of you than you know of yourself. You must know that I am the Sea King, and that we know full well the doings of the stars which shine in the heaven above, for they continually visit us on light evenings. Well, you were once a star. Many say a beautiful one. [There was another star you loved] more than the others, and, in your attentions to him, you abused your office as cup-bearer to the King of Heaven, and let your lover have free access to all of the choice wines of the palace. In this way, before you were aware of it, the peculiar and choice brands that the King especially liked were consumed, and, upon examination, your fault became known. As punishment, the King decided to banish you to earth, but fearing to send you both at once, lest you might be drawn together there, he sent your lover first, and after keeping you in prison for a long time, you were sent as daughter to your former lover. He is the man you claim as father. Heaven has seen your filial piety, however, and repents. You will be hereafter most highly favored, as a reward for your dutiful conduct. He then sent her to fine apartments prepared for her, where she was to rest and recuperate before going back to earth. . . .

After a due period of waiting and feasting on royal food, Sim Chung's beauty was more than restored. She had developed into a complete woman, and her beauty was dazzling; her cheeks seemed colored by the beautiful tints of the waters through which she moved with ease and comfort, while her mind blossomed forth like a flower in the rare society of the Sea King and his peculiarly gifted people. . . .

At night, when all was quiet, Sim Chung was wont to come forth and rest herself by walking in the moonlight. But, on one occasion, the King, being indisposed and restless, thought he would go to breathe the rich perfume of the strange flower and rest himself. In this way he chanced to see Sim Chung before she could conceal herself, and, of course, his surprise was unbounded. He accosted her, not without fear demanding who she might be. She, being also afraid, took refuge in her flower, when, to the amazement of both, the flower vanished, leaving her standing alone where it had been but a moment before. . . .

His Majesty very reluctantly went to see what it all meant. An officer versed in astronomy stated that they had, on the previous night, observed a brilliant star descend from heaven and alight upon the palace, and that they believed it boded good to the royal family. . . . It so happened that the queen was deceased, and it was soon decided that the King should take this remarkable maiden for his wife. . . .

After some time spent in such luxury, Sim Chung became lonely and mourned for her poor father, but despaired of being able to see him. She knew not if he were alive or dead, and the more she thought of it the more she mourned, till tears were in her heart continually, and not infrequently overflowed from her beautiful eyes. The King chanced to see her weeping, and was solicitous to know the cause of her sorrow, whereupon she answered that she was oppressed by a strange dream concerning a poor blind man, and was desirous of alleviating in some way the suffering of the many blind men in the country. Together they agreed that they would summon all the blind men of the country to a great feast, at which they should be properly clothed, amply fed, and treated each to a present of cash. . . .

When sufficient time had elapsed for the satisfying of his hunger, he was ordered brought to the Queen's pavilion, where Her Majesty scrutinized him closely for a few moments, and then, to the surprise and dismay of all her attendants, she screamed: "My father! My father!" and fell at his feet senseless. . . .

[T]he poor old blind man could barely collect his senses sufficiently to grasp the situation. As the full truth began to dawn upon him, he cried: "Oh! My child, can the dead come back to us? I hear your voice; I feel your form; but how can I know it is you, for I have no eyes? Away with these sightless orbs!" And he tore at his eyes with his nails, when to his utter amazement and joy, the scales fell away, and he stood rejoicing in his sight once more. . . .

His Majesty was overjoyed to have his lovely Queen restored to her wonted happy frame of mind. He made the old man an officer of high rank, appointed him a fine house, and had him married to the accomplished daughter of an officer of suitable rank, thereby fulfilling the last of the prophecy of both the aged priest and the King of the Sea.

Source: Allen, H. N. 1889. Pp. 152–169 in *Korean Tales: Being a Collection of Stories Translated from the Korean Folk Lore.* New York: Knickerbocker Press.

▣ Emily Dickinson, "Much Madness Is Divinest Sense" (1890)

With her usual economy of words and a confiding tone, Dickinson sketches the contextual nature of sanity and madness—what fits into the majority view is deemed fit, and the unusual is not only labeled but "handled with a Chain." Emily Dickinson, whose reclusive New England life remains the subject of much speculation, surely understood this harsh suspicion of difference from firsthand experience.

Much Madness is divinest Sense
To a discerning Eye;
Much Sense the starkest Madness.

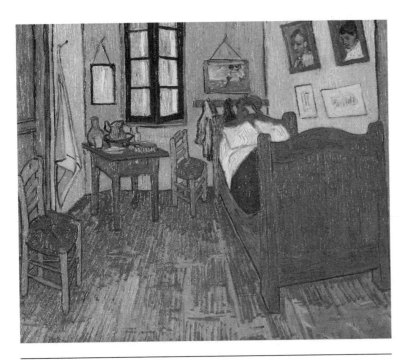

The Bedroom at Arles *(1889), by Vincent Van Gogh (1853–1890). Oil on canvas. Van Gogh's painting shows a bedroom in the Arles "Yellow House" that he decorated in preparation for visits from fellow artists and relatives. The rendition of the room is vivid in the artist's characteristic manner.*

Source: Musée d'Orsay, Paris, France.

'Tis the Majority
In this, as All, prevails.
Assent, and you are sane;
Demur—you're straightway dangerous,
And handled with a Chain.

Source: Dickinson, Emily. 1890. "Much Madness Is Divinest Sense." Available at: http://www.bartleby.com/113/1011.html

John Harvey Kellogg, from *Plain Facts* (1890)

John Harvey Kellogg is best known for his connection with the sanatorium in Battle Creek, Michigan, and the cereals he invented for his patients there. Kellogg's book Plain Facts *was one of hundreds of books about eugenics produced during the late nineteenth and early twentieth centuries. The author, like many eugenicists of his era, counsels against the freedom of disabled people to procreate. The argument participates in longstanding fallacies about the prevention of "defects" as a duty of American citizens.*

Persons having serious congenital deformities should not marry. The reason for this rule is obvious. Persons suffering with serious congenital defects, as natural blindness, deafness, deformity of the limbs, or defective development of any part, will be more or less likely to transmit the same deformities or deficiencies to their children. There are, of course, cases of natural blindness, as well as of disability in other respects, to which this rule does not apply, the natural process of development not being seriously defective. It has even been observed that there is a slight tendency to the reproduction in the offspring, of deformity which has been artificially produced in the parents, and has existed for a long time. Many ancient nations observe this rule. Infants born cripples were strangled at birth or left to die. A Spartan king was once required by his people to pay a heavy fine for taking a wife who was inferior in size.

Source: Kellogg, John Harvey. 1890. *Plain Facts for Old and Young: Embracing the Natural History and Hygiene of Organic Life.* Burlington, IA: I. F. Segner.

Walt Whitman, from *Collected Prose* (1891)

The poet's bravura inventory of his own physical and mental states touches on both the mundane and the spiritual aspects of his everyday experience. The housekeeper and nurse are mentioned by way of explaining the supports he depends upon to keep up his writing, his "buoyant spirits," and his "unmitigated faith."

But physical disability and the war-paralysis above alluded to have settled upon me more and more, the last year or so. Am now (1891) domicil'd, and have been, for some years, in this little old cottage and lot in Mickle Street, Camden, with a house-keeper and man nurse. Bodily I am completely disabled, but still write for publication. I keep generally buoyant spirits, write often as there comes any lull in physical sufferings, get in the sun and down to the river whenever I can, retain fair appetite, assimilation and digestion, sensibilities acute as ever, the strength and volition of my right arm good, eyesight dimming, but brain normal, and retain my heart's and soul's unmitigated faith not only in their own original literary plans, but in the essential bulk of American humanity east and west, north and south, city and country, through thick and thin, to the last.

Source: Whitman, Walt. 1982. Kaplan, Justin, ed. *Complete Poetry and Collected Prose.* New York: Library of America.

Friedrich Nietzsche, from *Thus Spoke Zarathustra* (1891)

In this excerpt from one of the German philosopher's most influential works, Nietzsche inverts the common biblical scenario of a prophet proving his powers by curing disabilities. Instead, when the group of disabled characters invites Zarathustra to show the legitimacy of his philosophy by healing them, he launches into a discussion about the centrality of disability to those who experience such conditions. Also in this section, Zarathustra evolves his theory of eternal return—the belief that one would willingly choose to repeat one's life in every detail again. The key to this radical proposal is the idea that those with disabilities would presumably do anything to avoid their conditions, and therefore Zarathustra's formulation is held out as the challenge to the cripples as a test for the ultimate claim of value made for even the most devalued lives.

From "On Redemption"

When Zarathustra went one day over the great bridge, then did the cripples and beggars surround him, and a hunchback spoke thus to him:

"Behold, Zarathustra! Even the people learn from you, and acquire faith in your teaching: but for them to believe fully in you, one thing is still needful—you must first of all convince us cripples! Here have you now a fine selection, and verily, an opportunity with more than one forelock! The blind can you heal, and make the lame run; and from him who has too much behind, could you well, also, take away a little;—that, I think, would be the right method to make the cripples believe in Zarathustra!"

Zarathustra, however, answered thus to him who so spoke: When one takes his hump from the hunchback, then does one take from him his spirit—so do the people teach. And when one gives the blind man eyes, then does he see too many bad things on the earth: so that he curses him who healed him. He, however, who makes the lame man run, inflicts upon him the greatest injury; for hardly can he run, when his vices run away with him—so do the people teach concerning cripples. And why should not Zarathustra also learn from the people, when the people learn from Zarathustra?

It is, however, the small thing to me since I have been amongst men, to see one person lacking an eye, another an ear, and a third a leg, and that others have lost the tongue, or the nose, or the head.

I see and have seen worse things, and divers things so hideous, that I should neither like to speak of all matters, nor even keep silent about some of them: namely, men who lack everything, except that they have too much of one thing—men who are nothing more than a big eye, or a big mouth, or a big belly, or something else big,—reversed cripples, I call such men.

And when I came out of my solitude, and for the first time passed over this bridge, then I could not trust my eyes, but looked again and again, and said at last: "That is an ear! An ear as big as a man!" I looked still more attentively—and actually there did move under the ear something that was pitiably small and poor and slim. And in truth this immense ear was perched on a small thin stalk—the stalk, however, was a man! A person putting a glass to his eyes, could even recognize further a small envious countenance, and also that a bloated little soul dangled at the stalk. The people told me, however, that the big ear was not only a man, but a great man, a genius. But I never believed in the people when they spoke of great men—and I hold to my belief that it was a reversed cripple, who had too little of everything, and too much of one thing.

When Zarathustra had spoken thus to the hunchback, and to those of whom the hunchback was the mouthpiece and advocate, then did he turn to his disciples in profound dejection, and said:

My friends, I walk amongst men as amongst the fragments and limbs of human beings!

This is the terrible thing to my eye, that I find man broken up, and scattered about, as on a battle—and butcher—ground.

And when my eye flees from the present to the bygone, it finds ever the same: fragments and limbs and fearful chances—but no men!

The present and the bygone upon earth—ah! my friends—that is my most unbearable trouble; and I should not know how to live, if I were not a seer of what is to come.

A seer, a purposer, a creator, a future itself, and a bridge to the future—and alas! also as it were a cripple on this bridge: all that is Zarathustra.

Source: Nietzsche, Friedrich. 1891. Common, Thomas, trans. *Thus Spoke Zarathustra.* Available at: http://morrandir.philosophy forums.com/e-books/Nietzsche/TSZ.txt

▣ "The Legend of Knockgrafton" (1892)

This Celtic fairy tale discusses disabled people who are appropriately deserving of cure in that they have taken up the proper attitude toward their bodily afflictions.

There was once a poor man who lived in the fertile glen of Aherlow, at the foot of the gloomy Galtee mountains, and he had a great hump on his back: he looked just as if his body had been rolled up and placed upon his shoulders; and his head was pressed down with the weight so much that his chin, when he was sitting, used to rest upon his knees for support. The country people were rather shy of meeting him in any lonesome place, for though, poor creature, he was as harm-less and as inoffensive as a new-born infant, yet his deformity was so great that he scarcely appeared to be a human creature, and some ill-minded persons had set strange stories about him afloat. He was said to have a great knowledge of herbs and charms; but certain it was that he had a mighty skilful hand in plaiting straw and rushes into hats and baskets, which was the way he made his livelihood.

Lusmore, for that was the nickname put upon him by reason of his always wearing a sprig of the fairy cap, or lusmore (the foxglove), in his little Straw hat, would ever get a higher penny for his plaited work than any one else, and perhaps that was the reason why some one, out of envy, had circulated the strange stories about him. Be that as it may, it happened that he was returning one evening from the pretty town of Cahir towards Cappagh, and as little Lusmore walked very slowly, on account of the great hump upon his back, it was quite dark when he came to the old moat of Knockgrafton, which stood on the right-band side of his road. Tired and weary was he, and noways

comfortable in his own mind at thinking how much farther he had to travel, and that he should be walking all the night; so he sat down under the moat to rest himself and began looking mournfully enough upon the moon.

Presently there rose a wild strain of unearthly melody upon the ear of little Lusmore; he listened, and he thought that he had never heard such ravishing music before. It was like the sound of many voices, each mingling and blending with the other so strangely that they seemed to be one, though all singing different strains, and the words of the song were these—

Da Luan, Da Mort ["Monday, Tuesday"], *Da Luan, Da Mort, Da Luan, Da Mort;*

when there would be a moment's pause, and then the round of melody went on again.

Lusmore listened attentively, scarcely drawing his breath lest he might lose the slightest note. He now plainly perceived that the singing was within the moat; and though at first it had charmed him so much, he began to get tired of hearing the same round sung over and over so often without any change; so availing himself of the pause when the *Da Luan, Da Mort,* had been sung three times, he took up the tune, and raised it with the words *augus Da Cadine* ["and Wednesday"], and then went on singing with the voices in side of the moat, *Da Luan, Da Mort,* finishing the melody, when the pause again came, with *augus Da Cadine.*

The fairies within Knockgrafton, for the song was a fairy melody, when they heard this addition to the tune, were so much delighted that, with instant resolve, it was determined to bring the mortal among them, whose musical skill so far exceeded theirs, and little Lusmore was conveyed into their company with the eddying speed of a whirlwind.

Glorious to behold was the sight that burst upon him as he came down through the moat, twirling round and round, with the lightness of a straw, to the sweetest music that kept time to his motion. The greatest honour was then paid him, for he was put above all the musicians, and he had servants tending upon him, and everything to his heart's content, and a hearty welcome to all; and, in short, he was made as much of as if he had been the first man in the land.

Presently Lusmore saw a great consultation going forward among the fairies, and, notwithstanding all their civility, he felt very much frightened, until one stepping out from the rest came up to him and said,

"Lusmore Lusmore!
Doubt not, nor deplore,
For the hump which you bore
On your back is no more;
Look down on the floor,
And view it, Lusmore !"

When these words were said, poor little Lusmore felt himself so light, and so happy, that he thought he could have bounded at one jump over the moon, like the cow in the history of the cat and the fiddle; and he saw, with inexpressible pleasure, his hump tumble down upon the ground from his shoulders. He then tried to lift up his head, and he did so with becoming caution, fearing that he might knock it against the ceiling of the grand hall, where he was; he looked round and round again with greatest wonder and delight upon everything, which appeared more and more beautiful; and, overpowered at beholding such a resplendent scene, his head grew dizzy, and his eyesight became dim. At last he fell into a sound sleep, and when he awoke he found that it was broad daylight, the sun shining brightly, and the birds singing sweetly; and that he was lying just at the foot of the moat of Knockgrafton, with the cows and sheep grazing peacefully round about him. The first thing Lusmore did, after saying his prayers, was to put his hand behind to feel for his hump, but no sign of one was there on his back, and he looked at himself with great pride, for he had now become a well-shaped dapper little fellow, and more than that, found himself in a full suit of new clothes, which he concluded the fairies had made for him.

Towards Cappagh he went, stepping out as lightly, and springing up at every step as if he had been all his life a dancing-master. Not a creature who met Lusmore knew him without his hump, and he had a great work to persuade every one that he was the same man—in truth he was not, so far as outward appearance went.

Of course it was not long before the story of Lusmore's hump got about, and a great wonder was made of it. Through the country, for miles round, it was the talk of every one, high and low.

One morning, as Lusmore was sitting contented enough, at his cabin door, up came an old woman to him, and asked him if he could direct her to Cappagh.

"I need give you no directions, my good woman," said Lusmore, "for this is Cappagh; and whom may you want here?"

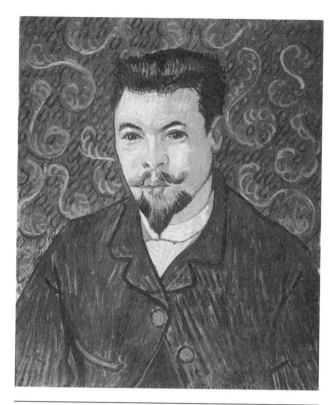

Portrait of Dr. Felix Rey, *by Vincent Van Gogh (1853–1890). After severing the lower half of his ear, Van Gogh was placed in a hospital in Arles, France, for medical and psychiatric care. His attending physician while at the hospital Hotel-Dieu was the physician portrayed here, Dr. Felix Rey. Rey remained Vincent's doctor for nearly a year, until the artist voluntarily admitted himself to the Saint-Paul-de-Mausole asylum.*

Source: Art Resource, New York.

"I have come," said the woman, "out of Decie's country, in the county of Waterford looking after one Lusmore, who, I have heard tell, had his hump taken off by the fairies for there is a son of a gossip of mine who has got a hump on him that will be his death; and maybe if he could use the same charm as Lusmore, the hump may be taken off him. And now I have told you the reason of my coming so far 'tis to find out about this charm, if I can."

Lusmore, who was ever a good-natured little fellow, told the woman all the particulars, how he had raised the tune for the fairies at Knockgrafton, how his hump had been removed from his shoulders, and how he had got a new suit of clothes into the bargain.

The woman thanked him very much, and then went away quite happy and easy in her own mind. When she came back to her gossip's house, in the county of Waterford, she told her everything that Lusmore had said, and they put the little hump-backed man, who was a peevish and cunning creature from his birth, upon a car, and took him all the way across the country. It was a long journey, but they did not care for that, so the hump was taken from off him; and they brought him, just at nightfall, and left him under the old moat of Knockgrafton.

Jack Madden, for that was the humpy man's name, had not been sitting there long when he heard the tune going on within the moat much sweeter than before; for the fairies were singing it the way Lusmore had settled their music for them, and the song was going on; *Da Luan, Da Mort, Da Luan, Da Mort, Da Luan, Da Mort, augus Da Cadine*, without ever stopping. Jack Madden, who was in a great hurry to get quit of his hump, never thought of waiting until the fairies had done, or watching for a fit opportunity to raise the tune higher again than Lusmore had; so having heard them sing it over seven times without stopping, out he bawls, never minding the time or the humour of the tune, or how he could bring his words in properly, *augus Da Cadine, augus Da Hena* ["and Wednesday and Thursday"], thinking that if one day was good, two were better; and that if Lusmore had one new suit of clothes given him, he should have two.

No sooner had the words passed his lips than he was taken up and whisked into the moat with prodigious force; and the fairies came crowding round about him with great anger, screeching, and screaming, and roaring out, "Who spoiled our tune? who spoiled our tune?" and one stepped up to him, above all the rest and said:

"Jack Madden! Jack Madden
Your words came so bad in
The tune we felt glad in;
This castle you're had in,
That your life we may sadden
Here's two humps for Jack Madden!"

And twenty of the strongest fairies brought Lusmore's hump and put it down upon poor Jack's back, over his own, where it became fixed as firmly as if it was nailed on with twelve-penny nails, by the best carpenter that ever drove one. Out of their castle they then kicked him; and, in the morning, when Jack Madden's mother and her gossip came to look after their little man, they found him half dead, lying at the foot of the moat, with the other hump upon his back. Well to be sure, how they did look at each other! but they were afraid to say anything, lest a hump might be put upon their own

shoulders. Home they brought the unlucky Jack Madden with them, as downcast in their hearts and their looks as ever two gossips were; and what through the weight of his other hump, and the long journey, he died soon after, leaving they say his heavy curse to any one who would go to listen to fairy tunes again.

Source: Jacobs, Joseph, trans. 1892. "The Legend of Knock grafton." Available at: http://www.public-domaincontent.com/books/legends_and_sagas/celt/flat/flat03.shtml

Walter E. Fernald, from *The History of the Treatment of the Feeble-Minded* (1893)

Walter Fernald, MD, director of the Waltham Institution for Feeblemindedness in Massachusetts, wrote one of the first U.S. histories on the topic of treatment methods. The essay promotes the need to continue institutionalization practices at a time when public unrest about their utility escalated. Fernald argues that the old objective of returning institutionalized residents to the community was a failure and that training has now largely transformed into permanent custodianship on behalf of the state.

The first recorded attempt to educate an idiot was made about the year 1800, by Itard, the celebrated physician-in-chief to the National Institution for the Deaf and Dumb at Paris, upon a boy found wild in a forest in the center of France, and known as the "savage of Aveyron." "This boy could not speak any human tongue, and was devoid of all understanding and knowledge." Believing him to be a savage, for five years Itard endeavored with great skill and perseverance to develop at the same time the intelligence of his pupil and the theories of the materialistic school of philosophy. Itard finally became convinced that this boy was an idiot, and abandoned the attempt to educate him. In the year 1818 and for a few years afterward, several idiotic children were received and given instruction at the American Asylum for the Deaf and Dumb at Hartford, and a fair degree of improvement in physical condition, habits, and speech was obtained.

In the year 1828 Dr. Ferret, physician at the Bicêtre in Paris, attempted to teach a few of the more intelligent idiots who were confined in this hospital to read and write and to train them to habits of cleanliness and order. In 1831 Dr. Fabret attempted the same work at the Salpêtrière; and in 1833 Dr. Voisin opened his private school for idiots in Paris. None of these attempts was successful enough to insure its continuance.

In 1837 Dr. E. Séguin, a pupil of Itard and Esquirol, began the private instruction of idiots at his own expense. In 1842 he was made the instructor of the school at the Bicêtre, which had been reopened by Dr. Voisin in 1839. Dr. Séguin remained at the Bicêtre only one year, retiring to continue the work in his private school in the Hospice des Incurables. After seven years of patient work and experiments and the publication of two or three pamphlets describing the work, a committee from the Academy of Sciences at Paris in 1844 examined critically and thoroughly his methods of training and educating idiot children, and reported to the Academy, giving it the highest commendation and declaring that, up to the time he commenced his labors in 1837, idiots could not be educated by any means previously known or practiced, but that he had solved the problem. His work thus approved by the highest authority, Dr. Séguin continued his private school in Paris until the Revolution in 1848, when he came to America, where he was instrumental in establishing schools for idiots in various States.

In 1846 Dr. Séguin published his classical and comprehensive "Treatise on Idiocy," which was crowned by the Academy and has continued to be the standard text-book for all interested in the education of idiots up to the present time. His elaborate system of teaching and training idiots consisted in the careful "adaptation of the principles of physiology, through physiological means and instruments, to the development of the dynamic, perceptive, reflective, and spontaneous functions of youth." This physiological education of defective brains as a result of systematic training of the special senses, the functions, and the muscular system, was looked upon as a visionary theory, but has been verified and confirmed by modem experiments and researches in physiological psychology.

Dr. Séguin's school was visited by scientists and philanthropists from nearly every part of the civilized world, and, his methods bearing the test of experience, other schools were soon established in other countries, based upon these methods.

In 1842 Dr. Guggenbühl established a school upon the slope of the Abendenberg in Switzerland, for the care and training of cretins, so many of whom are found in the dark, damp valleys of the Alps. This school was very successful in its results, and attracted

much attention throughout Europe. At Berlin, in 1842, a school for the instruction of idiots was opened by Dr. Saegert. In England the publication of the results of the work of Drs. Séguin, Guggenbühl, and Saegert, and the efforts of Drs. Connolly and Reed, led to the establishment of a private school at Bath in 1846, and later to the finely appointed establishments at Colchester and Earlswood.

The published description of the methods and results of these European schools attracted much interest and attention in America. In this country the necessity and humanity of caring for and scientifically treating the insane, the deaf and dumb, and the blind had become the policy of many of our most progressive States. The class of helpless and neglected idiots who had no homes, as a rule were cared for in jails and poorhouses. A few idiots who had been received at the special schools for the deaf and dumb and the blind showed considerable improvement after a period of training. Other cases who were especially troublesome had been sent to the insane hospitals, where it was shown that the habits and behavior of this class could be changed very much for the better. In their reports for 1845 Drs. Woodward and Brigham, superintendents of the State Insane Hospitals in Massachusetts and New York respectively, urged the necessity of making public provision for the education of idiots in those States. . . .

It was hoped and believed that a large proportion of this higher-grade or "improvable" class of idiots could be so developed and educated that they would be capable of supporting themselves and of creditably maintaining an independent position in the community. It was maintained that the State should not assume the permanent care of these defectives, but that they should be returned to their homes after they had been trained and educated. It was the belief of the managers that only a relatively small number of inmates could be successfully cared for in one institution. It was deemed unwise to congregate a large number of persons suffering under any common infirmity.

Nearly every one of these early institutions was opened at or near the capitals of their various States, in order that the members of the legislature might closely watch their operations and personally see their need and the results of the instruction and training of these idiots. No institution was ever abandoned or given up after having been established. In all of the institutions the applications for admission were far in excess of their capacity.

In the course of a few years, in the annual reports of these institutions we find the superintendents regretting that it was not expedient to return to the community a certain number of the cases who had received all the instruction the school had to offer. When the limit of age was reached, it was a serious problem to decide what should be done with the trained boy or girl. It was found that only a small proportion, even of these selected pupils, could be so developed and improved that they could go out into the world and support themselves independently. A larger number, as a result of the school discipline and training, could be taken home where they became comparatively harmless and unobjectionable members of the family, capable, under the loving and watchful care of their friends, of earning by their labor as much as it cost to maintain them. But in many cases the guardians of these children were unwilling to remove them from the institution, and begged that they might be allowed to remain where they could be made happy and kept from harm. Many of these cases were homeless and friendless, and, if sent away from the school, could only be transferred to almshouses where they became depraved and demoralized by association with adult paupers and vagrants of both sexes. It was neither wise nor humane to turn these boys and girls out to shift for themselves. The placing out of these feeble-minded persons always proved unsatisfactory. Even those who had suitable homes and friends able and willing to become responsible for them, by the death of these relatives were thrown on their own resources and drifted into pauperism and crime. It gradually became evident that a certain number of these higher-grade cases needed lifelong care and supervision, and that there was no suitable provision for this permanent custody outside these special institutions.

Once it was admitted that our full duty toward this class must include the retention and guardianship of some of these cases who had been trained in the schools, the wisdom and necessity of still further broadening the work became apparent. It was found that more than one-half of the applications for admission, and those by far the most insistent, were in behalf of the "unimprovables," as Dr. Howe described them. This lower class of idiots, many of them with untidy, disgusting, and disagreeable habits, feeble physically,

perhaps deformed and misshapen, often partially paralyzed or subject to epilepsy, cannot be given suitable care at home. There is no greater burden possible in a home or a neighborhood. It has been well said that by institution care, for every five idiots cared for we restore four productive persons to the community; for, whereas at home the care of each of these children practically requires the time and energies of one person, in an institution the proportion of paid employees is not over one to each five inmates. The home care of a low-grade idiot consumes so much of the working capacity of the wage-earner of the household that often the entire family become pauperized. Humanity and public policy demanded that these families should be relieved of the burden of these helpless idiots. From the nature of their infirmities it is evident that the care of this class must last as long as they live. As nearly every one of these low-grade idiots eventually becomes a public burden, it is better to assume this care when they are young and susceptible of a certain amount of training than to receive them later on, undisciplined, helpless, destructive, adult idiots.

The brighter class of the feeble-minded, with their weak will power and deficient judgment, are easily influenced for evil, and are prone to become vagrants, drunkards, and thieves. The modern scientific study of the deficient and delinquent classes as a whole has demonstrated that a large proportion of our criminals, inebriates, and prostitutes are really congenital imbeciles, who have been allowed to grow up without any attempt being made to improve or discipline them. Society suffers the penalty of this neglect in an increase of pauperism and vice, and finally, at a greatly increased cost, is compelled to take charge of adult idiots in almshouses and hospitals, and of imbecile criminals in jails and prisons, generally during the remainder of their natural lives. As a matter of mere economy, it is now believed that it is better and cheaper for the community to assume the permanent care of this class before they have carried out a long career of expensive crime....

The tendency to lead dissolute lives is especially noticeable in the females. A feeble-minded girl is exposed as no other girl in the world is exposed. She has not sense enough to protect herself from the perils to which women are subjected. Often bright and attractive, if at large they either marry and bring forth in geometrical ratio a new generation of defectives and dependants, or become irresponsible sources of corruption and debauchery in the communities where they live. There is hardly a poorhouse in this land where there are not two or more feeble-minded women with from one to four illegitimate children each. There is every reason in morality, humanity, and public policy that these feeble-minded women should be under permanent and watchful guardianship, especially during the child-bearing age. A feeble-minded girl of the higher grade was accepted as a pupil at the Massachusetts School for the Feeble-minded when she was fifteen years of age. At the last moment the mother refused to send her to the school, as she "could not bear the disgrace of publicly admitting that she had a feeble-minded child." Ten years later the girl was committed to the institution by the court, after she had given birth to six illegitimate children, four of whom were still living and all feeble-minded. The city where she lived had supported her at the almshouse for a period of several months at each confinement, had been compelled to assume the burden of the life-long support of her progeny, and finally decided to place her in permanent custody. Her mother had died broken-hearted several years previously.

Modern usage has sanctioned the use of the term "feeble-minded" to include all degrees and types of congenital defect, from that of the simply backward boy or girl but little below the normal standard of intelligence to the profound idiot, a helpless, speechless, disgusting burden, with every degree of deficiency between these extremes. The lack may be so slight as to involve only the ability to properly decide questions of social propriety or conduct, or simply questions of morality, or it may profoundly affect every faculty. In theory, the differences between these various degrees of deficiency are marked and distinct, while in practice the lines of separation are entirely indefinite, and individuals as they grow to adult life may be successively classed in different grades. "Idiocy," generically used, covers the whole range referred to, but is now specifically used to denote only the lowest grades. "Imbecility" has reference to the higher grades. "Feeble-Minded" is a less harsh expression, and satisfactorily covers the whole ground.

We have learned from the researches of modern pathology that in many cases the arrested or perverted development is not merely functional or a delayed infantile condition, but is directly due to the results of actual organic disease, or injury to the brain or nervous system, occurring either before birth or in early infancy.

The work of caring for this class in this country has been greatly aided by the active influence of the Association of Medical Officers of American Institutions for Idiotic and Feeble-minded Persons. This society was organized in 1876, during the Centennial Exposition at Philadelphia, and held its first meeting at the Pennsylvania Training School at Elwyn. The object of the Association is the consideration and discussion of all questions relating to the management, training, and education of idiots and feeble-minded persons. It also lends its influence to the establishment and fostering of institutions for this purpose. The Association meets annually for the reading of papers and the discussion of the various phases of this work. . . .

Source: Fernald, Walter E. 1893. *The History of the Treatment of the Feeble-Minded.* Boston: G. H. Ellis.

▣ Florence Kelley, "Injurious Employments" (1894)

In her first annual report as an Illinois factory inspector, Kelley focused on child labor as a practice that both disabled poor immigrant minors and exploited those who were already disabled. The story of Jaroslav Huptuk is especially revealing of its era; we see the various Progressive experts taking a hand in moving Huptuk from the community and unsafe work to the state institution (a resolution Kelley finds proper, in this instance).

The reckless employment of children in injurious occupations also is shown in the record of these medical examinations. A glaring example of this is Jaroslav Huptuk, a feeble-minded dwarf, whose affidavit shows him to be nearly sixteen years of age. This child weighs and measures almost exactly the same as a normal boy aged eight years and three months. Jaroslav Huptuk cannot read nor write in any language, not speak a consecutive sentence. Besides being dwarfed, he is so deformed as to be a monstrosity. Yet, with all these disqualifications for any kind of work, he has been employed for several years at an emery wheel, in a cutlery works, finishing knife-blades and bone handles, until, in addition to his other misfortunes, he is now suffering from [tuberculosis]. Dr. Holmes, having examined this boy, pronounced him unfit for work of any kind. His mother appealed from this to a medical college, where, however, the examining physician not only refused the lad a medical certificate, but exhibited him to the students as a monstrosity worthy of careful observation. He was finally taken in charge by an [orthopedist], and after careful treatment will be placed in a school for the feeble-minded. The kind of grinding at which this boy was employed has been prohibited in England for minors since 1883, by reason of the prevalence of "grinders' pthisis" among those who begin this work young.

Another occupation conspicuously injurious to children is the running of button-hole machines by foot-power. As a typical case: Joseph Poderovsky, aged fourteen years, was found by a deputy inspector running a heavy button-holer at 204 West Taylor street, in the shop of Michael Freeman. The child was required to report for medical examination, and pronounced by the examining physician rachitic and afflicted with a double lateral curvature of the spine. He was ordered discharged, and prohibited from working in any tailor shop. A few days later he was found at work at the same machine. A warrant was sworn out for the arrest of the employer, under Section Four of the law, but before it could be served the man left the State. This boy has a father in comfortable circumstances, and two adult able-bodied brothers.

Bennie Kelman, Russian Jew, four years in Chicago, fifteen years and four months old, father a glazier, found running a heavy sewing machine in a knee-pants shop. A health certificate was required, and the examination revealed a severe rupture. Careful questioning of the boy and his mother elicited the fact that he had been put to work in a boiler factory, two years before, when just thirteen years old, and had injured himself by lifting heavy masses of iron. Nothing had been done for the case, no one in the family spoke any English, or knew how help could be obtained. The sight test showed that he did not know his letters in English, though he claimed that he can read Jewish jargon. He was sent to the College of Physicians and Surgeons for treatment, and forbidden work until cured.

When the law went into operation, every tin-can and stamping works in Illinois was employing minors under sixteen years of age, at machines known to be liable to destroy the fingers, hands, and even the whole arm of the operator. The requirement of a medical certificate

for all minors so employed has materially reduced their number, but the law should be so amended as to give the inspector power to prohibit the employment of minors at this and all kindred occupations. Until such power is conferred, the mutilation of children will continue to be a matter of daily [occurrence].

The working of the law, even in its present inadequate form, is exemplified in its application to the tin-can industry by Norton's tin-can factory at Maywood. Here a very large number of boys are employed, a score having been found under fourteen years of age. In one part of the factory twenty to thirty boys work upon a shelf suspended between the first and second floors of the building. These unfortunate lads crouch, lie on their sides, sit on their feet, kneel, in short, assume every possible attitude except the normal, straight, sitting or standing posture of healthful employment. Their work consists in receiving pieces of tin sent to them by boys on the second floor, sorting them and poking them into slits in the shelf, whence the pieces of tin are conveyed to the machines on the ground floor for which they are destined. The atmosphere of the room at the height of the shelf is such that the inspector could endure it but a few minutes at a time. The noise of the machinery was so overpowering that it was impossible to make the boys hear questions until after two or three repetitions. The pieces of tin being sharp, the lad's fingers were bound up in cloths to prevent cutting, but in many cases these cloths were found to be saturated with blood. Altogether, the situation of these tin can boys was among the most deplorable discovered. Four inspections were made, and literal compliance with the wording of the law in all respects required. When the season ended, it was with the assurance upon the part of the Norton Bros. that they will open next year with no minors employed on their Maywood premises under sixteen years of age.

Source: Kelley, Florence. 1894. "Injurious Employments." Pp. 10–13 in *First Annual Report of the Factory Inspectors of Illinois.* Springfield, IL: H. W. Rokker.

▣ Cesare Lombroso and William Ferrero, from *The Female Offender* (1895)

In keeping with the late-nineteenth-century interest in "social Darwinism," which looks at societal phenomena from the perspective of Darwinian theory, this work examines criminality, prostitution, and lesbianism in women with reference to inborn or physical characteristics.

Although I argue that the female equivalent of the male born criminal is the prostitute and that she shares the same atavistic origin, I certainly need to state, very clearly, that she is less perverse and less harmful to society. While every crime involves calamity, prostitution can be a moral safety valve. In any case, it would not exist without male vice, for which it is a useful, if shameful, outlet. One might say that the more women degrade themselves, and the more they sin, the more they are helping society.

Thus, if I must show that in mind and body, woman is a male of arrested development, the fact that she is somewhat less criminal than he, and a little more pitiful, can compensate a thousandfold for her deficiency in the realm of intellect. Just as musical harmony and beauty conquer all social classes, the respect that all people have for women's intensity of feeling and maternal sentiment more than makes up for women's deficiency of intellect. A scientist will have a hundred admirers who quickly disappear, but women are saints who have a million admirers, forever.

Not one line of work justifies the great tyranny that continues to victimize women, from the taboo which forbids them to eat meat or touch a coconut, to that which impedes them from studying, and worse, from practicing a profession once they are educated. These ridiculous and cruel constraints, still widely accepted, are used to maintain or (sadder still) increase women's inferiority, exploiting them to our advantage. The same happens when we shower a docile victim with hypocritical elegies and, while pretending that she is an ornament, ready her for new sacrifices. (P. 37)

While these accumulated findings do not amount to much, this result is only natural. For if external differences between male criminals and normal men are few, they must be fewer still between female criminals and normal women. We noted earlier that stability of type is much greater in woman and differentiation much less, even when her skull is anomalous.

The following are our most important conclusions:

- Female criminals are shorter than normal women; and in proportion to their stature, prostitutes and female murderers weigh more than honest women
- Prostitutes have bigger calves than honest women
- Female thieves and above all prostitutes are inferior to honest women in cranial capacity and cranial circumference

- Criminals have darker hair than normal women, and this also holds good to a certain extent for prostitutes. Several studies have found that in these women rates of fair and red hair equal and sometimes exceed those of normal women.
- Grey hair, which is rare in the normal woman, is more than twice as frequent in the criminal woman. On the other hand, in both young and mature criminal women, baldness is less common than in normal women. Wrinkles are markedly more frequent in criminals of ripe years. Little of all this can be positively affirmed for prostitutes, who are painted and made up when not (as is usual) very young; but so far as it is possible to judge, prostitutes are as little subject to precocious greynes and baldness as are congenital male criminals. (Pp. 125–126)

The Nature and Causes of Lesbianism

Parent-Duchatelet, who is not always as correct in his analysis as he is precise in his information, explains lesbianism in terms of forced abstinence from men and residing with other women in prisons and brothels. But he does not take into consideration the fact that lesbianism also occurs in the broader world, which has little in common with prisons and brothels. To show this point, we have only to point out, as Sighele has sensibly noted, that a great many novels allude to this vice.

Lesbianism has various causes, the first and most significant of which is an excessive lustfulness, which seeks outlets in all directions, even in the most unnatural. In prisons, some women, being unable to satisfy themselves with a man, throw themselves on other women and become a center of corruption that spreads from the prisoners all the way to the nuns. This is why the majority of prisoners, even though they are only criminaloids and thus not oversexed, will become lesbians under the influence of extremely lascivious born criminals. As Parent-Duchatelet noted, prison is the great school for lesbianism. There even the most reluctant women, if they remain for eighteen or twenty months, end up giving in to the vice. In this respect women prisoners resemble animals; when unable to satisfy their sexual needs with the opposite sex, they attempt to do so with their own. The same thing occurs in madhouses, in which the appearance of a single lesbian is sufficient to infect all the other inmates, even if none of them earlier showed signs of this tendency (Lombroso, *Il tribadismo nei manicomi,* 1888).

A third cause of lesbianism is the way in which the gathering of many women, especially if the group includes prostitutes or lascivious women, provokes imitative behavior, intensifying the vices of each individual and increasing collective vice. Prostitutes often pass their days in the nude, in constant contact with another and often sleeping two or three in one bed. In the outer world, too, gatherings of women occur in boarding schools, during carnival orgies, and even during religious festivals. In brothels women hold competitions, betting on who has the most beautiful sexual organs; naturally this ends up in lesbianism. There are girls who at first resist, disgusted by this vice; they are therefore not born lesbians. Yet they succumb in a state of intoxication, or else they familiarize themselves with the practice little by little, eventually becoming occasional lesbians.

Fourth, maturity and old age tend to invert sexual characteristics, which further encourages sexual inversions among women. Natural history (as we saw earlier) demonstrates that among animals there is a tendency for elderly females to adopt masculine sexual habits. In fact, aging itself is a form of degeneration. While it is true that lesbianism can be found among many young women, most of them live in brothels, where they succumb when tempted by provocative companions.

Fifth, among prostitutes and also some women of easy morals, another cause of lesbianism is apathy and disgust for men produced by physical and sexual mistreatment. Abused by men, they may turn to women when they feel sexual passion (fishermen do not eat fish, as the saying goes). Then, too, women who truly love their paramours may from time to time experience male mistreatment, at which point they give themselves to women, hoping for more faithfulness and certainly kinder treatment. Thus did Nana throw herself at women out of disgust for men's filthy lusts and the way fickle lovers abandoned her.

"One of the causes of lesbianism," Sighle writes in "Coppia criminale" (Archivio di psichiatria, XII, P. 53), "is doubtless men's sexual perversions. Sadists (a term under which Sighele includes all men who practice sex unnaturally) force prostitutes into repugnant acts that exhaust and nauseate them. These women, even though they hardly seem feminine, can feel only disgust for men who are not completely masculine. And thus is born lesbianism—a logical and natural outcome. To escape one dreadful situation, prostitutes

fall on one another." The same thing happens with women who are not prostitutes. (Pp. 176–178)

Source: Lombroso, Cesare, and William Ferrero. 1895. *The Female Offender.* New York: D. Appleton.

Max Nordau, from *Degeneration* (1895)

Nordau argues that the frenzied and crowded conditions of modern life, especially in urban centers, produce a degeneration of the human mind and body that may be transmitted genetically to subsequent generations. Among the symptoms of this degeneration are moral insanity, nervous disorders, and susceptibility to false beliefs. Nordau's theories were later embraced by the Nazis to attack racially undesirable groups, especially urban Jews.

The clearest notion we can form of degeneracy is to regard it as a *morbid deviation from an original type.* This deviation, even if, at the outset, it was ever so slight, contained transmissible elements of such a nature that anyone bearing in him the germs becomes more and more incapable of fulfilling his functions in the world; and mental progress, already checked in his own person, finds itself menaced also in its descendants.

When under any kind of noxious influence an organism becomes debilitated, its successors will not resemble the healthy, normal type of the species, with capacities for development, but will form a new subspecies, which, like all others, possesses the capacity of transmitting to its offspring, in a continuously increasing degree, its peculiarities, these being morbid deviations from the normal form—gaps in development, malformations, and infirmities. That which distinguishes degeneracy from the formation of new species (phylogeny) is, that the morbid variation does not continually subsist and propagate itself, like one that is healthy, but, fortunately, is soon rendered sterile, and after a few generations often dies out before it reaches the lowest grade of organic degradation.

Degeneracy betrays itself among men in certain physical characteristics, which are denominated 'stigmata,' or brandmarks—an unfortunate term derived from a false idea, as if [degeneracy] were necessarily the consequences of a fault, and the indication of it a punishment. Such stigmata consist of deformities, multiple and stunted growths in the first line of asymmetry, the unequal development of the two halves of the face and cranium; then imperfections in the development of the external ear, which is conspicuous for its enormous size, or protrudes from the head, like a handle, and the lobe of which is either lacking or adhering to the head, and the helix of which is not involuted; further, squint-eyes, haire lips, irregularities in the form and position of the teeth; pointed or flat palates, webbed or supernumerary fingers (syn- and poly-dactylia), etc. In this book from which I have quoted, Morel gives a list of the anatomic phenomena of degeneracy, which later observers have largely extended. In particular, Lombroso has conspicuously broadened our knowledge of stigmata, but he apportions them merely to his 'born criminals'—a limitation which from the very scientific standpoint of Lombroso himself cannot be justified, his 'born criminals' being nothing but a subdivision of degenerates. Fere expresses this very emphatically when he says 'Vice, crime and madness are only distinguished from each other by social prejudices.'

There might be a sure means of proving that the application of the term 'degenerates' to the origination of all the *fin-de-siecle* movements in art and literature is not arbitrary, that is no baseless conceit, but a fact; and that would be a careful physical examination of the persons concerned and an inquiry into their pedigree. In almost all cases, relatives would be met with who were undoubtedly degenerate, and one or more stigmata discovered which would indisputably establish the 'Degeneration.' Of course, from human consideration, the result of such an inquiry could often not be made public; and he alone would be convinced who should be able to undertake it himself.

Science, however, has found, together with these physical stigmata, others of a mental order, which betoken degeneracy quite as clearly as the former; and they allow of an easy demonstration from all the works of degenerates, so that it is not necessary to measure the cranium of an author, or to see the lobe of a painter's ear, in order to recognize the fact that he belongs to the class of degenerates.

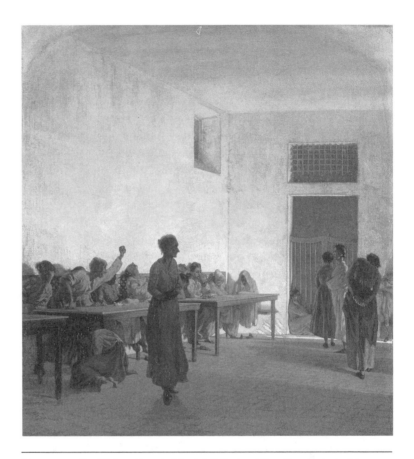

Department for Violent Female Mental Patients at San Bonafacio in Florence, Italy, *by Telemaco Signorini (1835–1901). This image portrays a locked ward for women diagnosed as "mental patients" within the Italian justice system. Nineteenth-century legal historians have discussed the ways in which psychiatry legitimated its professional necessity by providing expert professional opinions on the competency of those standing trial within the judicial system.*

Source: Art Resource, New York.

Quite a number of different designations have been found for these persons. Maudsley and Ball call them 'borderland dwellers'—that is to say, dwellers on the borderland between reason and pronounced madness. Magnan gives to them the name of 'higher degenerates' (*degeneres de superieurs),* and Lombroso speaks of '*mattoids*' (from *matto,* the Italian for insane), and 'graphomaniacs,' under which he classifies those semi insane persons who feel a strong impulse to write. In spite, however, of this variety of nomenclature, it is a question simply of one single species of individuals, who betray their fellowship by the similarity of their mental physiognomy.

In the mental development of degenerates, we meet with the same irregularity that we have observed in their physical growth. The asymmetry of face and cranium finds, as it were, its counterpart in their mental faculties. Some of the latter are completely stunted, others morbidly exaggerated. That which nearly all degenerates lack is the sense of morality and of right and wrong. For them there exists no law, no decency, no modesty. In order to satisfy any momentary impulse, or inclination, or caprice, they commit crimes and trespasses with the greatest calmness and self-complacency, and do not comprehend that other persons take offense thereat. When this phenomenon is present in a high degree, we speak of 'moral insanity' with Maudsley; there are, nevertheless, lower stages in which the degenerate does not, perhaps, himself commit any act which will bring him into conflict with the criminal code, but at least asserts the theoretical legitimacy of crime; seeks, with philosophically sounding fustian, to prove that 'good' and 'evil,' virtue and vice, are arbitrary distinctions; goes into raptures over evildoers and their deeds; professes to discover beauties in the lowest and most repulsive things; and tries to awaken interest in and so-called 'comprehension' of every bestiality. The two psychological roots of moral insanity, in all its degrees of development, are firstly unbounded egoism, and, secondly, impulsiveness—i.e., inability to resist a sudden impulse to any deed; and these characteristics also constitute the chief intellectual stigmata of degenerates. In the following sections of this work, I shall find occasion on which to show on what organic grounds, and in consequence of what peculiarities of their brain and nervous system, degenerates are necessarily egotistical and impulsive. In these introductory remarks, I would wish only to point out the stigma itself.

Another mental stigma of degenerates is their emotionalism. Morel has even wished to make this peculiarity their chief characteristic—erroneously, it seems to me, for it is present in the same degree among hysterics, and, indeed, is to be found in perfectly healthy persons, who, from any transient cause, such as illness, exhaustion, or from any mental shock, have been temporarily weakened. Nevertheless, it is a phenomenon rarely absent in a degenerate. He laughs until he sheds tears, or weeps copiously without adequate occasion; a commonplace line of poetry or of prose sends a shudder down his back; he falls into raptures before indifferent pictures or statues; and music especially, even the most insipid and least commendable, arouses in him the most vehement emotions. He is quite proud of being so vibrant a musical instrument, and boasts that where the Philistine remains completely cold, he feels his inner self confounded, the depths of his being broken up, and the bliss of the Beautiful pressing him

to the tips of his fingers. His excitability appears to him a mark of superiority; he believes himself to be possessed by a peculiar insight lacking in other mortals, and he is fain to despise the vulgar herd for the dullness and narrowness of their minds. The unhappy creature does not suspect that he is conceited about a disease and boasting about a derangement of the mind; and silly critics, when, through fear of being pronounced deficient in comprehension, they make desperate efforts to share the emotions of a degenerate in regard to some insipid or ridiculous production, or when they praise in exaggerated expressions the beauties which the degenerate asserts he finds therein, are unconsciously simulating one of the stigmata of semi-insanity.

Besides moral realm and emotionalism, there is to be observed in the degenerate a condition of mental weakness and dependency, which according to the circumstances of his life, assumes the form of pessimism, a vague fear of all men, and of the entire phenomenon of the universe, or self-abhorrence. 'These patients,' says Morel, 'feel perpetually compelled . . . to commiserate themselves, to sob, to repeat with the most desperate monotony the same questions and words. They have delirious presentations of ruin and damnation, and all sorts of imaginary fears.' 'Ennui never quits me' said a patient of this kind, whose case Roubinovitch describes, 'ennui of myself.' 'Among moral stigmata,' says the same author 'there are also to be specified those undefinable apprehensions manifested by degenerates when they see, smell, or touch any object.' And he further calls to notice 'their unconscious fear of everything and everyone.' In this picture of the sufferer from melancholia; downcast, somber, despairing of himself and the world, tortured by fear of the Unknown, menaced by undefined but dreadful dangers, we recognise in every detail the man of the Dusk of the Nations and the *fin-de-siecle* frame of mind, described in the first chapter.

With this characteristic dejectedness of the degenerate, there is combined, as a rule, a disinclination to action of any kind, attaining possibly to abhorrence of activity and powerlessness to will (*aboulia*). Now, it is a peculiarity of the human mind, known to every psychologist, that, inasmuch as the law of causality governs a man's whole thought, he imputes a rational basis to all his own decisions. This was prettily expressed by Spinoza when he said : 'If a stone flung by a human hand could think, it would certainly imagine that it flew because it wished to fly.' Many mental conditions and operations of which we become conscious are the result of causes which do not reach our consciousness. In this case we fabricate causes *a posteriori* for them, satisfying our mental need of distinct causality, and we have no trouble in persuading ourselves that we have truly explained them. The degenerate who shuns action is a consequence of his inherited deficiency of brain. He deceives himself into believing that he despises action from free determination, and takes pleasure in inactivity; and, in order to justify himself in his own eyes, he constructs a philosophy of renunciation and of contempt for the world and men, asserts that he has convinced himself of the excellence of Quietism, calls himself with consummate self-consciousness a Buddhist, and praises Nirvana in poetically eloquent phrases as the highest and worthiest ideal of the human mind. The degenerate and insane are the predestined disciples of Schopenhauer and Hartmann, and need only to acquire a knowledge of Buddhism to become converts to it.

With the incapacity for action there is connected the predilection for insane reverie. The degenerate is not in a condition to fix his attention long, or indeed at all, on any subject, and is equally incapable of correctly grasping, ordering, or elaborating into ideas and judgments the impressions of the internal world conveyed to his distracted consciousness by his defectively operating senses. It is easier and more convenient for him to allow his brain-centres to produce semi-lucid, nebulously blurred ideas and inchoate embryonic thoughts, and to surrender himself to the perpetual obfuscation of a boundless, aimless, and shoreless stream of fugitive ideas; and he rarely rouses himself to the painful attempt to check or counteract the capricious, and, as a rule, purely mechanical associations of ideas and succession of images, and bring under discipline the extraordinary tumult of his fluid presentations. On the contrary, he rejoices in his faculty of imagination, which he contrasts with the insipidity of the Philistine, and devotes himself with predilection to all sorts of unlicensed pursuits permitted by the unshackled vagabond of his mind; while he cannot endure well-ordered civil occupations, requiring attention and constant heed to reality. He calls this 'having an idealist temperament,' ascribes to himself irresistible aesthetic propinquities, and proudly styles himself an artist.

We will briefly mention some peculiarities frequently manifested by a degenerate. He is tormented by doubts, seeks for the basis of all phenomena, especially those whose first causes are completely inaccessible to us, and he is unhappy when his inquiries

and ruminations lead, as is natural, to no result. He is ever supplying new recruits to the army of system-inventing metaphysicians, profound expositors of the riddle of the universe, seekers for the philosopher's stone, the squaring of the circle and perpetual motion. These last three subjects have such a special attraction for him, that the Patent Office at Washington is forced to keep on hand printed replies to the numberless memorials in which patents are constantly demanded for the solution of these chimerical problems. In view of Lombroso's researches, it can scarcely be doubted that the writings and acts of revolutionists and anarchists are also attributable to degeneracy. The degenerate is incapable of adapting himself to existing circumstances. This incapacity, indeed, is an indication of morbid variation in every species, and probably a primary cause of their sudden extinction. He therefore rebels against conditions and views of things which he necessarily feels to be painful, chiefly because they impose upon him the duty of self-control, of which he is incapable on account of his organic weakness of will. Thus he becomes an improver of the world, and devises plans for making mankind happy, which, without exception are conspicuous quite as much by their fervent philanthropy, and often pathetic insincerity, as by their absurdity and monstrous ignorance of all real relations.

Finally, a cardinal mark of degenerates which I have reserved to the last, is mysticism. Colin says 'Of all the delirious manifestations peculiar to the hereditarily-afflicted, none indicates the condition more clearly, we think, than mystical delirium, or, when the malady has not reached this point, the being constantly occupied with mystical and religious questions, and exaggerated piety, etc.' In the following books, where the art and poetry of the times are treated of, I shall find occasion to show the reader that no difference exists between these tendencies and the religious manias observed in nearly all degenerates and sufferers from hereditary mental taint.

I have enumerated the most important features characterizing the mental condition of the degenerate. The reader can now judge for himself whether or not the diagnosis 'degeneration' is applicable to the originators of the new aesthetic tendencies. It must not for that matter be supposed that degeneration is synonymous with absence of talent. Nearly all the inquirers who have had degenerates under their observation expressly establish the contrary. A badly balanced mind is susceptible of the highest conceptions, while, on the other hand, one meets in the same mind with traits of meanness and pettiness all the more striking from the fact that they co-exist with the most brilliant qualities.' We shall find this reservation in all authors who have contributed to the natural history of the degenerate. 'As regards their intellect, they can,' says Roubinovitch, 'attain to a high degree of development, but from a moral point of view their existence is completely deranged. . . . A degenerate will employ his brilliant faculties as well in the service of some grand object as in the satisfaction of the basest propensities.' Lombroso has cited a large number of undoubted geniuses who were equally undoubted mattoids, graphomaniacs, or pronounced lunatics; and the utterance of a French savant, Guerinsen, 'Genius is a disease of the nerves,' has become a 'winged word.' This expression was imprudent, for it gave ignorant babblers a pretext, and apparently a right, to talk of exaggeration, and to contemn experts in nervous and mental diseases, because they professedly saw a lunatic in everyone who ventured to be something more than the most characterless, average being. Science does not assert that every genius is a lunatic; there are some geniuses of superabundant power whose high privilege consists in the possession of one or other extraordinarily developed faculty, without the rest of their faculties falling short of the average standard. Just as little, naturally, is every lunatic a genius; most of them, even if we disregard idiots of different degrees, are much rather pitiably stupid and incapable; but in many, nay, in abundant cases, the 'higher degenerate' of Magnan, just as he occasionally exhibits gigantic bodily stature or the disproportionate growth of particular parts, has some mental gift exceptionally developed at the cost, it is true, of the remaining faculties, which are wholly or partially atrophied. It is this which enables the well-informed to distinguish at the first glance between the sane genius, and the highly, or even the most highly, gifted degenerate. Take from the former the special capacity through which he becomes a genius, and there still remains a capable, often conspicuously intelligent, clever, moral, and judicious man, who will hold his ground with propriety in our social mechanism. Let the same be tried with the case of a degenerate, and there remains only a criminal or madman, for whom healthy humanity can find no use. If Goethe had never written a line of verse, he would, all the same, have still remained a man of the world, of good principles, a fine art connoisseur, a judicious collector, a keen observer of nature. Let us on the contrary, imagine a Schopenhauer who had written no

[astounding] books, and we should have before us only a repulsive *lusus naturae,* whose morals would necessarily exclude him from all respectable society, and whose fixed idea that he was a victim of persecution would point him out as a subject for a madhouse. The lack of harmony, the absence of balance, the singular incapacity of useful applying, or deriving satisfaction from, their own special faculty among highly gifted degenerates, strikes every healthy censor who does not allow himself to be prejudiced by the noisy admiration of critics, themselves degenerates: and will always prevent his mistaking the mattoid for the same exceptional man who opens out new paths for humanity and leads it to higher developments. I do not share Lombroso's opinion that highly-gifted degenerates are an active force in the progress of mankind. They corrupt and delude; they do, alas! frequently exercise deep influence, but this is always a baneful one. It may not be at once remarked, but it will reveal itself subsequently. If contemporaries do not recognise it, the historian of morals will point it out *a posteriori.* They, likewise, are leading men along the paths they themselves have found to new goals; but these goals are abysses or waste places. They are guides to swamps like will-o'-the-wisps, or to ruin like the ratcatcher of Hammelin. Observers lay stress on their unnatural sterility. 'They are,' says Tarabund, 'cranks; wrongheaded, unbalanced, incapable creatures; they belong to the class of whom it may not be said that they have no mind, but whose mind produces nothing.' 'A common type' writes Legrain, 'unites them:—weakness of judgment and unequal development of mental powers. . . . Their conceptions are never of a high order. They are incapable of great thoughts and prolific ideas. This fact forms a peculiar contrast to the frequently excessive development of their powers of imagination.' 'If they are painters,' we read in Lombroso, 'then their predominant attribute will be their colour-sense; they will be decorative. If they are poets, they will be rich in rhyme, brilliant in style, but barren of thought; sometimes they will be "decadents."

Such are the qualities of the most gifted of those who are discovering new paths, and are proclaimed by enthusiastic followers as the guides to the promised land of the future. Among them degenerates and mattoids predominate. The second of the above-mentioned diagnoses, on the contrary, applies for the most part to the multitude who admire these individuals and swear by them, who imitate the fashions they design, and take delight in the extravagances described in the previous chapter. In their case we have to deal chiefly with hysteria, or neurasthenia.

For reasons which will be elucidated in the next chapter, hysteria has hitherto been less studied in Germany than in France, where, more than elsewhere, it has formed a subject of earnest inquiry. We owe what we know of it almost exclusively to French investigators. The copious treatises of Axenfield, Richer, and in particular Gilles de la Tourette, adequately comprise our present knowledge of this malady; and I shall refer to these works when I enumerate the symptoms chiefly indicative of hysteria.

Among the hysterical—and it must not be thought that these are met with exclusively, or even preponderantly, among females, for they are quite as often, perhaps oftener, found among males—among the hysterical, as among the degenerate, the first thing which strikes us is an extraordinary emotionalism. 'The leading characteristic of the hysterical,' says Colin, 'is the disproportionate impressionability of their psychic centres. . . . They are, above all things, impressionable.' From this primary peculiarity proceeds a second quite as remarkable and important—the exceeding ease with which they can be made to yield to suggestion. The earlier observers always mentioned the boundless mendacity of the hysterical; growing, indeed, quite indignant at it, and making it the most prominent mark of the mental condition of such patients. They were mistaken. The hysterical subject does not consciously lie. He believes in the truth of his craziest inventions. The morbid mobility of his mind, the excessive excitability of his imagination, conveys to his consciousness all sorts of queer and senseless ideas. He suggests to himself that these ideas are founded on true perceptions, and believes in the truth of his foolish inventions until a new suggestion—perhaps his own, perhaps that of another person—has ejected the earlier one. A result of the susceptibility of the hysterical subject to suggestion is his irresistible passion for imitation, and the eagerness with which he yields to all the suggestions of writers and artists. When he sees a picture, he wants to become like it in attitude and dress; when he reads a book, he adopts its views blindly. He takes as a pattern the heroes of the novels which he has in his hand at the moment, and infuses himself into the characters moving before him on stage.

Added to this emotionalism and susceptibility to suggestion is a love of self never met in a sane person in anything like the same degree. The hysterical person's own 'I' towers up before his inner vision, and so completely fills his mental horizon that it conceals the whole of the remaining universe. He cannot endure that others should ignore him. He desires to be as important to his fellow-men as he is to himself. 'An incessant need pursues and governs the hysterical—to busy those about them with themselves. A means of satisfying this need is the fabrication of stories by which they become interesting. Hence come the adventurous occurrences which often enough occupy the police and the reports of the daily press. In the busiest thoroughfare the hysterical person is set upon, robbed, maltreated and wounded, dragged to a distant place, and left to die. He picks himself up painfully, and informs the police. He can show the wounds on his body. He gives all the details. And there is not a single word of truth in the whole story; it is all dreamt and imagined. He has himself inflicted his wounds in order for a short time to become the centre of public attention. In the lower stages of hysteria this need of making a sensation sometimes assumes more harmless forms. It displays itself in eccentricities of dress and behaviour. 'Other hysterical subjects are passionately fond of glaring colours and extravagant forms; they wish to attract attention and make themselves talked about.'

Source: Nordau, Max. 1895. Pp. 16–26 in *Degeneration*. New York: D. Appleton and Company.

▣ Charlotte Perkins Gilman, from *Women and Economics* (1898)

Charlotte Perkins Gilman was an accomplished writer and a feminist theorist. Although she was not widely recognized in her day as a sociologist, she also contributed to the field of sociology through her analysis of gender inequality. The intersection of eugenic thought and Progressive Era feminism is seen here in an excerpt from Gilman's best-known work of nonfiction. According to Gilman, Western women as a group are disabled by the culture, which overemphasizes their sexual appeal and maternal functions, to the detriment of their strength, coordination, and intelligence. This culturally produced weakness is in turn transmitted to their children, according to Gilman, and thus a feminism that restores and celebrates women's "natural" physical and mental gifts is also in the best interests of the race.

In this, in a certain over-coarseness and hardness, a too great belligerence and pride, a too great subservience to the power of sex-attraction, we find the main marks of excessive sex-distinction in men. It has been always checked and offset in them by the healthful activities of racial life. Their energies have been called out and their faculties developed along the lines of human progress. In the growth of industry, commerce, science, manufacture, government, art, religion, the male of our species has become human, far more than male. Strong as this passion is in him, inordinate as is his indulgence, he is a far more normal animal than the female of his species,—far less over-sexed. To him this field of special activity is but part of life,—an incident. The whole world remains besides. To her it is the world.

To make clear by an instance the difference between normal and abnormal sex-distinction, look at the relative condition of a wild cow and a "milch cow" such as we have made. The wild cow is a female. She has healthy calves, and milk enough for them; and that is all the femininity she needs. Otherwise than that she is bovine rather than feminine. She is a light, strong, swift, sinewy creature, able to run, jump and fight if necessary. We, for economic uses, have artificially developed the cow's capacity for producing milk. She has become a walking milk machine, bred and tended to that express end, her value measured in quarts. The secretion of milk is a maternal function—a sex function. The cow is oversexed. Turn her loose in natural conditions and, if she survives the change, she would revert in a very few generations to the plain cow, with her energies used in the general activities of her race, and not all running to milk.

Physically, woman belongs to a tall, vigorous, beautiful animal species, capable of great and varied exertion. In every race and time when she has opportunity for racial activity, she develops accordingly and is no less a woman for being a healthy human creature. In every race and time when she is denied this opportunity,—and few indeed, have been her years of freedom,—she has developed in the lines of action to which she was confined; and those were always the lines of sex-activity. In consequence the body of woman, speaking in the largest generalization, manifests sex-distinction predominantly.

Woman's femininity—and the "eternal feminine" means simply the eternal sexual—is more apparent in proportion to her humanity than the femininity of other animals in proportion to their caninity or felinity or equinity. "A feminine hand" or "a feminine foot" is distinguishable anywhere. We do not hear of " a feminine paw" or a "feminine hoof." A hand is an organ of prehension, a foot an organ of locomotion: they are not secondary sexual characteristics. The comparative smallness and feebleness of woman is a sex distinction. We have carried it to such an excess that women are commonly known as "the weaker sex." There is no such glaring difference between male and female in other advanced species. In the long migration of birds, in the careless motion of the grazing herds that used to swing up and down over the continent each year, in the wild steep journeys of the breeding salmon, nothing is heard of the weaker sex. And among the higher carnivore, where longer maintenance of the younger brings their condition nearer ours, the hunter dreads the attack of the female more than that of the male. The disproportionate weakness is an excessive sex-distinction. Its injurious effect may be broadly shown in Oriental nations, where the female in curtained harems is confined most exclusively to sex-functions and denied most fully the exercise of race-functions. In such peoples the weakness, the tendency to small bones and adipose tissue of the oversexed female, is transmitted to the male with a retarding effect on the development of the race. Conversely in early Germanic tribes, the comparatively free and humanly developed women—tall, strong and brave—transmitted to their sons a greater proportion of human power and much less of morbid sex-tendency.

The degree of feebleness and clumsiness common to women, the comparative inability to stand, walk, run, jump, climb and perform other race-functions common to both sexes, is an excessive sex distinction; and the ensuing transmission of this relative feebleness to their children, boys and girls alike, retards human development. Strong, free, active women, the sturdy, field-working peasant, the burden-bearing savage, are no less good mothers for their human strength. But our civilized "feminine delicacy," which appears somewhat less delicate when recognized as an expression of sexuality in excess,—makes us no better mothers, but worse. The relative weakness of women is a sex-distinction. It is apparent in her to a degree that injures motherhood, that injures wifehood, that injures the individual. The sex-usefulness and the human usefulness of women, their general duty to their kind, are greatly injured by this degree of distinction. In every way the over-sexed condition of the human female reacts unfavorably upon herself, her husband, her children, and the race.

Source: Gilman, Charlotte Perkins. 1966. Pp. 43–47 in *Women and Economics*. New York: Harper & Row. (Originally published 1898)

Charlotte Perkins Gilman, from "The Yellow Wallpaper" (1899)

Charlotte Perkins Gilman was herself prescribed the "rest cure" by its greatest proponent, Dr. Samuel Weir Mitchell. The oppressive gender assumptions implicit in the treatment of "invalid women"—with near-complete confinement to the home and bed, alone, without reading or other activity—were not lost on Gilman. "The Yellow Wallpaper," widely read as a feminist classic, is a semiautobiographical account of a woman's descent into madness.

John laughs at me, of course, but one expects that in marriage.

John is practical in the extreme. He has no patience with faith, an intense horror of superstition, and he scoffs openly at any talk of things not to be felt and seen and put down in figures.

John is a physician, and *perhaps*—(I would not say it to a living soul, of course, but this is dead paper and a great relief to my mind)—*perhaps* that is one reason I do not get well faster.

You see he does not believe I am sick!

And what can one do?

If a physician of high standing, and one's own husband, assures friends and relatives that there is really nothing the matter with one but temporary nervous depression—a slight hysterical tendency—what is one to do?

My brother is also a physician, and also of high standing, and he says the same thing.

So I take phosphates or phosphites—whichever it is, and tonics, and journeys, and air, and exercise, and am absolutely forbidden to "work" until I am well again. . . .

So I walk a little in the garden or down that lovely lane, sit on the porch under the roses, and lie down up here a good deal.

I'm getting really fond of the room in spite of the wall-paper. Perhaps *because* of the wall-paper.

It dwells in my mind so!

I lie here on this great immovable bed—it is nailed down, I believe—and follow that pattern about by the hour. It is as good as gymnastics, I assure you. I start, we'll say, at the bottom, down in the corner over there where it has not been touched, and I determine for the thousandth time that I *will* follow that pointless pattern to some sort of a conclusion. . . .

There is one end of the room where it is almost intact, and there, when the crosslights fade and the low sun shines directly upon it, I can almost fancy radiation after all,—the interminable grotesques seem to form around a common centre and rush off in headlong plunges of equal distraction.

It makes me tired to follow it. I will take a nap I guess.

I don't know why I should write this.

I don't want to.

I don't feel able. And I know John would think it absurd. But I must say what I feel and think in some way—it is such a relief!

But the effort is getting to be greater than the relief.

Half the time now I am awfully lazy, and lie down ever so much.

John says I mustn't lose my strength, and has me take cod liver oil and lots of tonics and things, to say nothing of ale and wine and rare meat.

Dear John! He loves me very dearly, and hates to have me sick. I tried to have a real earnest reasonable talk with him the other day, and tell him how I wish he would let me go and make a visit to Cousin Henry and Julia.

But he said I wasn't able to go, nor able to stand it after I got there; and I did not make out a very good case for myself, for I was crying before I had finished.

It is getting to be a great effort for me to think straight. Just this nervous weakness I suppose.

And dear John gathered me up in his arms, and just carried me upstairs and laid me on the bed, and sat by me and read to me till it tired my head.

He said I was his darling and his comfort and all he had, and that I must take care of myself for his sake, and keep well.

He says no one but myself can help me out of it, that I must use my will and self-control and not let any silly fancies run away with me.

There's one comfort, the baby is well and happy, and does not have to occupy this nursery with the horrid wall-paper.

If we had not used it, that blessed child would have! What a fortunate escape! Why, I wouldn't have a child of mine, an impressionable little thing, live in such a room for worlds.

I never thought of it before, but it is lucky that John kept me here after all, I can stand it so much easier than a baby, you see.

Of course I never mention it to them any more—I am too wise,—but I keep watch of it all the same.

There are things in that paper that nobody knows but me, or ever will.

Behind that outside pattern the dim shapes get clearer every day.

It is always the same shape, only very numerous.

And it is like a woman stooping down and creeping about behind that pattern. I don't like it a bit. I wonder—I begin to think—I wish John would take me away from here!

Source: Gilman, Charlotte Perkins. 1899. "The Yellow Wallpaper." Available at: http://www.pagebypagebooks.com/ Charlotte_Perkins_ Gilman/The_Yellow_Wallpaper/

▣ Stephen Crane, from *The Monster* (1899)

Levi Hume, a resident of Port Jervis, New York, became the model for Henry Johnson, the main character in Crane's novel The Monster, *about a black man who must face the ridicule of the townspeople. In real life, Hume was a physically disabled man who was employed as an ash man. Hume's physical imperfections, coupled with the layers of black soot he wore as a result of his labors, caused the townspeople to be less than kind. Furthermore, The Monster is said to have parallels to one of the town's most shameful historic events, the only public lynching in New York State. Interestingly enough, the lynching is said to have occurred in Orange Square—the very same square in which Crane used to sit with the orange blossoms. In the novel, a small-town doctor's son is saved from a burning house by Henry Johnson, a black man. In gratitude, the doctor takes it upon himself to salvage the life of the badly burned and disfigured hero. Others warn him that he is doing no service to the patient, but the physician cannot let go of one to whom he owes such a profound debt. The town begins to fear the newly created "monster." The burned man's life becomes a nightmare of rejection; the physician and his family are progressively rejected by the community.*

V.

Jake Rogers was the first man to reach the home of Tuscarora Hose Company Number Six. He had wrenched his key from his pocket as he tore down the street, and he jumped at the spring-lock like a demon.

As the doors flew back before his hands he leaped and kicked the wedges from a pair of wheels, loosened a tongue from its clasp, and in the glare of the electric light which the town placed before each of his hose-houses the next comers beheld the spectacle of Jake Rogers bent like hickory in the manfulness of his pulling, and the heavy cart was moving slowly towards the doors. Four men joined him at the time, and as they swung with the cart out into the street, dark figures sped towards them from the ponderous shadows back of the electric lamps. Some set up the inevitable question, "What district?"

"Second," was replied to them in a compact howl. Tuscarora Hose Company Number Six swept on a perilous wheel into Niagara Avenue, and as the men, attached to the cart by the rope which had been paid out from the windlass under the tongue, pulled madly in their fervor and abandon, the gong under the axle clanged incitingly. And sometimes the same cry was heard, "What district?"

"Second."

On a grade Johnnie Thorpe fell, and exercising a singular muscular ability, rolled out in time from the track of the on-coming wheel, and arose, dishevelled and aggrieved, casting a look of mournful disenchantment upon the black crowd that poured after the machine. The cart seemed to be the apex of a dark wave that was whirling as if it had been a broken dam. Back of the lad were stretches of lawn, and in that direction front doors were banged by men who hoarsely shouted out into the clamorous avenue, "What district?"

At one of these houses a woman came to the door bearing a lamp, shielding her face from its rays with her hands. Across the cropped grass the avenue represented to her a kind of black torrent, upon which, nevertheless, fled numerous miraculous figures upon bicycles. She did not know that the towering light at the corner was continuing its nightly whine.

Suddenly a little boy somersaulted around the corner of the house as if he had been projected down a flight of stairs by a catapultian boot. He halted himself in front of the house by dint of a rather extraordinary evolution with his legs. "Oh, ma," he gasped, "can I go? Can I, ma?"

She straightened with the coldness of the exterior mother-judgment, although the hand that held the lamp trembled slightly. "No, Willie; you had better come to bed."

Instantly he began to buck and fume like a mustang. "Oh, ma," he cried, contorting himself—"oh, ma, can't I go? Please, ma, can't I go? Can't I go, ma?"

"It's half past nine now, Willie."

He ended by wailing out a compromise: "Well, just down to the corner, ma? Just down to the corner?"

From the avenue came the sound of rushing men who wildly shouted. Somebody had grappled the bell-rope in the Methodist church, and now over the town rang this solemn and terrible voice, speaking from the clouds. Moved from its peaceful business, this bell gained a new spirit in the portentous night, and it swung the heart to and fro, up and down, with each peal of it.

"Just down to the corner, ma?"

"Willie, it's half past nine now."

VI.

The outlines of the house of Dr. Trescott had faded quietly into the evening, hiding a shape such as we call Queen Anne against the pall of the blackened sky. The neighborhood was at this time so quiet, and seemed so devoid of obstructions, that Hannigan's dog thought it a good opportunity to prowl in forbidden precincts, and so came and pawed Trescott's lawn, growling, and considering himself a formidable beast. Later, Peter Washington strolled past the house and whistled, but there was no dim light shining from Henry's loft, and presently Peter went his way. The rays from the street, creeping in silvery waves over the grass, caused the row of shrubs along the drive to throw a clear, bold shade.

A wisp of smoke came from one of the windows at the end of the house and drifted quietly into the branches of a cherry-tree. Its companions followed it in slowly increasing numbers, and finally there was a current controlled by invisible banks which poured into the fruit-laden boughs of the cherry-tree. It was no more to be noted than if a troop of dim and silent gray monkeys had been climbing a grape-vine into the clouds.

After a moment the window brightened as if the four panes of it had been stained with blood, and a quick ear might have been led to imagine the fire-imps calling and calling, clan joining clan, gathering to the colors. From the street, however, the house maintained its dark quiet, insisting to a passer-by that it was the safe dwelling of people who chose to retire early to tranquil dreams. No one could have heard this low droning of the gathering clans.

Suddenly the panes of the red window tinkled and crashed to the ground, and at other windows there suddenly reared other flames, like bloody spectres at the apertures of a haunted house. This outbreak had been well planned, as if by professional revolutionists.

A man's voice suddenly shouted: "Fire! Fire! Fire!" Hannigan had flung his pipe frenziedly from him because his lungs demanded room. He tumbled down from his perch, swung over the fence, and ran shouting towards the front door of the Trescotts.' Then he hammered on the door, using his fists as if they were mallets. Mrs. Trescott instantly came to one of the windows on the second floor. Afterwards she knew she had been about to say, "The doctor is not at home, but if you will leave your name, I will let him know as soon as he comes."

Hannigan's bawling was for a minute incoherent, but she understood that it was not about croup.

"What?" she said, raising the window swiftly.

"Your house is on fire! You're all ablaze! Move quick if—" His cries were resounding in the street as if it were a cave of echoes. Many feet pattered swiftly on the stones. There was one man who ran with an almost fabulous speed. He wore lavender trousers. A straw hat with a bright silk band was held half crumpled in his hand.

As Henry reached the front door, Hannigan had just broken the lock with a kick. A thick cloud of smoke poured over them, and Henry, ducking his head, rushed into it. From Hannigan's clamor he knew only one thing, but it turned him blue with horror. In the hall a lick of flame had found the cord that supported "Signing the Declaration." The engraving slumped suddenly down at one end, and then dropped to the floor, where it burst with the sound of a bomb. The fire was already roaring like a winter wind among the pines.

At the head of the stairs Mrs. Trescott was waving her arms as if they were two reeds. "Jimmie! Save Jimmie!" she screamed in Henry's face. He plunged past her and disappeared, taking the long-familiar routes among these upper chambers, where he had once held office as a sort of second assistant house-maid.

Hannigan had followed him up the stairs, and grappled the arm of the maniacal woman there. His face was black with rage. "You must come down," he bellowed.

She would only scream at him in reply: "Jimmie! Jimmie! Save Jimmie!" But he dragged her forth while she babbled at him.

As they swung out into the open air a man ran across the lawn, and seizing a shutter, pulled it from its hinges and flung it far out upon the grass. Then he frantically attacked the other shutters one by one. It was a kind of temporary insanity.

"Here, you," howled Hannigan, "hold Mrs. Trescott—And stop—"

The news had been telegraphed by a twist of the wrist of a neighbor who had gone to the fire-box at the corner, and the time when Hannigan and his charge struggled out of the house was the time when the whistle roared its hoarse night call, smiting the crowd in the park, causing the leader of the band, who was about to order the first triumphal clang of a military march, to let his hand drop slowly to his knees.

VII.

Henry pawed awkwardly through the smoke in the upper halls. He had attempted to guide himself by the walls, but they were too hot. The paper was crimpling, and he expected at any moment to have a flame burst from under his hands.

"Jimmie!"

He did not call very loud, as if in fear that the humming flames below would overhear him.

"Jimmie! Oh, Jimmie!"

Stumbling and panting, he speedily reached the entrance to Jimmie's room and flung open the door. The little chamber had no smoke in it at all. It was faintly illumined by a beautiful rosy light reflected circuitously from the flames that were consuming the house. The boy had apparently just been aroused by the noise. He sat in his bed, his lips apart, his eyes wide, while upon his little white-robed figure played caressingly the light from the fire. As the door flew open he had before him this apparition of his pal, a terror-stricken negro, all tousled and with wool scorching, who leaped upon him and bore him up in a blanket as if the whole affair were a case of kidnapping by a dreadful robber chief. Without waiting to go through the usual short but complete process of wrinkling up his face, Jimmie let out a gorgeous bawl, which resembled the expression of a calf's deepest terror. As Johnson, bearing him, reeled into the smoke of the hall, he flung his arms about his neck and buried his face in the blanket. He called twice in muffled tones: "Mam-ma! Mam-ma!"

When Johnson came to the top of the stairs with his burden, he took a quick step backwards. Through the smoke that rolled to him he could see that the lower hall was all ablaze. He cried out then in a howl that resembled Jimmie's former achievement. His legs gained a frightful faculty of bending sideways. Swinging about precariously on these reedy legs, he made his way back slowly, back along the upper hall. From the way of him then, he had given up almost all idea of escaping from the burning house, and with it the desire. He was submitting, submitting because of his fathers, bending his mind in a most perfect slavery to this conflagration.

He now clutched Jimmie as unconsciously as when, running toward the house, he had clutched the hat with the bright silk band.

Suddenly he remembered a little private staircase which led from a bedroom to an apartment which the doctor had fitted up as a laboratory and work-house, where he used some of his leisure, and also hours when he might have been sleeping, in devoting himself to experiments which came in the way of his study and interest.

When Johnson recalled this stairway the submission to the blaze departed instantly. He had been perfectly familiar with it, but his confusion had destroyed the memory of it.

In his sudden momentary apathy there had been little that resembled fear, but now, as a way of safety came to him, the old frantic terror caught him. He was no longer creature to the flames, and he was afraid of the battle with them. It was a singular and swift set of alternations in which he feared twice without submission, and submitted once without fear.

"Jimmie!" he wailed, as he staggered on his way. He wished this little inanimate body at his breast to participate in his tremblings. But the child had lain limp and still during these headlong charges and countercharges, and no sign came from him.

Johnson passed through two rooms and came to the head of the stairs. As he opened the door great billows of smoke poured out, but gripping Jimmie closer, he plunged down through them. All manner of odors assailed him during this flight. They seemed to be alive with envy, hatred, and malice. At the entrance to the laboratory he confronted a strange spectacle. The room was like a garden in the region where might be burning flowers. Flames of violet, crimson, green, blue, orange, and purple were blooming everywhere. There was one blaze that was precisely the hue of a delicate coral. In another place was a mass that lay merely in phosphorescent inaction like a pile of emeralds. But all these marvels were to be seen dimly through clouds of heaving, turning, deadly smoke.

Johnson halted for a moment on the threshold. He cried out again in the negro wail that had in it the sadness of the swamps. Then he rushed across the room. An orange-colored flame leaped like a panther at the lavender trousers. This animal bit deeply into Johnson. There was an explosion at one side, and suddenly before him there reared a delicate, trembling sapphire shape like a fairy lady. With a quiet smile she blocked his path and doomed him and Jimmie. Johnson shrieked, and then ducked in the manner of his race in fights. He aimed to pass under the left guard of the sapphire lady. But she was swifter than eagles, and her talons caught in him as he plunged past her. Bowing his head as if his neck had been struck, Johnson lurched forward, twisting this way and that way. He fell on his back. The still form in the blanket flung from his arms, rolled to the edge of the floor and beneath the window.

Johnson had fallen with his head at the base of an old-fashioned desk. There was a row of jars upon the top of this desk. For the most part, they were silent amid this rioting, but there was one which seemed to hold a scintillant and writhing serpent.

Suddenly the glass splintered, and a ruby-red snakelike thing poured its thick length out upon the top of the old desk. It coiled and hesitated, and then began to swim a languorous way down the mahogany slant. At the angle it waved its sizzling molten head to and fro over the closed eyes of the man beneath it. Then, in a moment, with mystic impulse, it moved again, and the red snake flowed directly down into Johnson's upturned face.

Afterwards the trail of this creature seemed to reek, and amid flames and low explosions drops like red-hot jewels pattered softly down it at leisurely intervals.

VIII.

Suddenly all roads led to Dr. Trescott's. The whole town flowed toward one point. Chippeway Hose Company Number One toiled desperately up Bridge Street Hill even as the Tuscaroras came in an impetuous sweep down Niagara Avenue. Meanwhile the machine of the hook-and-ladder experts from across the creek was spinning on its way. The chief of the fire department had been playing poker in the rear room of Whiteley's cigar-store, but at the first breath of the

alarm he sprang through the door like a man escaping with the kitty.

In Whilomville, on these occasions, there was always a number of people who instantly turned their attention to the bells in the churches and school-houses. The bells not only emphasized the alarm, but it was the habit to send these sounds rolling across the sky in a stirring brazen uproar until the flames were practically vanquished. There was also a kind of rivalry as to which bell should be made to produce the greatest din. Even the Valley Church, four miles away among the farms, had heard the voices of its brethren, and immediately added a quaint little yelp.

Doctor Trescott had been driving homeward, slowly smoking a cigar, and feeling glad that this last case was now in complete obedience to him, like a wild animal that he had subdued, when he heard the long whistle, and chirped to his horse under the unlicensed but perfectly distinct impression that a fire had broken out in Oakhurst, a new and rather high-flying suburb of the town which was at least two miles from his own home. But in the second blast and in the ensuing silence he read the designation of his own district. He was then only a few blocks from his house. He took out the whip and laid it lightly on the mare. Surprised and frightened at this extraordinary action, she leaped forward, and as the reins straightened like steel bands, the doctor leaned backward a trifle. When the mare whirled him up to the closed gate he was wondering whose house could be afire. The man who had rung the signal-box yelled something at him, but he already knew. He left the mare to her will.

In front of his door was a maniacal woman in a wrapper. "Ned!" she screamed at sight of him. "Jimmie! Save Jimmie!"

Trescott had grown hard and chill.

"Where?" he said. "Where?"

Mrs. Trescott's voice began to bubble. "Up—up—up—" She pointed at the second-story windows.

Hannigan was already shouting: "Don't go in that way! You can't go in that way!"

Trescott ran around the corner of the house and disappeared from them. He knew from the view he had taken of the main hall that it would be impossible to ascend from there. His hopes were fastened now to the stairway which led from the laboratory. The door which opened from this room out upon the lawn was fastened with a bolt and lock, but he kicked close to the lock and then close to the bolt. The door with a loud crash flew back. The doctor recoiled from the roll of smoke, and then bending low, he stepped into the garden of burning flowers. On the floor his stinging eyes could make out a form in a smouldering blanket near the window. Then, as he carried his son toward the door, he saw that the whole lawn seemed now alive with men and boys, the leaders in the great charge that the whole town was making. They seized him and his burden, and overpowered him in wet blankets and water.

But Hannigan was howling: "Johnson is in there yet! Henry Johnson is in there yet! He went in after the kid! Johnson is in there yet!"

These cries penetrated to the sleepy senses of Trescott, and he struggled with his captors, swearing unknown to him and to them, all the deep blasphemies of his medical-student days. He arose to his feet and went again toward the door of the laboratory. They endeavored to restrain him, although they were much affrighted at him.

But a young man who was a brakeman on the railway, and lived in one of the rear streets near the Trescotts, had gone into the laboratory and brought forth a thing which he laid on the grass.

IX.

There were hoarse commands from in front of the house. "Turn on your water, Five!" "Let 'er go, One!" The gathering crowd swayed this way and that way. The flames, towering high, cast a wild red light on their faces. There came the clangor of a gong from along some adjacent street. The crowd exclaimed at it. "Here comes Number Three!" "That's Three a-comin'!" A panting and irregular mob dashed into view, dragging a hose-cart. A cry of exultation arose from the little boys. "Here's Three!" The lads welcomed Never-Die Hose Company Number Three as if it was composed of a chariot dragged by a band of gods. The perspiring citizens flung themselves into the fray. The boys danced in impish joy at the displays of prowess. They acclaimed the approach of Number Two. They welcomed Number Four with cheers. They were so deeply moved by this whole affair that they bitterly guyed the late appearance of the hook and ladder company, whose heavy apparatus had almost stalled them on the Bridge Street hill. The lads hated and feared a fire, of course. They did not particularly want to have anybody's house burn, but still it was fine to see the gathering of the companies, and amid a great noise to watch their heroes perform all manner of prodigies.

They were divided into parties over the worth of different companies, and supported their creeds with no small violence. For instance, in that part of the little city where Number Four had its home it would be most daring for a boy to contend the superiority of any other company. Likewise, in another quarter, when a strange boy was asked which fire company was the best in Whilomville, he was expected to answer "Number One." Feuds, which the boys forgot and remembered according to chance or the importance of some recent event, existed all through the town.

They did not care much for John Shipley, the chief of the department. It was true that he went to a fire with the speed of a falling angel, but when there he invariably lapsed into a certain still mood, which was almost a preoccupation, moving leisurely around the burning structure and surveying it, puffing meanwhile at a cigar. This quiet man, who even when life was in danger seldom raised his voice, was not much to their fancy. Now old Sykes Huntington, when he was chief, used to bellow continually like a bull and gesticulate in a sort of delirium. He was much finer as a spectacle than this Shipley, who viewed a fire with the same steadiness that he viewed a raise in a large jackpot. The greater number of the boys could never understand why the members of these companies persisted in re-electing Shipley, although they often pretended to understand it, because "My father says" was a very formidable phrase in argument, and the fathers seemed almost unanimous in advocating Shipley.

At this time there was considerable discussion as to which company had gotten the first stream of water on the fire. Most of the boys claimed that Number Five owned that distinction, but there was a determined minority who contended for Number One. Boys who were the blood adherents of other companies were obliged to choose between the two on this occasion, and the talk waxed warm.

But a great rumor went among the crowds. It was told with hushed voices. Afterward a reverent silence fell even upon the boys. Jimmie Trescott and Henry Johnson had been burned to death, and Dr. Trescott himself had been most savagely hurt. The crowd did not even feel the police pushing at them. They raised their eyes, shining now with awe, toward the high flames.

The man who had information was at his best. In low tones he described the whole affair. "That was the kid's room—in the corner there. He had measles or somethin,' and this coon—Johnson—was a-settin' up with 'im, and Johnson got sleepy or somethin' and upset the lamp, and the doctor he was down in his office, and he came running up, and they all got burned together till they dragged 'em out."

Another man, always preserved for the deliverance of the final judgment, was saying: "Oh, they'll die sure. Burned to flinders. No chance. Hull lot of 'em. Anybody can see." The crowd concentrated its gaze still more closely upon these flags of fire which waved joyfully against the black sky. The bells of the town were clashing unceasingly.

A little procession moved across the lawn and toward the street. There were three cots, borne by twelve of the firemen. The police moved sternly, but it needed no effort of theirs to open a lane for this slow cortege. The men who bore the cots were well known to the crowd, but in this solemn parade during the ringing of the bells and the shouting, and with the red glare upon the sky, they seemed utterly foreign, and Whilomville paid them a deep respect. Each man in this stretcher party had gained a reflected majesty. They were footmen to death, and the crowd made subtle obeisance to this august dignity derived from three prospective graves. One woman turned away with a shriek at sight of the covered body on the first stretcher, and people faced her suddenly in silent and mournful indignation. Otherwise there was barely a sound as these twelve important men with measured tread carried their burdens through the throng.

The little boys no longer discussed the merits of the different fire companies. For the greater part they had been routed. Only the more courageous viewed closely the three figures veiled in yellow blankets.

X.

Old Judge Denning Hagenthorpe, who lived nearly opposite the Trescotts, had thrown his door wide open to receive the afflicted family. When it was publicly learned that the doctor and his son and the negro were still alive, it required a specially detailed policeman to prevent people from scaling the front porch and interviewing these sorely wounded. One old lady appeared with a miraculous poultice, and she quoted most damning scripture to the officer when he said that she could not pass him. Throughout the night some lads old enough to be given privileges or to compel them from their mothers remained vigilantly upon the kerb in anticipation of a death or some such event. The reporter of the *Morning Tribune* rode thither on his bicycle every hour until three o'clock.

Six of the ten doctors in Whilomville attended at Judge Hagenthorpe's house.

Almost at once they were able to know that Trescott's burns were not vitally important. The child would possibly be scarred badly, but his life was undoubtedly safe. As for the negro Henry Johnson, he could not live. His body was frightfully seared, but more than that, he now had no face. His face had simply been burned away.

Trescott was always asking news of the two other patients. In the morning he seemed fresh and strong, so they told him that Johnson was doomed. They then saw him stir on the bed, and sprang quickly to see if the bandages needed readjusting. In the sudden glance he threw from one to another he impressed them as being both leonine and impracticable.

The morning paper announced the death of Henry Johnson. It contained a long interview with Edward J. Hannigan, in which the latter described in full the performance of Johnson at the fire. There was also an editorial built from all the best words in the vocabulary of the staff. The town halted in its accustomed road of thought, and turned a reverent attention to the memory of this hostler. In the breasts of many people was the regret that they had not known enough to give him a hand and a lift when he was alive, and they judged themselves stupid and ungenerous for this failure.

The name of Henry Johnson became suddenly the title of a saint to the little boys. The one who thought of it first could, by quoting it in an argument, at once overthrow his antagonist, whether it applied to the subject or whether it did not.

Nigger, nigger, never die,
Black face and shiny eye.

Boys who had called this odious couplet in the rear of Johnson's march buried the fact at the bottom of their hearts.

Later in the day Miss Bella Farragut, of No. 7 Watermelon Alley, announced that she had been engaged to marry Mr. Henry Johnson.

XIV.

Reifsnyder's assistant had gone to his supper, and the owner of the shop was trying to placate four men who wished to be shaved at once. Reifsnyder was very garrulous—a fact which made him rather remarkable among barbers, who, as a class, are austerely speechless, having been taught silence by the hammering reiteration of a tradition. It is the customers who talk in the ordinary event.

As Reifsnyder waved his razor down the cheek of a man in the chair, he turned often to cool the impatience of the others with pleasant talk, which they did not particularly heed.

"Oh, he should have let him die," said Bainbridge, a railway engineer, finally replying to one of the barber's orations. "Shut up, Reif, and go on with your business!"

Instead, Reifsnyder paused shaving entirely, and turned to front the speaker. "Let him die?" he demanded. "How vas that? How can you let a man die?"

"By letting him die, you chump," said the engineer. The others laughed a little, and Reifsnyder turned at once to his work, sullenly, as a man overwhelmed by the derision of numbers.

"How vas that?" he grumbled later. "How can you let a man die when he vas done so much for you?"

"'When he vas done so much for you?'" repeated Bainbridge. "You better shave some people. How vas that? Maybe this ain't a barber shop?"

A man hitherto silent now said, "If I had been the doctor, I would have done the same thing."

"Of course," said Reifsnyder. "Any man vould do it. Any man that vas not like you, you—old—flint-hearted—fish." He had sought the final words with painful care, and he delivered the collection triumphantly at Bainbridge. The engineer laughed.

The man in the chair now lifted himself higher, while Reifsnyder began an elaborate ceremony of anointing and combing his hair. Now free to join comfortably in the talk, the man said: "They say he is the most terrible thing in the world. Young Johnnie Bernard— that drives the grocery wagon—saw him up at Alek Williams's shanty, and he says he couldn't eat anything for two days."

"Chee!" said Reifsnyder.

"Well, what makes him so terrible?" asked another.

"Because he hasn't got any face," replied the barber and the engineer in duet.

"Hasn't got any face?" repeated the man. "How can he do without any face!" "He has no face in the front of his head, in the place where his face ought to grow."

Bainbridge sang these lines pathetically as he arose and hung his hat on a hook. The man in the chair was about to abdicate in his favor. "Get a gait on you now," he said to Reifsnyder. "I go out at 7.31."

As the barber foamed the lather on the cheeks of the engineer he seemed to be thinking heavily. Then suddenly he burst out. "How would you like to be with no face?" he cried to the assemblage.

"Oh, if I had to have a face like yours—" answered one customer.

Bainbridge's voice came from a sea of lather. "You're kicking because if losing faces becomes popular, you'd have to go out of business."

"I don't think it will become so much popular," said Reifsnyder.

"Not if it's got to be taken off in the way his was taken off," said another man. "I'd rather keep mine, if you don't mind."

"I guess so!" cried the barber. "Just think!"

The shaving of Bainbridge had arrived at a time of comparative liberty for him. "I wonder what the doctor says to himself?" he observed. "He may be sorry he made him live."

"It was the only thing he could do," replied a man. The others seemed to agree with him.

"Supposing you were in his place," said one, "and Johnson had saved your kid. What would you do?"

"Certainly!"

"Of course! You would do anything on earth for him. You'd take all the trouble in the world for him. And spend your last dollar on him. Well, then?"

"I wonder how it feels to be without any face?" said Reifsnyder, musingly.

The man who had previously spoken, feeling that he had expressed himself well, repeated the whole thing. "You would do anything on earth for him. You'd take all the trouble in the world for him. And spend your last dollar on him. Well, then?"

"No, but look," said Reifsnyder; "supposing you don't got a face!"

XV.

As soon as Williams was hidden from the view of the old judge he began to gesture and talk to himself. An elation had evidently penetrated to his vitals, and caused him to dilate as if he had been filled with gas. He snapped his fingers in the air, and whistled fragments of triumphal music. At times, in his progress toward his shanty, he indulged in a shuffling movement that was really a dance. It was to be learned from the intermediate monologue that he had emerged from his trials laurelled and proud. He was the unconquerable Alexander Williams. Nothing could exceed the bold self-reliance of his manner. His kingly stride, his heroic song, the derisive flourish of his hands—all betokened a man who had successfully defied the world.

On his way he saw Zeke Paterson coming to town. They hailed each other at a distance of fifty yards.

"How do, Broth' Paterson?"

"How do, Broth' Williams?"

They were both deacons.

"Is you' folks well, Broth' Paterson?"

"Middlin,' middlin.' How's you' folks, Broth' Williams?"

Neither of them had slowed his pace in the smallest degree. They had simply begun this talk when a considerable space separated them, continued it as they passed, and added polite questions as they drifted steadily apart. Williams's mind seemed to be a balloon. He had been so inflated that he had not noticed that Paterson had definitely shied into the dry ditch as they came to the point of ordinary contact.

Afterward, as he went a lonely way, he burst out again in song and pantomimic celebration of his estate. His feet moved in prancing steps.

When he came in sight of his cabin, the fields were bathed in a blue dusk, and the light in the window was pale. Cavorting and gesticulating, he gazed joyfully for some moments upon this light. Then suddenly another idea seemed to attack his mind, and he stopped, with an air of being suddenly dampened. In the end he approached his home as if it were the fortress of an enemy.

Some dogs disputed his advance for a loud moment, and then discovering their lord, slunk away embarrassed. His reproaches were addressed to them in muffled tones.

Arriving at the door, he pushed it open with the timidity of a new thief. He thrust his head cautiously sideways, and his eyes met the eyes of his wife, who sat by the table, the lamp-light defining a half of her face. "Sh!" he said, uselessly. His glance travelled swiftly to the inner door which shielded the one bed-chamber. The pickaninnies, strewn upon the floor of the living-room, were softly snoring. After a hearty meal they had promptly dispersed themselves about the place and gone to sleep. "Sh!" said Williams again to his motionless and silent wife. He had allowed only his head to appear. His wife, with one hand upon the edge of the table and the other at her knee, was regarding him with wide eyes and parted lips as if he were a spectre. She looked to be one who was living in terror, and even the familiar face at the door had thrilled her because it had come suddenly.

Williams broke the tense silence. "Is he all right?" he whispered, waving his eyes toward the inner door. Following his glance timorously, his wife nodded, and in a low tone answered,

"I raikon he's done gone t'sleep."

Williams then slunk noiselessly across his threshold.

He lifted a chair, and with infinite care placed it so that it faced the dreaded inner door. His wife moved slightly, so as to also squarely face it. A silence came upon them in which they seemed to be waiting for a calamity, pealing and deadly.

Williams finally coughed behind his hand. His wife started, and looked upon him in alarm. "'Pears like he done gwine keep quiet ter-night," he breathed. They continually pointed their speech and their looks at the inner door, paying it the homage due to a corpse or a phantom. Another long stillness followed this sentence. Their eyes shone white and wide. A wagon rattled down the distant road. From their chairs they looked at the window, and the effect of the light in the cabin was a presentation of an intensely black and solemn night. The old woman adopted the attitude used always in church at funerals. At times she seemed to be upon the point of breaking out in prayer.

"He mighty quiet ter-night," whispered Williams. "Was he good ter-day?" For answer his wife raised her eyes to the ceiling in the supplication of Job. Williams moved restlessly. Finally he tip-toed to the door. He knelt slowly and without a sound, and placed his ear near the key-hole. Hearing a noise behind him, he turned quickly. His wife was staring at him aghast. She stood in front of the stove, and her arms were spread out in the natural movement to protect all her sleeping ducklings.

But Williams arose without having touched the door. "I raikon he er-sleep," he said, fingering his wool. He debated with himself for some time. During this interval his wife remained, a great fat statue of a mother shielding her children.

It was plain that his mind was swept suddenly by a wave of temerity. With a sounding step he moved toward the door. His fingers were almost upon the knob when he swiftly ducked and dodged away, clapping his hands to the back of his head. It was as if the portal had threatened him. There was a little tumult near the stove, where Mrs. Williams's desperate retreat had involved her feet with the prostrate children.

After the panic Williams bore traces of a feeling of shame. He returned to the charge. He firmly grasped the knob with his left hand, and with his other hand turned the key in the lock. He pushed the door, and as it swung portentously open he sprang nimbly to one side like the fearful slave liberating the lion. Near the stove a group had formed, the terror-stricken mother with her arms stretched, and the aroused children clinging frenziedly to her skirts.

The light streamed after the swinging door, and disclosed a room six feet one way and six feet the other way. It was small enough to enable the radiance to lay it plain. Williams peered warily around the corner made by the door-post.

Suddenly he advanced, retired, and advanced again with a howl. His palsied family had expected him to spring backward, and at his howl they heaped themselves wondrously. But Williams simply stood in the little room emitting his howls before an open window. "He's gone! He's gone! He's gone!" His eye and his hand had speedily proved the fact. He had even thrown open a little cupboard.

Presently he came flying out. He grabbed his hat, and hurled the outer door back upon its hinges. Then he tumbled headlong into the night. He was yelling: "Docteh Trescott! Docteh Trescott!" He ran wildly through the fields, and galloped in the direction of town. He continued to call to Trescott as if the latter was within easy hearing. It was as if Trescott was poised in the contemplative sky over the running negro, and could heed this reaching voice—"Docteh Trescott!"

In the cabin, Mrs. Williams, supported by relays from the battalion of children, stood quaking watch until the truth of daylight came as a re-enforcement and made them arrogant, strutting, swashbuckler children, and a mother who proclaimed her illimitable courage.

XVI.

Theresa Page was giving a party. It was the outcome of a long series of arguments addressed to her mother, which had been overheard in part by her father. He had at last said five words, "Oh, let her have it." The mother had then gladly capitulated.

Theresa had written nineteen invitations, and distributed them at recess to her schoolmates. Later her mother had composed five large cakes, and still later a vast amount of lemonade.

So the nine little girls and the ten little boys sat quite primly in the dining-room, while Theresa and her mother plied them with cake and lemonade, and also with ice-cream. This primness sat now quite strangely upon them. It was owing to the presence of Mrs. Page. Previously in the parlor alone with their games they had overturned a chair; the boys had let more or less of their hoodlum spirit shine forth. But when circumstances could be possibly magnified to warrant it, the girls made the boys victims of an insufferable pride, snubbing them mercilessly. So in the dining-room they resembled a class at Sunday-school, if it were not for the subterranean smiles, gestures, rebuffs, and poutings which stamped the affair as a children's party.

Two little girls of this subdued gathering were planted in a settle with their backs to the broad window. They were beaming lovingly upon each other with an effect of scorning the boys.

Hearing a noise behind her at the window, one little girl turned to face it. Instantly she screamed and sprang away, covering her face with her hands. "What was it? What was it?" cried every one in a roar. Some slight movement of the eyes of the weeping and shuddering child informed the company that she had been frightened by an appearance at the window. At once they all faced the imperturbable window, and for a moment there was a silence. An astute lad made an immediate census of the other lads. The prank of slipping out and looming spectrally at a window was too venerable. But the little boys were all present and astonished.

As they recovered their minds they uttered warlike cries, and through a side-door sallied rapidly out against the terror. They vied with each other in daring.

None wished particularly to encounter a dragon in the darkness of the garden, but there could be no faltering when the fair ones in the dining-room were present. Calling to each other in stern voices, they went dragooning over the lawn, attacking the shadows with ferocity, but still with the caution of reasonable beings. They found, however, nothing new to the peace of the night. Of course there was a lad who told a great lie. He described a grim figure, bending low and slinking off along the fence. He gave a number of details, rendering his lie more splendid by a repetition of certain forms which he recalled from romances. For instance, he insisted that he had heard the creature emit a hollow laugh.

Inside the house the little girl who had raised the alarm was still shuddering and weeping. With the utmost difficulty was she brought to a state approximating calmness by Mrs. Page. Then she wanted to go home at once.

Page entered the house at this time. He had exiled himself until he concluded that this children's party was finished and gone. He was obliged to escort the little girl home because she screamed again when they opened the door and she saw the night.

She was not coherent even to her mother. Was it a man? She didn't know. It was simply a thing, a dreadful thing.

XVII.

In Watermelon Alley the Farraguts were spending their evening as usual on the little rickety porch. Sometimes they howled gossip to other people on other rickety porches. The thin wail of a baby arose from a near house. A man had a terrific altercation with his wife, to which the alley paid no attention at all.

There appeared suddenly before the Farraguts a monster making a low and sweeping bow. There was an instant's pause, and then occurred something that resembled the effect of an upheaval of the earth's surface. The old woman hurled herself backward with a dreadful cry. Young Sim had been perched gracefully on a railing. At sight of the monster he simply fell over it to the ground. He made no sound, his eyes stuck out, his nerveless hands tried to grapple the rail to prevent a tumble, and then he vanished. Bella, blubbering, and with her hair suddenly and mysteriously dishevelled, was crawling on her hands and knees fearsomely up the steps.

Standing before this wreck of a family gathering, the monster continued to bow. It even raised a deprecatory claw. "Don' make no botheration 'bout me, Miss Fa'gut," it said, politely. "No, 'deed. I jes drap in ter ax if yer well this evenin,' Miss Fa'gut. Don' make no botheration. No, 'deed. I gwine ax you to go to er daince with me, Miss Fa'gut. I ax you if I can have the magnifercent gratitude of you' company on that 'casion, Miss Fa'gut."

The girl cast a miserable glance behind her. She was still crawling away. On the ground beside the porch young Sim raised a strange bleat, which expressed both his fright and his lack of wind. Presently the monster, with a fashionable amble, ascended the steps after the girl.

She grovelled in a corner of the room as the creature took a chair. It seated itself very elegantly on the edge. It held an old cap in both hands. "Don' make no

botheration, Miss Fa'gut. Don' make no botherations. No, 'deed. I jes drap in ter ax you if you won' do me the proud of acceptin' ma humble invitation to er daince, Miss Fa'gut."

She shielded her eyes with her arms and tried to crawl past it, but the genial monster blocked the way. "I jes drap in ter ax you 'bout er daince, Miss Fa'gut. I ax you if I kin have the magnifercent gratitude of you' company on that 'casion, Miss Fa'gut."

In a last outbreak of despair, the girl, shuddering and wailing, threw herself face downward on the floor, while the monster sat on the edge of the chair gabbling courteous invitations, and holding the old hat daintily to its stomach.

At the back of the house, Mrs. Farragut, who was of enormous weight, and who for eight years had done little more than sit in an arm-chair and describe her various ailments, had with speed and agility scaled a high board fence.

XVIII.

The black mass in the middle of Trescott's property was hardly allowed to cool before the builders were at work on another house. It had sprung upward at a fabulous rate. It was like a magical composition born of the ashes. The doctor's office was the first part to be completed, and he had already moved in his new books and instruments and medicines.

Trescott sat before his desk when the chief of police arrived. "Well, we found him," said the latter.

"Did you?" cried the doctor. "Where?"

"Shambling around the streets at daylight this morning. I'll be blamed if I can figure on where he passed the night."

"Where is he now?"

"Oh, we jugged him. I didn't know what else to do with him. That's what I want you to tell me. Of course we can't keep him. No charge could be made, you know."

"I'll come down and get him."

The official grinned retrospectively. "Must say he had a fine career while he was out. First thing he did was to break up a children's party at Page's. Then he went to Watermelon Alley. Whoo! He stampeded the whole outfit. Men, women, and children running pellmell, and yelling. They say one old woman broke her leg, or something, shinning over a fence. Then he went right out on the main street, and an Irish girl threw a fit, and there was a sort of riot. He began to run, and a big crowd chased him, firing rocks. But he gave them the slip somehow down there by the foundry and in the railroad yard. We looked for him all night, but couldn't find him."

"Was he hurt any? Did anybody hit him with a stone?"

"Guess there isn't much of him to hurt any more, is there? Guess he's been hurt up to the limit. No. They never touched him. Of course nobody really wanted to hit him, but you know how a crowd gets. It's like—it's like—"

"Yes, I know."

For a moment the chief of the police looked reflectively at the floor. Then he spoke hesitatingly. "You know Jake Winter's little girl was the one that he scared at the party. She is pretty sick, they say."

"Is she? Why, they didn't call me. I always attend the Winter family."

"No? Didn't they?" asked the chief, slowly. "Well—you know—Winter is—well, Winter has gone clean crazy over this business. He wanted—he wanted to have you arrested."

"Have me arrested? The idiot! What in the name of wonder could he have me arrested for?"

"Of course. He is a fool. I told him to keep his trap shut. But then you know how he'll go all over town yapping about the thing. I thought I'd better tip you."

"Oh, he is of no consequence; but then, of course, I'm obliged to you, Sam."

"That's all right. Well, you'll be down to-night and take him out, eh? You'll get a good welcome from the jailer. He don't like his job for a cent. He says you can have your man whenever you want him. He's got no use for him."

"But what is this business of Winter's about having me arrested?"

"Oh, it's a lot of chin about your having no right to allow this—this—this man to be at large. But I told him to tend to his own business. Only I thought I'd better let you know. And I might as well say right now, doctor, that there is a good deal of talk about this thing. If I were you, I'd come to the jail pretty late at night, because there is likely to be a crowd around the door, and I'd bring a—er—mask, or some kind of a veil, anyhow."

XIX.

Martha Goodwin was single, and well along into the thin years. She lived with her married sister in Whilomville. She performed nearly all the house-work in exchange for the privilege of existence. Every one tacitly recognized her labor as a form of penance for the early end of her betrothed, who had died of small-pox, which he had not caught from her.

But despite the strenuous and unceasing workaday of her life, she was a woman of great mind. She had adamantine opinions upon the situation in Armenia, the condition of women in China, the flirtation between Mrs. Minster of Niagara Avenue and young Griscom, the conflict in the Bible class of the Baptist Sunday-school, the duty of the United States toward the Cuban insurgents, and many other colossal matters. Her fullest experience of violence was gained on an occasion when she had seen a hound clubbed, but in the plan which she had made for the reform of the world she advocated drastic measures. For instance, she contended that all the Turks should be pushed into the sea and drowned, and that Mrs. Minster and young Griscom should be hanged side by side on twin gallows. In fact, this woman of peace, who had seen only peace, argued constantly for a creed of illimitable ferocity. She was invulnerable on these questions, because eventually she overrode all opponents with a sniff. This sniff was an active force. It was to her antagonists like a bang over the head, and none was known to recover from this expression of exalted contempt. It left them windless and conquered. They never again came forward as candidates for suppression. And Martha walked her kitchen with a stern brow, an invincible being like Napoleon.

Nevertheless her acquaintances, from the pain of their defeats, had been long in secret revolt. It was in no wise a conspiracy, because they did not care to state their open rebellion, but nevertheless it was understood that any woman who could not coincide with one of Martha's contentions was entitled to the support of others in the small circle. It amounted to an arrangement by which all were required to disbelieve any theory for which Martha fought. This, however, did not prevent them from speaking of her mind with profound respect.

Two people bore the brunt of her ability. Her sister Kate was visibly afraid of her, while Carrie Dungen sailed across from her kitchen to sit respectfully at Martha's feet and learn the business of the world. To be sure, afterwards, under another sun, she always laughed at Martha and pretended to deride her ideas, but in the presence of the sovereign she always remained silent or admiring. Kate, the sister, was of no consequence at all. Her principal delusion was that she did all the work in the upstairs rooms of the house, while Martha did it downstairs. The truth was seen only by the husband, who treated Martha with a kindness that was half banter, half deference. Martha herself had no suspicion that she was the only pillar of the domestic edifice. The situation was without definitions. Martha made definitions, but she devoted them entirely to the Armenians and Griscom and the Chinese and other subjects. Her dreams, which in early days had been of love of meadows and the shade of trees, of the face of a man, were now involved otherwise, and they were companioned in the kitchen curiously, Cuba, the hot-water kettle, Armenia, the washing of the dishes, and the whole thing being jumbled. In regard to social misdemeanors, she who was simply the mausoleum of a dead passion was probably the most savage critic in town. This unknown woman, hidden in a kitchen as in a well, was sure to have a considerable effect of the one kind or the other in the life of the town. Every time it moved a yard, she had personally contributed an inch. She could hammer so stoutly upon the door of a proposition that it would break from its hinges and fall upon her, but at any rate it moved. She was an engine, and the fact that she did not know that she was an engine contributed largely to the effect. One reason that she was formidable was that she did not even imagine that she was formidable. She remained a weak, innocent, and pig-headed creature, who alone would defy the universe if she thought the universe merited this proceeding.

One day Carrie Dungen came across from her kitchen with speed. She had a great deal of grist. "Oh," she cried, "Henry Johnson got away from where they was keeping him, and came to town last night, and scared everybody almost to death."

Martha was shining a dish-pan, polishing madly. No reasonable person could see cause for this operation, because the pan already glistened like silver. "Well!" she ejaculated. She imparted to the word a deep meaning. "This, my prophecy, has come to pass." It was a habit.

The overplus of information was choking Carrie. Before she could go on she was obliged to struggle for a moment. "And, oh, little Sadie Winter is awful sick, and they say Jake Winter was around this morning trying to get Doctor Trescott arrested. And poor old Mrs. Farragut sprained her ankle in trying to climb a fence. And there's a crowd around the jail all the time. They put Henry in jail because they didn't know what else to do with him, I guess. They say he is perfectly terrible."

Martha finally released the dish-pan and confronted the headlong speaker. "Well!" she said again, poising a great brown rag. Kate had heard the excited new-comer, and drifted down from the novel in her room. She was a shivery little woman. Her shoulder-blades seemed to be two panes of ice, for she was constantly shrugging and shrugging. "Serves him right if he was to lose all his patients," she said suddenly, in bloodthirsty tones. She snipped her words out as if her lips were scissors.

"Well, he's likely to," shouted Carrie Dungen. "Don't a lot of people say that they won't have him any more? If you're sick and nervous, Doctor Trescott would scare the life out of you, wouldn't he? He would me. I'd keep thinking."

Martha, stalking to and fro, sometimes surveyed the two other women with a contemplative frown.

XX.

After the return from Connecticut, little Jimmie was at first much afraid of the monster who lived in the room over the carriage-house. He could not identify it in any way. Gradually, however, his fear dwindled under the influence of a weird fascination. He sidled into closer and closer relations with it.

One time the monster was seated on a box behind the stable basking in the rays of the afternoon sun. A heavy crêpe veil was swathed about its head.

Little Jimmie and many companions came around the corner of the stable. They were all in what was popularly known as the baby class, and consequently escaped from school a half-hour before the other children. They halted abruptly at sight of the figure on the box. Jimmie waved his hand with the air of a proprietor.

"There he is," he said.

"O-o-o!" murmured all the little boys—"o-o-o!" They shrank back, and grouped according to courage or experience, as at the sound the monster slowly turned its head. Jimmie had remained in the van alone. "Don't be afraid! I won't let him hurt you," he said, delighted.

"Huh!" they replied, contemptuously. "We ain't afraid."

Jimmie seemed to reap all the joys of the owner and exhibitor of one of the world's marvels, while his audience remained at a distance—awed and entranced, fearful and envious.

One of them addressed Jimmie gloomily. "Bet you dassent walk right up to him." He was an older boy than Jimmie, and habitually oppressed him to a small degree. This new social elevation of the smaller lad probably seemed revolutionary to him.

"Huh!" said Jimmie, with deep scorn. "Dassent I? Dassent I, hey? Dassent I?"

The group was immensely excited. It turned its eyes upon the boy that Jimmie addressed. "No, you dassent," he said, stolidly, facing a moral defeat. He could see that Jimmie was resolved. "No, you dassent," he repeated, doggedly.

"Ho!" cried Jimmie. "You just watch!—you just watch!"

Amid a silence he turned and marched toward the monster. But possibly the palpable wariness of his companions had an effect upon him that weighed more than his previous experience, for suddenly, when near to the monster, he halted dubiously. But his playmates immediately uttered a derisive shout, and it seemed to force him forward. He went to the monster and laid his hand delicately on its shoulder. "Hello, Henry," he said, in a voice that trembled a trifle. The monster was crooning a weird line of negro melody that was scarcely more than a thread of sound, and it paid no heed to the boy.

Jimmie strutted back to his companions. They acclaimed him and hooted his opponent. Amidst this clamor the larger boy with difficulty preserved a dignified attitude.

"I dassent, dassent I?" said Jimmie to him. "Now, you're so smart, let's see you do it!"

This challenge brought forth renewed taunts from the others. The larger boy puffed out his cheeks. "Well, I ain't afraid," he explained, sullenly. He had made a mistake in diplomacy, and now his small enemies were tumbling his prestige all about his ears. They crowed like roosters and bleated like lambs, and made many other noises which were supposed to bury him in ridicule and dishonor. "Well, I ain't afraid," he continued to explain through the din.

Jimmie, the hero of the mob, was pitiless. "You ain't afraid, hey?" he sneered. "If you ain't afraid, go do it, then."

"Well, I would if I wanted to," the other retorted. His eyes wore an expression of profound misery, but he preserved steadily other portions of a pot-valiant air. He suddenly faced one of his persecutors. "If you're so smart, why don't you go do it?" This persecutor sank promptly through the group to the rear. The incident gave the badgered one a breathing-spell, and for a moment even turned the derision in another

direction. He took advantage of his interval. "I'll do it if anybody else will," he announced, swaggering to and fro.

Candidates for the adventure did not come forward. To defend themselves from this counter-charge, the other boys again set up their crowing and bleating. For a while they would hear nothing from him. Each time he opened his lips their chorus of noises made oratory impossible. But at last he was able to repeat that he would volunteer to dare as much in the affair as any other boy.

"Well, you go first," they shouted.

But Jimmie intervened to once more lead the populace against the large boy. "You're mighty brave, ain't you?" he said to him. "You dared me to do it, and I did—didn't I? Now who's afraid?" The others cheered this view loudly, and they instantly resumed the baiting of the large boy.

He shamefacedly scratched his left shin with his right foot. "Well, I ain't afraid." He cast an eye at the monster. "Well, I ain't afraid." With a glare of hatred at his squalling tormentors, he finally announced a grim intention. "Well, I'll do it, then, since you're so fresh. Now!"

The mob subsided as with a formidable countenance he turned toward the impassive figure on the box. The advance was also a regular progression from high daring to craven hesitation. At last, when some yards from the monster, the lad came to a full halt, as if he had encountered a stone wall. The observant little boys in the distance promptly hooted. Stung again by these cries, the lad sneaked two yards forward. He was crouched like a young cat ready for a backward spring. The crowd at the rear, beginning to respect this display, uttered some encouraging cries. Suddenly the lad gathered himself together, made a white and desperate rush forward, touched the monster's shoulder with a far-outstretched finger, and sped away, while his laughter rang out wild, shrill, and exultant.

The crowd of boys reverenced him at once, and began to throng into his camp, and look at him, and be his admirers. Jimmie was discomfited for a moment, but he and the larger boy, without agreement or word of any kind, seemed to recognize a truce, and they swiftly combined and began to parade before the others.

"Why, it's just as easy as nothing," puffed the larger boy. "Ain't it, Jim?"

"Course," blew Jimmie. "Why, it's as e-e-easy."

They were people of another class. If they had been decorated for courage on twelve battle-fields, they could not have made the other boys more ashamed of the situation.

Meanwhile they condescended to explain the emotions of the excursion, expressing unqualified contempt for any one who could hang back. "Why, it ain't nothin.' He won't do nothin' to you," they told the others, in tones of exasperation.

One of the very smallest boys in the party showed signs of a wistful desire to distinguish himself, and they turned their attention to him, pushing at his shoulders while he swung away from them, and hesitated dreamily. He was eventually induced to make furtive expedition, but it was only for a few yards. Then he paused, motionless, gazing with open mouth. The vociferous entreaties of Jimmie and the large boy had no power over him.

Mrs. Hannigan had come out on her back porch with a pail of water. From this coign she had a view of the secluded portion of the Trescott grounds that was behind the stable. She perceived the group of boys, and the monster on the box. She shaded her eyes with her hand to benefit her vision. She screeched then as if she was being murdered. "Eddie! Eddie! You come home this minute!"

Her son querulously demanded, "Aw, what for?"

"You come home this minute. Do you hear?"

The other boys seemed to think this visitation upon one of their number required them to preserve for a time the hang-dog air of a collection of culprits, and they remained in guilty silence until the little Hannigan, wrathfully protesting, was pushed through the door of his home. Mrs. Hannigan cast a piercing glance over the group, stared with a bitter face at the Trescott house, as if this new and handsome edifice was insulting her, and then followed her son.

There was wavering in the party. An inroad by one mother always caused them to carefully sweep the horizon to see if there were more coming. "This is my yard," said Jimmie, proudly. "We don't have to go home."

The monster on the box had turned his black crêpe countenance toward the sky, and was waving its arms in time to a religious chant. "Look at him now," cried a little boy. They turned, and were transfixed by the solemnity and mystery of the indefinable gestures. The wail of the melody was mournful and slow. They drew back. It seemed to spellbind them with the power of a funeral. They were so absorbed that they did not hear the doctor's buggy drive up to the stable. Trescott got out, tied his horse, and approached the group. Jimmie saw him first, and at his look of dismay the others wheeled.

"What's all this, Jimmie?" asked Trescott, in surprise.

The lad advanced to the front of his companions, halted, and said nothing. Trescott's face gloomed slightly as he scanned the scene.

"What were you doing, Jimmie?"

"We was playin,'" answered Jimmie, huskily.

"Playing at what?"

"Just playin.'"

Trescott looked gravely at the other boys, and asked them to please go home. They proceeded to the street much in the manner of frustrated and revealed assassins. The crime of trespass on another boy's place was still a crime when they had only accepted the other boy's cordial invitation, and they were used to being sent out of all manner of gardens upon the sudden appearance of a father or a mother. Jimmie had wretchedly watched the departure of his companions. It involved the loss of his position as a lad who controlled the privileges of his father's grounds, but then he knew that in the beginning he had no right to ask so many boys to be his guests.

Once on the sidewalk, however, they speedily forgot their shame as trespassers, and the large boy launched forth in a description of his success in the late trial of courage. As they went rapidly up the street, the little boy, who had made the furtive expedition cried out confidently from the rear, "Yes, and I went almost up to him, didn't I, Willie?"

The large boy crushed him in a few words. "Huh!" he scoffed. "You only went a little way. I went clear up to him."

The pace of the other boys was so manly that the tiny thing had to trot, and he remained at the rear, getting entangled in their legs in his attempts to reach the front rank and become of some importance, dodging this way and that way, and always piping out his little claim to glory.

XXI.

"By-the-way, Grace," said Trescott, looking into the dining-room from his office door, "I wish you would send Jimmie to me before school-time."

When Jimmie came, he advanced so quietly that Trescott did not at first note him. "Oh," he said, wheeling from a cabinet, "here you are, young man."

"Yes, sir."

Trescott dropped into his chair and tapped the desk with a thoughtful finger. "Jimmie, what were you doing in the back garden yesterday—you and the other boys—to Henry?"

"We weren't doing anything, pa."

Trescott looked sternly into the raised eyes of his son. "Are you sure you were not annoying him in any way? Now what were you doing, exactly?"

"Why, we—why, we—now—Willie Dalzel said I dassent go right up to him, and I did; and then he did; and then—the other boys were 'fraid; and then—you comed."

Trescott groaned deeply. His countenance was so clouded in sorrow that the lad, bewildered by the mystery of it, burst suddenly forth in dismal lamentations. "There, there. Don't cry, Jim," said Trescott, going round the desk. "Only—" He sat in a great leather reading-chair, and took the boy on his knee. "Only I want to explain to you—"

After Jimmie had gone to school, and as Trescott was about to start on his round of morning calls, a message arrived from Doctor Moser. It set forth that the latter's sister was dying in the old homestead, twenty miles away up the valley, and asked Trescott to care for his patients for the day at least. There was also in the envelope a little history of each case and of what had already been done. Trescott replied to the messenger that he would gladly assent to the arrangement.

He noted that the first name on Moser's list was Winter, but this did not seem to strike him as an important fact. When its turn came, he rang the Winter bell. "Good-morning, Mrs. Winter," he said, cheerfully, as the door was opened. "Doctor Moser has been obliged to leave town to-day, and he has asked me to come in his stead. How is the little girl this morning?"

Mrs. Winter had regarded him in stony surprise. At last she said: "Come in! I'll see my husband." She bolted into the house. Trescott entered the hall, and turned to the left into the sitting-room.

Presently Winter shuffled through the door. His eyes flashed toward Trescott. He did not betray any desire to advance far into the room. "What do you want?" he said.

"What do I want? What do I want?" repeated Trescott, lifting his head suddenly. He had heard an utterly new challenge in the night of the jungle.

"Yes, that's what I want to know," snapped Winter. "What do you want?"

Trescott was silent for a moment. He consulted Moser's memoranda. "I see that your little girl's case

is a trifle serious," he remarked. "I would advise you to call a physician soon. I will leave you a copy of Doctor Moser's record to give to any one you may call." He paused to transcribe the record on a page of his note-book. Tearing out the leaf, he extended it to Winter as he moved toward the door. The latter shrunk against the wall. His head was hanging as he reached for the paper. This caused him to grasp air, and so Trescott simply let the paper flutter to the feet of the other man.

"Good-morning," said Trescott from the hall. This placid retreat seemed to suddenly arouse Winter to ferocity. It was as if he had then recalled all the truths, which he had formulated to hurl at Trescott. So he followed him into the hall, and down the hall to the door, and through the door to the porch, barking in fiery rage from a respectful distance. As Trescott imperturbably turned the mare's head down the road, Winter stood on the porch, still yelping. He was like a little dog.

XXII.

"Have you heard the news?" cried Carrie Dungen, as she sped toward Martha's kitchen. "Have you heard the news?" Her eyes were shining with delight.

"No," answered Martha's sister Kate, bending forward eagerly. "What was it? What was it?"

Carrie appeared triumphantly in the open door. "Oh, there's been an awful scene between Doctor Trescott and Jake Winter. I never thought that Jake Winter had any pluck at all, but this morning he told the doctor just what he thought of him."

"Well, what did he think of him?" asked Martha.

"Oh, he called him everything. Mrs. Howarth heard it through her front blinds. It was terrible, she says. It's all over town now. Everybody knows it."

"Didn't the doctor answer back?"

"No! Mrs. Howarth—she says he never said a word. He just walked down to his buggy and got in, and drove off as co-o-o-l. But Jake gave him jinks, by all accounts."

"But what did he say?" cried Kate, shrill and excited. She was evidently at some kind of a feast.

"Oh, he told him that Sadie had never been well since that night Henry Johnson frightened her at Theresa Page's party, and he held him responsible, and how dared he cross his threshold—and—and—and—"

"And what?" said Martha.

"Did he swear at him?" said Kate, in fearsome glee.

"No—not much. He did swear at him a little, but not more than a man does anyhow when he is real mad, Mrs. Howarth says."

"O-oh!" breathed Kate. "And did he call him any names?"

Martha, at her work, had been for a time in deep thought. She now interrupted the others. "It don't seem as if Sadie Winter had been sick since that time Henry Johnson got loose. She's been to school almost the whole time since then, hasn't she?"

They combined upon her in immediate indignation. "School? School? I should say not. Don't think for a moment. School!"

Martha wheeled from the sink. She held an iron spoon, and it seemed as if she was going to attack them. "Sadie Winter has passed here many a morning since then carrying her school-bag. Where was she going? To a wedding?"

The others, long accustomed to a mental tyranny, speedily surrendered.

"Did she?" stammered Kate. "I never saw her."

Carrie Dungen made a weak gesture.

"If I had been Doctor Trescott," exclaimed Martha, loudly, "I'd have knocked that miserable Jake Winter's head off."

Kate and Carrie, exchanging glances, made an alliance in the air. "I don't see why you say that, Martha," replied Carrie, with considerable boldness, gaining support and sympathy from Kate's smile. "I don't see how anybody can be blamed for getting angry when their little girl gets almost scared to death and gets sick from it, and all that. Besides, everybody says—"

"Oh, I don't care what everybody says," said Martha.

"Well, you can't go against the whole town," answered Carrie, in sudden sharp defiance.

"No, Martha, you can't go against the whole town," piped Kate, following her leader rapidly.

"'The whole town,'" cried Martha. "I'd like to know what you call 'the whole town.' Do you call these silly people who are scared of Henry Johnson 'the whole town'?"

"Why, Martha," said Carrie, in a reasoning tone, "you talk as if you wouldn't be scared of him!"

"No more would I," retorted Martha.

"O-oh, Martha, how you talk!" said Kate. "Why, the idea! Everybody's afraid of him."

Carrie was grinning. "You've never seen him, have you?" she asked, seductively.

"No," admitted Martha.

"Well, then, how do you know that you wouldn't be scared?"

Martha confronted her. "Have you ever seen him? No? Well, then, how do you know you *would* be scared?"

The allied forces broke out in chorus: "But, Martha, everybody says so. Everybody says so."

"Everybody says what?"

"Everybody that's seen him say they were frightened almost to death. 'Tisn't only women, but it's men too. It's awful."

Martha wagged her head solemnly. "I'd try not to be afraid of him."

"But supposing you could not help it?" said Kate.

"Yes, and look here," cried Carrie. "I'll tell you another thing. The Hannigans are going to move out of the house next door."

"On account of him?" demanded Martha.

Carrie nodded. "Mrs. Hannigan says so herself."

"Well, of all things!" ejaculated Martha. "Going to move, eh? You don't say so! Where they going to move to?"

"Down on Orchard Avenue."

"Well, of all things! Nice house?"

"I don't know about that. I haven't heard. But there's lots of nice houses on Orchard."

"Yes, but they're all taken," said Kate. "There isn't a vacant house on Orchard Avenue."

"Oh yes, there is," said Martha. "The old Hampstead house is vacant."

"Oh, of course," said Kate. "But then I don't believe Mrs. Hannigan would like it there. I wonder where they can be going to move to?"

"I'm sure I don't know," sighed Martha. "It must be to some place we don't know about."

"Well," said Carrie Dungen, after a general reflective silence, "it's easy enough to find out, anyhow."

"Who knows—around here?" asked Kate.

"Why, Mrs. Smith, and there she is in her garden," said Carrie, jumping to her feet. As she dashed out of the door, Kate and Martha crowded at the window. Carrie's voice rang out from near the steps. "Mrs. Smith! Mrs. Smith! Do you know where the Hannigans are going to move to?"

XXIII.

The autumn smote the leaves, and the trees of Whilomville were panoplied in crimson and yellow.

The winds grew stronger, and in the melancholy purple of the nights the home shine of a window became a finer thing. The little boys, watching the sear and sorrowful leaves drifting down from the maples, dreamed of the near time when they could heap bushels in the streets and burn them during the abrupt evenings.

Three men walked down the Niagara Avenue. As they approached Judge Hagenthorpe's house he came down his walk to meet them in the manner of one who has been waiting.

"Are you ready, judge?" one said.

"All ready," he answered.

The four then walked to Trescott's house. He received them in his office, where he had been reading. He seemed surprised at this visit of four very active and influential citizens, but he had nothing to say of it.

After they were all seated, Trescott looked expectantly from one face to another. There was a little silence. It was broken by John Twelve, the wholesale grocer, who was worth $400,000, and reported to be worth over a million.

"Well, doctor," he said, with a short laugh, "I suppose we might as well admit at once that we've come to interfere in something which is none of our business."

"Why, what is it?" asked Trescott, again looking from one face to another. He seemed to appeal particularly to Judge Hagenthorpe, but the old man had his chin lowered musingly to his cane, and would not look at him.

"It's about what nobody talks of—much," said Twelve. "It's about Henry Johnson."

Trescott squared himself in his chair. "Yes?" he said.

Having delivered himself of the title, Twelve seemed to become more easy. "Yes," he answered, blandly, "we wanted to talk to you about it."

"Yes?" said Trescott.

Twelve abruptly advanced on the main attack. "Now see here, Trescott, we like you, and we have come to talk right out about this business. It may be none of our affairs and all that, and as for me, I don't mind if you tell me so; but I am not going to keep quiet and see you ruin yourself. And that's how we all feel."

"I am not ruining myself," answered Trescott.

"No, maybe you are not exactly ruining yourself," said Twelve, slowly, "but you are doing yourself a great deal of harm. You have changed from being the leading doctor in town to about the last one. It is mainly because there are always a large number of people who are very thoughtless fools, of course, but then that doesn't change the condition."

A man who had not heretofore spoken said, solemnly, "It's the women."

"Well, what I want to say is this," resumed Twelve: "Even if there are a lot of fools in the world, we can't see any reason why you should ruin yourself by opposing them. You can't teach them anything, you know."

"I am not trying to teach them anything." Trescott smiled wearily. "I—It is a matter of—well—"

"And there are a good many of us that admire you for it immensely," interrupted Twelve; "but that isn't going to change the minds of all those ninnies."

"It's the women," stated the advocate of this view again.

"Well, what I want to say is this," said Twelve. "We want you to get out of this trouble and strike your old gait again. You are simply killing your practice through your infernal pig-headedness. Now this thing is out of the ordinary, but there must be ways to—to beat the game somehow, you see. So we've talked it over—about a dozen of us—and, as I say, if you want to tell us to mind our own business, why, go ahead; but we've talked it over, and we've come to the conclusion that the only way to do is to get Johnson a place somewhere off up the valley, and—"

Trescott wearily gestured. "You don't know, my friend. Everybody is so afraid of him, they can't even give him good care. Nobody can attend to him as I do myself."

"But I have a little no-good farm up beyond Clarence Mountain that I was going to give to Henry," cried Twelve, aggrieved. "And if you—and if you—if you—through your house burning down, or anything—why, all the boys were prepared to take him right off your hands, and—and—"

Trescott arose and went to the window. He turned his back upon them. They sat waiting in silence. When he returned he kept his face in the shadow. "No, John Twelve," he said, "it can't be done."

There was another stillness. Suddenly a man stirred on his chair.

"Well, then, a public institution—" he began.

"No," said Trescott; "public institutions are all very good, but he is not going to one."

In the background of the group old Judge Hagenthorpe was thoughtfully smoothing the polished ivory head of his cane.

XXIV.

Trescott loudly stamped the snow from his feet and shook the flakes from his shoulders. When he entered the house he went at once to the dining-room, and then to the sitting-room. Jimmie was there, reading painfully in a large book concerning giraffes and tigers and crocodiles.

"Where is your mother, Jimmie?" asked Trescott.

"I don't know, pa," answered the boy. "I think she is upstairs."

Trescott went to the foot of the stairs and called, but there came no answer. Seeing that the door of the little drawing-room was open, he entered. The room was bathed in the half-light that came from the four dull panes of mica in the front of the great stove. As his eyes grew used to the shadows he saw his wife curled in an arm-chair. He went to her. "Why, Grace," he said, "didn't you hear me calling you?"

She made no answer, and as he bent over the chair he heard her trying to smother a sob in the cushion.

"Grace!" he cried. "You're crying!"

She raised her face. "I've got a headache, a dreadful headache, Ned."

"A headache?" he repeated, in surprise and incredulity.

He pulled a chair close to hers. Later, as he cast his eye over the zone of light shed by the dull red panes, he saw that a low table had been drawn close to the stove, and that it was burdened with many small cups and plates of uncut tea-cake. He remembered that the day was Wednesday, and that his wife received on Wednesdays.

"Who was here to-day, Gracie?" he asked.

From his shoulder there came a mumble, "Mrs. Twelve."

"Was she—um," he said. "Why—didn't Anna Hagenthorpe come over?"

The mumble from his shoulder continued, "She wasn't well enough."

Glancing down at the cups, Trescott mechanically counted them. There were fifteen of them. "There, there," he said. "Don't cry, Grace. Don't cry."

The wind was whining round the house, and the snow beat aslant upon the windows. Sometimes the coal in the stove settled with a crumbling sound, and the four panes of mica flashed a sudden new crimson. As he sat holding her head on his shoulder, Trescott found himself occasionally trying to count the cups. There were fifteen of them.

Source: Crane, Stephen. 1899. *The Monster*. Available at: http://www.underthesun.cc/Classics/Crane/THEMONSTER

◉ Walt Whitman, from "The Wound-Dresser" (1900)

The American poet Walt Whitman found himself working in hospitals as a nurse during the Civil War, when his brother George appeared on a listing of the wounded at the Battle of Fredericksburg. Whitman's description of one new amputee records his nursing duties as well as his sensitivity to the physical details of human pain.

From the stump of the arm, the amputated hand,

I undo the clotted lint, remove the slough, wash off the matter and blood,

Back on his pillow the soldier bends with curv'd neck and side-falling head,

His eyes are closed, his face is pale, he dares not look on the bloody stump,

And has not yet looked on it.

Source: Whitman, Walt. 1900. "The Wound-Dresser." Available at: http://www.princeton.edu/~batke/logr/log_159.html

◉ Helen Keller, from *The Story of My Life* (1902)

Helen Keller's education moves increasingly from learning based on sensation to knowledge of abstraction as her acquisition of language grows. Here Keller explains how she acquires the building blocks for an understanding of such abstract ideas as love on the basis of her experience of the natural world.

Chapter V

I recall many incidents of the summer of 1887 that followed my soul's sudden awakening. I did nothing but explore with my hands and learn the name of every object that I touched; and the more I handled things and learned their names and uses, the more joyous and confident grew my sense of kinship with the rest of the world.

When the time of daisies and buttercups came Miss Sullivan took me by the hand across the fields, where men were preparing the earth for the seed, to the banks of the Tennessee River, and there, sitting on the warm grass, I had my first lessons in the beneficence of nature. I learned how the sun and the rain make to grow out of the ground every tree that is pleasant to the sight and good for food, how birds build

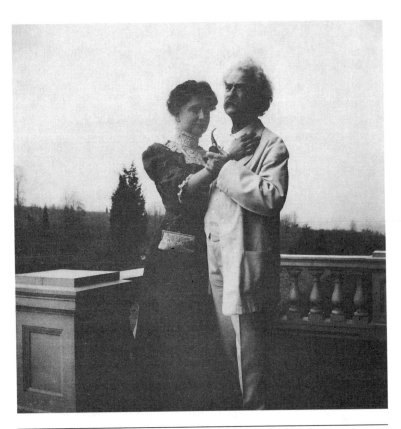

Mark Twain and Helen Keller *(ca. 1908), by Isabelle B. Lyon (1868–1958). The U.S. humorist Mark Twain is photographed here with Helen Keller. Keller was photographed with many other celebrity figures, and here she is positioned in a characteristic pose that emphasizes her deaf-blindness for viewers.*

Source: Art Resource, New York.

their nests and live and thrive from land to land, how the squirrel, the deer, the lion and every other creature finds food and shelter. As my knowledge of things grew I felt more and more the delight of the world I was in. Long before I learned to do a sum in arithmetic or describe the shape of the earth, Miss Sullivan had taught me to find beauty in the fragrant woods, in every blade of grass, and in the curves and dimples of my baby sister's hand. She linked my earliest thoughts with nature, and made me feel that "birds and flowers and I were happy peers."

But about this time I had an experience which taught me that nature is not always kind. One day my teacher and I were returning from a long ramble. The morning had been fine, but it was growing warm and sultry when at last we turned our faces homeward. Two or three times we stopped to rest under a tree by the wayside. Our last halt was under a wild cherry tree a short distance from the house. The shade was grateful, and the tree was so easy to climb that with my

teacher's assistance I was able to scramble to a seat in the branches. It was so cool up in the tree that Miss Sullivan proposed that we have our luncheon there. I promised to keep still while she went to the house to fetch it.

Suddenly a change passed over the tree. All the sun's warmth left the air. I knew the sky was black, because all the heat, which meant light to me, had died out of the atmosphere. A strange odour came up from the earth. I knew it, it was the odour that always precedes a thunderstorm, and a nameless fear clutched at my heart. I felt absolutely alone, cut off from my friends and the firm earth. The immense, the unknown, enfolded me. I remained still and expectant; a chilling terror crept over me. I longed for my teacher's return; but above all things I wanted to get down from that tree.

There was a moment of sinister silence, then a multitudinous stirring of the leaves. A shiver ran through the tree, and the wind sent forth a blast that would have knocked me off had I not clung to the branch with might and main. The tree swayed and strained. The small twigs snapped and fell about me in showers. A wild impulse to jump seized me, but terror held me fast. I crouched down in the fork of the tree. The branches lashed about me. I felt the intermittent jarring that came now and then, as if something heavy had fallen and the shock had traveled up till it reached the limb I sat on. It worked my suspense up to the highest point, and just as I was thinking the tree and I should fall together, my teacher seized my hand and helped me down. I clung to her, trembling with joy to feel the earth under my feet once more. I had learned a new lesson—that nature "wages open war against her children, and under softest touch hides treacherous claws."

After this experience it was a long time before I climbed another tree. The mere thought filled me with terror. It was the sweet allurement of the mimosa tree in full bloom that finally overcame my fears. One beautiful spring morning when I was alone in the summer-house, reading, I became aware of a wonderful subtle fragrance in the air. I started up and instinctively stretched out my hands. It seemed as if the spirit of spring had passed through the summer-house. "What is it?" I asked, and the next minute I recognized the odour of the mimosa blossoms. I felt my way to the end of the garden, knowing that the mimosa tree was near the fence, at the turn of the path. Yes, there it was, all quivering in the warm sunshine, its blossom-laden branches almost touching the long grass. Was there ever anything so exquisitely beautiful in the world before! Its delicate blossoms shrank from the slightest earthly touch; it seemed as if a tree of paradise had been transplanted to earth. I made my way through a shower of petals to the great trunk and for one minute stood irresolute; then, putting my foot in the broad space between the forked branches, I pulled myself up into the tree. I had some difficulty in holding on, for the branches were very large and the bark hurt my hands. But I had a delicious sense that I was doing something unusual and wonderful so I kept on climbing higher and higher, until I reached a little seat which somebody had built there so long ago that it had grown part of the tree itself. I sat there for a long, long time, feeling like a fairy on a rosy cloud. After that I spent many happy hours in my tree of paradise, thinking fair thoughts and dreaming bright dreams.

Chapter VI

I had now the key to all language, and I was eager to learn to use it. Children who hear acquire language without any particular effort; the words that fall from others' lips they catch on the wing, as it were, delightedly, while the little deaf child must trap them by a slow and often painful process. But whatever the process, the result is wonderful. Gradually from naming an object we advance step by step until we have traversed the vast distance between our first stammered syllable and the sweep of thought in a line of Shakespeare.

At first, when my teacher told me about a new thing I asked very few questions. My ideas were vague, and my vocabulary was inadequate; but as my knowledge of things grew, and I learned more and more words, my field of inquiry broadened, and I would return again and again to the same subject, eager for further information. Sometimes a new word revived an image that some earlier experience had engraved on my brain.

I remember the morning that I first asked the meaning of the word, "love." This was before I knew many words. I had found a few early violets in the garden and brought them to my teacher. She tried to kiss me: but at that time I did not like to have any one kiss me except my mother. Miss Sullivan put her arm gently round me and spelled into my hand, "I love Helen."

"What is love?" I asked.

She drew me closer to her and said, "It is here," pointing to my heart, whose beats I was conscious of for the first time. Her words puzzled me very much because I did not then understand anything unless I touched it.

I smelt the violets in her hand and asked, half in words, half in signs, a question which meant, "Is love the sweetness of flowers?"

"No," said my teacher.

Again I thought. The warm sun was shining on us. "Is this not love?" I asked, pointing in the direction from which the heat came. "Is this not love?"

It seemed to me that there could be nothing more beautiful than the sun, whose warmth makes all things grow. But Miss Sullivan shook her head, and I was greatly puzzled and disappointed. I thought it strange that my teacher could not show me love.

A day or two afterward I was stringing beads of different sizes in symmetrical groups—two large beads, three small ones, and so on. I had made many mistakes, and Miss Sullivan had pointed them out again and again with gentle patience. Finally I noticed a very obvious error in the sequence and for an instant I concentrated my attention on the lesson and tried to think how I should have arranged the beads. Miss Sullivan touched my forehead and spelled with decided emphasis, "Think."

In a flash I knew that the word was the name of the process that was going on in my head. This was my first conscious perception of an abstract idea.

For a long time I was still—I was not thinking of the beads in my lap, but trying to find a meaning for "love" in the light of this new idea. The sun had been under a cloud all day, and there had been brief showers; but suddenly the sun broke forth in all its southern splendour.

Again I asked my teacher, "Is this not love?"

"Love is something like the clouds that were in the sky before the sun came out," she replied. Then in simpler words than these, which at that time I could not have understood, she explained: "You cannot touch the clouds, you know; but you feel the rain and know how glad the flowers and the thirsty earth are to have it after a hot day. You cannot touch love either;

but you feel the sweetness that it pours into everything. Without love you would not be happy or want to play."

The beautiful truth burst upon my mind—I felt that there were invisible lines stretched between my spirit and the spirits of others.

From the beginning of my education Miss Sullivan made it a practice to speak to me as she would speak to any hearing child; the only difference was that she spelled the sentences into my hand instead of speaking them. If I did not know the words and idioms necessary to express my thoughts she supplied them, even suggesting conversation when I was unable to keep up my end of the dialogue.

This process was continued for several years; for the deaf child does not learn in a month, or even in two or three years, the numberless idioms and expressions used in the simplest daily intercourse. The little hearing child learns these from constant repetition and imitation. The conversation he hears in his home stimulates his mind and suggests topics and calls forth the spontaneous expression of his own thoughts. This natural exchange of ideas is denied to the deaf child. My teacher, realizing this, determined to supply the kinds of stimulus I lacked. This she did by repeating to me as far as possible, verbatim, what she heard, and by showing me how I could take part in the conversation. But it was a long time before I ventured to take the initiative, and still longer before I could find something appropriate to say at the right time.

The deaf and the blind find it very difficult to acquire the amenities of conversation. How much more this difficulty must be augmented in the case of those who are both deaf and blind! They cannot distinguish the tone of the voice or, without assistance, go up and down the gamut of tones that give significance to words; nor can they watch the expression of the speaker's face, and a look is often the very soul of what one says.

Source: Keller, Helen. 1902. *The Story of My Life.* Available at: http://digital.library.upenn.edu/women/keller/life/part-I.html

▣ W. E. B. Du Bois, from "The Talented Tenth" (1903)

In one of the most famous essays in African American literature, Du Bois champions his vision of an exceptional group of individuals who might set the tone and *educate the great majority of African American citizens. The "talented tenth" would represent a notion of intellectual superiority parallel to that espoused by Galton in Hereditary Genius.*

The Negro race, like all races, is going to be saved by its exceptional men. The problem of education, then, among Negroes must first of all deal with the Talented Tenth; it is the problem of developing the Best of this race that they may guide the Mass away from the contamination and death of the Worst, in their own and other races. Now the training of men is a difficult and intricate task. Its technique is a matter for educational experts, but its object is for the vision of seers. If we make money the object of man-training, we shall develop money-makers but not necessarily men; if we make technical skill the object of education, we may possess artisans but not, in nature, men. Men we shall have only as we make manhood the object of the work of the schools—intelligence, broad sympathy, knowledge of the world that was and is, and of the relation of men to it—this is the curriculum of that Higher Education which must underlie true life. On this foundation we may build bread winning, skill of hand and quickness of brain, with never a fear lest the child and man mistake the means of living for the object of life.

If this be true—and who can deny it—three tasks lay before me; first to show from the past that the Talented Tenth as they have risen among American Negroes have been worthy of leadership; secondly to show how these men may be educated and developed; and thirdly to show their relation to the Negro problem.

You misjudge us because you do not know us. From the very first it has been the educated and intelligent of the Negro people that have led and elevated the mass, and the sole obstacles that nullified and retarded their efforts were slavery and race prejudice; for what is slavery but the legalized survival of the unfit and the nullification of the work of natural internal leadership? Negro leadership therefore sought from the first to rid the race of this awful incubus that it might make way for natural selection and the survival of the fittest. In colonial days came Phillis Wheatley and Paul Cuffe striving against the bars of prejudice; and Benjamin Banneker, the almanac maker, voiced their longings when he said to Thomas Jefferson, "I freely and cheerfully acknowledge that I am of the African race and in colour which is natural to them, of the deepest dye; and it is under a sense of the most profound gratitude to the Supreme Ruler of the Universe, that I now confess to you that I am not under that state of tyrannical thraldom and inhuman captivity to which too many of my brethren are doomed, but that I have abundantly tasted of the fruition of those blessings which proceed from that free and unequalled liberty with which you are favored, and which I hope you will willingly allow, you have mercifully received from the immediate hand of that Being from whom proceedeth every good and perfect gift.

"Suffer me to recall to your mind that time, in which the arms of the British crown were exerted with every powerful effort, in order to reduce you to a state of servitude; look back, I entreat you, on the variety of dangers to which you were exposed; reflect on that period in which every human aid appeared unavailable, and in which even hope and fortitude wore the aspect of inability to the conflict, and you cannot but be led to a serious and grateful sense of your miraculous and providential preservation, you cannot but acknowledge, that the present freedom and tranquility which you enjoy, you have mercifully received, and that a peculiar blessing of heaven.

"This, sir, was a time when you clearly saw into the injustice of a state of Slavery, and in which you had just apprehensions of the horrors of its condition. It was then that your abhorrence thereof was so excited, that you publicly held forth this true and invaluable doctrine, which is worthy to be recorded and remembered in all succeeding ages: 'We hold these truths to be self evident, that all men are created equal; that they are endowed with certain inalienable rights, and that among these are life, liberty and the pursuit of happiness.'"

Then came Dr. James Derham, who could tell even the learned Dr. Rush something of medicine, and Lemuel Haynes, to whom Middlebury College gave an honorary A. M. in 1804. These and others we may call the Revolutionary group of distinguished Negroes—they were persons of marked ability, leaders of a Talented Tenth, standing conspicuously among the best of their time. They strove by word and deed to save the color line from becoming the line between the bond and free, but all they could do was nullified by Eli Whitney and the Curse of Gold. So they passed into forgetfulness.

But their spirit did not wholly die; here and there in the early part of the century came other exceptional men. Some were natural sons of unnatural fathers and were given often a liberal training and thus a race of

educated mulattoes sprang up to plead for black men's rights. There was Ira Aldridge, whom all Europe loved to honor; there was that Voice crying in the Wilderness, David Walker, and saying:

"I declare it does appear to me as though some nations think God is asleep, or that he made the Africans for nothing else but to dig their mines and work their farms, or they cannot believe history sacred or profane. I ask every man who has a heart, and is blessed with the privilege of believing—Is not God a God of justice to all his creatures? Do you say he is? Then if he gives peace and tranquility to tyrants and permits them to keep our fathers, our mothers, ourselves and our children in eternal ignorance and wretchedness to support them and their families, would he be to us a God of Justice? I ask, O, ye Christians, who hold us and our children in the most abject ignorance and degradation that ever a people were afflicted with since the world began—I say if God gives you peace and tranquility, and suffers you thus to go on afflicting us, and our children, who have never given you the least provocation—would He be to us a God of Justice? If you will allow that we are men, who feel for each other, does not the blood of our fathers and of us, their children, cry aloud to the Lord of Sabaoth against you for the cruelties and murders with which you have and do continue to afflict us?"

This was the wild voice that first aroused Southern legislators in 1829 to the terrors of abolitionism.

In 1831 there met that first Negro convention in Philadelphia, at which the world gaped curiously but which bravely attacked the problems of race and slavery, crying out against persecution and declaring that "Laws as cruel in themselves as they were unconstitutional and unjust, have in many places been enacted against our poor, unfriended and unoffending brethren (without a shadow of provocation on our part), at whose bare recital the very savage draws himself up for fear of contagion—looks noble and prides himself because he bears not the name of Christian." Side by side this free Negro movement, and the movement for abolition, strove until they merged in to one strong stream. Too little notice has been taken of the work which the Talented Tenth among Negroes took in the great abolition crusade. From the very day that a Philadelphia colored man became the first subscriber to Garrison's "Liberator," to the day when Negro soldiers made the Emancipation Proclamation possible, black leaders worked shoulder to shoulder with white men in a movement, the success of which would have been impossible without them. There was Purvis and Remond, Pennington and Highland Garnett, Sojourner Truth and Alexander Crummel, and above, Frederick Douglass—what would the abolition movement have been without them? They stood as living examples of the possibilities of the Negro race, their own hard experiences and well wrought culture said silently more than all the drawn periods of orators— they were the men who made American slavery impossible. As Maria Weston Chapman said, from the school of anti-slavery agitation, "a throng of authors, editors, lawyers, orators and accomplished gentlemen of color have taken their degree! It has equally implanted hopes and aspirations, noble thoughts, and sublime purposes, in the hearts of both races. It has prepared the white man for the freedom of the black man, and it has made the black man scorn the thought of enslavement, as does a white man, as far as its influence has extended. Strengthen that noble influence! Before its organization, the country only saw here and there in slavery some faithful Cudjoe or Dinah, whose strong natures blossomed even in bondage, like a fine plant beneath a heavy stone. Now, under the elevating and cherishing influence of the American Anti-slavery Society, the colored race, like the white, furnishes Corinthian capitals for the noblest temples."

Where were these black abolitionists trained? Some, like Frederick Douglass, were self-trained, but yet trained liberally; others, like Alexander Crummell and McCune Smith, graduated from famous foreign universities. Most of them rose up through the colored schools of New York and Philadelphia and Boston, taught by college-bred men like Russworm, of Dartmouth, and college-bred white men like Neau and Benezet.

After emancipation came a new group of educated and gifted leaders: Langston, Bruce and Elliot, Greener, Williams and Payne. Through political organization, historical and polemic writing and moral regeneration, these men strove to uplift their people. It is the fashion of to-day to sneer at them and to say that with freedom Negro leadership should have begun at the plow and not in the Senate—a foolish and mischievous lie; two hundred and fifty years that black serf toiled at the plow and yet that toiling was in vain till the Senate passed the war amendments; and two hundred and fifty years more the half-free serf of to-day may toil at his plow, but unless he have political rights

and righteously guarded civic status, he will still remain the poverty-stricken and ignorant plaything of rascals, that he now is. This all sane men know even if they dare not say it.

And so we come to the present—a day of cowardice and vacillation, of strident wide-voiced wrong and faint hearted compromise; of double-faced dallying with Truth and Right. Who are to-day guiding the work of the Negro people? The "exceptions" of course. And yet so sure as this Talented Tenth is pointed out, the blind worshippers of the Average cry out in alarm: "These are exceptions, look here at death, disease and crime—these are the happy rule." Of course they are the rule, because a silly nation made them the rule: Because for three long centuries this people lynched Negroes who dared to be brave, raped black women who dared to be virtuous, crushed dark-hued youth who dared to be ambitious, and encouraged and made to flourish servility and lewdness and apathy. But not even this was able to crush all manhood and chastity and aspiration from black folk. A saving remnant continually survives and persists, continually aspires, continually shows itself in thrift and ability and character. Exceptional it is to be sure, but this is its chiefest promise; it shows the capability of Negro blood, the promise of black men. Do Americans ever stop to reflect that there are in this land a million men of Negro blood, well-educated, owners of homes, against the honor of whose womanhood no breath was ever raised, whose men occupy positions of trust and usefulness, and who, judged by any standard, have reached the full measure of the best type of modern European culture? Is it fair, is it decent, is it Christian to ignore these facts of the Negro problem, to belittle such aspiration, to nullify such leadership and seek to crush these people back into the mass out of which by toil and travail, they and their fathers have raised themselves?

Can the masses of the Negro people be in any possible way more quickly raised than by the effort and example of this aristocracy of talent and character? Was there ever a nation on God's fair earth civilized from the bottom upward? Never; it is, ever was and ever will be from the top downward that culture filters. The Talented Tenth rises and pulls all that are worth the saving up to their vantage ground. This is the history of human progress; and the two historic mistakes which have hindered that progress were the thinking first that no more could ever rise save the few already risen; or second, that it would better the unrisen to pull the risen down. . . .

The problem of training the Negro is to-day immensely complicated by the fact that the whole question of the efficiency and appropriateness of our present systems of education, for any kind of child, is a matter of active debate, in which final settlement seems still afar off. Consequently it often happens that persons arguing for or against certain systems of education for Negroes, have these controversies in mind and miss the real question at issue. The main question, so far as the Southern Negro is concerned, is: What under the present circumstance, must a system of education do in order to raise the Negro as quickly as possible in the scale of civilization? The answer to this question seems to me clear: It must strengthen the Negro's character, increase his knowledge and teach him to earn a living. Now it goes without saying that it is hard to do all these things simultaneously or suddenly and that at the same time it will not do to give all the attention to one and neglect the others; we could give black boys trades, but that alone will not civilize a race of ex-slaves; we might simply increase their knowledge of the world, but this would not necessarily make them wish to use this knowledge honestly; we might seek to strengthen character and purpose, but to what end if this people have nothing to eat or to wear? A system of education is not one thing, nor does it have a single definite object, nor is it a mere matter of schools. Education is that whole system of human training within and without the school house walls, which molds and develops men. If then we start out to train an ignorant and unskilled people with a heritage of bad habits, our system of training must set before itself two great aims—the one dealing with knowledge and character, the other part seeking to give the child the technical knowledge necessary for him to earn a living under the present circumstances. These objects are accomplished in part by the opening of the common schools on the one, and of the industrial schools on the other. But only in part, for there must also be trained those who are to teach these schools—men and women of knowledge and culture and technical skill who understand modern civilization, and have the training and aptitude to impart it to the children under them.

Source: Du Bois, W. E. B. 1903. "The Talented Tenth." In Washington, Booker T., ed. *The Negro Problem: A Series of Articles by Representative Negroes of Today.* New York: Pott and Company.

Carry A. Nation, from *The Use and Need of the Life of Carry A. Nation* (1905)

Carry Nation, who is best known for her radical advocacy of temperance, included in her autobiography a discussion of her child's chronic health issues (and her interpretation of them as "the result of a drunken father and a distracted mother"). The Campbellite religious dimension of this excerpt is particularly strong, and probably strange to many, but it is quite in line with the temperance rhetoric of the time.

About this time my little Charlien, who had been such a help to me, began to go into a decline, until she was taken down with typhoid fever. Her case was violent and she was delirious from the first. This my only child was peculiar. She was the result of a drunken father and a distracted mother. The curse of heredity is one of the most heart-breaking results of the saloon. Poor little children are brought into the world, cursed by disposition and disease, entailed on them. How can mothers be true to their offspring with a constant dread of the nameless horrors wives are exposed to by being drunkards' wives. Men will not raise domestic animals under conditions where the mothers may bring forth weak or deformed offspring. My precious child seemed to have taken a perfect dislike to Christianity. This was a great grief to me, and I used to pray to God to save her soul at any cost; I often prayed for bodily affliction on her, if that was what would make her love and serve God. Anything for her eternal salvation.

Her right cheek was very much swollen, and on examination we found there was an eating sore inside her cheek. This kept up in spite of all remedies, and at last the whole of her right cheek fell out, leaving the teeth bare. My friends and boarders were very angry at the physician, saying she was salivated. From the first something told me this is an answer to your prayer. At this time, when her life was despaired of, I had an intense longing to save my child, who was so dear to me. I said: "Oh, God, let me keep a piece of my child." A minister said: "Don't pray for the life of your child; she will be so deformed it were better she were dead." I could not feel this way. After being at death's door for nine days, she began to recover. The wound in her face healed up to a hole about the size of a twenty-five cent piece. Her jaws closed and remained so for eight years. The sickness of my daughter and the keeping up of the hotel was such a tax on my mind, that for six months all transactions would recede from my memory. For instance, if anyone told me something, in an hour afterwards, I could not tell whether it had been hours, days or months since it was told me. I never entirely recovered from this, still being forgetful of names, dates and circumstances, unless they are particularly impressed upon my mind. When I could afford it, I took my child, then twelve years old, down to Galveston, put her under the care of Dr. Dowell for the purpose of closing the hole in her cheek. I had to leave the little one down there among strangers, for I could not afford to stay with her. A mother only will know what this means. After four operations the place was closed up in her cheek, still her mouth was closed, her teeth close together. I suffered torture all these years for fear she might strangle to death. I took her to San Antonio, Texas, to Dr. Herff, and he and his two sons removed a section of the jawbone, expecting to make an artificial joint, enabling her to use the other side of her jaw. After all this, the operation was a failure, and her jaws closed up again.

Source: Nation, Carry A. 1905. The Use and Need of the Life of Carry A. Nation. Available at: www.e-bookshop.gr/gutenberg/files/crntn10.pdf

▣ Upton Sinclair, from *The Jungle* (1906)

Sinclair's novel about the ravages of the meatpacking industry in Chicago on the lives of nonunionized labor was instrumental in leading to reforms. The first excerpt below discusses the ubiquitous prevalence of disability among children of the working classes. The second excerpt discusses the descent of the out-of-work protagonist, Jurgis, into abject poverty and a life of begging for work that he can no longer perform physically.

From Chapter 13

During this time that Jurgis was looking for work occurred the death of little Kristoforas, one of the children of Teta Elzbieta. Both Kristoforas and his brother, Juozapas, were cripples, the latter having lost one leg by having it run over, and Kristoforas having congenital dislocation of the hip, which made it

impossible for him ever to walk. He was the last of Teta Elzbieta's children, and perhaps he had been intended by nature to let her know that she had had enough. At any rate he was wretchedly sick and undersized; he had the rickets, and though he was over three years old, he was no bigger than an ordinary child of one. All day long he would crawl around the floor in a filthy little dress, whining and fretting; because the floor was full of drafts he was always catching cold, and snuffling because his nose ran. This made him a nuisance, and a source of endless trouble in the family. For his mother, with unnatural perversity, loved him best of all her children, and made a perpetual fuss over him—would let him do anything undisturbed, and would burst into tears when his fretting drove Jurgis wild.

And now he died. Perhaps it was the smoked sausage he had eaten that morning—which may have been made out of some of the tubercular pork that was condemned as unfit for export. At any rate, an hour after eating it, the child had begun to cry with pain, and in another hour he was rolling about on the floor in convulsions. Little Kotrina, who was all alone with him, ran out screaming for help, and after a while a doctor came, but not until Kristoforas had howled his last howl. No one was really sorry about this except poor Elzbieta, who was inconsolable. Jurgis announced that so far as he was concerned the child would have to be buried by the city, since they had no money for a funeral; and at this the poor woman almost went out of her senses, wringing her hands and screaming with grief and despair. Her child to be buried in a pauper's grave! And her stepdaughter to stand by and hear it said without protesting! It was enough to make Ona's father rise up out of his grave to rebuke her! If it had come to this, they might as well give up at once, and be buried all of them together! . . . In the end Marija said that she would help with ten dollars; and Jurgis being still obdurate, Elzbieta went in tears and begged the money from the neighbors, and so little Kristoforas had a mass and a hearse with white plumes on it, and a tiny plot in a graveyard with a wooden cross to mark the place. The poor mother was not the same for months after that; the mere sight of the floor where little Kristoforas had crawled about would make her weep. He had never had a fair chance, poor little fellow, she would say. He had been handicapped from his birth. If only she had heard about it in time, so that she might have had that great doctor to cure him of his lameness! . . . Some time ago, Elzbieta was told, a Chicago billionaire had paid a fortune to bring a great European surgeon over to cure his little daughter of the same disease from which Kristoforas had suffered. And because this surgeon had to have bodies to demonstrate upon, he announced that he would treat the children of the poor, a piece of magnanimity over which the papers became quite eloquent. Elzbieta, alas, did not read the papers, and no one had told her; but perhaps it was as well, for just then they would not have had the carfare to spare to go every day to wait upon the surgeon, nor for that matter anybody with the time to take the child. . . .

From Chapter 27

Poor Jurgis was now an outcast and a tramp once more. He was crippled—he was as literally crippled as any wild animal which has lost its claws, or been torn out of its shell. He had been shorn, at one cut, of all those mysterious weapons whereby he had been able to make a living easily and to escape the consequences of his actions. He could no longer command a job when he wanted it; he could no longer steal with impunity—he must take his chances with the common herd. Nay worse, he dared not mingle with the herd—he must hide himself, for he was one marked out for

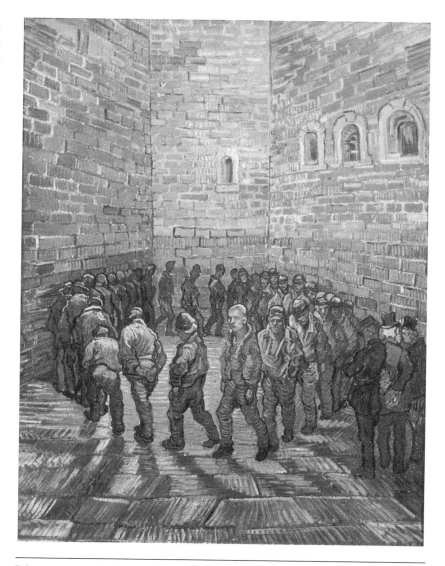

Prisoner's Walk *(1890), by Vincent Van Gogh (1853–1890). Painted while Van Gogh was an inmate at the asylum in San Remy, the painting captures the claustrophobia and despair that accompany individual loss of liberty at the hands of institutions.*

Source: Art Resource, New York.

destruction. His old companions would betray him, for the sake of the influence they would gain thereby; and he would be made to suffer, not merely for the offense he had committed, but for others which would be laid at his door, just as had been done for some poor devil on the occasion of that assault upon the "country customer" by him and Duane.

And also he labored under another handicap now. He had acquired new standards of living, which were not easily to be altered. When he had been out of work before, he had been content if he could sleep in a doorway or under a truck out of the rain, and if he could get fifteen cents a day for saloon lunches. But now he desired all sorts of other things, and suffered

because he had to do without them. He must have a drink now and then, a drink for its own sake, and apart from the food that came with it. The craving for it was strong enough to master every other consideration—he would have it, though it were his last nickel and he had to starve the balance of the day in consequence.

Jurgis became once more a besieger of factory gates. But never since he had been in Chicago had he stood less chance of getting a job than just then. For one thing, there was the economic crisis, the million or two of men who had been out of work in the spring and summer, and were not yet all back, by any means. And then there was the strike, with seventy thousand men and women all over the country idle for a couple of months—twenty thousand in Chicago, and many of them now seeking work throughout the city. It did not remedy matters that a few days later the strike was given up and about half the strikers went back to work; for every one taken on, there was a "scab" who gave up and fled. The ten or fifteen thousand "green" Negroes, foreigners, and criminals were now being turned loose to shift for themselves. Everywhere Jurgis went he kept meeting them, and he was in an agony of fear lest some one of them should know that he was "wanted." He would have left Chicago, only by the time he had realized his danger he was almost penniless; and it would be better to go to jail than to be caught out in the country in the winter time.

At the end of about ten days Jurgis had only a few pennies left; and he had not yet found a job—not even a day's work at anything, not a chance to carry a satchel. Once again, as when he had come out of the hospital, he was bound hand and foot, and facing the grisly phantom of starvation. Raw, naked terror possessed him, a maddening passion that would never leave him, and that wore him down more quickly than the actual want of food. He was going to die of hunger! The fiend reached out its scaly arms for him—it touched him, its breath came into his face; and he would cry out for the awfulness of it, he would wake up in the night, shuddering, and bathed in perspiration, and start up and flee. He would walk, begging for work, until he was exhausted; he could not remain still—he would wander on, gaunt and haggard, gazing about him with restless eyes. Everywhere he went, from one end of the vast city to the other, there were hundreds of others like him; everywhere was the sight of plenty and the merciless hand of authority waving them away. There is one kind of prison where the man is behind bars, and everything that he desires is outside; and there is another kind where the things are behind the bars, and the man is outside. . . .

Source: Sinclair, Upton. 1906. *The Jungle.* New York: The Jungle Publishing Company.

◉ Joseph Conrad, from *The Secret Agent* (1907)

The mind is hierarchically superior to the body in the Western tradition; it follows from this that human beings whose minds are weak are not wise enough to restrain their bodily passions. Here Conrad displays

Stevie's inability to control himself, but he also illustrates the split between mind and body in the characters of Mrs. Verloc and Stevie. The question is, how long will Mrs. Verloc be able to exercise mental control over Stevie's powerful physical inclinations?

Stevie, left alone beside the private lamp-post of the Charity, his hands thrust deep into his pockets, glared with vacant sulkiness. At the bottom of his pockets his incapable, weak hands were clenched hard into a pair of angry fists. In the face of anything which affected directly or indirectly his morbid dread of pain, Stevie ended by turning vicious. A magnanimous indignation swelled his frail chest to bursting, and caused his candid eyes to squint. Supremely wise in knowing his own powerlessness, Stevie was not wise enough to restrain his passions. The tenderness of his universal charity had two phases as indissolubly joined and connected as the reverse and obverse sides of a medal. The anguish of immoderate compassion was succeeded by the pain of an innocent but pitiless rage. Those two states expressing themselves outwardly by the same signs of futile bodily agitation, his sister Winnie soothed his excitement without ever fathoming its twofold character. Mrs Verloc wasted no portion of this transient life in seeking for fundamental information. This is a sort of economy having all the appearances and some of the advantages of prudence. Obviously it may be good for one not to know too much. And such a view accords very well with constitutional indolence.

On that evening on which it may be said that Mrs Verloc's mother having parted for good from her children had also departed this life, Winnie Verloc did not investigate her brother's psychology. The poor boy was excited, of course. After once more assuring the old woman on the threshold that she would know how to guard against the risk of Stevie losing himself for very long on his pilgrimages of filial piety, she took her brother's arm to walk away. Stevie did not even mutter to himself, but with the special sense of sisterly devotion developed in her earliest infancy, she felt that the boy was very much excited indeed. Holding tight to his arm, under the appearance of leaning on it, she thought of some words suitable to the occasion.

"Now, Stevie, you must look well after me at the crossings, and get first into the bus, like a good brother."

This appeal to manly protection was received by Stevie with his usual docility. It flattered him. He raised his head and threw out his chest.

"Don't be nervous, Winnie. Mustn't be nervous! Bus all right," he answered in a brusque, slurring stammer partaking of the timorousness of a child and the resolution of a man. He advanced fearlessly with the woman on his arm, but his lower lip drooped. Nevertheless, on the pavement of the squalid and wide thoroughfare, whose poverty in all the amenities of life stood foolishly exposed by a mad profusion of gas-lights, their resemblance to each other was so pronounced as to strike the casual passers-by.

Before the doors of the public-house at the corner, where the profusion of gas-light reached the height of positive wickedness, a four-wheeled cab standing by the kerbstone, with no one on the box, seemed cast out into the gutter on account of irremediable decay. Mrs Verloc recognized the conveyance. Its aspect was so profoundly lamentable, with such a perfection of grotesque misery and weirdness of macabre detail, as if it were the Cab of Death itself that Mrs Verloc, with that ready compassion of a woman for a horse (when she is not sitting behind him), exclaimed vaguely!

"Poor brute."

Hanging back suddenly, Stevie inflicted an arresting jerk upon his sister.

"Poor! Poor!" he ejaculated appreciatively. "Cabman poor, too. He told me himself."

The contemplation of the infirm and lonely steed overcame him. Jostled, but obstinate, he would remain there, trying to express the view newly opened to his sympathies of the human and equine misery in close association. But it was very difficult. "Poor brute, poor people!" was all he could repeat. It did not seem forcible enough, and he came to a stop with an angry splutter. "Shame!" Stevie was no master of phrases, and perhaps for that very reason his thoughts lacked clearness and precision. But he felt with great completeness and some profundity. That little word contained all his sense of indignation and horror at one sort of wretchedness having to feed upon the anguish of the other—as the poor cabman beating the poor horse in the name, as it were, of his poor kids at home. And Stevie knew what it was to be beaten. He knew it from experience. It was a bad world. Bad! Bad!

Mrs Verloc, his only sister, guardian, and protector, could not pretend to such depths of insight. Moreover, she had not experienced the magic of the cabman's eloquence. She was in the dark as to the inwardness of the word "Shame." And she said placidly:

"Come along, Stevie. You can't help that."

The docile Stevie went along; but now he went along without pride, shamblingly, and muttering half words, and even words that would have been whole if they had not been made up of halves that did not belong to each other. It was as though he had been trying to fit all the words he could remember to his sentiments in order to get some sort of corresponding idea. And, as a matter of fact, he got it at last. He hung back to utter it at once.

"Bad world for poor people."

Directly he had expressed that thought he became aware that it was familiar to him already in all its consequences. This circumstance strengthened his conviction immensely, but also augmented his indignation. Somebody, he felt, ought to be punished for it—punished with great severity. Being no sceptic, but a moral creature, he was in a manner at the mercy of his righteous passions.

"Beastly!" he added, concisely.

It was clear to Mrs Verloc that he was greatly excited.

"Nobody can help that," she said. "Do come along. Is that the way you're taking care of me?"

Stevie mended his pace obediently. He prided himself on being a good brother. His morality, which was very complete, demanded that from him. Yet he was pained at the information imparted by his sister Winnie—who was good. Nobody could help that! He came along gloomily, but presently he brightened up. Like the rest of mankind, perplexed by the mystery of the universe, he had his moments of consoling trust in the organized powers of the earth.

"Police," he suggested, confidently.

"The police aren't for that," observed Mrs Verloc, cursorily, hurrying on her way.

Stevie's face lengthened considerably. He was thinking. The more intense his thinking, the slacker was the droop of his lower jaw. And it was with an aspect of hopeless vacancy that he gave up his intellectual enterprise.

"Not for that?" he mumbled, resigned but surprised. "Not for that?" He had formed for himself an ideal conception of the metropolitan police as a sort of benevolent institution for the suppression of evil. The notion of benevolence especially was very closely associated with his sense of the power of the men in blue. He had liked all police constables tenderly, with a guileless trustfulness. And he was pained. He was irritated, too, by a suspicion of duplicity in the members of the force. For Stevie was frank and as open as the day himself. What did they mean by pretending then? Unlike his sister, who put her trust in face values, he wished to go to the bottom of the matter. He carried on his inquiry by means of an angry challenge.

"What are they for then, Winn? What are they for? Tell me."

Winnie disliked controversy. But fearing most a fit of black depression consequent on Stevie missing his mother very much at first, she did not altogether decline the discussion. Guiltless of all irony, she answered yet in a form which was not perhaps unnatural in the wife of Mr Verloc, Delegate of the Central Red Committee, personal friend of certain anarchists, and a votary of social revolution.

"Don't you know what the police are for, Stevie? They are there so that them as have nothing shouldn't take anything away from them who have."

She avoided using the verb "to steal," because it always made her brother uncomfortable. For Stevie was delicately honest. Certain simple principles had been instilled into him so anxiously (on account of his "queerness") that the mere names of certain transgressions filled him with horror. He had been always easily impressed by speeches. He was impressed and startled now, and his intelligence was very alert.

"What?" he asked at once, anxiously. "Not even if they were hungry? Mustn't they?"

The two had paused in their walk.

"Not if they were ever so," said Mrs Verloc, with the equanimity of a person untroubled by the problem of the distribution of wealth and exploring the perspective of the roadway for an omnibus of the right colour. "Certainly not. But what's the use of talking about all that? You aren't ever hungry."

She cast a swift glance at the boy, like a young man, by her side. She saw him amiable, attractive, affectionate and only a little, a very little peculiar. And she could not see him otherwise, for he was connected with what there was of the salt of passion in her tasteless life—the passion of indignation, of courage, of pity, and even of self-sacrifice. She did not add: "And you aren't likely ever to be as long as I live." But she might very well have done so, since she had taken effectual steps to that end. Mr Verloc was a very good husband. It was her honest impression that nobody could help liking the boy. She cried out suddenly:

"Quick, Stevie. Stop that green bus."

And Stevie, tremulous and important with his sister Winnie on his arm, flung up the other high above his head at the approaching bus, with complete success.

Source: Conrad, Joseph. 1907. *The Secret Agent: A Simple Tale.* Available at: http://www.online-literature.com/conrad/secret_agent/

Clifford Beers, from *A Mind That Found Itself* (1910)

The story of Clifford Beers's hallucinations and suicide attempts, which led to his being committed to an asylum, provides the author with an opportunity to reflect upon care methods in U.S. asylums. In this excerpt, he examines the abuse applied to patients by their personal attendants and the way in which such abuse can be fostered by the institutions in which the attendants work.

XXIX

The central problem in the care of the insane is the elimination of actual physical abuse. What I have narrated from my own experience and from the experiences of others makes clear enough the nature of the average attendant. Under a bad regime their baser natures gradually gain the mastery. Surprising as it may seem, many an assault is due in the last analysis to a wanton desire to satisfy what amounts to a craving for human blood. This fact is well illustrated in the remark of an attendant, in the Kentucky institution already referred to, who said, "When I came here if any one had told me that I would be guilty of striking a patient I would have called him crazy himself, but now I take delight in punching hell out of them."

What is responsible for the development of the brutal attendant and his continued existence?

In the first place, not only do locks and bars *protect* men mean enough to abuse the helpless, the sense of security itself really *inspires* them to wicked deeds. And this feeling of security is strengthened by the knowledge that chance witnesses can but rarely testify convincingly in a court of law. Being removed from the restraining influence of sane eyes, the attendant does not fear to abuse, or (the vicious type) even sometimes to kill a patient. At the worst he sees no greater penalty in store for him than the loss of his position. The chance of arrest and trial is so remote as to escape consideration; and a trial has few terrors for such attendants as are arrested, for acquittal is almost certain. Indeed, on those rare occasions when attendants happen to be indicted for murder or manslaughter, the public generally gives them the benefit of the doubt, assuming that their work is highly dangerous, and arguing that the occasional sacrifice of the life of an insane patient is unavoidable, therefore justifiable. In this the public is in error, for, though the work in question may be, and at times *is,* harassing, it is, by no means, peculiarly hazardous. The number of unprovoked attacks made upon attendants by insane patients is, in fact, small, and would become almost negligible were all patients treated kindly from the moment of commitment.

But can we put all the blame on attendants for assaulting patients when the management shows no aggressive disposition to protect the latter? Such indifference is far more reprehensible than the cowardly conduct of ill-paid men, the majority of whom have had few advantages of education. The professional thug-attendant who, when a fellow-attendant is assaulting a patient, deliberately turns his back so that he may say, if ever questioned, that he saw no assault, is, in my opinion, less deserving of censure than those doctors who, knowing that brutality is common in their institution, weakly resign themselves to what they call "conditions."

Much of the suffering among the insane to-day is, in my opinion, due to the giving of too much authority to assistant physicians. Many of them, especially the young and inexperienced, are not to be trusted implicitly. Or, if they are to be given almost absolute authority over the patients in wards assigned to their care, let the superintendent exercise his authority to set aside any order which he may deem inexpedient or unjust. All superintendents have such authority. What I wish to emphasize is that they too often fail to exercise it. As a result of their laxness, or timidity—a timidity perhaps inspired by a misconception of the ethics of their profession—the helpless patient is permitted unnecessarily to suffer; and, I regret to record, frequently is this suffering of the patient due to what seems a selfish desire of the superintendent to preserve peace in his official family—the medical staff. Official peace at such a price amounts to crime.

But quite as culpable as lax discipline is the selfish desire on the part of doctors in authority to escape annoying investigations. When it does happen that they cannot avoid reporting felonious assaults or suspected

murders to the proper authorities, their action, I regret to say, is too often in mere self-defense, and not from a righteous desire to protect their patients. Knowing that the battered and mutilated condition of the corpse, or a living victim of abuse, for that matter, will arouse suspicion on the part of the relatives of the victim, those in authority sometimes take the initiative in order to "save their face." In making this assertion I am well within the bounds of charity and truth, and the conduct of this type of doctor at the subsequent trial invariably is such as to support my contention. This behavior is quite human; for, let it be borne in mind that almost every honest investigation into these suspicious deaths reveals a greater or less degree—sometimes a criminal degree—of neglect on the part of the doctors themselves. If cornered at last by an aroused public opinion they are too ready to shift the responsibility upon the ignorant and untrained attendants whose brutality is but the reflex of the doctors' indifference, neglect, or cowardice. But this is the last resort. Usually they will first equivocate to the verge of deliberate falsehood. They will outrun the public by giving the benefit of all doubts to the attendants. Not to do so would in many cases cause the accused to turn on them and reveal conditions they would prefer to hide. Human nature, like Nature herself, is influenced by immutable laws. Self-interest is apt to kill one's higher feelings. To fight the fight of the oppressed, the outraged, the dead, too frequently forces one to abandon a chosen career. Therefore, the still voice of a timid conscience whispers (in a perverted sense): "Let the dead bury their dead."

I cannot lay too much stress on this absolute fact: that hospital managements deliberately, wilfully, and selfishly suppress evidence which, if presented to the proper authorities, would lead to the conviction of guilty attendants, and eventually to their almost complete elimination from asylums. Several instances of such suppression have come to my attention since my discharge, two of which I shall now cite. During the summer of 1907, a Committee of Investigation appointed by the Legislature of the State of New Jersey, uncovered, several months after the commission of the crime, the suppressed evidence of the murder of a patient by attendants at the Trenton State Hospital. On the witness-stand the hospital official in authority admitted that the attendants had killed the patient and that their only punishment had been their prompt discharge as employees. He further admitted that the "scandal" had been deliberately suppressed, and that no evidence or report of the crime had been submitted to the proper authorities as is, of course, required by law. So skilfully was this crime concealed that even the wife of the victim was unable to learn the cause of her husband's death until the investigators laid bare the facts. And this same Committee of Investigation uncovered another alleged and, to my mind, proved murder in another State Hospital for the Insane—at Morris Plains, New Jersey. Here, again, the "scandal" (a hospital euphemism for "murder" and lesser crimes) was "hushed-up" or "whitewashed." When it was finally dragged into the light of day, what happened? Those in authority, making characteristic use of the ignorance of the public regarding such matters, brazenly, I think, denied in sweeping terms, and under oath, the incriminating evidence of supposedly credible witnesses. If an investigation in New Jersey can reveal two unreported murders that occurred within a year in two State Hospitals, how many such crimes would be unearthed should the two hundred and twenty-six public and one hundred and two private hospitals for the insane in this country be *honestly* investigated? The probable figure is too appalling to print. . . .

We must admit that the problem of securing efficiency among attendants is not an easy one. To make it easier several improvements must be made in the lot of the attendants themselves. For one thing, the niggardly salaries now offered make it extremely difficult for a management to secure or keep the right type. Competent men and women can earn two or three times as much in other and more congenial lines of endeavor. The average scale of wages for attendants in hospitals for the insane ranges from sixteen to twenty-four dollars a month, with room and board. Women usually receive sixteen or eighteen dollars at the beginning; men from eighteen to twenty, though the rates vary throughout the country. There is a slight margin, too, for an increase in salary, but even the exceptionally able attendants seldom receive more than thirty dollars a month. This bespeaks a false, a vicious economy. Not that the average attendant deserves a cent more than he receives; but would it not be wiser, more humane, and, in the end, cheaper, to offer inducements calculated to attract to this neglected field of service a higher type of character?— nay, and keep him there, for nothing is more demoralizing than the constant changing that goes on in the ranks of the present attendants. To offer a wage of, say, forty, with a maximum of fifty dollars a month,

including board and room, would, no doubt, be a move in the right direction.

However, such a merely pecuniary inducement would not, of itself, accomplish the purpose. Indeed, alone, it might defeat the purpose. For, after discussing this problem with doctors who have employed attendants, I am brought to the conclusion that increased wages, unaccompanied by increased and deserved privileges, and more wholesome and refined surroundings, would probably appeal only to burly workers in rougher fields. Wages high enough to attract a more refined type are, at the present stage of hospital development, out of the question; whereas privileges and refining influences might even now be brought to bear with excellent effect. Model dormitories, and separate cottages for married employees, instead of mere sleeping places, shorter and less exhausting hours, and proper places in which the extra leisure could be enjoyed—a library, billiard room, etc.,— these would go farther than money toward the great task of refinement. It is unfair to keep an attendant on duty twelve or fifteen hours a day (these are now the common working hours) and for the balance of his time confine him to his ward under restrictions nearly as irksome as those to which the patients themselves must perforce submit. A few States, notably New York and Massachusetts, have granted appropriations for the creation of such conditions as I am describing. If these appropriations were enlarged, and if other States followed the same policy, it is safe to predict that thousands of refined men and women would enter this field who are now debarred. And once in the work they should be offered the same chances for advancement as are offered to employees in any well conducted commercial establishment. Such a policy, carried to its logical conclusion, would include also a system of pensions for those attendants who should devote the better part of their lives to this noble service.

Still another effective means of eliminating brutality by the introduction of refining influences would consist in the wider employment of women nurses in men's wards. To the uninitiated this suggestion will no doubt seem ill-advised; yet, at this moment, there are in this country—and abroad, as well,—some hospitals for the insane where women nurses, assisted, of course, by orderlies, as are nurses in general hospitals, are managing men's wards with gratifying success. What is needed is a general adoption of this humane practice. Not all classes of male patients can safely or advantageously be placed in charge of women nurses; but other classes—the more intelligent and less disturbed—comprising thousands, can, if anything, be managed better by women of capacity than by men of any sort. The superior tact and quicker sympathy of women—God-given qualities—work wonders among insane men quite as readily as in the sane world. It cannot be denied that under the present regime women nurses in charge of troublesome women patients have not been entirely free from charges of cruelty; indeed, the contrary has been proved, as the results of investigations show—but they are far less subject to this charge than men attendants. According to those superintendents who have successfully placed women nurses in charge of men's wards, thousands of male patients who now suffer at the hands of unfeeling and incompetent male attendants could be brought under remedial and uplifting influences simply by having women placed over them in positions of authority. And the salutary influence of women in wards where they are available would have a tendency, as experience has demonstrated, to spread throughout all other wards where their immediate presence is impracticable or unsafe. It would therefore seem desirable to substitute female for male nurses wherever possible.

Such a course, too, would further simplify the problem of securing an adequate number of attendants. The services of women are easier to secure, and women readily take up nursing as a profession—as a life-work; whereas men naturally look upon such work simply as a means of providing a livelihood until they can secure work more to their liking.

There are in this country about twenty thousand men and women working as attendants in our asylums and hospitals for the insane. Of this number several thousand are, without doubt, individuals of refinement. Now, if a few thousand persons of refinement can work under such conditions as obtain so generally to-day in our hospitals and asylums, is it not reasonable to suppose that improved conditions would eventually attract a full complement of workers of the same type? Strange as it may seem, many attendants now so employed, enjoy their work and would not of their own choice relinquish it. And I make bold to appeal to those grinding thousands now eking out a livelihood in work apparently more attractive, but, in truth, less endurable, to seek improved conditions and increased usefulness in those hospitals where the application of the Golden Rule to insanity is now

possible. In such places a feeling of security and interest soon overcomes the instinctive timidity or repugnance felt by many when, in the capacity of attendants, they first come in contact with the insane. Such contact, barring exceptional cases influenced by a too impressionable temperament on the part of the nurse, renders one, as it were, immune. It would surprise (perhaps annoy) many sane persons, were they to realize how slightly many of the inmates of asylums differ from their more fortunate brothers at large. Yet among those who have been brought into close contact with the insane this is a trite observation; and it is the key to the problem which causes so many to wonder how and why it is that men and women, at liberty to choose their vocations, deliberately cast their lot with that portion of humanity which the average person seems so willing to shun.

Source: Beers, Clifford. 1910. *A Mind That Found Itself.* New York: Longman, Greens, and Company.

◉ Konrad Biesalski, from *Manual for the Care of Cripples* (1911)

The pediatrician, surgeon, and orthopedic specialist Konrad Biesalski (1868–1930) can be regarded as a founder of German rehabilitation and disability policy. Above all, he looked after the care of physically disabled people, who at the beginning of the twentieth century were still called "cripples." In 1906, he initiated the first registry and census of physically disabled children and youth in the German empire; the census produced the proof that disability constituted a major problem with respect to the poor population. In addition, Biesalski defined physical disability as an illness in the medical-orthopedic sense, after which he was able to establish treatment and social policies for physically disabled people.

I. What Is a Cripple?

This question has been answered variously depending on the specific profession or position of the person answering with respect to the cripple's care. In 1906 all crippled youth were officially counted in Germany. As a result of this census, a definition has been established. . . .

It states: 'A cripple in need of institutional care is (as a result of a congenital or acquired nerve or bone and joint condition) a sick person, who is disabled in the use of his trunk or limbs. The interaction between the degree of his ailment (including other illnesses and defects) and the cost of living in his surroundings is so unfavorable that his remaining mental and physical strength can only be developed to the highest possible economic independence in an institution that can offer a variety of medical and pedagogic measures that are necessary for this aim.'

The entire public system of cripples' care [*Krüppelfürsorge*] in Germany deals only with the cripples amongst the poor population. Cripples of affluent parents are not counted in these official statistics.

The above definition emphasizes that the cripple is an ill person, for whose care the doctor is ultimately responsible. The definition goes on to divide the cripple's care into two large groups: the first, in which the level of care requires placement in a special institution—a so-called cripple home—the elaboration of which is included in the above definition, and the second, in which the cripples can also become 'de-crippled' [*entkrüppelt*] without home care. Therefore, the main division is between the 'Institutional' [*Heimbedürftige*] and the 'Non-Institutional' [*Nichtheimbedürftige*].

If a child with a congenitally defective arm is born the son of an affluent father, this child is not subject to the public system of cripples' care, because the father will raise the boy to reach his highest potential work capacity through the father's own fortunes. If a child suffers from a moderate ailment, e.g. from a middle-degree curvature of the spine, however, and is at the same time an orphan or illegitimate child, and feeble-minded, deaf-mute, or blind and poor, this child needs our help. Without it, the child would be neglected physically, morally, and economically.

The uppermost *purpose of all well-ordered cripples' care,* is to make the cripple fit for work, or in short, as expressed in a catchphrase, to change him from an alms recipient into a taxpayer. To achieve this purpose, three separate groups of professionals are active in the cripples' care. The *doctor* cures the cripple's ailment or at least improves it as much as possible. The *teacher* provides the cripple with the necessary school education, the *master craftsman* teaches him a trade. Although these three fields are independent of one another, they do not stand next to each other as strangers, but instead work at the same time with and in one another, so that out of these three

occupations a completely new field emerges, namely, that of cripples' care. . . .

Source: Biesalski, Konrad. 1911. Pp. 13–15, 18, in *Leitfaden der Krüppelfürsorge: Im Auftrag der Deutschen Vereinigung für Krüppelfürsorge.* Leipzig and Hamburg, Germany: Leopold Voss. [*Manual for the Care of Cripples: In Contract with the German Organization for Cripples' Care.* Vogt, Sara, trans.].

▣ Randolph Bourne, "The Handicapped" (1911)

In John Dos Passos's sprawling epic U.S.A., *social critic and writer Randolph Bourne (1886–1918) is described as "a tiny twisted unscared ghost in a black cloak hopping along the grimy old brick and brownstone streets still left in New York, crying out in a shrill soundless giggle: War is the health of the state." Bourne's opposition to World War I, his understanding of the changes it would bring, and his appreciation of the role of youth in social movements are usually seen as his primary intellectual contributions. However, he has recently been receiving more attention for his writing about disability. His essay "The Handicapped" originally appeared in the* Atlantic Monthly *in 1911. Bourne died in 1918 in the influenza epidemic that followed in the wake of World War I.*

It would not perhaps be thought, ordinarily, that the man whom physical disabilities have made so helpless that he is unable to move around among his fellows, can bear his lot more happily, even though he suffer pain, and face life with a more cheerful and contented spirit, than can the man whose handicaps are merely enough to mark him out from the rest of his fellows without preventing him from entering with them into most of their common affairs and experiences. But the fact is that the former's very helplessness makes him content to rest and not to strive. I know a young man so helplessly disabled that he has to be carried about, who is happy in reading a little, playing chess, taking a course or two in college, and all with the sunniest good-will in the world, and a happiness that seems strange and unaccountable to my restlessness. He does not cry for the moon.

When the handicapped youth, however, is in full possession of his faculties, and can move about freely, he is perforce drawn into all the currents of life. Particularly if he has his own way in the world to make, his road is apt to be hard and rugged, and he will penetrate to an unusual depth in his interpretation both of the world's attitude toward such misfortunes, and of the attitude toward the world which such misfortunes tend to cultivate in men like him. For he has all the battles of a stronger man to fight, and he is at a double disadvantage in fighting them. He has constantly with him the sense of being obliged to make extra efforts to overcome the bad impression of his physical defects, and he is haunted with a constant feeling of weakness and low vitality which makes effort more difficult and renders him easily fainthearted and discouraged by failure. He is never confident of himself, because he has grown up in an atmosphere where nobody has been very confident of him; and yet his environment and circumstances call out all sorts of ambitions and energies in him which, from the nature of his case, are bound to be immediately thwarted. This attitude is likely to keep him at a generally low level of accomplishment unless he have an unusually strong will, and a strong will is perhaps the last thing to develop under such circumstances.

The handicapped man is always conscious that the world does not expect very much from him. And it takes him a long time to see in this a challenge instead of a firm pressing down to a low level of accomplishment. As a result, he does not expect very much of himself; he is timid in approaching people, and distrustful of his ability to persuade and convince. He becomes extraordinarily sensitive to other people's first impressions of him. Those who are to be his friends he knows instantly, and further acquaintance adds little to the intimacy and warm friendship that he at once feels for them. On the other hand, those who do not respond to him immediately cannot by any effort either on his part or theirs overcome that first alienation.

This sensitiveness has both its good and its bad sides. It makes friendship the most precious thing in the world to him, and he finds that he arrives at a much richer and wider intimacy with his friends than do ordinary men with their light, surface friendships, based on good fellowship or the convenience of the moment. But on the other hand this sensitiveness absolutely unfits him for business and the practice of a profession, where one must be "all things to all men," and the professional manner is indispensable to success. For here, where he has to meet a constant stream of men of all sorts and conditions, his sensitiveness to these first impressions will make his case hopeless. Except with those few who by some secret

sympathy will seem to respond, his physical deficiencies will stand like a huge barrier between his personality and other men's. The magical good fortune of attractive personal appearance makes its way almost without effort in the world, breaking down all sorts of walls of disapproval and lack of interest. Even the homely person can attract by personal charm.

The doors of the handicapped man are always locked, and the key is on the outside. He may have treasures of charm inside, but they will never be revealed unless the person outside cooperates with him in unlocking the door. A friend becomes, to a much greater degree than with the ordinary man, the indispensable means of discovering one's own personality. One only exists, so to speak, with friends. It is easy to see how hopelessly such a sensitiveness incapacitates a man for business, professional or social life, where the hasty and superficial impression is everything, and disaster is the fate of the man who has not all the treasures of his personality in the front window, where they can be readily inspected and appraised.

It thus takes the handicapped man a long time to get adjusted to his world. Childhood is perhaps the hardest time of all. As a child he is a strange creature in a strange land. It was my own fate to be just strong enough to play about with the other boys, and attempt all their games and "stunts," without being strong enough actually to succeed in any of them. It never used to occur to me that my failures and lack of skill were due to circumstances beyond my control, but I would always impute them, in consequence of my rigid Calvinistic bringing-up, I suppose, to some moral weakness of my own. I suffered tortures in trying to learn to skate, to climb trees, to play ball, to conform in general to the ways of the world. I never resigned myself to the inevitable, but overexerted myself constantly in a grim determination to succeed. I was good at my lessons, and through timidity rather than priggishness, I hope, a very well-behaved boy at school; I was devoted, too, to music, and learned to play the piano pretty well. But I despised my reputation for excellence in these things, and instead of adapting myself philosophically to the situation, I strove and have been striving ever since to do the things I could not.

As I look back now it seems perfectly natural that I should have followed the standards of the crowd, and loathed my high marks in lessons and deportment, and the concerts to which I was sent by my aunt, and the exhibitions of my musical skill that I had to give before admiring ladies. Whether or not such an experience is typical of handicapped children, there is tragedy there for those situated as I was. For had I been a little weaker physically, I should have been thrown back on reading omnivorously and cultivating my music, with some possible results; while if I had been a little stronger, I could have participated in the play on an equal footing with the rest. As it was, I simply tantalized myself, and grew up with a deepening sense of failure, and a lack of pride in that at which I really excelled.

When the world became one of dances and parties and social evenings and boy-and-girl attachments,— the world of youth,—I was to find myself still less adapted to it. And this was the harder to bear because I was naturally sociable, and all these things appealed tremendously to me. This world of admiration and gayety and smiles and favors and quick interest and companionship, however, is only for the well-begotten and the debonair. It was not through any cruelty or dislike, I think, that I was refused admittance; indeed they were always very kind about inviting me. But it was more as if a ragged urchin had been asked to come and look through the window at the light and warmth of a glittering party; I was truly in the world, but not of the world. Indeed there were times when one would almost prefer conscious cruelty to this silent, unconscious, gentle oblivion. And this is the tragedy, I suppose, of all the ill-favored and unattractive to a greater or less degree; the world of youth is a world of so many conventions, and the abnormal in any direction is so glaringly and hideously abnormal.

Although it took me a long time to understand this, and I continued to attribute my failure mostly to my own character, trying hard to compensate for my physical deficiencies by skill and cleverness, I suffered comparatively few pangs, and got much better adjusted to this world than to the other. For I was older, and I had acquired a lively interest in all the social politics; I would get so interested in watching how people behaved, and in sizing them up, that only at rare intervals would I remember that I was really having no hand in the game. This interest just in the ways people are human, has become more and more a positive advantage in my life, and has kept sweet many a situation that might easily have cost me a pang. Not that a person with disabilities should be a sort of detective, evil-mindedly using his social opportunities for spying out and analyzing his friends' foibles, but that, if he does acquire an interest in

people quite apart from their relation to him, he may go into society with an easy conscience and a certainty that he will be entertained and possibly entertaining, even though he cuts a poor enough social figure. He must simply not expect too much.

Perhaps the bitterest struggles of the handicapped man come when he tackles the business world. If he has to go out for himself to look for work, without fortune, training, or influence, as I personally did, his way will indeed be rugged. His disability will work against him for any position where he must be much in the eyes of men, and his general insignificance has a subtle influence in convincing those to whom he applies that he is unfitted for any kind of work. As I have suggested, his keen sensitiveness to other people's impressions of him makes him more than usually timid and unable to counteract that fatal first impression by any display of personal force and will. He cannot get his personality over across that barrier. The cards seem stacked against him from the start. With training and influence something might be done, but alone and unaided his case is almost hopeless. The attitude toward him ranges from, "You can't expect us to create a place for you," to, "How could it enter your head that we should find any use for you?" He is discounted at the start: it is not business to make allowances for anybody; and while people are not cruel or unkind, it is the hopeless finality of the thing that fills one's heart with despair.

The environment of a big city is perhaps the worst possible that a man in such a situation could have. For the thousands of seeming opportunities lead one restlessly on and on, and keep one's mind perpetually unsettled and depressed. There is a poignant mental torture that comes with such an experience,—the urgent need, the repeated failure, or rather the repeated failure even to obtain a chance to fail, the realization that those at home can ill afford to have you idle, the growing dread of encountering people,—all this is something that those who have never been through it can never realize. Personally I know of no particular way of escape. One can expect to do little by one's own unaided efforts. I solved my difficulties only by evading them, by throwing overboard some of my responsibility, and taking the desperate step of entering college on a scholarship. Desultory work is not nearly so humiliating when one is using one's time to some advantage, and college furnishes an ideal environment where the things at which a man handicapped like myself can succeed really count. One's self-respect can begin to grow like a weed.

For at the bottom of all the difficulties of a man like me is really the fact that his self-respect is so slow in growing up. Accustomed from childhood to being discounted, his self-respect is not naturally very strong, and it would require pretty constant success in a congenial line of work really to confirm it. If he could only more easily separate the factors that are due to his physical disability from those that are due to his weak will and character, he might more quickly attain self-respect, for he would realize what he is responsible for, and what he is not. But at the beginning he rarely makes allowances for himself; he is his own severest judge. He longs for a "strong will," and yet the experience of having his efforts promptly nipped off at the beginning is the last thing on earth to produce that will.

If the handicapped youth is brought into harsh and direct touch with the real world, life proves a much more complex thing to him than to the ordinary man. Many of his inherited platitudes vanish at the first touch. Life appears to him as a grim struggle, where ability does not necessarily mean opportunity and success, nor piety sympathy, and where helplessness cannot count on assistance and kindly interest. Human affairs seem to be running on a wholly irrational plan, and success to be founded on chance as much as on anything. But if he can stand the first shock of disillusionment, he may find himself enormously interested in discovering how they actually do run, and he will want to burrow into the motives of men, and find the reasons for the crass inequalities and injustices of the world he sees around him. He has practically to construct anew a world of his own, and explain a great many things to himself that the ordinary person never dreams of finding unintelligible at all. He will be filled with a profound sympathy for all who are despised and ignored in the world. When he has been through the neglect and struggles of a handicapped and ill-favored man himself, he will begin to understand the feelings of all the horde of the unpresentable and the unemployable, the incompetent and the ugly, the queer and crotchety people who make up so large a proportion of human folk.

We are perhaps too prone to get our ideas and standards of worth from the successful, without reflecting that the interpretations of life which patriotic legend, copy-book philosophy, and the sayings of the wealthy give us, are pitifully inadequate for those who fall behind in the race. Surely there are enough people to whom the task of making a decent living and maintaining themselves and their families in their social class, or of winning and keeping the respect of their fellows, is a hard and bitter task, to make a philosophy gained through personal disability and failure as just and true a method of appraising the life around us as the cheap optimism of the ordinary professional man. And certainly a kindlier, for it has no shade of contempt or disparagement about it.

It irritates me as if I had been spoken of contemptuously myself, to hear people called "common" or "ordinary," or to see that deadly and delicate feeling for social gradations crop out, which so many of our upper middle-class women seem to have. It makes me wince to hear a man spoken of as a failure, or to have it said of one that he "doesn't amount to much." Instantly I want to know why he has not succeeded, and what have been the forces that have been working against him. He is the truly interesting person, and yet how little our eager-pressing, on-rushing world cares about such aspects of life, and how hideously though unconsciously cruel and heartless it usually is!

Often I had tried in argument to show my friends how much of circumstance and chance go to the making of success; and when I reached the age of sober reading, a long series of the works of radical social philosophers, beginning with Henry George, provided me with the materials for a philosophy which explained why men were miserable and overworked, and why there was on the whole so little joy and gladness among us, and which fixed the blame. Here was suggested a goal, and a definite glorious future, toward which all good men might work. My own working hours became filled with visions of how men could be brought to see all that this meant, and how I in particular might work some great and wonderful thing for human betterment. In more recent years, the study of history and social psychology and ethics has made those crude outlines sounder and more normal, and brought them into a saner relation to other aspects of life and thought, but I have not lost the first glow of enthusiasm, nor my belief in social progress as the first right and permanent interest for every thinking and true-hearted man or woman.

I am ashamed that my experience has given me so little chance to count in any way either toward the spreading of such a philosophy or toward direct influence and action. Nor do I yet see clearly how I shall be able to count effectually toward this ideal. Of one thing I am sure, however: that life will have little meaning for me except as I am able to contribute toward some such ideal of social betterment, if not in deed, then in word. For this is the faith that I believe we need to-day, all of us,—a truly religious belief in human progress, a thorough social consciousness, an eager delight in every sign and promise of social improvement, and best of all, a new spirit of courage that will dare. I want to give to the young men whom I see,—who, with fine intellect and high principles, lack just that light of the future on their faces that would give them a purpose and meaning in life,—to them I want to give some touch of this philosophy, that will energize their lives, and save them from the disheartening effects of that poisonous counsel of timidity and distrust of human ideals which pours out in steady stream from reactionary press and pulpit.

It is hard to tell just how much of this philosophy has been due to handicap. If it is solely to that that I owe its existence, the price has not been a heavy one to pay. For it has given me something that I should not know how to be without. For, however gained, this radical philosophy has not only made the world intelligible and dynamic to me, but has furnished me with the strongest spiritual support. I know that many people, handicapped by physical weakness and failure, find consolation and satisfaction in a very different sort of faith,—in an evangelical religion, and a feeling of close dependence on God and close communion with him. But my experience has made my ideal of character militant rather than long-suffering.

Source: Bourne, Randolph. 1911. "The Handicapped." *The Atlantic Monthly* 111:320–329.

W. Y. Evans Wentz on Changelings and Fairy Faith (1911)

The Fairy-Faith in Celtic Countries was the first book by W. Y. Evans Wentz, who later went on to translate the essential texts of Tibetan Buddhism, such as The Book of the Dead. *In this work, science meets superstition: Evans Wentz interprets fairy tales in order to explain the treatment of disabled children and beliefs about them. The work grows out of Modernist Primitivism, which emphasized the need to take seriously what earlier generations had dismissed as "primitive." Evans Wentz does this by showing how apparently "superstitious" healing practices actually were real "medicine" in former cultural beliefs and by discussing Celtic stories about changelings.*

Our examination of living children said to have been changed by fairies shows . . . (a) that many changelings are so called merely because of some bodily deformity or because of some abnormal mental or pathological characteristics capable of an ordinary rational explanation, (b) but that other changelings who exhibit a change of personality, such as is recognized by psychologists, are in many cases best explained on the Demon-Possession Theory, which is a well-established scientific hypothesis.

Therefore, since the residuum or x-quantity of the Fairy-Faith, the folk-religion of the Celtic peoples, cannot be explained away by any known scientific laws, it must for the present stand, and the Psychological Theory of the Nature and Origin of the Belief in Fairies in Celtic Countries is to be considered as hypothetically established in the eyes of Science. Hence we must cease to look upon the term *fairy* as being always a synonym for something fanciful, non-real, absurd. We must also cease to think of the Fairy-Faith as being no more than a fabric of groundless beliefs. In short, the ordinary non-Celtic mind must readjust itself to a new set of phenomena that through ignorance on its part it has been content to disregard, and to treat with ridicule and contempt as so much outworn 'superstition.'

Source: Evans Wentz, W. Y. 1911. *The Fairy-Faith in Celtic Countries.* Available at: http://www.public-domain-content.com/books/legends_and_sagas/celt/ffcc/ffcc411.shtml

Charles B. Davenport, "Marriage Laws and Customs" (1912)

Charles Benedict Davenport (1866–1944) was born in Stamford, Connecticut, and received a PhD in biology from Harvard in 1892. He became director of Cold Springs Harbor Laboratory, where he founded the U.S. Eugenics Record office. In his 1912 essay, "Marriage Laws and Customs," Davenport warns that escalating numbers of immigrants will result in a rampant increase in feebleminded, insane, sexually deviant, and impoverished people.

The subject matter of eugenics is offspring and offspring imply parents. For legal and other reasons society regards a knowledge of parentage as very important. Marriage is society's method of securing that knowledge. Incidentally the arrangement of marriage is of

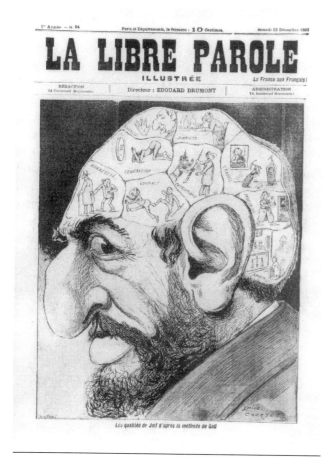

LA LIBRE PAROLE
ILLUSTRÉE
La France aux Français!

Directeur : EDOUARD DRUMONT

Les qualités de Juif d'après la méthode de Gall

The Qualities of the Jew After Gall's Method *(1893), by Emile Courtet (1857–1938). The "inferiority" of Jewish people and other minorities were often emphasized in caricatures that exaggerated physical features presumed to deviate from those of the dominant culture.*

Source: Art Resource, New York.

value for eugenical studies, in fact the principles of eugenics could hardly be established in its absence.

But society asks not only for a registry of matings but seeks to control, in some degree, the nature of the matings. On the one hand it seeks to protect monogamy and the young from the legal consequences of marriage. On the other hand, the nature of control measures, roughly, the result of society's experience that certain matings result in undesirable offspring. Let us, accordingly, examine some of these laws.

The most widespread marriage regulation of biological import in modern civilized states is that which limits the relationship of those whose mating may receive a legal sanction. In practically all of the States of the Union marriage of brother and sister, of parent and child, even of grandparent and grandchild is forbidden, and it is sometimes expressly stated that such

marriages have no legal standing. In most States the marriage of uncle and niece, or of aunt and nephew, are forbidden. When it comes to the mating of cousins, legislators have been in much greater doubt. About a third of the States forbid such marriages, and these are chiefly in the western, or more recently settled, territory. In most European States, I am informed, no legal limitation to the marriage of cousins exists.

Let us now consider in how far there is a biological justification for these laws. I know that there are those who hold that the mating even of brother and sister for generations may result in offspring without blemish. We are referred to the Incas of Peru, about whom we know little in detail, and to the Ptolomies, of whom we know a little more, but not as much as a well-trained field worker of the Eugenics Record Office would discover in two or three days. The last Cleopatra, the daughter of a brother and sister, is pointed out to us as the great argument against the evil effects of incestuous marriages. That she was the crowning flower of a beautiful race may be admitted, but is there any doubt that, were she living to-day, she would be placed in the manic-depressive ward of a hospital for the insane, with further history of paranoia and erotomania? But we, too, have histories of incest, brought in by our field workers, histories of families brought up, not in palaces, but in hovels in the woods. For example, a criminalistic man had, by an unknown woman, a number of boys and girls. One of the boys, who was a drunken, feeble-minded fellow with criminalistic tendencies, has had by his own sister a daughter who is a drunken epileptic. This daughter by her own father has had four children of whom one is epileptic, two are imbecile, and the fourth was an encephalic monster who died at birth. I would undertake to produce two cases of this general sort for each case that may be offered of the "romantic," "vivacious" product of a brother and sister mating. And can we doubt that a sober minded people have been impressed by such cases as I have cited, have stored them up in their memory as part of experience, and have crystallized that experience in laws against incest?

And how about the marriage of first cousins? Are the laws that forbid such marriages justifiable? Our modern knowledge of heredity leads to the conclusion that cousin marriages (like the marriage of sibs, possibly) [are] not injurious per se, but because such marriages enhance the probability that the same defect shall inhere in each of the two germ-cells that unite to start the development of the child. While the prohibition of cousin marriages is doubtless a rough eugenic measure, it were better if the prohibition were qualified somewhat as follows: "The marriage of cousins is forbidden when in the parental fraternity that is common to both, there is a case of inability to learn at school, of dementia precox or manic depressive insanity in any of their forms, of epilepsy, of congenital deafness, of albinism, or of cleft palate." Such a restriction in the application of the law might well increase the difficulty of administering it, but the law would be rendered more significant and less unjust. . . .

If [laws forbidding cousin marriages under certain conditions] could not be enforced, of what use would they be? Their value would be primarily educational, and this value would be enhanced by a penalty for every enfringement of the law, such as more or less prolonged deprivation of some of the rights of citizenship. In time the reasonableness of the legislation would make a strong appeal.

The second legal limitation of a biological sort is that concerning the physical (including the mental) condition of those who contemplate marriage. Many States provide that if either party is an idiot or insane, the marriage is void, on the legal ground that such persons are incapable of making a valid contract. In not a few States paupers are permitted to marry only under restrictions, the limitation having an economic basis, namely that a male pauper cannot support a wife. In few, if any, of the States of the Union have the legislators or the people grasped the idea of restricting the marriage of the mentally or physically defective in order to diminish the procreation of more defectives. Laws against the marriage of the feebleminded are futile in any case. For so long as a feeble-minded person is at large he will find another feeble-minded person who will live with him and have children by him. It would be as sensible to hope to control by legislation the mating of rabbits. The only way to prevent the reproduction of the feeble-minded is to sterilize or segregate them. As to the marriage of the insane, it seems doubtful if it is wise to refuse this without qualification. Two mentally normal persons who have each an insane parent are more apt to have insane offspring than an insane person who marries one in whom there is no taint of insanity. I think it might be unwise to deny to every person who has shown a tendency to manic depressive insanity in its lighter forms marriage into mentally sound stock. Further study of this matter is needed. The requirement of a physician's certificate as to bodily soundness, which some clergymen are requiring in the States, is primarily directed toward venereal disease and certainly has eugenical bearings. When a requirement is made of a certificate that both parties come of mentally and physically satisfactory stock, a still more important step in eugenics will have been taken.

Finally, the third legal limitation of a biological sort is that concerning the mixture of races. Most of the States of the Union have laws declaring marriages void when contracted between a white person and a negro or the descendants of a negro for a certain number of generations, usually three; i.e., "having one-eighth of negro blood." But the law of the State of Georgia prohibits for ever and declares null and void any marriage between a white person and one of "African descent." The Oregon law renders void any marriage of a white person with a person having one-fourth or more of negro, Chinese or Kanaka blood, or any person having more than one-half Indian blood.

The biological basis for such laws is doubtless an appreciation of the fact that negroes and the other races carry traits that do not go well with our social organization. For the Ethiopian has not undergone that selection that in Europe weeded out the traits that failed to recognize property rights, or that failed to give industry, ambition and sex control. The Southerner looks aghast at the possibility that these traits shall become disseminated throughout his social organization and become part and parcel of the make up of his descendants. So with the cruelty of the Indian. These fears are justified, but the cure is inadequate. Already the south is full of persons of one-eighth negro blood, whose (illegitimate) children may legally marry with whites. The Georgia law which denies marriage of white persons to descendants of blacks, however remote, is equally futile. Many a child arises in the third or later generations that by no test shows evidence of "African descent." How unjust the Missouri law that provides that the proportion of negro blood is to be determined by the jury from the appearance of the person! The south, indeed, has a problem in its huge "feeble-minded" coloured population; but the problem is of the same order as that in the north and in England, and the solution is this: Forget unessentials, like skin colour, and focus attention on socially important defects. Then, by sterilization or segregation, prevent the reproduction of the socially inadequate. Thus will the mentally incompetent strains be eliminated and the good physical traits of some of the black races be added, as a valued heritage to enhance the physical manhood of the south.

I feel sure that if law will take lessons from biology many of the disasters that have been feared may be averted.

Source: Davenport, Charles B. 1912. "Marriage Laws and Customs." Pp. 153–155 in *Problems in Eugenics: Papers Communicated to the First International Eugenics Congress.* London: Eugenics Education Society.

▣ Maria Montessori on the Orthophrenic School (1912)

In 1896, Maria Montessori (1870–1952) became one of the first female physicians in Italy. During her tenure at the psychiatric clinic of the University of Rome, Montessori developed an interest in disabled children. In 1899, she and Giuseppe Montesano founded the Scuola Magistrale Ortofrenica, which was both an educational institute for disabled children and a training institute for instructors. Montessori was a lecturer of disability pedagogy from 1900 to 1918 at the Regio Instituto Superiore Femminile di Magistero in Rome. Montessori traveled extensively and presented her work in order to disseminate her ideas. Maria Montessori was nominated three times for the Nobel Peace Prize. The excerpt below from her book, The Montessori Method *(1912), provides an overview of the methods she developed for educating disabled children*

From Chapter 2. "History of Methods"

About fifteen years ago, being assistant doctor at the Psychiatric Clinic of the University of Rome, I had occasion to frequent the insane asylums to study the sick and to select subjects for the clinics. In this way I became interested in the idiot children who were at that time housed in the general insane asylums. In those days thyroid organotherapy was in full development, and this drew the attention of physicians to deficient children. I myself, having completed my regular hospital services, had already turned my attention to the study of children's diseases.

It was thus that, being interested in the idiot children, I became conversant with the special method of education devised for these unhappy little ones by Edward Seguin, and was led to study thoroughly the idea, then beginning to be prevalent among the physicians, of the efficacy of 'pedagogical

treatment' for various morbid forms of disease such as deafness, paralysis, idiocy, rickets, etc. The fact that pedagogy must join with medicine in the treatment of disease was the practical outcome of the thought of the time. And because of this tendency the method of treating disease by gymnastics became widely popular. I, however, differed from my colleagues in that I felt that mental deficiency presented chiefly a pedagogical, rather than mainly a medical, problem. Much was said in the medical congresses of the medico-pedagogic method for the treatment and education of the feebleminded, and I expressed my differing opinion in an address on *Moral Education* at the Pedagogical Congress of Turin in 1898. I believe that I touched a chord already vibrant, because the idea, making its way among the physicians and elementary teachers, spread in a flash as presenting a question of lively interest to the school.

In fact, I was called upon by my master, Guido Baccelli, the great Minister of Education, to deliver to the teachers of Rome a course of lectures on the education of feeble-minded children. This course soon developed into the State Orthophrenic School, which I directed for more than two years.

In this school we had an all-day class of children composed of those who in the elementary schools were considered hopelessly deficient. Later on, through the help of a philanthropic organisation, there was founded a Medical Pedagogic Institute where, besides the children from the public schools, we brought together all of the idiot children from the insane asylums in Rome.

I spent these two years with the help of my colleagues in preparing the teachers of Rome for a special method of observation and education of feeble-minded children. Not only did I train teachers, but what was much more important, after I had been to London and Paris for the purpose of studying in a practical way the education of deficients, I gave myself over to the actual teaching of the children, directing at the same time the work of the other teachers in our institute.

I was more than an elementary teacher, for I was present, or directly taught the children, from eight in the morning to seven in the evening without interruption. These two years of practice are my first and indeed my true degree in pedagogy. From the very beginning of my work with deficient children (1898 to 1900) I felt that the methods which I used had in them nothing peculiarly limited to the instruction of idiots. I believed that they contained educational principles *more rational* than those in use, so much more so, indeed, that through their means an inferior mentality would be able to grow and develop. This feeling, so deep as to be in the nature of an intuition, became my controlling idea after I had left the school for deficients, and, little by little, I became convinced that similar methods applied to normal children would develop or set free their personality in a marvellous and surprising way.

Source: Montessori, Maria. 1912. George, Anne E., trans. *The Montessori Method.* New York: Frederick Stokes Company. Available at: http://www.moteaco.com/method/method.html

▣ Isabelle Thompson Smart, from *Studies in the Relation of Physical Inability and Mental Deficiency to the Body Social* (1912)

Isabelle Thompson Smart, MD, was the Medical Examiner of Mentally Defective Children to the Department of Education in New York City. Smart wrote numerous eugenics tracts seeking to enlist pediatricians in the task of identifying and reporting potentially "defective" children to social work agencies. Her work demonstrates the prominent role of female professionals in the eugenics intelligentsia. The excerpt below demonstrates efforts in the medical arena by women to apply a more empirical and hard-hitting diagnostic gaze; this involvement by women differs radically from that of the more maternal social workers whom H. H. Goddard believed to be the most effective for assessments and information-gathering tasks.

Emerson once said that "Nothing great was ever achieved without enthusiasm" and perhaps we have here the crux of our problem for the care and training of the mental defective. Certainly, up to within a very short time ago there was no very definite or marked enthusiasm over either the physical or mental qualifications of the ament. The less said about this class of society the better pleased people seemed to be, and, as for our lawmakers and those whose duty it was to make adequate provision for these unfortunates and protect them by the much vaunted "strong arm of the law," they have time and again turned a deaf ear to any plea which was made in their behalf, and we are now

reaping in a large harvest of shame and crime as a just reward for the general ignorance and neglect of them.

I have chosen, somewhat at random, a group of 10,000 cases which have been presented to me for medical examination, to determine their physical and mental fitness for the work required of them in the school grades. In every instance the child had fallen behind others of his or her age and grade and had continued to retrogress for some terms. In every instance I found positive physical defects, and, with many, combination of physical unfitness with a serious mental defect, which demanded a proper segregation of the case in question. Oft times the improvable cases had become discouraged because of the ever constant inability to cope with the tasks set by the curriculum, discouragement when the little brother or sister, perhaps years younger than our weakling, was able to reach the same grade with our defective and in a term pass ahead to a higher grade, receiving the praise of parents and teachers, while our unfortunate received the on demand berating which he should never have been called upon to bear. Today the outlook for such a child is a little more favorable, for the sleepiest teachers now have had borne in upon them the fact that there are children who are wholly incapable of doing grade work, and that very many are unable to do even the manual work.

Ten thousand cases! Ten thousand little human beings so seriously handicapped that they will never be able to enter fully into competition in order to earn a livelihood—so seriously handicapped that the major number should be segregated, and marriage and procreation be absolutely denied them.

The greater number of the physical defects could be very much bettered—many of them cured—but the mental unfitness is irreparable. Up to a certain point, all of these cases could be trained to become useful units in a colony life, suited to their individual needs and under proper supervision; but if left to drift, after their brief term of school life ends, will in large measure become derelicts, and will, in time, fill our penal institutions and our homes for fallen women or worse, live at large and procreate their kind in large numbers.

Not a single low-grade case of imbecility or idiocy has been included in the number of cases presented; all would fall within the limits of middle grade and morons.

All of the low-grade cases of idiocy, imbecility, and Mongolianism should, without any question, be placed where they may be protected from society and from themselves; but the number is so great in the city and State of New York that adequate provision is, at present, and for some years to come entirely out of the question. . . .

Perhaps one of the most interesting phases of my work has been the attempt to tabulate the nations represented by the children sent up to me for these special examinations. It is only in the natural sequence of the manner of growth of our population that a very large percentage of the cases of mental defect should be found among our alien population, for in such a cosmopolitan city as New York nearly all nations send representatives—one might say misrepresentatives, for, surely, no mental derelict can truly be said to represent his or her native land. Up to the present and, at this time, one cannot tell what changes may occur—the two nations which may be said to lead all others are Russia and Italy. For a long time Russia was first on the list, but now Italy has come up to her and has even surpassed her by a fraction of 1 percent. The German Empire and Austria have contributed no small number, while Britain sends her quota, Ireland leading, followed by England and Scotland; Wales has not contributed any subject for my study. The other countries contributing their quota have been Poland, Scandinavia, France, Bohemia, Romania, Spain, Turkey, Switzerland, Syria, Greece, Arabia, Canada, West Indies, and, of the South American countries, Brazil.

These studies of our urban population are in no way complete, nor can they become so for a very long time, because of the inadequacy of the number employed in making these investigations. The need for more physicians who are specializing in this particular field of research is great, and their work should be augmented by that of an earnest, intelligent corps of social workers, whose time would be entirely devoted to the ferreting out of the kind of statistics which will prove of paramount value.

The hygienic relation of persons of such lowered physical and mental stamina to the body social, it seems to me, is so apparent as to make a summing up practically unnecessary. Surely no one in this audience needs to be prodded to do his duty in seeking the proper housing, proper segregation, and right and just laws for the unfortunate class of individuals we have had under consideration.

What we need in the United States of America is a realizing sense by our thinking people of the enormity of the problem which confronts us. Our immigration problem is tremendous. Gladly do we welcome the poor amid the downtrodden of other nations, but we must be firm in our exclusion of the mentally unfit. Our work there must go on not only at our ports of entry, but

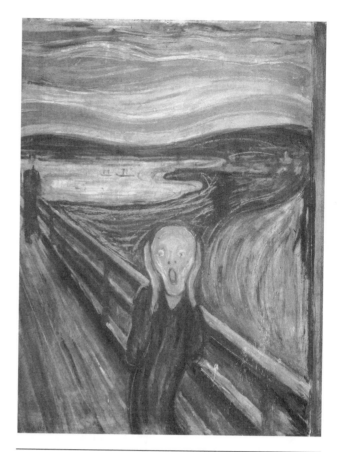

The Scream *(1893), by Edvard Munch (1863–1944). Munch's painting* The Scream *portrays a figure that is often taken as a quintessential expression of modernity. Munch himself writes that he experienced intense fear during a moment of isolation while on an evening walk: "My friends walked on—I stood there, trembling with fear. And I sensed a great, infinite scream pass through nature." Wavy lines and a red sky capture the sensation of terror he describes, and Munch's effort to capture his own feelings of besiegement by emotions struck a cord of sentiment for many at the time.*

Source: Art Resource, New York.

at the points of embarking, and the steamship companies must be held responsible for their unprincipled part in the bringing over, under much hardship, of so many cases of mental and physical unfitness.

Without a doubt we will always have the "ament" and the physical defective with us, for so long as we disobey the laws of hygiene and of health we must expect at least a part of the punishment meted out on the innocent offspring. It is largely dependent on those of us who are alive to the immenseness of the problem and who are in vital touch with it to make our voices heard whenever and wherever we find opportunity to do so. We must even make these opportunities, and we must have our law makers become familiar with the class of cases herein described.

They must be made cognizant of the conditions producing such defectives, and then made intelligent as to the direful consequences of legalizing the propagation of the unfit.

The task is stupendous, but if all interested will loyally pull together for the common good of humanity I am hopeful that we may accomplish much. "Nothing great was ever achieved without enthusiasm."

Percental chart of 10,000 cases showing relative physical defects.

Chorea	4.0
Epilepsy	5.1
Heart	29.9
Nose	34.9
Throat	42.6
Neurotic	37.0
Sex	41.5
Speech	42.0
Ears	48.3
Dental	71.4
Indicating general medical care	74.3
Eyes	95.3
Needing residential hospital care	6.9
Needing special open-air school	3.5

Percental chart of 10,000 cases children born in foreign countries.

Italy	15.3
Russia	15.1
Germany	7.7
Austria	3.5
Ireland	3.3
England	.9
Roumania	.8
Scandinavia	.7
Polish Jews	.5
Bohemia	.5
France	.1
Scotland	.1
Greece	.07
West Indies	.07
Turkey	.07
Spain	.06
Syria	.06
Canada	.04
Switzerland	.03
Holland	.03
Brazil	.03
Cuba	.01
Arabia	.01
Unknown or mixed parentage	8.3

Percental chart of 10,000 cases children born in the United States.

Russian parentage	20.5
Italian parentage	18.9
German parentage	13.9
Irish parentage	7.1
Austro-Hungarian parentage	5.8
English parentage	1.9
Scandinavian parentage	1.4
Roumanian parentage	1.1
Bohemian parentage	1.0
Polish parentage	.7
Scotch parentage	.3
French parentage	.2
Spanish parentage	.1
Swiss parentage	.1
West Indian parentage	.1
Turkish parentage	.07
Dutch parentage	.07
Greek parentage	.07
Syrian parentage	.07
Brazilian parentage	.04
Cuban parentage	.04
Arabian parentage	.01
American (whites and negroes)	17.3

Note: 25.42 percent of all cases were of foreign extraction; 48.05 percent of all cases were American born of mixed foreign parentage.

Source: Smart, Isabelle Thompson. 1912. *Studies in the Relation of Physical Inability and Mental Deficiency to the Body Social.* From the Smith Ely Jeliffe Collection, proprietor Dr. David Braddock, University of Colorado, Boulder.

▣ Henry H. Goddard, "The Improvability of Feeble-Minded Children" (1913)

Henry H. Goddard (1866–1957) served as director of the Vineland Training Center for Feebleminded Boys and Girls in New Jersey between 1906 and 1918. An ardent eugenicist who believed that "feeblemindedness" was hereditary, Goddard believed that intelligence could be scientifically measured, because mental capacity was fixed and finite. To measure intelligence, he translated and adapted Binet's Intelligence Test in order to diagnose adolescent residents under his charge at Vineland. However, in order to show the test's wider validity, he also applied it to immigrants at Ellis Island and to U.S. army recruits. He was hired as a consultant by the New York Public Schools regarding the placement of students into special learning tracks. Ultimately, Goddard renounced many of the positions he had touted for decades in various eugenics contexts.

How improvable is a feeble-minded child? This question is so fundamental, and so much depends upon the answer to it, that it is no wonder it has been the burning question since the care of the feeble-minded became common. Historically it has played no small part in the progress of the institutional care of these defectives. For years and years it was believed that nothing could be done for them and consequently nothing was done. Then, under the inspiration of the immortal Séguin it was discovered much could be done, and it is no wonder that in the enthusiasm of that discovery many went to the opposite extreme and believed that they could even be cured.

It is somewhat unfortunate that today there are certain belated travelers along the road who will talk of curing feeble-mindedness, while the impossibility of the cure of this condition has long been demonstrated. The question of improvability has had its ups and downs from the time of Séguin until the present. Today we might be said to be in the blackness of confusion. We think feeble-mindedness is improvable, from one standpoint; considering it in another way, we conclude it is not.

We know that there is a time when the feeble-minded have reached their limit, and our institutions are largely filled with individuals who are known to have long since passed their limit of improvement. In the case of younger children we still talk about improvable and unimprovable cases. In the case of any particular individual there is or has been in the past, very little dispute among those who know the case. More recently we have been led to question this, and we at Vineland, have had some dispute as to whether a group of children was improving or not improving.

Viewed from the standpoint of our usual definition of arrested development, the question is: are these persons already arrested in their development, or are they only in the process of arrest? And if the latter, how long does this process continue, and what is its method? Does a child develop at a normal rate up to a certain point and then suddenly stop, or does he develop slowly from birth up to a certain age, and then stop? Or again, does he develop at a normal rate for a few years, and then take a few years in which he keeps getting more and more backward, continually slowing down and finally stopping?

Whatever theories there may have been in answer to these questions, there have never been so far as the writer knows, many facts to substantiate the position until the present time. The reason for this lack of data is, that we never had any adequate means of measuring the mental development of a child at any one time. That difficulty has now been remedied through the Binet-Simon Measuring Scale of Intelligence, and on the basis of this we are now able to present data which seem to go a long way toward answering the question. This scale of intelligence has been in use at Vineland for two years, thereby giving us three annual testings. Upon a study of these results we ought to be able to answer the question, "How many children are improving and how many are standing still?" We had hoped to be able to do this after one year, but we found that there was considerable variability, which experience taught us was entirely normal with feeble-minded children, they doing one day what they cannot do the next, or vice versa; so that we are compelled to wait for the end of the second year giving us the third testing before we could draw any definite conclusion. The facts here presented are based upon the examination of three hundred forty-six children of both sexes, of mental ages from one to twelve, and physical ages from five to forty, with a few beyond this upper limit.

We have had three annual testings by the Binet scale, the result is that from the first to the last testing, two years apart, one hundred and nine persons have made no variation whatever not even a point. This is thirty-two per cent. If we add to this those who have gained or lost one or two points, we have two hundred thirty-two individuals, or about sixty-seven percent whose variation is so slight that it must be considered accidental. The remaining 33 percent have gained or lost three points or more. If we subtract those who have lost, we have left ninety-six persons or twenty-eight percent who at first sight seem to have made some definite progress. Closer examination, however convinces us that some part of this is due to what we have sometimes called the normal variation of the abnormal mind; in other words, that it is somewhat an accident, perhaps of attention, as to whether a child answers one question more or one question less than he did on a former occasion.

A fact which makes us believe that much of this is due to accidental variation, is that these changes occur quite as often in the older persons, who, no one of experience, believes is actually increasing in mentality, as they do among those of the younger years where we might more naturally expect it. These data wait further analysis and study, and the application of further studies, but it seems to be pretty clearly indicated that the vast majority of feeble-minded children are not changing and are not improving in their intellectual level; if there is an improvement it seems to be during the mental ages of three to nine inclusive. Among the idiots, for example, it is very low indeed; here are the figures for the idiots, that is, those having a mentality of one or two.

1. Of twenty-one idiots testing one year mentally, only one is able to do any of the Binet. He (a boy of fifteen) has from the first testing, known his eyes and mouth but has made no improvement. All have stood still. That is, twenty-one idiots, mentality one, age eight to thirty-eight, have made no progress.

2. Of thirty idiots testing two years mentally, twenty-seven, ages ten to thirty six, have not changed; three, aged respectively eleven, twelve and seventeen have learned one point in the Binet.

Of twenty-five idiots testing 2 1–5 to 2 4–5, fifteen have not varied except when the test was given by inexperienced persons and a retesting brought back the former grading. These fifteen range in age from seventeen to thirty six. One, aged thirty, has lost one point, 2 2–5 to 2 1–5, and five aged fourteen to twenty-one, have gained one to three points, none reaching higher than 2 4–5 by this gain. [Goddard's application of IQ scoring was intended to assess the mental age of the person examined, as distinct from chronological age. According to his theory, the mental capacities of "subnormals" became prematurely arrested and no amount of training/education could improve them.]

The remaining four started two years ago with a "potentiality" for three years mentality and have advanced as follows:

F. 14—2 2–5 to 3 2–5.
F. 15—2 3–5 to 3.
F. 16—2 3–5 to 3.
M. 12—2 4–5 to 3 1–5.

The conclusion that we are thus forced to accept, namely, that a very small percentage of feeble-minded children is making any mental improvement, is both surprising and somewhat discouraging, and will even be rejected by some as certainly fallacious; for do we not know that they are improving? Do we not see them improving every day? Are they not learning to do things?

The great group of the so called improvable children are doing things to-day that they could not have done a year ago. This is most certainly true, and in this fact lies our excuse for our institutions with their training departments. Nevertheless it is not difficult to show that this is not incompatible with the conclusion drawn from our data. To make this clear it is only necessary to call attention to the difference between what we may call trainability and raising the intellectual level.

A normal boy of eight, for example, has what we may call for convenience, eight-year-old intelligence; his intelligence is not yet as high as that of a normal boy of nine, still less of ten, but he can do certain things, namely those things which involve nothing more than eight-year-old intelligence. He cannot do anything that involves nine-year-old intelligence or anything higher. Now the normal boy is of eight-year intelligence only one year, and then he becomes nine years old and does the things that involve nine-year intelligence. Then he becomes ten years, and so on, until he reaches his complete development. But the feeble-minded boy who is arrested in his development at the age of eight remains with a mentality of eight year after year. As the years go by he can never learn to do things that require nine or ten-year-old intelligence because he never has that much intelligence, but there is no limit to the number of eight-year-old things that he can learn to do. It is this trainability to do anything and everything that involves only eight-year-old intelligence that is generally mistaken for increase in intelligence itself; and this is the explanation of the misunderstanding when the psychologist says the child has not improved and the teacher says he has; the former means that he has not increased his mental level, the latter means that he has learned to do a number of things that he could not do a year ago. Both are correct. He has learned to do these things and he will continue to learn to do new things for a good many years, but he can never learn to do anything that requires a higher intelligence than that at which he was arrested in his development.

So far we have not answered the question, "How does the child reach his point of arrested development?" Is it by a gradual slowing down or by a sudden stop? Nor can we answer this question surely, as yet. Perhaps it is a matter of the individual. Some develop one way and some another. The full answer to this part of the question must wait further study.

There are some indications, however, that some children arc pretty nearly normal until about eight or nine or ten years of age, and then they stop rather suddenly. For example, children test normal at six, and defective at ten never having developed beyond seven. Or defective at twelve, not having developed beyond nine. Others seem to have always been a little backward, but kept getting more and more backward until the age perhaps of nine or ten, when they seem to have entirely stopped. It must be possible to measure the rate of progress sometime when our psychological methods become more complete. . . .

The capacity for learning at the different ages during the evolutionary period might be likened to tin cups of uniform diameter but varying in height. The short cup can not be made to hold more than its capacity, so no amount of training will enable the child of a low mental age—the short cup—to perform the things which only a person of higher mental age—the long cup—can learn. On the other hand there are things that a child of any given mental age can learn to do,—the number increasing with the advance of mental age to the end of the period of mental evolution.

Source: Goddard, Henry H. 1913. "The Improvability of Feeble-Minded Children." *Journal of Psycho-Asthenics* 17(4). From the Smith Ely Jeliffe Collection, proprietor Dr. David Braddock, University of Colorado, Boulder.

▣ Sigmund Freud, from "On Narcissism: An Introduction" (1914)

Freud develops his concept of narcissism, the pathological focus on one's own person to the exclusion of others, through the example of pain. Pain and suffering supposedly steal a person's interest in other people, thereby approximating the pathological selfishness called narcissism.

It is universally known, and we take it as a matter of course, that a person who is tormented by organic pain and discomfort gives up his interest in the things of the external world, in so far as they do not concern his suffering. Closer observation teaches us that he also withdraws *libidinal* interest from his love-objects: so long as he suffers, he ceases to love. The commonplace nature of this fact is no reason why we should be deterred from translating it into terms of the libido theory. We should then say: the sick man withdraws his libidinal cathexes back upon his own ego, and

sends them out again when he recovers. 'Concentrated is his soul,' says Wilhelm Busch of the poet suffering from toothache, 'in his molar's narrow hole.' Here libido and ego-interest share the same fate and are once more indistinguishable from each other. The familiar egoism of the sick person covers both. We find it so natural because we are certain that in the same situation we should behave in just the same way. The way in which a lover's feelings, however strong, are banished by bodily ailments, and suddenly replaced by complete indifference, is a theme which has been exploited by comic writers to an appropriate extent.

Source: Freud, Sigmund. 1953–1964. "On Narcissism: An Introduction." Pp. 82–83 in Strachey, James, ed. *Psychological Works of Sigmund Freud, Vol. 14*. London: Hogarth Press. (Originally published 1914)

▣ Sigmund Freud, from *Some Character-Types Met with in Psycho-Analytic Work* (1916)

Freud explains that pain and physical deformity produce a feeling of extraordinariness in people with disabilities to the point where they may believe that moral laws obeyed by other people do not apply to them. Freud offers the example of Richard III as a disabled person who believes that life's rules do not govern his behavior because he deserves compensation for his suffering. Feelings of being disadvantaged, Freud argues, lead to pathological egotism.

Psycho-analytic work is continually confronted with the task of inducing the patient to renounce an immediate and directly attainable yield of pleasure. He is not asked to renounce all pleasure; that could not, perhaps, be expected of any human being. . . . No, the patient is only asked to renounce such satisfactions as will inevitably have detrimental consequences. His privation is only to be temporary; he has only to learn to exchange an immediate yield of pleasure for a better assured, even though a postponed one. Or, in other words, under the doctor's guidance he is asked to make the advance from the pleasure principle to the reality principle by which the mature human being is distinguished from the child. . . .

When in this way one asks the patient to make a provisional renunciation of some pleasurable satisfaction, to make a sacrifice, to show his readiness to accept some temporary suffering for the sake of a better end, or even merely to make up his mind to submit to a necessity which applies to everyone, one comes upon individuals who resist such an appeal on a special ground. They say they have renounced enough and suffered enough, and have a claim to be spared any further demands; they will submit no longer to any disagreeable necessity, for they are exceptions and, more over, intend to remain so. . . .

Now it is no doubt true that everyone would like to consider himself an 'exception' and claim privileges over others. But precisely because of this there must be a particular reason, and one not universally present, if someone actually proclaims himself an exception and behaves as such. This reason may be of more than one kind; in the cases I investigated I succeeded in discovering a common peculiarity in the earlier experiences of these patients' lives. Their neuroses were connected with some experience or suffering to which they had been subjected in their earliest childhood, one in respect of which they knew themselves to be guiltless, and which they could look upon as an unjust disadvantage imposed upon them. . . . In one of these patients, a woman, the attitude towards life which I am discussing came to a head when she learnt that a painful organic trouble, which had hindered her from attaining her aims in life, was of congenital origin. So long as she looked upon this trouble as an accidental and late acquisition, she bore it patiently; as soon as she found that it was part of an innate inheritance, she became rebellious. The young man who believed that he was watched over by a special providence had in his infancy been the victim of an accidental infection from his wet-nurse, and had spent his whole later life making claims for compensation, an accident pension, as it were, without having any idea on what he based those claims. In this case the analysis, which constructed this event out of obscure mnemic residues and interpretations of the symptoms, was confirmed objectively by information from his family.

For reasons which will be easily understood I cannot communicate very much about these or other case histories. Nor do I propose to go into the obvious analogy between deformities of character resulting from protracted sickliness in childhood and the behaviour of whole nations whose past history has been full of suffering. Instead, however, I will take the opportunity of pointing to a figure created by the greatest of poets—a figure in whose character the claim to be an exception is closely bound up with and is motivated by the circumstance of congenital disadvantage.

In the opening soliloquy to Shakespeare's *Richard III*, Gloucester, who subsequently becomes King, says:

> But I, that am not shaped for sportive tricks,
> Nor made to court an amorous looking-glass;
> I that am rudely stamp'd, and want love's majesty
> To strut before a wanton ambling nymph;
> I, that am curtail'd of this fair proportion,
> Cheated of feature by dissembling Nature,
> Deform'd, unfinish'd, sent before my time
> Into this breathing world, scarce half made up,
> And that so lamely and unfashionable,
> That dogs bark at me as I halt by them;
> . . . .
> And therefore, since I cannot prove a lover,
> To entertain these fair well-spoken days,
> I am determined to prove a villain,
> And hate the idle pleasures of those days.

At a first glance this tirade may perhaps seem unrelated to our present theme. Richard seems to say nothing more than: 'I find these idle times tedious, and I want to enjoy myself. As I cannot play the lover on account of my deformity, I will play the villain; I will intrigue, murder and do anything else I please.' Such a frivolous motivation could not but stifle any stirring of sympathy in the audience, if it were not a screen for something much more serious. Otherwise the play would be psychologically impossible, for the writer must know how to furnish us with a secret background of sympathy for his hero, if we are to admire his boldness and adroitness without inward protest; and such sympathy can only be based on understanding or on a sense of a possible inner fellow-feeling for him.

I think, therefore, that Richard's soliloquy does not say everything; it merely gives a hint, and leaves us to fill in what it hints at. When we do so, however, the appearance of frivolity vanishes, the bitterness and minuteness with which Richard has depicted his deformity make their full effect, and we clearly perceive the fellow-feeling which compels our sympathy even with a villain like him. What the soliloquy thus means is: 'Nature has done me a grievous wrong in denying me the beauty of form which wins human love. Life owes me reparation for this, and I will see that I get it. I have a right to be an exception, to disregard the scruples by which others let themselves be held back. I may do wrong myself, since wrong has been done to me.' And now we feel that we ourselves might become like Richard, that on a small scale, indeed, we are already like him. Richard is an enormous magnification of something we find in ourselves as well. We all think we have reason to reproach Nature and our destiny for congenital and infantile disadvantages; we all demand reparation for early wounds to our narcissism, our self-love. Why did not Nature give us the golden curls of Balder or the strength of Siegfried or the lofty brow of genius or the noble profile of aristocracy? Why were we born in a middle-class home instead of a royal palace? We could carry off beauty and distinction quite as well as any of those whom we are now obliged to envy for these qualities.

Source: Freud, Sigmund. 1953–1964. Ch. 1, "The Exceptions," in *Some Character-Types Met with in Psycho-Analytic Work.* Pp. 311–315 in Strachey, James, ed. *Psychological Works of Sigmund Freud, Vol. 14.* London: Hogarth Press. (Originally published 1916)

▣ D. Amaury Talbot, from *Woman's Mysteries of a Primitive People: The Ibibios of Southern Nigeria* (1915)

This is an ethnography of the Ibibio, a Nigerian tribe. Written by a pioneering Englishwoman in the early twentieth century, this book focuses on the ritual life of women. Despite the naive colonialist attitude, it presents a female perspective that was seldom seen in the ethnographic literature of the period.

From Chapter III. "Birth Customs"

In that part of the district which lies round Awa a reason is given for the killing of twins which is quite unconnected with any idea as to demoniacal origin. The following is the local account of the cause of the custom:

> The first pair of twins sent to Earth, so our mothers tell, unfortunately came to the dwelling of a family poor and of little account. When news of their arrival reached the neighbouring chiefs and members of great houses, these gathered together in much anxiety at such an unprecedented occurrence, and consulted as to what should be done. "Behold," said they, "this woman first bore one child. Now she has given birth to two together; should she continue to go on in the way in which she has begun, next time she may bear four, and after that six or even eight, and so on until her family surpasses any of ours. If poor people are allowed to grow 'strong' at such a rate, what will become of us? We shall have no chance to seize their property on the death of the head of their house, nor to force them to serve us as before when their family was small and of little account and there was none to take their part."

That, so our grandmothers tell, is the reason why the murder of twins was started in the Awa country. Had the first twins come to a rich or powerful family there would have been no killing.

> Not long afterwards the king's head wife also gave birth to a boy and a girl, and a meeting of the townsfolk was called to discuss the matter. The king and his relatives tried their utmost to save the lives of the babes, but the poor folk combined and said, "They shall be killed, as were those of our women." The more the rich strove to save the chief's twin children, the more did the poor insist upon their death, crying, "As you did to us and our babes, so will we do also unto you and yours." That is the reason why twin children were killed even unto our own day. In the country round Awa, however, no "twin mother" is ever put to death, only driven forth from her town.

With this fear before their eyes, it is natural that women about to become mothers should consult a native doctor some time before the expected birth of their babes in order to learn from him if there is any probability of the arrival of twins. Should he answer in the affirmative, medicine is given by which the danger may be averted.

Next to the dread of becoming a mother of twins looms that of bearing a child into whose body some evil spirit has entered. This may be that of ancestor or kinsman undesirable on account of bodily or mental deformity, or because they come from a family tainted with "witchcraft."

So-called "birth-marks" seem to be quite common among this people, although such are here attributed to causes different from those assigned them in northern climes. An Ibibio baby is eagerly scanned for any sign that may reveal the identity of the indwelling Ego. Parents often notice some likeness to a dead friend, or trick of speech or movement in a child that to their minds shows that it is an old spirit reborn in some new body. A striking example of the way in which such deductions are made happened at Ndiya about ten years ago, and was told as follows:

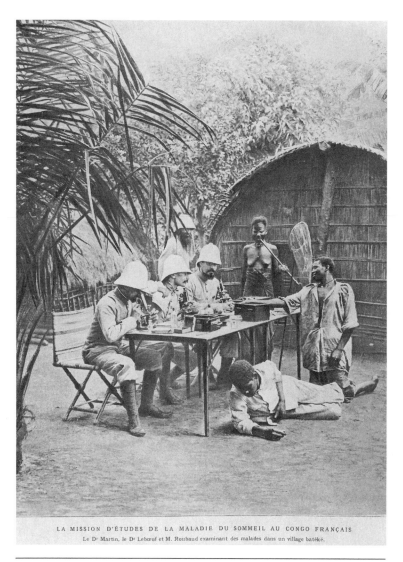

LA MISSION D'ÉTUDES DE LA MALADIE DU SOMMEIL AU CONGO FRANÇAIS
Le Dr Martin, le Dr Lebœuf et M. Roubaud examinant des malades dans un village batéké.

"Patients' Examination" during a mission studying sleeping sickness in French Congo (1907). Colonial infiltration by European powers around the globe was often accompanied by medical studies of native populations. Of particular interest were indigenous diseases that also affected European immigrants residing in these locations. Here, resident people are examined by medical authorities to better understand the nature of sleeping sickness among residents of the Congo.

Source: Art Resource, New York.

A man named Osim Essiet married a wife, and a little while before the birth of their first child he was attacked by an enemy and left lying in the bush with his head severed from his body. When he did not return, friends set out to look for him. After some time they found the corpse, bore it home and laid it upon a native bed. When the young wife saw this horrible sight, she cried out and flung herself down by the side of the body, calling upon the name of her husband and entreating him not to leave her.

Some weeks afterwards the child was born. Round his neck was the mark as of a line at the place where his father's head had been severed, and, indeed, his neck is still shorter than that of most people. The townsfolk noticed this peculiarity, and felt sure, because of it, that the boy was really Osim Essiet himself come back to life again because he loved his wife very dearly and in answer to her entreaties that she might not be left alone. They therefore gave him, in his new incarnation, the same name as he had borne before.

A somewhat similar case happened at Ikott Atako, near Eket, and is thus related:

There was once a woman of this town, Etuk Nkokk by name, who, not long after she had left the Fatting-house, bore a boy. At first the babe was like other children save that he was very weak, but as the years went on he hardly seemed to grow at all, and by the age of twenty was not quite four feet high. One day his mother went out and noticed the fine strong children born to her neighbors. When she came home, she looked gloweringly at her sickly son and said, "No other woman has a child like you! I wish you might die that I may be no more shamed by the sight of you!" Not long afterwards the boy sickened and died, and before they brought the coffin in which to lay him for burial the mother said to herself: "This piccan gave me too much trouble! I wish to find some way of punishing him and preventing him from returning to life." So she took thought, and at length cut off his right hand, saying to herself, "Now he will surely be ashamed, and not come back into my family any more."

A few months later another child was born, but lo! it was the same boy come back again, as was plain to be seen because he had only one hand. When the people went to see the mother and the new-born babe, they recognized him at once for the one who had died, and, seeing the handless wrist, asked "How could you do such a cruel thing to your firstborn?" She answered, "It was because I did not want him to come back again, and thought he would be ashamed to show himself among us thus maimed." The people said, "It is a misfortune, but it cannot be helped! This is your punishment, and you must just do your best for him." So the woman took their advice and did everything possible for the child, in consequence of which he grew up and is still alive, a little taller than during his first earth-life, but smaller than other men.

The mother of Chief Henshaw of Oron regards him as an example of reincarnation. The name Nyung, by which he is everywhere known among black people, means "thrice born"—an appellation which she gave him because her two first babes had died, and she believed that at his birth the same spirit came back once more; this time, not in vain.

The dread of the return of "wandering souls," who reincarnate only to bring trouble upon the family into which they have chosen to come, is common over the greater part of West Africa. Mary Kingsley thus describes the way in which parents seek to protect themselves against the infliction of these annoying spirits:

> When two babes in a family have previously died in suspicious circumstances the father takes the body of the third baby which has also died in the same way and smashes one of its leg bones before it is thrown away into the bush; for he knows he has got a wanderer soul—namely a *sisa.* . . . He just breaks the leg so as to warn the soul he is not a man to be trifled with, and will not have his family kept in a state of perpetual uproar and expense. It sometimes happens, however, in spite of this that when his fourth baby arrives that too goes off in convulsions. Thoroughly roused now, paterfamilias sternly takes a chopper, and chops that infant's remains extremely small, and it is scattered broadcast. Then he holds he has eliminated that sisa from his family.

I am informed, however, that the fourth baby to arrive in a family afflicted by a *sisa* does not usually go off in convulsions, but that fairly frequently it is born lame, which shows that it is that wanderer soul back with its damaged leg.

Source: Talbot, D. Amaury. 1915. Pp. 36–41 in *Woman's Mysteries of a Primitive People: The Ibibios of Southern Nigeria.* Available at: http://www.sacred-texts.com/afr/wmp/wmp00.htm

▣ Frank B. Linderman, from *Indian Why Stories* (1915)

Indian "Why Stories" were collected, translated, and written down by European missionaries and early ethnographers. They presumably helped to capture what was often pejoratively thought of as aboriginal folklore by Native American tribes in North America. The stories attempt to explain physical or cognitive differences that exist among people and other species.

How The Ducks Got Their Fine Feathers

Another night had come, and I made my way toward War Eagle's lodge. In the bright moonlight the dead leaves of the quaking-aspen fluttered down whenever the wind shook the trees; and over the village great flocks of ducks and geese and swan passed in a never-ending procession, calling to each other in strange tones as they sped away toward the waters that never freeze.

In the lodge War Eagle waited for his grandchildren, and when they had entered, happily, he laid aside his pipe and said:

"The Duck-people are travelling to-night just as they have done since the world was young. They are going away from winter because they cannot make a living when ice covers the rivers.

"You have seen the Duck-people often. You have noticed that they wear fine clothes but you do not know how they got them; so I will tell you to-night.

"It was in the fall when leaves are yellow that it happened, and long, long ago. The Duck-people had gathered to go away, just as they are doing now. The buck-deer was coming down from the high ridges to visit friends in the lowlands along the streams as they have always done. On a lake Old-man saw the Duck-people getting ready to go away, and at that time they all looked alike; that is, they all wore the same colored clothes. The loons and the geese and the ducks were there and playing in the sunlight. The loons were laughing loudly and the diving was fast and merry to see. On the hill where Old-man stood there was a great deal of moss, and he began to tear it from the ground and roll it into a great ball. When he had gathered all he needed he shouldered the load and started for the shore of the lake, staggering under the weight of the great burden. Finally the Duck-people saw him coming with his load of moss and began to swim away from the shore.

"'Wait, my brothers!' he called, 'I have a big load here, and I am going to give you people a dance. Come and help me get things ready.'

"'Don't you do it,' said the gray goose to the others; 'that's Old-man and he is up to something bad, I am sure.'

"So the loon called to Old-man and said they wouldn't help him at all.

"Right near the water Old-man dropped his ball of moss and then cut twenty long poles. With the poles he built a lodge which he covered with the moss, leaving a doorway facing the lake. Inside the lodge he built a fire and when it grew bright he cried:

"'Say, brothers, why should you treat me this way when I am here to give you a big dance? Come into the lodge,' but they wouldn't do that. Finally Old-man began to sing a song in the duck-talk, and keep time with his drum. The Duck-people liked the music, and swam a little nearer to the shore, watching for trouble all the time, but Old-man sang so sweetly that pretty soon they waddled up to the lodge and went inside. The loon stopped near the door, for he believed that what the gray goose had said was true, and that Old-man was up to some mischief. The gray goose, too, was careful to stay close to the door but the ducks reached all about the fire. Politely, Old-man passed the pipe, and they all smoked with him because it is wrong not to smoke in a person's lodge if the pipe is offered, and the Duck-people knew that.

"'Well,' said Old-man, 'this is going to be the Blind-dance, but you will have to be painted first.

"'Brother Mallard, name the colors—tell how you want me to paint you.'

"'Well,' replied the mallard drake, 'paint my head green, and put a white circle around my throat, like a necklace. Besides that, I want a brown breast and yellow legs: but I don't want my wife painted that way.'

"Old-man painted him just as he asked, and his wife, too. Then the teal and the wood-duck (it took a long time to paint the wood-duck) and the spoonbill and the blue-bill and the canvasback and the goose and the brant and the loon—all chose their paint. Old-man painted them all just as they wanted him to, and kept singing all the time. They looked very pretty in the firelight, for it was night before the painting was done.

"'Now,' said Old-man, 'as this is the Blind-dance, when I beat upon my drum you must all shut your eyes tight and circle around the fire as I sing. Every one that peeks will have sore eyes forever.'

"Then the Duck-people shut their eyes and Old-man began to sing: 'Now you come, ducks, now you come—tum-tum, tum; tum-tum, tum.'

"Around the fire they came with their eyes still shut, and as fast as they reached Old-man, the rascal would seize them, and wring their necks. Ho! things were going fine for Old-man, but the loon peeked a little, and saw what was going on; several others heard the fluttering and opened their eyes, too. The loon cried out, 'He's

killing us—let us fly,' and they did that. There was a great squawking and quacking and fluttering as the Duck-people escaped from the lodge. Ho! but Old-man was angry, and he kicked the back of the loon-duck, and that is why his feet turn from his body when he walks or tries to stand. Yes, that is why he is a cripple to-day.

"And all of the Duck-people that peeked that night at the dance still have sore eyes—just as Old-man told them they would have. Of course they hurt and smart no more but they stay red to pay for peeking, and always will. You have seen the mallard and the rest of the Duck-people. You can see that the colors Old-man painted so long ago are still bright and handsome, and they will stay that way forever and forever. Ho!"

Source: Linderman, Frank, B. [Co Skee See Co Cot]. 1915. "How the Ducks Got Their Fine Feathers." In *Indian Why Stories: Sparks from War Eagle's Lodge-Fire.* Available at: www.e-book shop.gr/gutenberg/files/inwhy10.pdf

◙ Franz Kafka, from *The Metamorphosis* (1915)

Franz Kafka (1883–1924) was born in Prague, Czechoslovakia, to a middle-class Jewish family. His works are often characterized as expressing the essential alienation of the human condition at the beginning of the twentieth century. His experience of tuberculosis played a key role in the cultivation of his distinctive absurdist fictional style, in which characters suffer profoundly from social neglect. The excerpt here from one of his most celebrated stories, The Metamorphosis, *demonstrates his profound identification with individuals whose divergent bodies and minds result in their isolation from the rest of society. Kafka spent his final years moving in and out of sanatoriums that were often indicative of the impersonal bureaucracies of modern life that he critiqued.*

As Gregor Samsa awoke one morning from uneasy dreams he found himself transformed in his bed into a gigantic insect. He was lying on his hard, as it were armor-plated, back and when he lifted his head a little he could see his domelike brown belly divided into stiff arched segments on top of which the bed quilt could hardly stay in place and was about to slide off completely. His numerous legs, which were pitifully thin compared to the rest of his bulk, waved helplessly before his eyes. . . .

First of all he wanted to get up quietly, without any excitement; get dressed; and, the main thing, have breakfast, and only then think about what to do next, for he saw clearly that in bed he would never think things through to a rational conclusion. He remembered how even in the past he had often felt some kind of slight pain, possibly caused by lying in an uncomfortable position, which, when he got up, turned out to be purely imaginary, and he was eager to see how today's fantasy would gradually fade away. That the change in his voice was nothing more than the first sign of a bad cold, an occupational ailment of the traveling salesman, he had no doubt in the least.

It was very easy to throw off the cover; all he had to do was puff himself up a little, and it fell off by itself. But after this, things got difficult, especially since he was so unusually broad. He would have needed hands and arms to lift himself up, but instead of that he had only his numerous little legs, which were in every different kind of perpetual motion and which, besides, he could not control. If he wanted to bend one, the first thing that happened was that it stretched itself out; and if he finally succeeded in getting this leg to do what he wanted, all the others in the meantime, as if set free, began to work in the most intensely painful agitation. "Just don't stay in bed being useless," Gregor said to himself.

First he tried to get out of bed with the lower part of his body, but this lower part—which by the way he had not seen yet and which he could not form a clear picture of—proved too difficult to budge; it was taking so long; and when finally, almost out of his mind, he lunged forward with all his force, without caring, he had picked the wrong direction and slammed himself violently against the lower bedpost, and the searing pain he felt taught him exactly the lower part of his body was, for the moment anyway, the most sensitive.

He therefore tried to get the upper part of his body out of bed first and warily turned his head toward the edge of the bed. This worked easily, and in spite of its width and weight, the mass of his body finally followed, slowly, the movement of his head. But when at last he stuck his head over the edge of the bed into the air, he got too scared to continue any further, since if he finally let himself fall in this position, it would be a miracle if he didn't injure his head. And just now he had better not for the life of him lose consciousness; he would rather stay in bed.

But when, once again, after the same exertion, he lay in his original position, sighing, and again

watched his little legs struggling, if possible more fiercely, with each other and saw no way of bring peace and order into this mindless motion, he again told himself that it was impossible for him to stay in bed and that the most rational thing was to make any sacrifice for even the smallest hope of freeing himself from bed. But at the same time he did not forget to remind himself occasionally that thinking things over calmly—indeed, as calmly as possible—was much better than jumping to desperate decisions. At such moments he fixed his eyes as sharply as possible on the window, but unfortunately there was little confidence and cheer to be gotten from the view of the morning fog, which shrouded even the other side of the narrow street. "Seven o'clock already" he said to himself as the alarm clock struck again, "seven o'clock already and still such a fog."

Source: Kafka, Franz. 1948. Muir, Edwin, and Willa Muir, trans. *The Metamorphosis*. In *The Penal Colony: Stories and Short Pieces*. New York: Schocken. (Originally published 1915)

Ada M. Fitts, "Classes and Institutions" (1916)

This excerpt comes from a paper read at the National Conference of Charities and Correction, Indianapolis, Indiana, May 1916, and at the National Educational Association, New York City, July 1916. Ada M. Fitts was the Supervisor of Special Classes for Boston, Massachusetts. The essay identifies various scenarios for educating children diagnosed as feebleminded.

The problem of feeble-mindedness is very much before the public, and everywhere in this country, community surveys, the use of mental tests and studies of family histories are furnishing evidence that the feeble-minded are an increasingly important factor in all forms of social and educational work.

Along with the other agencies that are interested in finding a solution to this far reaching problem, the public school authorities have become aroused and are providing classes which it is hoped will furnish training for pupils who are not able to make good in the regular grades. Before discussing my subject: "How to Fill the Gap Between the Special Classes and Institutions," I wish to review what the public schools have attempted to do in preparation for this time of leaving school. It is generally believed that the special

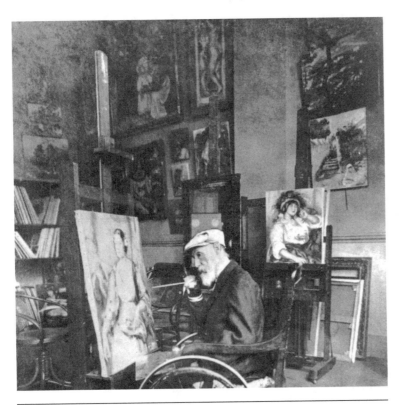

Photograph of Auguste Renoir at his easel (1914). From 1898 onward, Renoir (1841–1919) experienced bouts of rheumatoid arthritis, which ultimately worked its way to his legs and hands. He continued to paint, often in his studio from his bed, while wedging his brushes between his fingers or binding them with tape. As his paralysis increased, he turned from painting to sculpture, where he would employ an assistant to form the clay to his specifications.

Source: Art Resource, New York.

class is the first step in the attempt to solve the problem. Its function is first: to educate the community and the teachers of normal children to realize the situation; second: to seek out the feeble-minded children and help them, and by so doing, help the normal children who have been retarded; third: to relieve the teacher who gives perhaps thirty percent, of her energy to the few feeble-minded pupils she may have. This energy is taken from her normal pupils and does not materially benefit the feeble-minded, as only in the special class can we do our best for these children; fifth, to secure justice to society, for it is a matter of social justice that the feeble-minded be recognized and trained as far as it is possible to do so.

The pupils should be selected by a trained expert who uses a combination of tests and who will win the confidence of parents as well as give a diagnosis of the child's mental and physical condition. In many places the high grade improvable feeble-minded children have been selected by such experts and then placed in classes under the direction of trained teachers. The number of pupils in a class is wisely limited to fifteen to a teacher, and through individual work she tries to fit her pupils for adult life. Special classes take feeble-minded children as early as possible—say—from seven to eight years of age. Some eventually return to grade and are able to complete a part of the fourth grade work; a few more are transferred directly to the institution; but the majority should remain in special classes till they reach the school age limit.

Three methods have been adopted: first, to have the special class occupy a room in an elementary school building and care for the mentally defective children of that immediate district; second, to group these pupils in a central school; and third, a combination of both individual classes and centers. In Massachusetts until recently, children were allowed to leave school at fourteen, but with the raising of the compulsory school age limit to sixteen, we found ourselves (two years ago) face to face with the problem of what to do with the special class children who must remain in school until they are sixteen years of age. In Boston in order to provide the next necessary step beyond the individual class, the regular grade pupils occupying two six-room buildings, were accommodated elsewhere and these buildings were used as centers: one for special class girls and another for special class boys. Pupils for these centers were selected from individual classes all over the city (one or two from each) as their fitness to profit by this special advantage was recognized. The separation of the sexes has proved to be of distinct advantage both to pupils and teachers, thus adding to the efficiency of the work. Little difficulty has been experienced thus far in transportation over long distances, the city paying the car fares.

At the centers advanced manual work is begun and grading and classification are possible. The program is so arranged that each child has one and one-half hours physical, one and one-half hours academic, and two hours manual work each day. The girls are given a trained teacher to instruct them in domestic science, millinery, sewing, embroidery, crocheting, knitting, mending and preserving. The boys are taught brush making, boot blacking, woodworking, serving of lunches, dish washing, simple tailoring, gardening, assistant janitor work, and other forms of comparatively unskilled labor. In this way we attempt to carry on the training of special class children from seven to sixteen years of age.

The special class, in my opinion, should be still further supplemented by workrooms where, under favorable conditions, pupils over sixteen may be provided with work for which they would be paid. Cobbling, chair caning, tool sharpening, brush and mat making, are industries which might be carried on profitably. They could thus be guarded and controlled in part without being taken from their homes. This brings up the question of how long the public schools should assume the responsibility of these children beyond the school age limit. It seems to me that it should do so for another year or two at least, unless there is some other agency ready to do the work. The school funds are used for work with adults in continuation and evening schools and centers—why not for the much needed work with the feeble-minded?

The most important factor is the teacher who presides over the special class. She must be one who is quick to perceive, able to adapt, whose sympathies are keen and whose outlook is broad, but who combines with these gifts, steadiness of purpose and the power to raise and hold her pupil to his best. A sense of humor will help out in many a situation. In Boston the teachers are given time in which to visit the children's homes, learn the conditions and confer with the parents. The teacher knows how much freedom can safely be given the child; she knows his limitations and when work is undertaken for which he is not adapted, she is able to suggest other lines. She could keep in touch with him and advise him as need arose, if she had the time; but the demands of her classroom are all that should be asked of her strength. In some cities, visiting teachers whose function is that of social workers have done this work most acceptably.

Most will agree that the ideal condition would be for many of the mentally defective to go from the school directly to the institution, and thus safeguard the public from inefficiency, unemployment, pauperism, vagrancy, degeneracy, and all the other social consequences of feeblemindedness. Since this is impossible, we must attempt to fill the gap between the special class and the institution by providing a system of after-care for the feeble-minded who are forced to compete with the normal in the working world. As has been said "It is not sufficient for society that the subnormal should be properly trained in school; it is the business of someone to see that they meet the difficulties of the earn-a-living world. It is of small use to train laboriously in school for shop or farm and then see the graduate enter messenger service or other unskilled and spasmodic labor. Pioneers are needed to make this new adjustment, to study the situation, plan for it, and to enter into it. It is time for them to think together, plan together, and for others to help put the results of the deliberation into operation."

The child may have been prepared for appropriate employment, but he cannot be given the necessary power of self-direction. The subnormal person (young or old) does not have that guiding power within; he must have outside control that should never be relaxed. The need is for a person or persons who will provide this oversight and follow the career of each individual, continuing the guidance begun by the teacher. He should be closely connected with the representatives of various educational, religious, philanthropic, civic and medical organizations. This person should be strong, tactful, persistent one who has been a teacher of mentally defective children and also, if possible, with training as a social worker. The after-care work would naturally divide into two parts: first, the obtaining of information about pupils; second, oversight of pupils at work and knowledge of where suitable positions can be secured. In order to do this it would be necessary to canvass the employers of comparatively unskilled labor to arrange to have notifications sent the officer when there are vacancies to be filled. . . .

At the Massachusetts School for the Feeble-Minded at Waverley, Dr. Fernald is making a careful after-care study of all the patients who have been discharged from the school for the past twenty-five years. He says: "Wherever it is possible our field-workers have visited these patients and the fullest inquiry has been made as to the kind of life they have lived since leaving the institution. The inquiry was planned primarily to furnish a basis of evolution as to the practical results given at the school. The inquiry also sought information as to the social, economic and moral life of the feeble-minded individual in the community."

Source: Fitts, Ada, M. 1916. "Classes and Institutions." From the Smith Ely Jeliffe Collection, proprietor Dr. David Braddock, University of Colorado, Boulder.

▣ Carl Sandburg, "Cripple" (1916)

Carl Sandburg (1878–1967) was a Chicago-based poet well known for his depictions of midwestern life. In poems such as "Cripple," he metaphorized disability as a sign of the ravages of industrialization on the body. Additionally, Sandburg used images of Nature as a sign of robust health compared to the decrepitude of the life of an individual with disability.

Once when I saw a cripple
Gasping slowly his last days with the white plague,
Looking from hollow eyes, calling for air,
Desperately gesturing with wasted hands
In the dark and dust of a house down in a slum,
I said to myself
I would rather have been a tall sunflower
Living in a country garden
Lifting a golden-brown face to the summer,
Rain-washed and dew-misted,
Mixed with the poppies and ranking hollyhocks,
And wonderingly watching night after night
The clear silent processionals of stars.

Source: Sandburg, Carl. 1916. "Cripple." In *Chicago Poems.* New York: Henry Holt and Company. Available at: http://www.bartleby.com/165/26.html

▣ Captain Arthur H. Samuels on Disabled Veterans (1918)

The author of this piece argues that what the general public, and particularly businessmen and employers, owe disabled veterans is not charity, but a job, and a continuing commitment in the postwar period to see to it that the private sector does its part to reintegrate these men, after government programs have rehabilitated and retrained them.

"After the war, if a cripple stops me on the street and asks for help," said a philanthropic business man in New York recently, "how can I tell whether he is a real veteran or just an impostor? Of course, I always want to give something to the boys who went over the top. Will they wear a button to show that they've been soldiers?"

And the answer was this: "Any man who stops you and asks for alms is a beggar whether he was in the war or not. No buttons or insignia will be necessary."

This New Yorker had naïvely got at the very roots of reconstruction. Thousands of men and women everywhere are puzzled over the same thing, for the public does not yet understand the distinction between the cripple who can make good if he wants to, and the beggar who *could* make good but *doesn't* want to.

The gap is wide; and one of the most difficult and vital tasks confronting the Government and the other forces involved in the problem is to reconstruct the public attitude: to destroy utterly the worn-out notion about the cripple and to teach the new.

Picture a soldier who has lost both legs walking—he *will* walk—into the president's office of an industrial plant, where he is received cordially and with honor.

"It happened in the Toul sector," he says "about a year and a half ago and it was nine months before I was discharged from the hospital with these artificial legs. But early in the game I made up my mind to make good. I couldn't go back to railroading—I used to be a conductor—so I decided to take up stenography and typewriting. The Government gave me a fine course, everything I needed. I am qualified to hold down a secretarial job and I need one right now. I can't afford to be idle."

The president who really admired his caller, listened politely. He liked the man's personality. He reached for his check book.

"We are proud of men like you," he said as he wrote, "and you deserve to succeed. Here's fifty dollars. I'm sorry I haven't a position open. Good luck to you. You deserve success."

Now the ex-soldier was human and he accepted the money. He shouldn't have done so. But he is not the one to be blamed. The president, unwittingly, did a vicious thing by offering it to him and every man or woman who gives alms but not opportunity to the disabled man—soldier, sailor, or civilian—is an enemy of reconstruction. One gift of money that is not actually earned may utterly stifle the ambition of the handicapped man.

Business men must be told this again and again. The American public must know that their Government has provided a fair compensation and insurance for the wounded, which, with vocational training, provide our returned soldiers and sailors with adequate means to re-enter civil life. There is a general appreciation of the fact that our men will not be turned loose and allowed to drift as after former wars, but it is natural that a subject so new and complicated has got to be explained, iterated, and reiterated.

This is being done today in an infinite number of ways. The various forces that create and guide public opinion in America are at work enthusiastically and wholeheartedly, offering every possible means of cooperation. For after all, reconstruction is not a matter of propaganda to be jammed through: it is news—one of the biggest pieces of news that has yet found its way into the channels of national publicity.

Newspapers, magazines, motion pictures, pamphlets, speeches—these and other mediums are bringing reconstruction and its significance into the American home and American industry. The Office of the Surgeon General, the American Red Cross, and the Federal Board for Vocational Education are small portion of the factors making it known.

The success of this great plan will depend on the attitude of the public. Public opinion is a pretty loose term as it is generally applied. In this instance, however, it is pat, because it represents several very definite and concrete elements—the man himself, his family, his friends, and his employers. Sympathy and encouragement are plentiful these days while we are in the throes of the conflict, but they will be difficult to maintain when the thrill of battle has passed and the nation has settled down to its normal activities. And after the war—long after—they will be needed most.

Men and women of America by word-of-mouth, house-to-house publicity based on what they read and hear are rapidly developing a new psychology toward the handicapped. Gradually they are reconstructing themselves. And the more thoughtful are beginning to comprehend that physical reconstruction and vocational training will not stop with the coming of peace, but will become powerful and permanent factors in American society and industry.

Source: Samuels, Captain Arthur H. 1918. "Reconstructing the Public." *Carry-On* 1:15–16. [The editors acknowledge the assistance of John Kinder of the University of Minnesota in sharing this document.]

◉ Violet Jacob, "Kirsty's Opeenion" (1918)

In this Scots dialect poem, Violet Jacob (1863–1946) portrays the changed domestic arrangements of the disabled World War I veteran after his return home. In the last lines, the reader is assured that the wife has not become less quarrelsome in consideration of her husband's lost limb; instead, the poet declares that his military experience itself has simply made him less susceptible to nagging.

Fine div I ken what ails yon puddock, Janet,
That aince wad hae her neb set up sae hie;
There's them that disna seem to understaun it,
I'se warrant ye it's plain eneuch to me!

Mibbie ye'll mind her man-a fine wee cratur,
Ower blate to speak (puir thing, he didna daur);
What garred him fecht was jist his douce-like natur;
Gairmans is bad, but Janet's tongue was waur.

But noo he's hame again, ye wadna ken her,
He isna feared to contradick her flet;
He smokes a' day, comes late to get his denner,
(I mind the time she'd sort him weel for that!)

What's garred her turn an tak a road divairgint?
Ye think she's wae because he wants a limb?
Ach! haud yer tongue, ye fuil—the man's a sair-gint,
An there's nae argy-bargyin wi him!

Source: Jacob, Violet. 1918. "Kirsty's Opeenion." In *More Songs of Angus and Others.* Available at: http://www.scotstext.org/makars/violet_jacob/poems.asp

◉ Office of the Surgeon General, "War Cripple Axioms and Fundamentals" (1918)

This document summarizes the influential views of Douglas C. McMurtrie, the director of the Red Cross Institute for Crippled and Disabled Men and editor of the American Journal of Care for Cripples, on the proper assumptions to adopt in order to direct the work of rehabilitation and reintegration of disabled World War I veterans. McMurtrie, along with rehabilitation professionals in every major nation at war at the time, believed that aggressive normalization through systematic vocational retraining must be the basis of any program for rehabilitation of men injured or made chronically ill in consequence of service during the war.

Part 1. Public Policy: The Modern Program of Assistance and Benefit Disabled Veterans in the Twentieth Century

21. To complete physical rehabilitation in amputation cases, artificial limbs must be supplied. That a stump shrinks for some time after amputation introduces one

element of difficulty, in that a limb that fits six months after amputation may come far from doing so after twelve months. For this reason it may be wise to provide the soldier at first with a simple temporary limb, and later with a more elaborate and permanent one. He must be quite explicitly assured of this plan, however, as he will otherwise become suspicious of being put off with an inferior article.

22. Employment of the graduates must be closely integrated with [that] secured for the re-educated soldier, but he must be placed as intelligently as possible. To the man the work must be satisfactory and the environment agreeable; to the employer the personality of the soldier must be acceptable and his product sufficient to the requirements. Of course, this ideal can only be approximated, but a trained and capable employment officer can do much in this direction. Only by skilled and thorough work can permanent results be obtained—and nothing is more costly to all parties concerned than short-time employment and frequent change of job.

23. The first job for the man returned from the front is easy to secure—so easy that we should not be misled by the superficial indications. The employer is patriotic and anxious to help the crippled soldiers. But when the war shall have been over a few years, these motives will be no longer effective. The man taken on in a time of national stress will be just one of the employees, and his retention in service will depend upon performance alone. If the original placement was intelligent the man will have made progress, gained confidence and experience and made his position sure. If, on the other hand, he was ill-fitted for the job, he will have grown progressively less efficient and in consequent discouraged, and his status will be precarious indeed. A permanent injury might thus result from an employment bungle in the first instance. All this simply means that effective placement is not an amateur job.

24. The support and direction of after-care for the war cripple is most emphatically a national one. This can be demonstrated not only as a matter of principle but also by actual experiential results.

From the viewpoint of principle, it may be concluded that the returned soldier should not be dependent for one of his most vital necessities on the dole of private charity, for which is expected a grateful appreciation.

25. The training schools should be under public control and have the advantage of central direction by expert and capable executives. There is also no riper field for the expression of mawkish sentimentality than in caring for the crippled or blind, and the injured soldier must be protected from becoming its victim. With schools operated under local auspices there would be a few good ones, and many of the indifferent variety. And there is no problem more delicate than that of coping with ill-directed and silly charitable enterprises.

26. The chief advantage accruing from centralized public control is the character the work then assumes in its relation to the individual war cripples. It is regarded much as is the public school system; the solder is thus entitled to training by virtue of his rights as a citizen and an honorable public servant. There is of charity no taint whatever.

With an acknowledged national responsibility, the facilities provided can keep pace with—or, indeed, ahead of—the requirements. The work can be carried out on a plan fixed in advance, and its standards be consistent country-wide.

27. Another advantage of federal control lies in the simplicity of integration between the medical and educational interests. The former is under military and, therefore, national authority, and simplification of procedure cannot but result from having the latter of less scope. The training classes must in many instances be carried on in medical institutions, as there is a considerable period of convalescence in which the men should be under re-education.

28. One of the principal methods of restoring disabled soldiers to health is the prescription of specified exercise, and it has been found that this is best gained in workshops rather than with mechanotherapeutic apparatus. Finding that they can do some practical thing, however simple, is immensely encouraging to men who may have lost hope of future usefulness. Occupational therapy plays now one of the leading roles in the convalescent treatment of the wounded, and this makes all the more desirable a close relation between the two branches of the work.

29. A central and national direction of the work for war cripples does not in the least prelude the utilization of volunteer effort and facilities. In fact, voluntary contribution of time and money is highly desirable, particularly in committing more people to a first-hand interest in the enterprise, and in giving the schools root in their local communities. Buildings can be loaned, trade school classrooms and equipment made available, machinery and apparatus for instruction

donated, funds contributed, and personal service volunteered. Existing organizations can offer to provide the necessary social service work in the homes of the men; local employment agencies can be of help by acting [as] links in the national chain.

30. Such private assistance will be more than desirable; it will be essential. Because provision for war cripples is a temporary problem and it would not be wise to erect new buildings, equip expensive machine shops, and build up a complete and self-sufficient organization for a few years' work. For trade classes it will be better to obtain the use for part time of shops in existing schools—institutions which will be in position to afford such facilities on account of the number of their regular students who will have been called to arms. In England, the technical institutes are being wisely used; in France, many war cripples are being instructed in the regular schools of agriculture.

Source: U.S. War Department, Office of the Surgeon General. 1918. "War Cripple Axioms and Fundamentals." Record Group 112, U.S. National Archives.

▣ Alice Duer Miller, "How Can a Woman Best Help?" (1918)

Rehabilitation professionals were keenly aware that a particularly important private agent in the reintegration of the disabled veteran was his mother, wife, or girlfriend. By pampering him, a woman could sap his will to become self-supporting and encourage him to feel it was his right to be taken care of for the rest of his life. On the other hand, by accepting partnership with the government in encouraging him to help himself, a woman was an especially significant influence on the normalization of his postdisability life.

Practical experience of the war shows that the degree to which a soldier can recover is in a large measure a question of his state of mind; and his state of mind is usually a reflection of the state of mind of his wife or his mother. Women have always known in a general way that mental attitude has much to do with a patient's recovery in ordinary illness. Now we see that the same thing is true of the man who has contracted tuberculosis, has been blinded, has lost an arm or a leg, or is suffering from any of the physical or mental diseases that war leaves in its wake. The hope of his future lies in making him believe he has a future. His return to useful activity depends on his own conviction that he can be useful. The instant he is content to be an invalid he will become and remain an invalid.

To prevent his losing hope, to keep up his sense of responsibility is in the power of his womankind. That is why it is necessary that every woman who has a man on the other side should understand what the government is trying to do for him, why it is doing it, and how she can help.

First of all she ought to know that each man's pension will be continued however little or much he progresses on the road to health and self-support. The government does this not only from a sense of justice, but because, knowing that recovery is largely a mental state, it realizes that it would be setting up an obstacle, if it should penalize a man for recovering by taking away or even decreasing his pension.

Then, women should see that the government is doing this for the sake of the wounded men themselves. Protection of the health of soldiers while they are part of the fighting force, is for the sake of the army. But this re-education of wounded men for civil life is done in the interest of the individual. In past times, governments have found it cheaper to entomb such men in institutions for incurables and in soldiers' homes—to pay them their pensions and forget about them. The present idea is that the country owes them more than their pensions; it owes them the fullest possible return to a normal life.

But in order to return them to normal life it will be necessary to retain control of them beyond the military hospital. There must first come bedside treatment, of course—the direct medical or surgical treatment for the disease or wound; then the special treatment necessary to fit him for his selected occupation; then, outside the hospital, his training in a vocational school; and then at last his entrance upon his industrial job.

In every step the help of women is essential; not only in cheering him during the first stages, but in encouraging him to follow patiently and exactly the detail of his training—a routine more wearisome to many natures than fighting.

Our government asks that we use our love to strengthen the will of our wounded—not to weaken it. This may sound like a harsh thing to say to a woman who has sent out a strong healthy man and receives him back blinded or crippled, until we remember that the object of it is to save the soldier and to keep alive in him the courage that was by no means all expended at the front.

The shock to the man who wakes up after the operation to find that he has lost an arm or a leg is not only the shock of his own handicap, but the horror of being a dependent—something useless and abnormal. Too much sympathy of the wrong kind intensifies this feeling, instead of decreasing it. And as a matter of fact, it isn't true; with the help of modern science, the handicapped man can still attain a high degree of usefulness and activity.

The recovery of our disabled soldiers—their return to a useful life—is in the control of the women of this country. No war work that has ever been offered to us is as important—or perhaps as difficult.

But it can be done only with the help of women—only if wives and mothers and sisters will give as much pride and self-sacrifice to the return of their men to civil life as they gave to sending them away to the colors.

Source: Miller, Alice Duer. 1918. "How Can a Woman Best Help?" *Carry-On* 1:17–18. [The editors acknowledge the assistance of John Kinder of the University of Minnesota in sharing this document.]

◨ Two Cripples, "The Sluggard and the Ant" (1918)

Those advancing the new program of aggressive normalization knew that without the cooperation of the public and the disabled veterans themselves, they would not get very far in reintegrating men as self-supporting citizens in the economy and in society. In this selection, we see the effort to shift the terms of the discourse about the character of the ideal disabled veteran ("the ant") away from the tradition that conceived him as a warrior and hero and toward a vision of the veteran as uncomplaining, hardworking, resilient, and—perhaps above all else—industrious. By contrast, "the sluggard" wants to be taken care of by a government pension and to have his children work for him.

The Sluggard

One of my arms below the elbow was shot off in an accident. The other arm was shot off nearer the hand. I cannot and I have not been able to do any work myself. Fortunately for me, I was and am able to control my children who did my work as

I directed them. Otherwise I should have been an object of charity. That is how I made my success at farming.

Injured soldiers should live on a pension. Other people should follow gainful occupations.

The Ant

I have both arms off, my right arm is taken off at the shoulder joint and of the left arm I have a three-inch stump, and you have no idea how much this stump helps out. I am farming 180 acres; I have 80 in corn and 80 in oats every year. I have a married man working for me. I always pay my hired help well and keep them satisfied and interested in my work. I plow corn with a riding cultivator, haul corn, or anything, drive the binder when cutting oats, the mower when cutting hay; in fact, everything my hired man does but hitching and harnessing the horses, milking the cows, and a few odd jobs; but while he is doing the rest of the work I am feeding the hogs, horses, and cows and tending to business affairs. I do the feeding by taking a scoop shovel on my shoulder and holding it with my hand and chin and it does not hurt or bother me in the least.

I do my own planting of corn and sowing of oats. Of course, I have things fixed and made handy for me. All the doors and gates are made so I can open them.

I do all my driving with the lines over my shoulder. I drive four and five horses abreast by hitching them so I can drive them all with just two lines. I learn how to do new things every day. I can drive a Ford car as good as any one, cranking it with my feet. Since my accident I have bought 120 acres of land, have not quite paid for it yet, but expect to in three years.

I also have gotten married and, of course, a man in my condition needs a wife. We have a little boy four and a half years old who is also a great comfort to me. I never allow myself to get the blues or discouraged. I try to always look on the bright side of things. I find it helps me. I pay my bills and keep my credit good, and whenever I need money I can get it, and that is what it takes to make the farm go. I do all my own correspondence and write my checks with the pencil between my teeth. I think I have given you a-plenty but there are many things that I can do that I have not written, and if I can help you any in the future will be glad to do so.

Source: Anonymous ["by Two Cripples"]. 1918. "The Sluggard and the Ant," *Carry-On* 1:9.

Douglas C. McMurtrie, from *The Disabled Soldier* (1919)

During and the immediately after World War I, Douglas McMurtrie surveyed the emergence of programs of vocational rehabilitation in all of the major nations at war, including the enemy belligerents, Germany and its allies, whose efforts he admired greatly for their professionalism and dedication, even as he acknowledged the official state of animosity. In these three selections, McMurtrie traces the inception and development during the war of the idea that aggressive normalization is the best method of rehabilitation. He acknowledges the different mix of national and local factors in each example, accounting, to varying degrees in each case, for the relevance of prior programs of assistance to disabled soldiers, wartime contingencies such as labor shortages and fiscal difficulties, the nature of the industrial infrastructure, and the state of public opinion regarding both disability and veterans.

Chapter XIV

Kingdom and Dominion

When England sent her first "contemptible little army" to the continent in defense of the violated rights of Belgium, it was followed not alone by more British but by troops from every corner of the globe. In every dominion of the empire troops were enlisted to "fight for the right" as the home country had seen it, and were dispatched to the front as fast as circumstances allowed.

Great Britain and every one of her dominions, in consequence of their heroic stand for the benefit of civilization, have had to face the problem of the returning disabled soldier. In the solutions attained by these commonwealths, dealing as they have with Anglo-Saxons, men of similar traditions, habits, and impulses as ourselves, the United States must find peculiar interest and derive unusual profit from the showing of their experience.

When the first British disabled began to return to the streets of London, there was scant provision for their care.

Now to every British soldier who lies in the hospital ward three possibilities are open—a visit from the dark-winged Messenger, a period of convalescence and the buckling on again of the sword for another thrust at the Hun, or "Blighty," the old familiar haunts, an economic crutch in the shape of a pension, and a job suited to his physical limitations. As surely as the stricken deer seeks the familiar glades so does the discharged warrior turn his halting steps to the sheep downs of the south or the smoky towns of Lancashire, the heather hills of Scotland, the mines of Cardiff, or the long, long way to *Tipperary.*

If we could visualize the procession of maimed and disabled men in mufti as it leaves the discharge depot we would see it melt away into the economic horizon of every portion of the United Kingdom, to carry to each county, borough, and town the problem of the care of the disabled man as a legacy of the Great War for the stability of those free institutions the Anglo-Saxon prizes above life or sound limbs. And in each and every district he will find that provision has been made to continue his medical treatment, choose for him an occupation suited to the abridgement of his powers, and induct him into it after proper training. Should he be in doubt as to his rights under the new and unusual laws of the realm, the Local Pensions Committee stands ready to secure his rights, succor his family, and educate him to surmount the handicap the enemies of civilization have laid upon him. And this, not because England thought this out as the best way to care for her disabled heroes, but because it chimed in with her way of doing things in the past. Local government has always been a cherished prerogative of the English commonwealth since the days of the petty kingdoms. A representative government may sketch its plans in the large, but the English community must be given a free hand in filling in the local training of disabled soldiers.

So when the Disabled Sailors' and Soldiers' Committee reported to Parliament in 1915 that "the care of the sailors and soldiers, who have been disabled in the war, is an obligation which should fall primarily upon the state" and that body passed the Naval and Military War Pensions Act in 1915 to provide for "the care of officers and men disabled in consequence of the present war," the plan proposed to commit the disabled man to the care of a local committee of his own townsmen. To be sure, later developments of the plan necessitated modifications of this scheme in the interests of coordinated measures for the economic welfare of the realm, but this is essentially the genius of the English plan—local responsibility for bringing the opportunities afforded by the government to the door of each disabled man.

Specific instances of like care [are] not wanting. The Incorporated Soldiers' and Sailors' Help Society, which was established under royal patronage at the close of the South African War, had sought to aid the ex-service man in finding employment by furnishing him with the name of a "friend" in each parish or ward throughout the empire. The Old Age Pensions scheme of the state was administered by local committees in every borough and urban district having a population of 20,000 or over. The necessities of the families of the enlisted men had long been looked after by the Soldiers' and Sailors' Families Association by a ramification of local committees composed largely of clergymen and ladies of leisure in all parts of the country.

It was quite natural, therefore, that Parliament should look to a local committee to take the hand of the disabled man and lead him all the way back to a life of productive and contented activity. It was thought that the necessities of each man could best be assessed and provided for by a committee of his townsmen familiar with the conditions that environed him and his family. The soundness of this principle cannot be questioned, and while it may not make for uniformity it at least has the advantage of intimacy. It is the recognition of a principle, expressed many times in Parliamentary debate and charity organization, that in dealing with individuals in widely differing stations in life and with peculiar necessities, a human element must somehow be provided which the uniformity of governmental regulations does not permit. The human element—a quick sympathy, an intimate knowledge of a disabled man's circumstances, a way to help [those] unfamiliar to rules of a bureau—this can be supplied best by the local committees.

And so England followed the blazed trail of private philanthropic organizations and established Local Pensions Committees in every county, county borough, and urban district having a population of not less than 50,000. The committees are responsible to the Ministry of Pensions, which establishes rules and regulations to secure uniformity in the provisions they make for the men committed to their care. The appointment of these committees is largely left to the local authorities, but in general they must include some women, some representatives of labor, and members of the Soldiers' and Sailors' Families Association, and of the Soldiers' and Sailors' Help Society. A salaried secretary appointed by the Ministry of Pensions is a kind of liaison officer between the local body and the central office.

The duties of the Local Pensions Committee are broadly sketched in the instructions of the Ministry of Pensions: "The local committee should regard themselves as responsible for all discharged men of this class (i.e., disabled) living in their area. They should make it their business to get in touch with every such man, whether or not he has obtained employment or occupation since his discharge, and see that the treatment or training which his condition needs is secured for him when he needs it. . . . It is vitally important both in the man's interest and in that of the Nation that any case which needs either treatment or training should be taken in hand at once. Local committees must not be content with dealing only with the men who happen to present themselves to them for assistance; they must see that they have information as to the condition of all discharged pensioners in their areas, and make it a point of getting in touch with them directly they are discharged."

The committee is to be guided in its decisions in regard to suitable training for a man by several considerations. His previous occupation must have weight. The proposed occupation must be suitable to his age, disablement, and physical condition. If any recommendation as to his training has been indicated on his notification of award for pension or by a hospital visitor, this must be considered. Not least of the factors entering into a solution of the problem before the committee must be the opportunities for a living wage in the occupation chosen for him.

It must be quite clear that if the local committee were left to its own devices wholly in choosing an occupation for the man the result in the field of industry might be disastrous. The influx of a large number of disabled men into a particular occupation without some standard of training might arouse antagonisms that would be unfortunate. This necessitated some rulings by the central office in the interests of coordinated effort. Both the employers of labor and the work people must have some voice in the matter, especially in a country whose labor organization has made such strides. The necessary machinery was provided by the Ministry of Pensions cooperating with the ministry of Labor. Trade Advisory Committees have been appointed *for most of the principal trades*. Each committee is composed of an equal number of employers and work people. It is the duty of each committee to advise the Ministry of Pensions as to conditions under which the training of men in that trade can best be given, the best methods of training, the suitable centers for it, and in general to secure uniformity in the training. The numerous reports already issued contain a valuable fund of information regarding the trade from the viewpoint of the man who is physically handicapped. The analysis of an industry with the man with abridged powers in view is a phase of industrial efficiency that the war has developed. Never again can the old laissez faire policy of allowing the handicapped man to stumble along the industrial road undirected and unassisted prevail. Society cannot again close its eyes to this waste of human efficiency and the heartbreak of the man whose work powers are unappreciated because of some physical abridgement he has suffered.

The question of wages to be paid to a disabled man will always be a vexing problem. Where a disabled man can do his full stint of the work and compete with his normal fellows, he should plainly receive the equal wages whether he is receiving a pension or not. But there are grounds for debate when the man is physically unable to perform a full task either in hours or output. The inevitable tendency will be for the employer to depreciate the man's ability. The exploitation of the disabled man, especially when he is receiving a pension, is feared by organized labor, jealous of its wage standards. An effort has been made to provide machinery for obviating his difficulty. The Ministry of Labor has set up in the principal industrial centers advisory wages boards composed of representatives of employers and work people and three members of the Local Pensions Committee. This committee is to advise the local committee, or an employer desirous of employing a handicapped man, what would be an equitable wage in his particular case, taking into consideration the man's physical capacity and the current rate of wages for the industry in that locality. The question of a man's pension is not to be taken into account. The committee acts purely in an advisory capacity, but it is hoped by these means to provide against the exploitation of cripples or the lowering of trade standards.

It is the duty of the Local Pensions Committee to provide facilities for the training of its disabled ex-service men. It was soon seen that the training facilities of a larger area than that within the jurisdiction of most local committees must be made available if the variety of occupations demanded were to be provided. So Joint Advisory Committees, composed of the representatives of local committees, were formed in 1916 to arrange comprehensive schemes for utilizing the

facilities for technical education within whole counties or groups of counties. Twenty-two of these joint committees were formed in the United Kingdom. They surveyed the technical facilities in their respective districts and syndicated them in the interests of all.

For many years the British government has had local technical schools, and the result has been a surprisingly large number of institutions where one or more trades are taught. These trades cover the principal industries of the country. The number of technical schools in the industrial counties of Lancashire and Yorkshire is particularly noticeable. Both of these counties formulated ambitious schemes for the training of disabled men in every variety of industry pertaining to the soil, the mine, the factory, and the sea. The cooperation of all the principal technical schools in the training of disabled men was secured. The offer of facilities seems to have greatly exceeded the demand.

Not only have the technical schools been utilized for re-education but many men have been trained directly in workshops and factories. The plan advocated by several of the trades advisory committees provides that a man shall spend part of his time at a school and part of his time in actual work in a factory or workshop; by this means a balance is maintained between the theoretical and the practical.

It must not be supposed that every man returns to his home district absolutely unprepared for an altered industrial career. Many of the men avail themselves of the opportunities afforded by the workshops connected with the hospitals in which they have spent their period of convalescence. Early in the history of the war lucrative workshops were established in the hospitals of Roehampton and Brighton, whither men who have suffered some amputation are sent. Major Mitchell, the director of one of the leading technical institutes, was chosen to direct the courses. The therapeutic value of manual work has been fully recognized, and many a man, invited to busy himself in a workshop with the tools of a man's job ready to his hands, has not only found a stimulus to the functional activity of injured members but has actually learned a trade while waiting for nature to heal his wounds and the government to furnish him with an artificial limb. Not every man avails himself of the opportunities offered him in the hospital and must look to his local committee to furnish the opportunities for training he slighted or to supplement his training by continuations courses.

Upon his discharge from military service the disabled man is granted a pension based upon the degree of physical disability he has suffered and is free to return to his home locality. His future lies within the advisory jurisdiction of his Local Pensions Committee acting for the ministry of Pensions. He may choose to live a life of inactivity depending for a scanty subsistence upon the slender stipend granted him by the Ministry of Pensions. He may accept a job ready to his hand, because of acute industrial conditions caused by the war, from which he is likely to be ousted by the return of able-bodied men upon the demobilization of the army. Or, he may accept training at the expense of the state and become a skilled worker with better prospects of continued employment when normal times return. The good sense of the man and the persuasiveness of the local committee will largely determine what course he is to pursue.

If he elects to take training he will receive, during the time required for his re-education up to six months, his total disability pension together with a family allowance, all necessary fees will be paid for him and at the end of his course he will receive a bonus for each week of training. The state cares for both himself and his family during his period of re-education. At the end of his course he will be fortified against the exigencies of the future by the wages he can earn at a skilled trade and the regular pension to which his injuries entitle him. It is expressly stipulated that his pension shall never suffer diminution because of his increased earning capacity. Many disabled men are now receiving from this dual source larger incomes than they enjoyed before they entered the service of their country.

The demand for disabled men who have received training has been so great that no difficulty has been found in finding employment for them. The admirable system of state labor exchanges provides the facilities for placing disabled men in industry and their services will be in still greater demand when peace returns and conditions of employment are greatly altered by the return of men from the front.

While the preparation of disabled men to enter into competition with their normal fellows seems to promise the best results on the whole, still it must be recognized that many men with severe physical limitations must be provided for in special institutions under favorable work conditions. Specialized machinery and carefully planned team work can make productive units of badly handicapped men with whom

the average employer is not willing to bother. Large provision for this class of men has been made by the Lord Roberts' Workshops, which are being multiplied in different parts of the country. Some ten years before the war the Soldiers' and Sailors' Help Society opened workshops in London to provide employment for disabled ex-service men for whom it was extremely difficult to find work. The work has been greatly expanded since the war, and the enterprise has taken the name of the nation's military idol, who was greatly interested in the project. Toy-making, with the many processes involved, has been found a suitable industry for many types of disability, and the enterprise has been successfully conducted on a sound commercial basis. The plans of the society contemplate facilities in the eleven workshops in different parts of the country for the accommodation of between four and five thousand men.

Across the Firing Line

Prepared as she was for war, so also was Germany prepared for the consequences of war. At the outbreak of the war, she had of all other countries laid the most solid foundation for the care of the crippled soldier. The German National Federation for the Care of Cripples is an organization of long standing. There had been developed, during half a century's experience, fifty-eight cripple homes, under private auspices, ranging in size from six to three hundred beds. Some of them were already taking adults as well as children, and they had among them 221 workshops, teaching 51 trades. In addition, there were sanatoria and re-educational workshops for industrial cripples under the employers' accident insurance companies; there were orthopedic hospitals operated by municipalities, and there were trade schools and employment bureaus under various government auspices.

All these resources accumulated in peacetime for the rehabilitation of cripples were mobilized immediately after the outbreak of the war—almost simultaneously with the military mobilization. Eight days after the outbreak of hostilities, the Empress, at the instance of Dr. Biesalski, Germany's leading orthopedist and secretary of the National Federation for the Care of Cripples, address[ed] to existing institutions for the crippled a letter pointing out the necessities ahead and urging them to open their doors and provide facilities for the treatment and training of disabled soldiers. To this all the homes immediately consented. Dr. Biesalski undertook a tour of Germany and visited the principal cities urging the formation of voluntary committees for the care of war cripples. The immediate result was the formation of volunteer committees in many cities and of larger ones in some states and provinces. At the present time, Germany is thoroughly covered by a network of such organizations. A local committee usually comprises representatives of the municipality, of the military district command, the accident insurance associations, the Red Cross, the women's leagues, the employers, the chamber of commerce, the chamber of handwork, and the labor unions. In the fall of 1915, a national committee was formed with the object of coordinating the work and making investigations and plans for the future.

There are four stages in the treatment of the disabled soldier: (1) medical treatment; (2) provision of artificial limbs and functional re-education; (3) vocational advice and vocational re-education; and (4) placement. Of these activities, the first two are controlled by the imperial military authorities and are conducted on uniform lines. With regard to vocational and economic rehabilitation, on the contrary, there is no general direction given by any central authority; the re-education schools are of varying types and most unevenly distributed; the work is in the hands of local and private or semi-private agencies; it is done mostly by volunteers and is not even supervised by the imperial government.

However, in spite of the absence of any general system of organization, there is a complete unity of purpose and the work is everywhere carried on in accordance with certain universally accepted and officially sanctioned principles. These were formulated by Dr. Biesalski in this way:

1. No charity, but work for the war disabled.

2. Disabled soldiers must be returned to their homes and to their old conditions; as far as possible, to their old work.

3. The disabled soldier must be distributed among the mass of the people as though nothing had happened.

4. There is no such thing as being crippled, while there exists the iron will to overcome the handicap.

5. There must be the fullest publicity on this subject, first of all among the disabled men themselves.

The possibility of rehabilitation is accepted as a creed by all the institutions working to this end, it is put in practice, and the statement is that in ninety percent of the cases the desired results are attained.

There is a fairly complete network of orthopedic homes distributed all over the empire. Their number has been put at about two hundred. They are all under military discipline. The time for treatment for a man in the orthopedic hospital is from two to six months. Men are kept here until they are ready to go back to the army or are pronounced definitely unfit for service. Even if they are so unfit, the war department does not discharge them until they are pronounced by the physician physically fit to go back to civil life.

The best hospitals are excellently equipped. Complaints have been made, however, that the remote hospitals have very incomplete arrangements and that the great demand for orthopedists leaves some places unsupplied.

More and more emphasis is being placed on physical exercise as a means of bringing disabled men back to the standard. The plan is that a man shall begin very simple but systematic physical exercises even before he is out of bed. These are gradually increased until finally he has two or three hours a day under a regular gymnasium instructor. Games and outdoor sports are found to have an immense therapeutic value, both psychological and physiological, as compared with medico-mechanical treatment. Thus we find, at the different hospitals, as part of the regular regime, ball playing, spear throwing, bowling, shooting, quoits, handball, jumping, club swinging, and swimming. Finally, though the hospitals do not attempt to train a man to a trade, many of them have attached workshops for purposes of functional re-education. There is great emphasis placed on the fact that even this occupational therapy should be really useful and should lead the patient direct[ly] to some practical occupation.

All artificial limbs are furnished and kept in repair by the government. The government has prescribed maximum prices for prostheses of different types. Otherwise there is no official supervision. No standard pattern is prescribed, and the matter is left to the doctors and engineers of the country. The result is an immense stimulation of activity. The magazines are full of descriptions of new prostheses recommended by doctors and manual training teachers from all parts of the country. At an exhibition of artificial limbs, held at Charlottenburg, they were shown thirty kinds of artificial arms and fifty types of artificial legs in actual use.

The principle now thoroughly accepted is that the prosthesis should reproduce not the lost limb but the lost function. It should not be an imitation arm or leg, but a tool. The standard of merit is the number of activities it makes possible.

Re-education in Germany goes on at the same time as the medical treatment. This has two causes. First, there is the strong conviction among all cripple welfare workers that results can be obtained only by getting hold of a patient at the earliest possible moment of convalescence, and second, the fact that, since the government does not pay anything towards re-education, it is more economical for the care committees to attend to it while the men are in the hospitals and thus save themselves the expense of maintenance.

The local care committee usually appoints vocational advisers whose appointments have to be sanctioned by the local military authorities, who control the visits to the men in the hospitals. As soon as a soldier is well enough to be visited, the committee sends representative to get full data on his experience and his physical condition, and then advise him as to re-education or immediate return to work. The principle is fast held to that man must, if humanly possible, go back to his old trade, or, failing that, to an allied one.

The trade training is given while the men are still in the military hospital, beginning, in fact, as soon as they are able to be out of bed. The workshops are maintained by the local care committees; they can be located either in the hospital, or at an outside point to which the men go every day. The first plan is followed by but a few of the larger institutions; in most instances there are no workshops maintained at the hospitals. The local care committee may utilize the local trade schools. There are excellent facilities for this, since every town has at least one trade school. Some representative of the educational authorities generally serves on the local care committee and the schools are eager, in any case, to offer free instruction. German magazines are full of advertisements of free courses for war cripples, offered by schools of the most varying kind, public and private, from agricultural and commercial schools to professional schools and universities. On the other hand, in a large town, with a number of hospitals, the committee may create a school of its own. Thus, in Dusseldorf, for instance, where there are fifty hospitals, the committee has taken possession of a school building equipped with shops and tools and given twenty courses open to men from all the hospitals.

It is planned that none of the courses shall take more than six months, the maximum time for hospital care. These short courses are intended for men of experience who need further practice in their old trade or in an allied one. If a man needs further training after this short course, he becomes the charge of the local care committee, which supports him while he attends a technical school or pays the premium for apprenticing him to a master workman.

A special effort is being made to return to the land all who have any connection with it, such as farmers, farm laborers, and even hand-workers of country birth. All the hospitals that have any land give courses in farming and gardening for their patients. It is estimated that there are several hundred such hospital farms, small or large, operated by the wounded. In addition to this, there are definite summer farm courses at agricultural schools and universities, which are free to cripples. There are in the empire ten regular agricultural schools for war cripples.

Since the one-armed man has one of the gravest handicaps, special arrangements have been made in several places for his training. The purpose of these courses for the one-armed is to accustom the soldier to exercise the stump and the remaining member performing the daily duties such as eating, washing, dressing, tying knots, using simple tools, and the like. This is a preliminary to specialized trade training, and the process is said usually to require about six weeks.

An essential feature of the course is left-handed writing for those who have lost the right arm, not only for men in preparation for clerical work but for others as well. This training banishes to a marked degree the feeling of helplessness and likewise gives the hand greater flexibility and skill. German teachers have made a scientific study of this question and state that left-handed writing can be made as legible and characteristic as right-handed. Samples of left-handed writing from Nurnberg show excellent script after from twelve to twenty lessons.

Left-handed drawing, designing, and modeling are often added subjects of instruction. Men with clerical experience are taught to use the typewriter, sometimes using the stump, sometimes a special prosthesis, and sometimes with a shift key worked with the knee.

All the schools for one-armed put great emphasis on physical training. In the school at Heidelberg, under a regular gymnasium instructor, the men do almost all the athletic feats possible to two-armed men.

There is no uniform machinery for the placement of war cripples. The care committees, while interviewing the man in the hospital, also get in touch with his former employer. Sometimes a position is thus secured even before the man has started his training, and the latter is then adapted to the requirements of that particular position. But it is not always possible to place a man with his old employer. Some of the larger care committees run employment bureaus of their own. Others turn over to some other agency the man who cannot be taken back to his old position—usually to the regular employment bureaus. Germany has a system of public employment bureaus supported by the municipalities. The bureaus in each state or province are united under a state or provincial directorate, and the directorates in an imperial federation. Some of these had before the war, special divisions for the handicapped, and others have established them since the outbreak of hostilities. Employers' and workmen's associations are of considerable assistance in the placement of war cripples, especially the Federation of German Employers' Associations, which has been recently formed for this particular purpose, and the many master guilds of handworkers. There are also a number of agencies due to charitable or private initiative.

Finally, there are open to war cripples a very large number of positions in government service. The imperial government has promised that all former employees of the railways, post office, and civil service will be re-employed, if not in their old capacity, in a kindred position. These men are to be paid without consideration of their pensions. The post office department has decided to give all future agencies and sub-agencies in the rural districts to war cripples, provided they are fit for the positions and want to settle on the land. Many city governments make efforts to take in cripples. There are reserved for cripples a number of employments under the war department, which through its recently created welfare department attempts also to develop placement activity wherever there is no very active local care committee, publishing twice a week a journal which lists positions open for war cripples.

Chapter XVI: For the U.S. Forces

The situation of the United States with regard to making provision for the disabled soldier is perhaps slightly different from that of the other belligerents.

One of the principal causes of difference is the selective influence on the personnel of the military forces of the conscription law.

This legislation has specifically exempted, temporarily at any rate, agricultural workers, highly skilled mechanics, and those who, because of their special qualifications, are necessary to the maintenance of the national interest at home. In Italy and France the situation with regard to the make-up of the army is vastly different. There we find almost all the able-bodied agricultural workers in the service, and battalions of highly skilled mechanics and experienced workmen in uniform.

The problem of refitting for industry the disabled soldiers of the European forces is therefore very unlike that of the United States. Up to the present time the force sent to the front consists practically of men between the ages of twenty-one and thirty-one. This means that the majority of men disabled will not be highly skilled or long experienced in any occupation and thus will be more plastic from the vocational point of view. Past experience has in European practice been the main determinant of training for the future. It may be expected that in many of the American cases this will afford no definite criterion. Either the soldier may have entered the service direct from school or college or if he has been at work for some time, it is likely to have been in a dozen different jobs of varying character. Many of the men, therefore, can answer definitely to no "former occupation." As has been found in Canadian experience, the soldier when asked his trade will report that for three months prior to the war he worked on a railroad. "Then you are a railroad man?" is the question. "No," is the answer, "for the two months before that I was in a cotton mill, and still earlier drove a delivery wagon for a local firm." In such a case past experience is almost a negligible factor, and the man may properly be restudied vocationally in order that he may be trained in the skilled trade most suited to his qualifications and talents.

An interesting experiment in vocational analysis and allocation has been carried out by the military authorities in classifying drafted men for special lines of army service. The new recruits have been given simple psychological tests prior to their assignment to work as radio operators, oxy-acetylene welders, linemen in the signal corps, drivers or mechanicians in the motor transport service, and so forth. The results have been encouraging and the experience gained will undoubtedly be helpful in further vocational guidance of the men returning for discharge.

In the general process, it is likely that many men who were previously undifferentiated as to occupation, who possibly looked forward to careers as clerks or general utility men, may be directed into skilled trades which will afford to them a much greater financial opportunity, and will contribute more largely to the national stability and efficiency.

The recent wave of interest in the United States in vocational education has put the country in better shape to deal with the instructional requirements of the disabled soldier than would have been the case ten years ago. Although not claiming facilities to compare with those afforded by the fine system of technical institutes in Great Britain, there are in practically every important urban community of America, one or more vocational schools. Industrial education is well provided for by schools, the first of which were founded by private initiative but operated on a non-commercial basis. The later institutions have been established by local educational authorities as part of the public school systems.

Commercial education, to a noteworthy extent, is still in the hands of business colleges that are run as profit-making enterprises. But the work of many of them is efficient to a creditable degree.

Agricultural education has been splendidly provided for by the agricultural colleges and experiment stations maintained by the several states, with assistance, in some instances, from the national government. These institutions have the most modern equipment, expert teaching staffs, and the finest facilities for imparting a practical knowledge of agriculture.

And finally, it must be recalled that practically every American university has industrial departments with shop equipment, which afford to students not only the theoretical, but also the practical, type of instruction. As the war goes on the universities will be drained of students, while the vocational schools whose regular pupils are of younger age, will tend to continue full. In Canada the university plants have been put to good use in the training of disabled soldiers. Even more extensive facilities of this character are available in the United States.

Prior to the entry of America into the war there had been almost no provision for rehabilitation of the disabled adult. There had been several employment bureaus for cripples, in New York, Boston, Cincinnati, and Philadelphia. These agencies had been struggling bravely, without recourse to training facilities, and with scant public support, to solve the economic problems of the disabled, and were attaining an encouraging degree of success. About five years previous there had been started, but later discontinued, a training school for crippled men.

So in spite of the excellent foundation of general vocational education the United States, at her entrance into hostilities, stood practically without special facilities for the re-education of the disabled. The need of such special provision had been long recognized by workers with the handicapped and was repeatedly discussed in a special journal on cripples that was their organ.

The first move to meet this need was taken the second month after America's declaration of war, when a public-spirited citizen offered to the American Red Cross funds sufficient to establish and maintain in New York City a training school for crippled men. While an original motive of the fight was a desire to make provision that might be helpful to the disabled American soldier, the school was started for crippled men in general, without distinction as to their civilian or military affiliation. Thus came into being the Red Cross Institute for Crippled and Disabled Men.

It became soon evident that this organization had logical responsibilities much wider in scope than the conduct of a local school of re-education. Legislation making government provision for the training of disabled soldiers did not appear on the statute books until fourteen months after the inception of hostilities, so for a considerable period there was no official agency to which to turn for information and advice. Yet there was wide interest in provision for the disabled soldier. To meet demands from the public for data on the organization, methods, and principles of re-education, as derived from experience abroad, and to provide a scientific foundation for the development of its own activities, the Institute initiated in July 1917, a department of research. There was early issued a bibliography of the subject, followed by reports on activity in different countries, monographs, and translations, which have been freely distributed for the information of all interested in the subject.

This Institute, which undertook at once the training of crippled industrial workers, has established courses in the manufacture of artificial limbs, oxy-acetylene welding, printing, motion picture operating, jewelry-making, and mechanical drafting. There are also departments of employment, industrial surveys, and public education.

During the incubation of the national program the Red Cross Institute for Crippled and Disabled Men thus served as an experiment station and proving ground, and unofficially met demands upon it to the best of its ability.

In the formulation of the government plans there was considerable difference of opinion as to what authority or authorities should be charged with the responsibility of re-educating the disabled soldier. It was urged on the one hand that the entire task of rehabilitation in all its aspects should be entrusted to the Surgeon General of the Army; on the other hand that it might be handled by the Bureau of War Risk Insurance—a government department administering family allotments and allowances and the new life and disability insurance, privilege of which was offered to men entering upon military service. A later suggestion advanced by the Council of National Defense was that re-education be entrusted to a commission under the War Department, made up of representatives of all the official and non-official interests concerned. Another proposal which was approved by a conference called by the Surgeon General of the army at the instance of the Secretary of War, and which was embodied in the draft of a legislative proposal, called for an independent commission of five, composed of representatives of the Surgeon General of the Army, the Surgeon General of the Navy, the Treasury Department, the Department of Labor, and the Federal Board for Vocational Education.

The Administration felt, however, the unwisdom of erecting more independent boards or commissions unrelated to the regular executive mechanism. For this reason it was decided to fix the task on some already existing government department. The one designated in legislation introduced with executive approval, and later enacted, assigned the responsibility of providing for the rehabilitation of the disabled soldier and sailor to the Federal Board for Vocational Education, a body which had been created a year earlier to administer federal aid to vocational education by the states. The bill committing this new function to the Board became law on June 27, 1918.

Meantime, the Surgeon General of the Army had been establishing reconstruction hospitals for the intensive treatment of physical disablement. In connection with each of these medical centers educational work had been undertaken—with three ends in view. The first was to provide to convalescent patients occupation for therapeutic purposes; the second to provide educational opportunities during the period of invalidism to men who would be returned to the front or discharged without permanent disability; the third to train disabled men whom it was desired to retain in the military organization for special or limited service. In carrying out the two latter aims, the educational departments of the hospitals have entered well within the vocational field.

Important links in the military hospital chain are the reception hospitals at Fox Hills, Staten Island, N.Y.; at Ellis Island, in New York harbor and at Newport News, VA. At these institutions there are first received from hospital ships or transports all soldiers invalided home from overseas. The men are classified as to treatment need and district of residence, and promptly "cleared" to the appropriate institution.

During the period of hospital or convalescent care the soldier has advantage of physical and occupational therapy administered by a corps of trained workers known as "reconstruction aides" but more familiarly named "blue gowns" on account of their uniform.

Classes in the various military hospitals have already been established. The subjects taught at General Hospital No. 6, for McPherson, Atlanta, Ga., for example are motor mechanics, telegraphy, wireless telegraphy, typewriting, mechanical drafting, cabinet-making, carpentry, harness repairing, poultry raising, reading and writing English, penmanship and bookkeeping, and printing.

When a candidate for discharge from the military forces is so disabled as to entitle him to compensation for disability, his case is discussed with him, while he is still in the hospital, by a vocational adviser of the Federal Board for Vocational Education. He is told that the United States Government will train him free of charge for a new trade. It is entirely optional with the man whether he take advantage of this opportunity for training or not, but every influence is brought to bear to make his decision affirmative.

After the disabled man is discharged from the hospital, he becomes a civilian and his dealings are with the Federal Board and the Bureau of War Risk Insurance.

If the man decides to take a course of training, he is supported during the period of re-education through payment by the Bureau of War Risk Insurance of his compensation for disability or his former military pay, whichever is the greater. During this period the compulsory allotments and allowances to his dependents are continued just as if he were still in military service. He is given instruction that is paid for and supervised by the Federal Board for Vocational Education in one of the schools approved by that body.

The Federal Board for Vocational Education has announced that its provision of re-education will be made, so far as possible, through the use of existing schools, or by placement for training, under a modified system of apprenticeship, with manufacturing or commercial establishments. Special institutions will be founded only where absolutely necessary.

The Board is establishing district offices to decentralize the work, is making training arrangements for current cases, and is following up to their homes men who were discharged from the army prior to the inception of re-educational activity, and who stand in possible need of training. Local offices are already in operation in New York, Boston, Philadelphia, Cincinnati, Atlanta, Washington, D.C., New Orleans, Minneapolis, Chicago, St. Louis, Dallas, Denver, San Francisco, and Seattle.

After training is complete, the re-educated soldier will be placed in a job by the Federal Board, acting, as provided by the law, in cooperation with the United States Employment Service of the Department of Labor. The Board also includes in its placement function any man physically rehabilitated in an army or navy hospital, whether he be a candidate for retraining or not.

The American Red Cross has offered to the government authorities the facilities of its extensive home service organization throughout the country. This service, directed by the Department of Civilian Relief, can help to align the family as an encouraging force behind the re-education program, can keep the family wheels moving smoothly during the period of training, can provide to the vocational officers much useful information on the home conditions and community record of any individual soldiers, can follow up the case after return to employment, and help in many ways to make the re-education permanently effective.

The actual work of putting the disabled American soldier back on his feet is still in its infancy, and many details still remain to be worked out in experience. But in principle, the United States has followed the best example of her Allies—in accepting provision for the disabled soldiers as a national responsibility to be met at public expense. It is clear that no American soldier need be dependent upon the alms of charity for his rehabilitation.

But the complete success of the work rests with the people of the United States—upon whether we sympathetically grasp and effectively express in our relations with the graduates of re-education the new spirit of dealing with the disabled—upon whether we sense the glory of restoring the ex-soldier's ability to earn his own living, or whether we continue the old temporary hero worship and permanent pauperization. The self-respect of self-support or the ignominy of dependence—which shall the future hold for our disabled soldiers? The credit or the blame for the decision will largely rest with the American public.

The open road is before us.

Source: McMurtrie, Douglas C. 1919. Pp. 185–195, 209–217, and 223–232 in *The Disabled Soldier*. New York: Macmillan.

▣ Sherwood Anderson, from *Winesburg, Ohio* (1919)

In the preface to his story of oppressive midwestern small-town life, Sherwood Anderson discusses his narrator's obsession with disabled characters, or, as he calls them, "grotesques." The act of characterization requires a "deforming" precept in that characters are brought to life through their defining idiosyncrasies. In this excerpt, the narrator imagines a procession of such characters with their "misshapen bodies" parading before him in dreams.

The writer, an old man with a white mustache, had some difficulty in getting into bed. The windows of the house in which he lived were high and he wanted to look at the trees when he awoke in the morning. A carpenter came to fix the bed so that it would be on a level with the window.

Quite a fuss was made about the matter. The carpenter, who had been a soldier in the Civil War, came into the writer's room and sat down to talk of building a platform for the purpose of raising the bed. The writer had cigars lying about and the Carpenter smoked.

For a time the two men talked of the raising of the bed and then they talked of other things. The soldier got on the subject of the war. The writer, in fact, led him to that subject. The carpenter had once been a prisoner in Andersonville Prison and had lost a brother. The brother had died of starvation, and whenever the carpenter got upon that subject, he cried. He, like the old writer, had a white mustache, and when he cried he puckered up his lips and the mustache bobbed up and down. The weeping old man with the cigar in his mouth was ludicrous. The plan the writer had for the raising of his bed was forgotten and later the carpenter did it in his own way and the writer, who was past sixty, had to help himself with a chair when he went to bed at night.

In his bed, the writer rolled over on his side and lay quite still. For years he had been beset with notions concerning his heart. He was a hard smoker and his heart fluttered. The idea had got into his mind that he would come to die unexpectedly and always when he got into bed he thought of that. It did not alarm him. The effect in fact was quite a special thing and not easily explained. It made him more alive, there in bed, than any other time. Perfectly still, he lay and his body was old and not much use any more, but something inside him was altogether young. He was like a pregnant woman, only that thing inside him was not a baby but a youth. No it wasn't a youth, it was a woman, young, and wearing a coat of mail like a knight. It is absurd, you see, to try to tell what was inside the old writer as he lay on his high bed and listened to the fluttering of his heart. The thing to get at is what the writer, or the young thing within the writer, was thinking about.

The old writer, like all of the people in the world, had got, during his long life, a great many notions in his head. He had once been quite handsome and a number of women had been in love with him. And then, of course, he had known people, many people, known them in a peculiarly intimate way that was different from the way in which you and I know people. At least that is what the writer thought and the thought pleased him. Why quarrel with an old man concerning his thoughts?

In bed, the writer had a dream that was not a dream. As he grew somewhat sleepy but was still conscious, figures began to appear before his eyes. He imagined the young indescribable thing within himself was driving a long procession of figures before his eyes.

You see interest in all this lies in the figures that went before the eyes of the writer. They were all grotesques. All of the men and women the writer had ever known had become grotesques.

The grotesques were not all horrible. Some were amusing, some almost beautiful, and one, a woman all drawn out of shape, hurt the old man by her grotesqueness. When she passed he made a noise like a small dog whimpering. Had you come into the room you might have supposed the old man had unpleasant dreams or perhaps indigestion.

For an hour the procession of the grotesques passed before the eyes of the old man, and then, although it was a painful thing to do, he crept out of bed and began to write. Some one of the grotesques had made a deep impression on his mind and he wanted to describe it.

At his desk the writer worked for an hour. In the end he wrote a book which he called "The Book of the Grotesque." It was never published, but I saw it once and it made an indelible impression on my mind. The book had one central thought that is very strange and has always remained with me. By remembering it I have been able to understand many people and things that I was never able to understand before. The thought was involved but a simple statement of it would be something like this:

That in the beginning when the world was young there were a great many thoughts but no such thing as a truth. Man made the truths himself and each truth was a composite of a great many vague thoughts. All about in the world were the truths and they were all beautiful.

The old man had listed hundreds of the truths in his book. I will not try to tell you all of them. There was the truth of virginity and the truth of passion, the truth of wealth and of poverty, of thrift and of profligacy, of carelessness and of abandon. Hundreds and hundreds were the truths and they were all beautiful.

And then people came along. Each as he appeared snatched up one of the truths and some who were quite strong snatched up a dozen of them.

It was the truths that made the people grotesques. The old man had quite an elaborate theory concerning the matter. It was his notion that the moment one of the people took one of the truths to himself, called it his truth, and tried to live his life by it, he became a grotesque and the truth he embraced became a falsehood.

You can see for yourself how the old man, who had spent all his life writing and was filled with words, would writes hundreds of pages concerning this matter. The subject would become so big in his mind that he himself would be in danger of becoming a grotesque. He didn't, I suppose, for the same reason that he never published the book. It was the young thing inside him that saved the old man.

Concerning the old carpenter who fixed the bed for the writer, I only mentioned him because he, like many of what are called very common people, became the nearest thing to what is understandable and lovable of all the grotesques in the writer's book.

Source: Anderson, Sherwood. 1919. Pp. 21–24 in *Winesburg, Ohio*. New York: Penguin.

▣ John Dos Passos
on Randolph Bourne (1919)

In this obituary for Randolph Bourne, John Dos Passos identifies the profound lack of choices afforded to those with body differences, while also noting that choice persists as the American value par excellence. As a person with a disability, one's freedom to choose is already curtailed at birth, and one's body becomes a constant reminder of this foreclosure on bodily liberties. In addition, Dos Passos uses the occasion to comment upon the radical insights into war and the wages of social disenfranchisement possessed by disabled thinkers and writers.

Randolph Bourne

Randolph Bourne came as an inhabitant of this earth without the pleasure of choosing his dwelling or his career. He was a hunchback, grandson of a congregational minister, born in 1886 in Bloomfield, New Jersey; there he attended grammar school and high school. At the age of seventeen he went to work as a secretary to a Morristown businessman. He worked his way through Columbia working in a pianola record factory in Newark, working as proofreader, piano tuner, accompanist in a vocal studio in Carnegie Hall.

At Columbia he studied with John Dewey, got a traveling fellowship that took him to England Paris Rome Berlin Copenhagen, wrote a book on the Gary schools. In Europe he heard music, a great deal of Wagner and Scriabine and bought himself a black cape.

This little sparrowlike man
tiny twisted bit of flesh in a black cape,
always in pain and ailing,
put a pebble in his sling
and hit Goliath square in the forehead with it.
War, he wrote, is the health of the state.

Half musician, half educational theorist (weak health and being poor and twisted in body and on bad terms with his people hadn't spoiled the world for Randolph Bourne; he was a happy man, loved die Meistersinger and playing Bach with his long hands that stretched so easily over the keys and pretty girls and good food and evenings of talk. When he was dying of pneumonia a friend brought him an eggnog; Look at the yellow, its beautiful, he kept saying as his life ebbed into delirium and fever. He was a happy man.) Bourne seized with feverish intensity on the ideas then going around at Columbia he picked rosy glasses out of the turgid jumble of John Dewey's teaching through which he saw clear and sharp.

the shining capitol of reformed democracy,
Wilson's New Freedom;
but he was too good a mathematician;
he had to work the equations out;
with the result that in the crazy spring of 1917
he began to get unpopular where his bread was buttered at the New Republic;
for New Freedom read Conscription, for Democracy, Win the War, for Reform, Safeguard the Morgan Loans for Progress Civilization Education Service, Buy a Liberty Bond, Strafe the Hun, Jail the Objectors.

He resigned from the New Republic; only The Seven Arts had the nerve to publish his articles against the war. The backers of the Seven Arts took their money elsewhere; friends didn't like to be seen with Bourne, his father wrote him begging him not to disgrace the family name. The rainbowtinted future of reformed democracy went pop like a pricked soapbubble.

The liberals scurried to Washington; some of his friends pled with him to climb up on Schoolmaster Wilson's sharabang; the war was great fought from the swivel chairs of Mr. Creel's bureau in Washington.

He was cartooned, shadowed by the espionage service and the counter-espionage service; taking a walk with two girl friends at Wood's Hole he was arrested, a trunk full of manuscript and letters stolen from him in Connecticut. (Force to the utmost, thundered Schoolmaster Wilson).

He didn't live to see the big circus of the Peace of Versailles or the purplish normalcy of the Ohio Gang. Six weeks after the armistice he died planning an essay on the foundations of future radicalism in America.

If any man has a ghost
Bourne has a ghost,
a tiny twisted unscared ghost in a black cloak
hopping along the grimy old brick and brownstone streets still left in downtown New York,
crying out in a shrill soundless giggle;
War is the health of the state.

Source: Dos Passos, John. 1919. *U.S.A.* Available at: http://www .art4exec.org/who-was-bourne.htm

Karl Binding and Alfred Hoche, from *Permission for the Destruction of Worthless Life, Its Extent and Form* (1920)

Binding and Hoche's influential work argued that the German state was failing under the burden of caring for disabled people who were using up a disproportionate amount of resources. They referred to such individuals as "lives unworthy of life" and divided potential candidates for state-sponsored "euthanasia" into three groups: war wounded, patients in permanent comas, and "idiots" housed in psychiatric hospitals. The work proved critical in fashioning a medical industry that would recognize killing as a viable application of medical technology.

Are there humans who have lost their human characteristics to such an extent that their continued existence has lost all value for themselves and for society? One only needs to pose the question and a feeling of anxiety stirs in anyone who is used to assessing the value of individual lives both to the people themselves and to the community. He is painfully aware of how wasteful we are with the most valuable and self-sufficient lives which are full of energy and vigour and what labor, patience, and resources are squandered simply in order to try and sustain worthless lives until nature—often cruelly tardy—removes the last possibility of their continuation. If, at the same time, one thinks of a battlefield covered with thousands of young corpses, or of a mine in which hundreds of hard-working miners have been buried, and if one compares them to our institutions for idiots, with the care which is devoted to their inmates—one is deeply shocked by the sharp discrepancy between, on the one hand, the sacrifice of man's most precious resource and, on the other, the tremendous care devoted to creatures which are not only completely worthless but are of negative value.

It cannot be doubted that there are people for whom death would come as a release and, at the same time, for society and the state in particular, would represent liberation from a burden which, apart from being an example of a great self sacrifice, is not of the slightest use. . . .

However, I am firmly of the opinion that rational calculation should not be the sole basis on which to answer this question; the reply must win approval through a deep sense of correctness. Every killing which is permitted must be felt, at least by the person concerned, as a release; otherwise, such permission must be ruled out.

It follows from this, however, that it is absolutely vital to respect completely everybody's will to live, even that of the most sick, tortured, or useless people.

The legal order can never be allowed to operate as a murderer and a killer forcibly breaking the will to live of its victims. Naturally, there can be no question of permitting the killing of the feeble-minded person who feels happy with his life.

Source: Binding, Karl, and Alfred Hoche. 2001. *Permission for the Destruction of Worthless Life, Its Extent and Form.* In Noakes, Jeremy, and Geoffrey Pridham, eds. *Nazism 1919–1945: State, Economy and Society, 1933–1939: A Documentary Reader.* Exeter, UK: University of Exeter Press. (Originally published 1920)

W. E. B. Du Bois, "Race Intelligence" (1920)

In this comment, Du Bois attacks the legacy of scientific racism in efforts to find a physical source for proving African American inferiority.

For a century or more it has been the dream of those who do not believe Negroes are human that their wish should find some scientific basis. For years they depended on the weight of the human brain, trusting that the alleged underweight of less than a thousand Negro brains, measured without reference to age, stature, nutrition or cause of death, would convince the world that black men simply could not be educated. Today scientists acknowledge that there is no warrant for such a conclusion and that in any case absolute weight of the brain is no criterion for racial ability. Measurements of the bony skeleton followed and great hopes of the scientific demonstration of race inferiority were held for a while. But they had to be surrendered when Zulus and Englishmen were found in the same dolichocephalic class. Then came psychology: The children of the public schools were studied and it was discovered that some colored children ranked lower than white children. This gave wide satisfaction even though it pointed out that the average included most of both races and that considering the educational opportunities and social environment of the races the differences were measurements simply of the ignorance and poverty of the black child's surroundings.

Source: Du Bois, W. E. B. 1987. "Race Intelligence." In Huggins, Nathan I., ed. *Du Bois: Writings.* New York: Library of America. (Originally published 1920)

▣ O Hwa-Su, "The Bride Who Would Not Speak" (1920)

This tale was told by O Hwa-Su and collected by Zong In-Sob in Korea in 1920. The tale includes a common Korean saying given to a woman getting married: she should be "mute for three years, deaf for three years and blind for three years." This indicates women's difficult position in their parents-in-law's family and patriarchal culture. They were admonished to perform a disabled person, but they could never be actually disabled to remain in marriage.

Once upon a time a man said to his daughter when she was setting out to go for her wedding, 'A daughter-in-law's life is very hard. She must pretend that she does not see the things that are to be seen, that she does not hear the words spoken around her, and she must speak as little as possible.'

So for three years after her marriage the girl spoke never a word. Her husband's family thought she was deaf and dumb, and so they decided to send her back to her father's house.

As she went back riding in a palanquin she chanced to hear a mountain pheasant call, and she said, 'Dear pheasant! I have missed your voice these long years.' Her father-in-law, who was walking beside the palanquin, was overjoyed to hear her speak and took her back to her husband at once. Then he sent his servants to catch the pheasant.

As she cooked the pheasant the daughter-in-law sang, 'The wings that protected me I will serve to my father-in-law. And the rolling nagging beak I will serve to my mother-in-law. And the rolling eyes will do for my husband's sister.'

Source: Zong In-Sob. 1969. "The Bride Who Would Not Speak." In *Folk Tales from Korea*. New York: Greenwood Press.

▣ Ewald Meltzer, Survey Sent to German Parents of 162 Disabled Children (1920)

In 1920, Ewald Meltzer sent around the following survey to the parents of 162 disabled children in order to assess attitudes toward euthanasia. Nazi advocates of medical murder later referenced the poll as evidence that parents would not protest the death of their institutionalized disabled children. In fact, the architects of the children's "euthanasia" program employed parental

comments about how such killings might be carried out with their consent.

Meltzer Questionnaire

Given in 1920 to male parents or guardians of two hundred children living at the Katharinehof State Home for Non-Educable, Feeble-Minded Children in Grosshennersdorf, Germany.

Would you give your consent in every circumstance to a painless shortening of your child's life, after an expert had determined him incurably imbecilic?

Would you give your consent only if you could no longer care for your child, for example if you were about to pass away?

Would you give your consent if your child were suffering serious physical and mental anguish?

What is your wife's opinion of questions 1–3?

Source: Burleigh, Michael. 2000. *The Third Reich: A New History*. New York: Hill and Wang.

▣ Martin Barr, "Some Notes on Asexualization" (1920)

Martin Barr, MD, served as chief physician of the Pennsylvania Training School for Feeble-minded Children in Elwyn, Pennsylvania. He was one of the fiercest advocates of coerced sterilization of individuals diagnosed as feebleminded in the United States.

Asexualization is not a new subject. Indeed as practiced in many lands, in many forms, for thousands of years, it is almost as old as the world itself. In the Scriptures we find mention of it, notably in the Book of Job, and in some parts of the New Testament; and it is often referred to in other ancient writings: the Histories of Assyria, China, Egypt, India, Persia, Rome and Greece speak of it again and again. It was practiced before the reign of Semiramis; and Andramgtis, King of Lydia, sanctioned sterilization in both sexes. . . .

Goethe said: "Fools and sensible people are alike harmless. It is only the half-foolish and half-wise who are most dangerous." Surely this is a truth verified by the fact that the feeble-minded have so multiplied and increased as to become a distinct race, now beginning to be recognized as such; needing protection for themselves and the world from them. But what is not *fully recognized,* as yet, is the fact that mental defectives suffer not only from exaggerated sexual impulses; but from mental and moral debility, causing always a minimum of judgment and of will-power, leaving them greater slaves to the impulse of the moment, than are many normal children.

There is consequently little, if any, balance between the intellectual and moral faculties, and but a rudimentary idea of relative values, constituting inability to recognize or to resist coming in; rendering them therefore mere creatures of the moment and slaves of temptation. Indeed they are so crooked that they are parallel to nothing, and one can hardly fathom how protean are the vagaries of mental defect.

That the quieting of nervous and exaggerated emotional excitation is a primary and necessary factor in developing and training mental defectives, experience has proven; it further points to asexualization as a powerful agent; a measure therefore contributing to the protection and advancement of the individual, either within or without institution walls.

Moreover this quieting of, or power of holding in abeyance, the sexual impulses, is the surest weapon for combating prostitution, providing thus a protection to society as well as to the irresponsible who, recognized or unrecognized, proves either seducer or victim.

"Race betterment," thus once secured, insures not only diminution of the defective, but also of the criminal ranks, now continually recruited from that class.

The jails, penitentiaries, almshouses and reformatories are filled with defectives, many of whom are allowed to return unprotected to life outside, where—as before stated, with the sexual impulses ever exaggerated—they reproduce their kind from 2 to 6 times more rapidly than do normal people.

Heredity being the primary factor in production, the natural means of arrest is the removal of sexual desire in the unfit, and destruction of power to procreate.

A very conservative estimate places the number of mental defectives in the United States at between 300,000 and 400,000, while it is fairly computed that of these only 39,000 are cared for in institutions.

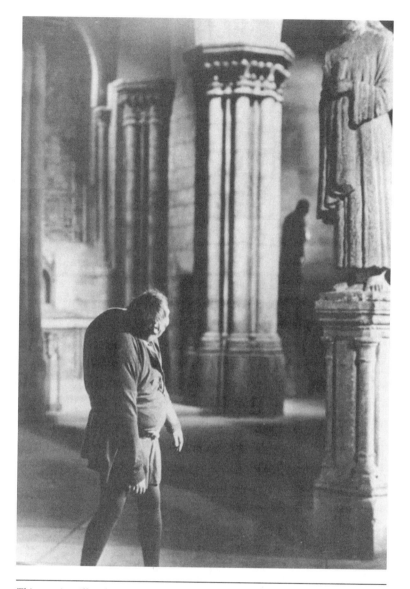

This movie still is from The Hunchback of Notre Dame, *Lon Chaney's first big-budget film and the one that made him a star of the cinema screen. Chaney delivers a remarkable performance as Quasimodo, using heavy weights to simulate a "crippled" gait but still managing to retain the expressive power of his body.*

Source: *The Hunchback of Notre Dame* (1923), directed by Wallace Worsley. B&W, 69 minutes. Reprinted by permission of Paul Darke.

There are 51,000 avowed cases of feeble-minded in the state of New York, over 14,000 in Massachusetts, and in Pennsylvania the number has been estimated at 20,000.

It has been conjectured that over 50 percent of the prostitutes in the United States are feeble-minded.

We quarantine influenza, leprosy and venereal diseases and have laws governing the use of alcohol and of narcotics; and, while we have some laws for the *protection* of the feeble-minded, we have accomplished but little to stem the tide of degeneracy, and pollution of our normal population.

In 1892 the Training School at Elwyn demonstrated the benefit of asexualization by the sterilization of two patients. When in 1894 Dr. P. Hoyt Pilcher, of Winfield, Kansas, reported that he had operated upon a number [of] boys (38 cases) with gratifying results, a howl went up throughout the length and breadth of our land, the like of which was never heard before or since. The political papers censured him, and the medical journals, in the main praised and upheld him.

Later, Dr. Everett Flood, in Massachusetts, operated upon 26 cases, with the result that sexual appetite disappeared absolutely in all but two, and in these was markedly reduced.

Necessity for the adoption of heroic measures has been found, in the experience of a large proportion of institutions, asylums and prisons, and is now being persistently urged by leaders in the work.

That mere sentimental prejudice is gradually succumbing to the promulgation of this prevention of "True Race Suicide" is shown in the action of the legislatures of some thirteen states legalizing the asexualization of imbeciles, criminals and rapists.

Pennsylvania, the first to demonstrate by operation the beneficial results attained by asexualization, was also the first to demand legislative authority in broadening the work. In this thrice have her efforts been defeated—each time suppressed by a single voice—the veto of two governors (1905–1909) and the influence of one legislator (1911).

In 1907 Indiana passed the first bill authorizing operations upon confirmed criminals, idiots, imbeciles and rapists in state institutions.

Some 800 were vasectomied; and of these 200 were operated upon at their own request.

California followed with a law to permit the asexualization of inmates of state hospitals for feeble-minded, and convicts in state institutions.

In 1909 Connecticut enacted a similar law, followed by New Jersey, Wisconsin and New Hampshire; the operations to be oophorectomy in the females and castration, or vasectomy, in the males.

We must face the fact that the very life-blood of the nation is being poisoned by the rapid production of mental and moral defectives, and the only thing that will dam the flood of degeneracy and insure the survival of the fittest, is abrogation of all power to procreate.

The shibboleth of the day is "lock up all degenerates once so proven." And this we do. But sooner or later the brighter ones, whose defects for a time are masked by the benefits received from training, are removed from the protection of sequestration, either by parents or guardians convinced of "cure" so-called; or again by the misdirected philanthropy of idle women; or some charitable societies, eager to set them at liberty "that they may have their chance." They have all right—and pressing forward they go out to meet the "Years to Come" and tramp through the black morasses of sexual filth until precipitated into the whirlpool of the stormy "Sea of Life" from which few, if any, ever return: and double prisoners and captives of the victims and their own passions, they sink lower and lower, consorting with the muck and filth, the scum and dregs of mankind. Then these hereditary irresponsibles—degenerates, imbeciles, defective delinquents and epileptics—the very nightmare of the human race, ever with sexual impulses exaggerated, find their "chance" in reproduction. Unconsciously innocent poisoners of a normal race, they are nevertheless its worst enemy.

In regard to the character of operations: Personally I prefer castration for the male, and oophorectomy for the female, as insuring security beyond adventure; and when performed on the young, desire almost entirely ceases, or is at least held in reasonable abeyance.

If for sentimental reasons the removal of the organs are objected to, vasectomy or fellectomy may be substituted.

Source: Barr, Martin W. 1920. "Some Notes on Asexualization, with a Report of Eighteen Cases." *Journal of Nervous and Mental Diseases* 51:231–241. From the Smith Ely Jeliffe Collection, proprietor Dr. David Braddock, University of Colorado, Boulder.

▣ Helen MacMurchy, from *The Almosts: A Study of the Feebleminded* (1920)

This excerpt provides an early example of literary analysis that considers artistic attention to disabled characters. While the author gives credit for this representational "kindness," she also affirms a eugenics divide between "normal" and "abnormal" citizens.

Chapter V. The Case for the Feeble-minded

Great writers have recognized the feeble-minded. They know that there are such people. When they painted the great world there was a place found on the canvas for the feeble-minded. Great writers discovered long before the modern "uplifter" was born that we must reckon with the mental defective as one of those many things in heaven and earth that are not dealt with by some philosophers, and yet that makes a great difference to the community and to social progress.

Kindness is the key that unlocks the problem of the feeble-minded—kindness and wisdom. The feeble-minded must have a permanent guide, philosopher and friend, so Wamba has Cedric and Gurth, Maggy has Little Dorrit, Billy has Dr. Amboyne, and Henry Little, and Barnaby Rudge has his mother. Mental defectives cannot manage by themselves, though we have tried to pretend to the contrary.

As to our attitude towards them: Nicholas Nickleby "treated Smike like a human creature." So he was. So was the Fool in "Lear." So with the rest. They are human creatures—human beings, and differ among themselves in reactions, in character, in endowment, in emotion, almost as much as the rest of us. Yet while this is true, there remains a world of difference even in fiction between the normal and the mentally defective. Little Dorrit and Maggy, Gurth and Wamba, Gabriel Varden and Barnaby Rudge—the verdict is never in doubt for a moment. The one makes upon the reader the definite impression of a normal person, but the other is "not all there."

Source: MacMurchy, Helen. 1920. Pp. 169–170 in *The Almosts: A Study of the Feebleminded*. Boston: Houghton Mifflin.

◙ T. S. Eliot, from *The Waste Land* (1922)

Eliot builds on the classical tradition that links disability to superhuman gifts through the figure of Tiresias, the blind seer. However, what the blind prophet foretells in The Waste Land is the banality and insignificance of modern existence.

From "The Fire Sermon"

At the violet hour, when the eyes and back
Turn upward from the desk, when the human engine
    waits
Like a taxi throbbing waiting,
I Tiresias, though blind, throbbing between two lives,
Old man with wrinkled female breasts, can see
At the violet hour, the evening hour that strives
Homeward, and brings the sailor home from sea,

The typist home at teatime, clears her breakfast, lights
Her stove, and lays out food in tins.
Out of the window perilously spread
Her drying combinations touched by the sun's
    last rays,
On the divan are piled (at night her bed)
Stockings, slippers, camisoles, and stays.
I Tiresias, old man with wrinkled dugs
Perceived the scene, and foretold the rest—
I too awaited the expected guest.
He, the young man carbuncular, arrives,
A small house agent's clerk, with one bold stare,
One of the low on whom assurance sits
As a silk hat on a Bradford millionaire.
The time is now propitious, as he guesses,
The meal is ended, she is bored and tired,
Endeavours to engage her in caresses
Which still are unreproved, if undesired.
Flushed and decided, he assaults at once;
Exploring hands encounter no defence;
His vanity requires no response,
And makes a welcome of indifference.
(And I Tiresias have foresuffered all
Enacted on this same divan or bed;
I who have sat by Thebes below the wall
And walked among the lowest of the dead.)
Bestows one final patronizing kiss,
And gropes his way, finding the stairs unlit . . .

Source: Eliot, T. S. 1922. *The Waste Land*. Available at: http://www.bartleby.com/201/1.html

◙ William Carlos Williams, "To Elsie" (1923)

Perhaps the premier imagist poet in the United States, William Carlos Williams also served as a physician in New Jersey. His poem "To Elsie" metaphorizes modernist concerns with collapsing social institutions in the figure of Elsie, the "broken-brained" maid who took care of his house. Enshrining a common eugenics theme of hereditary degeneration, Elsie represents both an infantilized disabled woman and a symbol of capitalism's unbridled pursuit of consumerist lifestyles.

The pure products of America
go crazy—
mountain folk from Kentucky

or the ribbed north end of
Jersey
with its isolate lakes and

valleys, its deaf-mutes, thieves
old names
and promiscuity between

devil-may-care men who have taken
to railroading
out of sheer lust of adventure—

and young slatterns, bathed
in filth
from Monday to Saturday

to be tricked out that night
with gauds
from imaginations which have no

peasant traditions to give them
character
but flutter and flaunt

sheer rags—succumbing without
emotion
save numbed terror

under some hedge of choke-cherry
or viburnum—
which they cannot express—

Unless it be that marriage
perhaps
with a dash of Indian blood

will throw up a girl so desolate
so hemmed round
with disease or murder

that she'll be rescued by an
agent—
reared by the state and

sent out at fifteen to work in
some hard-pressed
house in the suburbs—

some doctor's family, some Elsie—
voluptuous water
expressing with broken

brain the truth about us—
her great
ungainly hips and flopping breasts

addressed to cheap
jewelry
and rich young men with fine eyes

as if the earth under our feet
were
an excrement of some sky

and we degraded prisoners
destined
to hunger until we eat filth

while the imagination strains
after deer
going by in fields of goldenrod in

the stifling heat of September
Somehow
it seems to destroy us

It is only in isolate flecks that
something
is given off

No one
to witness
and adjust, no one to drive the car

Source: Williams, William Carlos. 1923. "To Elsie." Available at:
http://eir.library.utoronto.ca/rpo/display/poem2318.html

◉ Henry Edward Abt, from *The Care, Cure, and Education of the Crippled Child* (1924)

Henry Edward Abt was a progressive social reformer during the early twentieth century in the United States. This excerpt provides a good example of the ways in which Abt sought to champion the treatment and education of disabled children as a primary sign of modern U.S. enlightenment.

In the course of this book we shall first step back and examine those darker ages when physical imperfection was a horrible stigma. We shall examine in a cursory manner those physical conditions which cause children to be handicapped. We shall then follow the little cripple as he is carried to the modem clinic, subjected to modern miracles of surgery, brought to the cheerful convalescent home, where he perhaps stands erect for the first time in his life, and where he is brought from the darkness of ignorance and introduced to the delights of education; and we shall finally gaze upon him and his fellows as they step forth into life and find themselves fully able to cope with their problems as if they had never been prostrate. . . .

Chapter I: Introduction

On a hot summer afternoon in 1863, a foreign representative to the United States, several members of the Cabinet, and the President of the United States are said to have been traversing one of the broad avenues of Washington. They were discussing matters of international importance. It was, therefore, somewhat surprising to the others when Abraham Lincoln abruptly interrupted the conversation and left the group. Stooping at a nearby tree, the emancipator lifted a fallen baby bird to its nest. Returning to his associates, Lincoln remarked, "And now, gentlemen, continue."[1]

Although one of the greatest leaders the world has ever known found time to give his attention to an unfortunate little bird, until the past century all humanity has carelessly and consistently neglected its own unfortunate crippled children. For centuries of the Christian Era men have declared, like Mr. Scrooge in Charles Dickens' immortal *Christmas Carol,* "What then, if he be like to die, he had better do it, and decrease the surplus population." Hundreds of millions of those declaring themselves followers of the Master who said, "Suffer little children to come unto me, for such is the kingdom of God,"[2] and again, to the hunchback woman, "Woman, thou art loosed from thine infirmity,"[3] have made crippled children public jests, exiles from society.

---

[1] The author has searched unsuccessfully for the source of this anecdote. It is a story he heard as a young child, and is one which he has never forgotten. It is very appropriately illustrative of the spirit of the movement to aid crippled children.
[2] St. Mark, Chapter X, 14.
[3] St. Luke, Chapter XIII, 12.

The movement to care for and educate children, maimed or deformed by disease or accident, may be considered to have two aspects, the humanitarian and the sociological. This classification is recorded not because any such distinct cleavage exists, but to satisfy those who insist upon a mechanistic interpretation of life. Unless the "science" of sociology succeeds in making life more beautiful for its students, for the immediate spiritual happiness of the largest proportion of human beings, or for generations to come, it is an inexcusable waste of time. Were life really the dismal mechanical existence that some of our sociological scholars are pleased to interpret, it would seem that this information had best be transmitted to as few humans as possible. If life, properly understood, were truly nothing but a birth-to-death struggle, devoid of joy or pleasure, it would seem that the "laissez-faire" policy of those who interpret it in this manner had best be extended to education and study of the sort they pursue. The popular proverb, "ignorance is bliss" is easily extended to this sort of knowledge, for the ignorant might then grasp their few momentary transports of ecstasy without realizing their error.

As a matter of fact, no such situation exists. The study of crippled children brings to the right-minded man an appreciation of his own happy, healthy existence, a deeper understanding of the suffering and distress of his neighbors, leading to a deeper and finer emotional experience, as well as the knowledge of how to reduce and alleviate this suffering.

Source: Abt, Henry Edward. 1924. *The Care, Cure, and Education of the Crippled Child.* International Society for Crippled Children. Available at: http://www.disabilitymuseum.org/lib/docs/1449.htm

▣ Thomas Mann, from *The Magic Mountain* (1924)

Mann, for whom the modern world resembles a hospital, examines life at the microscopic level where matter experiences a ceaseless cycle of renewal and decay. Human life is the awakened consciousness of this relation between living and dying.

What then was life? It was warmth, the warmth generated by a form-preserving instability, a fever of matter, which accompanied the process of ceaseless decay and repair of albumen molecules that were too impossibly complicated, too impossibly ingenious in structure. It was the existence of the actually impossible-to-exist, of a half-sweet, half-painful balancing, or scarcely balancing, in this restricted and feverish process of decay, and renewal, upon the point of existence. It was not matter and it was not spirit, but something between the two, a phenomenon conveyed by matter, like the rainbow on the waterfall, and like the flame. Yet why not material—it was sentient to the point of desire and disgust, the shamelessness of matter become sensible of itself, the incontinent form of being. It was a secret and ardent stirring in the frozen chastity of the universal; it was a stolen and voluptuous impurity of sucking and secreting; an exhalation of carbonic acid gas and material impurities of mysterious origin and composition. It was a pullulation, an unfolding, a form-building (made possible by the over-balancing of its instability, yet controlled by the laws of growth inherent within it), of something brewed out of water, albumen, salt and fats, which was called flesh, and which became form, beauty, a lofty image, and yet all the time the essence of sensuality and desire. For this form and beauty were not spirit-borne; nor, like the form and beauty of sculpture, conveyed by a neutral and spirit-consumed substance, which could in all purity make beauty perceptible to the senses. Rather was it conveyed and shaped by the somehow awakened voluptuousness of matter, of the organic, dying-living substance itself, the reeking flesh.

Source: Mann, Thomas. 1927. Lowe-Porter, H. T., trans. *The Magic Mountain*. New York: Random House.

▣ Oliver Wendell Holmes, *Buck v. Bell,* 274 U.S. 200 (1927)

In one of the most notorious eugenics-based legal cases, U.S. Supreme Court Justice Oliver Wendell Holmes based his decision in support of sterilization on the longstanding prejudice that cognitively disabled women were more promiscuous than non-disabled women. Eugenics historians have since established that Carrie Buck—the woman targeted in the case because of a diagnosis of "feeblemindedness"—had been raped by a relative of her foster parents. Further study of the case has revealed that her lawyer in the case acted in collusion with the lawyer for the Virginia Colony to ensure that the sterilization law was upheld.

Mr. Justice Holmes delivered the opinion of the Court.

This is a writ of error to review a judgment of the Supreme Court of Appeals of the State of Virginia, affirming a judgment of the Circuit Court of Amherst County, by which the defendant in error, the superintendent of the State Colony for Epileptics and Feeble Minded, was ordered to perform the operation of salpingectomy upon Carrie Buck, the plaintiff in error, for the purpose of making her sterile. 143 Va. 310. The case comes here upon the contention that the statute authorizing the judgment is void under the Fourteenth Amendment as denying to the plaintiff in error due process of law and the equal protection of the laws.

Carrie Buck is a feeble minded white woman who was committed to the State Colony above mentioned in due form. She is the daughter of a feeble minded mother in the same institution, and the mother of an illegitimate feeble minded child. She was eighteen years old at the time of the trial of her case in the Circuit Court, in the latter part of 1924. An Act of Virginia, approved March 20, 1924 recites that the health of the patient and the welfare of society may be promoted in certain cases by the sterilization of mental defectives, under careful safeguard, &c.; that the sterilization may be effected in males by vasectomy and in females by salpingectomy, without serious pain or substantial danger to life; that the Commonwealth is supporting in various institutions many defective persons who if now discharged would become a menace but if incapable of procreating might be discharged with safety and become self-supporting with benefit to themselves and to society; and that experience has shown that heredity plays an important part in the transmission of insanity, imbecility, &c. The statute then enacts that whenever the superintendent of certain institutions including the above named State Colony shall be of opinion that it is for the best interests of the patients and of society than an inmate under his care should be sexually sterilized, he may have the operation performed upon any patient afflicted with hereditary forms of insanity, imbecility, &c., on complying with the very careful provisions by which the act protects the patients from possible abuse.

The superintendent first presents a petition to the special board of directors of his hospital or colony, stating the facts and the grounds for his opinion, verified by affidavit. Notice of the petition and of the time and place of the hearing in the institution is to be served upon the inmate, and also upon his guardian, and if there is no guardian the superintendent is to apply to the Circuit Court of the County to appoint one. If the inmate is a minor notice also is to be given to his parents if any with a copy of the petition. The board is to see to it that the inmate may attend the hearings if desired by him or his guardian. The evidence is all to be reduced to writing, after the board has made its order for or against the operation, the superintendent, or the inmate, or his guardian, may appeal to the Circuit Court of the County. The Circuit Court may consider the record of the board and the evidence before it and such other admissible evidence as may be offered, and may affirm, revise, or reverse the order of the board and enter such order as it deems just. Finally any party may apply to the Supreme Court of Appeals, which, if it grants the appeal, is to hear the case upon the record of the trial in the Circuit Court and may enter such order as it thinks the Circuit Court should have entered. There can be no doubt that so far as procedure is concerned the rights of the patient are most carefully considered, and as every step in this case was taken in scrupulous compliance with the statute and after months of observation, there is no doubt that in that respect the plaintiff in error has had due process of law.

The attack is not upon the procedure but upon the substantive law. It seems to be contended that in no circumstances could such an order be justified. It certainly is contended that the order cannot be justified upon the existing grounds. The judgment finds the facts that have been recited and that Carrie Buck "is the probable potential parent of socially inadequate offspring, likewise afflicted, that she may be sexually sterilized without detriment to her general health and that her welfare and that of society will be promoted by her sterilization," and thereupon makes the order. In view of the general declarations of the legislature and the specific findings of the Court, obviously we cannot say as matter of law that the grounds do not exist, and if they exist they justify the result. We have seen more than once that the public welfare may call upon the best citizens for their lives. It would be strange if it could not call upon those who already sap the strength of the State for these lesser sacrifices, often not felt to be such by those concerned, in order to prevent our being swamped with incompetence. It is better for all

the world, if instead of waiting to execute degenerate offspring for crime, or to let them starve for their imbecility, society can prevent those who are manifestly unfit from continuing their kind. The principle that sustains compulsory vaccination is broad enough to cover cutting the Fallopian tubes. *Jacobson* v. *Massachusetts,* 197 U.S. 11. Three generations of imbeciles are enough.

But, it is said, however it might be if this reasoning were applied generally, it fails when it is confined to the small number who are in the institutions named and is not applied to the multitudes outside. It is the usual last resort of constitutional arguments to point out shortcomings of this sort. But the answer is that the law does all that is needed when it does all that it can, indicates a policy, applies it to all within the lines, and seeks to bring within the lines all similarly situated so far and so fast as its means allow. Of course so far as the operations enable those who otherwise must be kept confined to be returned to the world, and thus open the asylum to others, the equality aimed at will be more nearly reached.

Judgment affirmed.
Mr. Justice Butler dissents.

◉ D. H. Lawrence, from *Lady Chatterley's Lover* (1928)

Lawrence uses Clifford, the cripple in the motor-chair, to criticize modernity's embrace of technology to the exclusion of love and the natural world. On the one hand, Clifford wants Connie to bear a son for him and to preserve the natural world from destruction. On the other hand, he wants a son only to carry forward his name, and he represents the forces of technology that attack nature. How easy would it be for Lawrence to embody these contradictory positions had Clifford not been disabled?

On a frosty morning with a little February sun, Clifford and Connie went for a walk across the park to the wood. That is, Clifford chuffed in his motor-chair, and Connie walked beside him.

The hard air was still sulphurous, but they were both used to it. Round the near horizon went the haze, opalescent with frost and smoke, and on the top lay the small blue sky; so that it was like being inside an enclosure, always inside. Life always a dream or a frenzy, inside an enclosure.

The sheep coughed in the rough, sere grass of the park, where frost lay bluish in the sockets of the tufts. Across the park ran a path to the wood-gate, a fine ribbon of pink. Clifford had had it newly gravelled with sifted gravel from the pit-bank. When the rock and refuse of the underworld had burned and given off its sulphur, it turned bright pink, shrimp-coloured on dry days, darker, crab-coloured on wet. Now it was pale shrimp-colour, with a bluish-white hoar of frost. It always pleased Connie, this underfoot of sifted, bright pink. It's an ill wind that brings nobody good.

Clifford steered cautiously down the slope of the knoll from the hall, and Connie kept her hand on the chair. In front lay the wood, the hazel thicket nearest, the purplish density of oaks beyond. From the wood's edge rabbits bobbed and nibbled. Rooks suddenly rose in a black train, and went trailing off over the little sky.

Connie opened the wood-gate, and Clifford puffed slowly through into the broad riding that ran up an incline between the clean-whipped thickets of the hazel. The wood was a remnant of the great forest where Robin Hood hunted, and this riding was an old, old thoroughfare coming across country. But now, of course, it was only a riding through the private wood. The road from Mansfield swerved round to the north.

In the wood everything was motionless, the old leaves on the ground keeping the frost on their underside. A jay called harshly, many little birds fluttered. But there was no game; no pheasants. They had been killed off during the war, and the wood had been left unprotected, till now Clifford had got his game-keeper again.

Clifford loved the wood; he loved the old oak-trees. He felt they were his own through generations. He wanted to protect them. He wanted this place inviolate, shut off from the world.

The chair chuffed slowly up the incline, rocking and jolting on the frozen clods. And suddenly, on the left, came a clearing where there was nothing but a ravel of dead bracken, a thin and spindly sapling leaning here and there, big sawn stumps, showing their tops and their grasping roots, lifeless. And patches of blackness where the woodmen had burned the brushwood and rubbish.

This was one of the places that Sir Geoffrey had cut during the war for trench timber. The whole knoll, which rose softly on the right of the riding, was denuded and strangely forlorn. On the crown of the knoll where the oaks had stood, now was bareness; and from there you could look out over the trees to the colliery railway, and the new works at Stacks Gate. Connie had stood and looked, it was a breach in the pure seclusion of the wood. It let in the world. But she didn't tell Clifford.

This denuded place always made Clifford curiously angry. He had been through the war, had seen what it meant. But he didn't get really angry till he saw this bare hill. He was having it replanted. But it made him hate Sir Geoffrey.

Clifford sat with a fixed face as the chair slowly mounted. When they came to the top of the rise he stopped; he would not risk the long and very jolty down-slope. He sat looking at the greenish sweep of the riding downwards, a clear way through the bracken and oaks. It swerved at the bottom of the hill and disappeared; but it had such a lovely easy curve, of knights riding and ladies on palfreys.

'I consider this is really the heart of England,' said Clifford to Connie, as he sat there in the dim February sunshine.

'Do you?' she said, seating herself in her blue knitted dress, on a stump by the path.

'I do! this is the old England, the heart of it; and I intend to keep it intact.'

'Oh yes!' said Connie. But, as she said it she heard the eleven-o'clock hooters at Stacks Gate colliery. Clifford was too used to the sound to notice.

'I want this wood perfect . . . untouched. I want nobody to trespass in it,' said Clifford.

There was a certain pathos. The wood still had some of the mystery of wild, old England; but Sir Geoffrey's cuttings during the war had given it a blow. How still the trees were, with their crinkly, innumerable twigs against the sky, and their grey, obstinate trunks rising from the brown bracken! How safely the birds flitted among them! And once there had been deer, and archers, and monks padding along on asses. The place remembered, still remembered.

Clifford sat in the pale sun, with the light on his smooth, rather blond hair, his reddish full face inscrutable.

'I mind more, not having a son, when I come here, than any other time,' he said.

'But the wood is older than your family,' said Connie gently.

'Quite!' said Clifford. 'But we've preserved it. Except for us it would go . . . it would be gone already, like the rest of the forest. One must preserve some of the old England!'

'Must one?' said Connie. 'If it has to be preserved, and preserved against the new England? It's sad, I know.'

'If some of the old England isn't preserved, there'll be no England at all,' said Clifford. 'And we who have this kind of property, and the feeling for it, must preserve it.'

There was a sad pause. 'Yes, for a little while,' said Connie.

'For a little while! It's all we can do. We can only do our bit. I feel every man of my family has done his bit here, since we've had the place. One may go against convention, but one must keep up tradition.' Again there was a pause.

'What tradition?' asked Connie.

'The tradition of England! of this!'

'Yes,' she said slowly.

'That's why having a son helps; one is only a link in a chain,' he said.

Connie was not keen on chains, but she said nothing. She was thinking of the curious impersonality of his desire for a son.

'I'm sorry we can't have a son,' she said.

He looked at her steadily, with his full, pale-blue eyes.

'It would almost be a good thing if you had a child by another man,' he said. 'If we brought it up at Wragby, it would belong to us and to the place. I don't believe very intensely in fatherhood. If we had the child to rear, it would be our own, and it would carry on. Don't you think it's worth considering?'

Connie looked up at him at last. The child, her child, was just an 'it' to him. It . . . it . . . it!

'But what about the other man?' she asked.

'Does it matter very much? Do these things really affect us very deeply? . . . You had that lover in Germany . . . what is it now? Nothing almost. It seems to me that it isn't these little acts and little connexions we make in our lives that matter so very much. They pass away, and where are they? Where . . . Where are the snows of yesteryear? . . . It's what endures through one's life that matters; my own life matters to me, in its long continuance and development. But what do the occasional connexions matter? And the occasional sexual connexions especially! If people don't exaggerate them ridiculously, they pass like the mating of birds. And so they should. What does it matter? It's the life-long companionship that matters. It's the living together from day to day, not the sleeping together once or twice. You and I are married, no matter

what happens to us. We have the habit of each other. And habit, to my thinking, is more vital than any occasional excitement. The long, slow, enduring thing . . . that's what we live by . . . not the occasional spasm of any sort. Little by little, living together, two people fall into a sort of unison, they vibrate so intricately to one another. That's the real secret of marriage, not sex; at least not the simple function of sex. You and I are interwoven in a marriage. If we stick to that we ought to be able to arrange this sex thing, as we arrange going to the dentist; since fate has given us a checkmate physically there.'

Connie sat and listened in a sort of wonder, and a sort of fear. She did not know if he was right or not. There was Michaelis, whom she loved; so she said to herself. But her love was somehow only an excursion from her marriage with Clifford; the long, slow habit of intimacy, formed through years of suffering and patience. Perhaps the human soul needs excursions, and must not be denied them. But the point of an excursion is that you come home again.

'And wouldn't you mind *what* man's child I had?' she asked.

'Why, Connie, I should trust your natural instinct of decency and selection. You just wouldn't let the wrong sort of fellow touch you.'

She thought of Michaelis! He was absolutely Clifford's idea of the wrong sort of fellow.

'But men and women may have different feelings about the wrong sort of fellow,' she said.

'No,' he replied. 'You care for me. I don't believe you would ever care for a man who was purely antipathetic to me. Your rhythm wouldn't let you.'

She was silent. Logic might be unanswerable because it was so absolutely wrong.

'And should you expect me to tell you?' she asked, glancing up at him almost furtively.

'Not at all, I'd better not know. . . . But you do agree with me, don't you, that the casual sex thing is nothing, compared to the long life lived together? Don't you think one can just subordinate the sex thing to the necessities of a long life? Just use it, since that's what we're driven to? After all, do these temporary excitements matter? Isn't the whole problem of life the slow building up of an integral personality, through the years? living an integrated life? There's no point in a disintegrated life. If lack of sex is going to disintegrate you, then go out and have a love-affair. If lack of a child is going to disintegrate you, then have a child if you possibly can. But only do these things so that you have an integrated life, that makes a long harmonious thing. And you and I can do that together . . . don't you think? . . . if we adapt ourselves to the necessities, and at the same time weave the adaptation together into a piece with our steadily-lived life. Don't you agree?'

Connie was a little overwhelmed by his words. She knew he was right theoretically. But when she actually touched her steadily-lived life with him she . . . hesitated. Was it actually her destiny to go on weaving herself into his life all the rest of her life? Nothing else?

Was it just that? She was to be content to weave a steady life with him, all one fabric, but perhaps brocaded with the occasional flower of an adventure. But how could she know what she would feel next year? How could one ever know? How could one say Yes? for years and years? The little yes, gone on a breath! Why should one be pinned down by that butterfly word? Of course it had to flutter away and be gone, to be followed by other yes's and no's! Like the straying of butterflies.

'I think you're right, Clifford. And as far as I can see I agree with you. Only life may turn quite a new face on it all.'

'But until life turns a new face on it all, you do agree?'

'Oh yes! I think I do, really.'

She was watching a brown spaniel that had run out of a side-path, and was looking towards them with lifted nose, making a soft, fluffy bark. A man with a gun strode swiftly, softly out after the dog, facing their way as if about to attack them; then stopped instead, saluted, and was turning downhill. It was only the new game-keeper, but he had frightened Connie, he seemed to emerge with such a swift menace. That was how she had seen him, like the sudden rush of a threat out of nowhere.

He was a man in dark green velveteens and gaiters . . . the old style, with a red face and red moustache and distant eyes. He was going quickly downhill.

'Mellors!' called Clifford.

The man faced lightly round, and saluted with a quick little gesture, a soldier!

'Will you turn the chair round and get it started? That makes it easier,' said Clifford.

The man at once slung his gun over his shoulder, and came forward with the same curious swift, yet soft movements, as if keeping invisible. He was moderately tall and lean, and was silent. He did not look at Connie at all, only at the chair.

'Connie, this is the new game-keeper, Mellors. You haven't spoken to her ladyship yet, Mellors?'

'No, Sir!' came the ready, neutral words.

The man lifted his hat as he stood, showing his thick, almost fair hair. He stared straight into Connie's eyes, with a perfect, fearless, impersonal look, as if he wanted to see what she was like. He made her feel shy. She bent her head to him shyly, and he changed his hat to his left hand and made her a slight bow, like a gentleman; but he said nothing at all. He remained for a moment still, with his hat in his hand.

'But you've been here some time, haven't you?' Connie said to him.

'Eight months, Madam . . . your Ladyship!' he corrected himself calmly.

'And do you like it?'

She looked him in the eyes. His eyes narrowed a little, with irony, perhaps with impudence.

'Why, yes, thank you, your Ladyship! I was reared here . . .'

He gave another slight bow, turned, put his hat on, and strode to take hold of the chair. His voice on the last words had fallen into the heavy broad drag of the dialect . . . perhaps also in mockery, because there had been no trace of dialect before. He might almost be a gentleman. Anyhow, he was a curious, quick, separate fellow, alone, but sure of himself.

Clifford started the little engine, the man carefully turned the chair, and set it nose-forwards to the incline that curved gently to the dark hazel thicket.

'Is that all then, Sir Clifford?' asked the man.

'No, you'd better come along in case she sticks. The engine isn't really strong enough for the uphill work.' The man glanced round for his dog . . . a thoughtful glance. The spaniel looked at him and faintly moved its tail. A little smile, mocking or teasing her, yet gentle, came into his eyes for a moment, then faded away, and his face was expressionless. They went fairly quickly down the slope, the man with his hand on the rail of the chair, steadying it. He looked like a free soldier rather than a servant. And something about him reminded Connie of Tommy Dukes.

When they came to the hazel grove, Connie suddenly ran forward, and opened the gate into the park. As she stood holding it, the two men looked at her in passing, Clifford critically, the other man with a curious, cool wonder; impersonally wanting to see what she looked like. And she saw in his blue, impersonal eyes a look of suffering and detachment, yet a certain warmth. But why was he so aloof, apart?

Clifford stopped the chair, once through the gate, and the man came quickly, courteously, to close it.

'Why did you run to open?' asked Clifford in his quiet, calm voice, that showed he was displeased. 'Mellors would have done it.'

'I thought you would go straight ahead,' said Connie.

'And leave you to run after us?' said Clifford.

'Oh, well, I like to run sometimes!'

Mellors took the chair again, looking perfectly unheeding, yet Connie felt he noted everything. As he pushed the chair up the steepish rise of the knoll in the park, he breathed rather quickly, through parted lips. He was rather frail really. Curiously full of vitality, but a little frail and quenched. Her woman's instinct sensed it.

Connie fell back, let the chair go on. The day had greyed over; the small blue sky that had poised low on its circular rims of haze was closed in again, the lid was down, there was a raw coldness. It was going to snow. All grey, all grey! the world looked worn out.

The chair waited at the top of the pink path. Clifford looked round for Connie.

'Not tired, are you?' he said.

'Oh, no!' she said.

But she was. A strange, weary yearning, a dissatisfaction had started in her. Clifford did not notice: those were not things he was aware of. But the stranger knew. To Connie, everything in her world and life seemed worn out, and her dissatisfaction was older than the hills.

They came to the house, and around to the back, where there were no steps. Clifford managed to swing himself over on to the low, wheeled house-chair; he was very strong and agile with his arms. Then Connie lifted the burden of his dead legs after him.

The keeper, waiting at attention to be dismissed, watched everything narrowly, missing nothing. He went pale, with a sort of fear, when he saw Connie lifting the inert legs of the man in her arms, into the other chair, Clifford pivoting round as she did so. He was frightened.

'Thanks, then, for the help, Mellors,' said Clifford casually, as he began to wheel down the passage to the servants' quarters.

'Nothing else, Sir?' came the neutral voice, like one in a dream.

'Nothing, good morning!'

'Good morning, Sir.'

'Good morning! it was kind of you to push the chair up that hill . . . I hope it wasn't heavy for you,' said Connie, looking back at the keeper outside the door.

His eyes came to hers in an instant, as if wakened up. He was aware of her.

'Oh no, not heavy!' he said quickly. Then his voice dropped again into the broad sound of the vernacular: 'Good mornin' to your Ladyship!'

'Who is your game-keeper?' Connie asked at lunch.

'Mellors! You saw him,' said Clifford.

'Yes, but where did he come from?'

'Nowhere! He was a Tevershall boy . . . son of a collier, I believe.'

'And was he a collier himself?'

'Blacksmith on the pit-bank, I believe: overhead smith. But he was keeper here for two years before the war . . . before he joined up. My father always had a good opinion of him, so when he came back, and went to the pit for a blacksmith's job, I just took him back here as keeper. I was really very glad to get him . . . its almost impossible to find a good man round here for a gamekeeper . . . and it needs a man who knows the people.'

'And isn't he married?'

'He was. But his wife went off with . . . with various men . . . but finally with a collier at Stacks Gate, and I believe she's living there still.'

'So this man is alone?'

'More or less! He has a mother in the village . . . and a child, I believe.'

Clifford looked at Connie, with his pale, slightly prominent blue eyes, in which a certain vagueness was coming. He seemed alert in the foreground, but the background was like the Midlands atmosphere, haze, smoky mist. And the haze seemed to be creeping forward. So when he stared at Connie in his peculiar way, giving her his peculiar, precise information, she felt all the background of his mind filling up with mist, with nothingness. And it frightened her. It made him seem impersonal, almost to idiocy.

And dimly she realized one of the great laws of the human soul: that when the emotional soul receives a wounding shock, which does not kill the body, the soul seems to recover as the body recovers. But this is only appearance. It is really only the mechanism of the re-assumed habit. Slowly, slowly the wound to the soul begins to make itself felt, like a bruise, which only slowly deepens its terrible ache, till it fills all the psyche. And when we think we have recovered and forgotten, it is then that the terrible after-effects have to be encountered at their worst.

So it was with Clifford. Once he was 'well,' once he was back at Wragby, and writing his stories, and feeling sure of life, in spite of all, he seemed to forget, and to have recovered all his equanimity. But now, as the years went by, slowly, slowly, Connie felt the bruise of fear and horror coming up, and spreading in him. For a time it had been so deep as to be numb, as it were non-existent. Now slowly it began to assert itself in a spread of fear, almost paralysis. Mentally he still was alert. But the paralysis, the bruise of the too-great shock, was gradually spreading in his affective self.

And as it spread in him, Connie felt it spread in her. An inward dread, an emptiness, an indifference to everything gradually spread in her soul. When Clifford was roused, he could still talk brilliantly and, as it were, command the future: as when, in the wood, he talked about her having a child, and giving an heir to Wragby. But the day after, all the brilliant words seemed like dead leaves, crumpling up and turning to powder, meaning really nothing, blown away on any gust of wind. They were not the leafy words of an effective life, young with energy and belonging to the tree. They were the hosts of fallen leaves of a life that is ineffectual. . . .

Source: Lawrence, D. H. 1928. *Lady Chatterley's Lover.* Available at: http://www.web-books.com/Classics/Lawrence/Chatterley/

▣ Nicholas O. Isaacson, "The Tie That Binds" (1928)

Disabled veterans are frequently seen exclusively as clients of the welfare state, whose identities and organizations are a product exclusively of their effort to exact benefits and assistance from governments. While this perspective does speak to an aspect of the experience of disabled veterans in the modern era, it fails to understand the larger sources of the disabled veterans' solidarity in such common experiences as war, incurring a disability, and rehabilitation. It also fails to account for idealism born of these common experiences and informing their solidarity. Founded in the wake of World War I, the Disabled American Veterans of the World War included men with the complete spectrum of service-related impairments and chronic illnesses; the organization had a membership of approximately 25,000 men in the interwar period.

Born in the tumult of bloody battle—brotherhood is a bond that has endured, and will endure on down from ages past to aeons yet to come—the tie of comradeship.

Men who have bared their breasts to the barbs of a common foe, who have taken in their bodies the lethal gas, the rending shot and the macerating shell of a national enemy are joined together in a union eternal.

Soldier organizations have that bond in common.

But only in the Disabled American Veterans of the World War is that bond sanctified by the blood sacrifice, welded by the heat of passion that rises as comrade sees the soul of comrade torn from body and sent to the haven of the souls of those gone West.

We stand, all for one, one for all.

We are the DAV.

For those who made the supreme sacrifice we have reverence and cherished memories.

For those who bled, but did not die, who won back some measure of their splendid young manhood offered so freely that the nation might not be crushed beneath the heel of foreign oppression, we hold comradeship, and the hand of congratulation.

For those who still fight on, weary, tired, but dauntless, who spend their days gazing at wall and ceiling in the hospitals, we have sympathy and extend the hand and pledge of eternal loyalty.

Some of us have fared well, in those days since the dawn of Armistice broke over a world soon to be at peace, a world in which no screaming shells flew through the air, seeking lodgement in the flesh of men. Some of us have fought a bitter fight, seeking to retrace that pathway to success. Some of us are still at the lower levels of that upward path.

But whatever our condition, whatever our present status, we are Comrades. We are, as ever and for always, one for all and all for one.

Much has been done, in the years that have passed, to better conditions. Far more is yet to be encompassed.

Together, in unison, constantly striving to attain our objectives, we can wear away the opposition that stands between us and our hopes. As a great, unified power we can go forward to that state where no veteran may suffer further as a result of sacrifices for his country.

Bring in the comrade who is not a member, that we may grow in power. Bring in the comrade who may need our combined power of organization to win that which may be his just due, but of which he has been deprived.

Live, think, talk the bond that binds us.

With that thought in mind, of loyalty, faith, and love for one another, as your commander for the glorious organization year that closes with this convention, I greet you.

NICHOLAS O. ISAACSON,
State Commander.

Source: Isaacson, Nicholas O. 1928. "The Tie That Binds." In the convention program for the State Convention of the Disabled American Veterans of the World War, Department of Illinois, May 24–26, 1928. The editors acknowledge the assistance of Dr. Jeffrey S. Resnick of the Orthotic and Prosthetic Assistance Fund, Inc., in sharing this document, which is part of his private collection. Permission granted by the Illinois Chapter of Disabled American Veterans.

▣ William Faulkner, from *The Sound and the Fury* (1929)

William Faulkner (1897–1962), one of the most celebrated writers of the American modernist period, created lasting stories about the experiences of people with disabilities in the early twentieth century. Sometimes these were deployed as metaphors of social decay, but Faulkner also wrote memorable portraits by imagining disabled people's subjective perspective of the world. This excerpt from The Sound and the Fury, *a novel narrated by multiple characters, opens with a first-person narrative of Benjamin Compson ("Benjy"), a 33-year-old man diagnosed with "idiocy" who was based on a neighbor of Faulkner's with Down syndrome. The second excerpt is narrated by Benjy's brother, Jason Compson, a violent eugenicist who would like to have his sibling institutionalized so he would no longer "disgrace" his fallen aristocratic Southern family. The dialectic between the two demonstrates the violence directed at cognitively disabled people during the eugenics period.*

Benjy Compson narrating the event leading up to his castration:

They came on. I opened the Gate and they stopped, turning. I was trying to say, and I caught her, trying to say, and she screamed and I was trying to say and trying and the bright shapes began to stop and the bright shapes began to stop and I tried to get out. I tried to get it off my face, but the bright shapes were going again. They were going up the hill to where it fell away and I tried to cry. But when I breathed in, I couldn't breathe out again to cry, and I tried to keep from falling off the hill and I fell off the hill into the bright, whirling shapes.

Jason Compson's internal narrative about his brother Benjamin:

How to stop my clock with a nose spray and then you can send Ben to the Navy I says or to the Calvary anyway, they use geldings in the Calvary. Then when she sent Quentin home for me to feed too I says I guess that's right too, instead of me having to go way up north for a job they sent the job down here to me and then Mother begun to cry and I says it's not that I have any objection to having it here; if it's any satisfaction to you I'll quit work and nurse it myself and let you and Dilsey keep the flour barrel full, or Ben, rent him out to a sideshow; there must be folks somewhere that would pay a dime to see him, then she cried more and kept saying my poor afflicted baby and I says yes he'll be quite a help to you when he gets his growth not being more than one and a half times high as me now and she says she'd be dead soon and then we'd all be better off and so I says all right, all right, have it your way.

Source: Faulkner, William. 1990. *The Sound and the Fury.* New York: Vintage. Originally published 1929. Copyright 1929 and renewed 1957 by William Faulkner. Used by permission of Random House, Inc.

▣ The Beginning of Korean Special Education (1929)

George Paik explains the origin of education for disabled children as American missionary Dr. Rosetta Hall's effort. In his description, blind people's traditional occupation is introduced. The Braille applied by Hall was later replaced with Pak Du Seong's Hunmaengjeongeum, the Korean alphabet.

All persons suffering from deformities claim our sympathy, but the blind in Korea deserve a double share, not only for their physical misfortune, but also because they are often forced to become sorcerers and exorcists. In order to make "the blind girls of Korea happy, useful members of the Christian home circle," Mrs. Rosetta S. Hall, M.D., initiated education for them. When Mrs. Hall was a girl she had learned, as an amusement, the use of the "New York point" system of raised letters. When she came to Korea as a missionary, she found that her casually acquired knowledge was most useful.

As early as the spring of 1894 she began to give instruction to the blind daughter of a Christian. When her husband died, in 1894, she returned to America. During her stay in the United States, she visited the

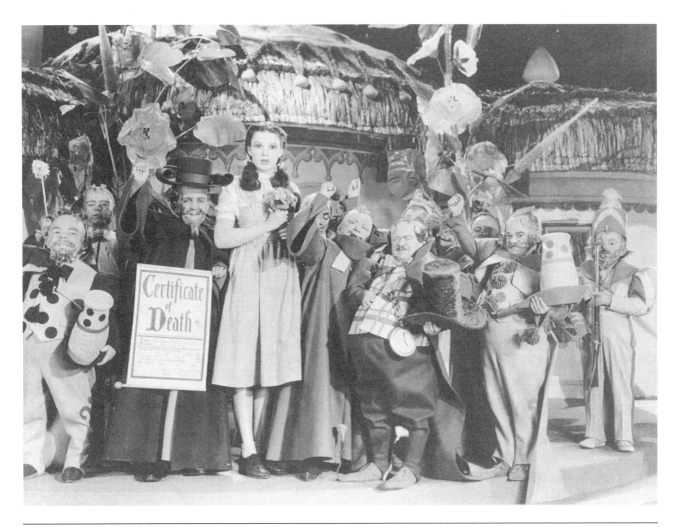

The Wizard of Oz is the classic fantasy of the girl Dorothy, from middle America (Kansas), who finds herself in a surreal world populated by Munchkins and anthropomorphized animals and inanimate figures.

Source: *The Wizard of Oz* (1939), directed by Victor Fleming. B&W/color, 100 minutes. Reprinted by permission of Paul Darke.

Institution for the Blind in New York and relearned the "Point" system. Upon her return to Korea in 1897, she adapted this to the Korean alphabet and syllabary, preparing part of a primer and the Ten Commandments, and taught the girl whom she had begun to instruct in 1894. The work thus commenced so attracted the attention of the people that by 1906 there were seven students. With money given her by friends in America, Mrs. Hall maintained a class-room in connection with her dispensary, where these girls were taught. They were not only given regular day school education, but also lessons in the practical arts.

Source: Paik, L. George. 1929. Pp. 324–325 in *The History of Protestant Missions in Korea 1832–1910*. Seoul, South Korea: Yonsei University Press.

▣ Thomas "Fats" Waller, Harry Brooks, and Andy Razaf, "What Did I Do To Be So Black and Blue" (1929)

The blues classic, recorded by Louis Armstrong, plays with the metaphor of bruising—black and blue marks—to explore racism in the United States.

Cold empty bed . . . springs hurt my head
Feels like ole Ned . . . wished I was dead
What did I do . . . to be so black and blue
Even the mouse . . . ran from my house
They laugh at you . . . and all that you do
What did I do . . . to be so black and blue

I'm white . . . inside . . . but, that don't help my case

> That's life . . . can't hide . . . what is in my face
> How would it end . . . ain't got a friend
> My only sin . . . is in my skin
> What did I do . . . to be so black and blue
> How would it end . . . I ain't got a friend
> My only sin . . . is in my skin
> What did I do . . . to be so black and blue

▣ "Where Work of Salvaging Human Beings Goes Forward" (1930)

The following article details the philosophy of 1930s-era segregated schooling for physically disabled children in the United States by describing the School for Crippled Children (later named Condon School) in Cincinnati, Ohio. These institutions were established as an alternative to hospital schools, but they were largely nonintegrated, both racially and in terms of developmental disability, until the 1960s. This particular school included a full therapeutic regimen—physical, occupational, speech, medical, and dental—that functioned parallel to academic and technical training.

Cincinnati is the scene of one of the greatest human experiments going on in the present-day world—the reconstruction of human salvage. While the best that Cincinnati affords [in] medical and surgical skill is concentrated in trying to make normal as possible, misshapen bodies and twisted limbs, the best educational thought of the city is directed to preparing them to cope with the problems of life in competition with the normal persons of the community.

The experiment is being conducted and conducted happily—in the School for Crippled Children, operated by the Board of Education on Rockdale avenue, near Burnet, Avondale. The school has just about everything needed to sustain life and keep residents happy. It's a self-contained structure, and inside its walls one might eat, sleep, work, play, see the doctor, read and learn without ever finding it necessary to leave.

Cincinnati treats its unfortunate children well here. They're taught to make the most of themselves. They're taught to forget that they're handicapped. They're taught to lead normal lives. They're taught to earn a living among normal persons.

It is this psychological background, this self-confidence, that is the school's primary objective, Mrs. Mary T. Betts, principal, explains. And, proudly she conducts visitors through the structure.

She shows them the modern pediatric orthopedic, cardiac and dental offices, each fitted with the latest and most perfect of instruments and other equipment, but it is with more pride that she shows the class rooms, where the students are given a cultural background, and the handicraft rooms, where they are given a vocational background.

Handicraft Rooms

There are two principal handicraft rooms and a number of smaller ones. The one for boys is fitted out exactly like those in schools for normal children. There are work benches, equipped with vises, and there are wood-working tools of every sort. Off on the side is a smaller room, where the finished products are painted.

The work of the students shows quite the professional touch. They produce everything from small bookends on up, and each piece is carefully tooled and decorated.

On the girls' side is a large sewing room and a large kitchen. The students here learn everything from lowering hems to delicate embroidery, and from frying eggs to preparing exotic salads.

"We attempt to teach them to do the unusual sort of work," Mrs. Bett explains, "The unusual provides them a better market and a better chance to make a living."

Even while they're in school the students may make part of their expenses, for much of the work they produce finds a ready market, not only in Cincinnati, but throughout the country.

For Regular Study

The classrooms for regular study, too, are like ordinary classrooms, except that the desks and chairs may be fitted with special apparatus to make the child more comfortable.

But in spite of all such things as these, most of the pupils must be treated for their afflictions, and the school provides for them thoroughly.

In one respect it differs from other such institutions. Most of them are either only one story high, or have ramps, instead of stairways, to link the several floors. The Cincinnati school has stairways.

"After all," Mrs. Betts says, "in ordinary conditions [the] children must climb stairs. Here we can teach them to do it, increase their confidence in their ability to do it."

The stairways are provided with banisters of several heights, to aid the children, and their instructors, of course help them further. And there are elevators for wheel-chair patients.

The various clinics are each considered complete. There [are] complete orthopedic and pediatric suites, where each case receives special attention and corrective treatment. Outstanding specialists contribute their services.

There is a large restroom, open in warm weather and gassed in in cold weather, where, on cloudy days the children lie on cots in a circle under a gargantuan ray machine which substitutes for the sun.

Source: "Where Work of Salvaging Human Beings Goes Forward." 1930, December 11. *Cincinnati Times Star* 18:1.

◎ Virginia Woolf, from *On Being Ill* (1930)

In this excerpt from an essay that was published as a slim book in 1930, Woolf proclaims the universal, the inescapable, the invisible, and the overwhelming nature of the embodied experience. Everyone has a body that endures illness and pain, and no one can be in the world separate from the body. However, the literary reflection of these truths is minimal (to Woolf's eye), because the whole idea of "this monster, the body, this miracle, its pain" is so fearsome to contemplate.

Considering how common illness is, how tremendous the spiritual change that it brings, how astonishing, when the lights of health go down, the undiscovered countries that are then disclosed, what wastes and deserts of the soul a light attack of influenza brings to view, what precipices and lawns sprinkled with bright flowers a little rise of temperature reveals, what ancient and obdurate oaks are uprooted in us by the act of sickness, how we go down into the pit of death and feel the waters of annihilation close above our heads and wake thinking to find ourselves in the presence of the angels and the harpers when we have a tooth out and come to the surface in the dentist's armchair and confuse his "Rinse the mouth—rinse the mouth" with the greetings of the Deity stooping from the floor of Heaven to welcome us—when we think of this, as we are so frequently forced to think of it, it becomes strange indeed that illness has not taken its place with love and battle and jealousy among the prime themes of literature. Novels, one would have thought, would have been devoted to influenza; epic poems to typhoid; odes to pneumonia; lyrics to toothache. But no; with a few exceptions—De Quincey attempted something of the sort in *The Opium Eater;* there must be a volume or two about disease scattered through the pages of Proust—literature does its best to maintain that its concern is with the mind; that the body is a sheet of plain glass through which the soul looks straight and clear, and, save for one or two passions such as desire and greed, is null, and negligible and non-existent. On the contrary, the very opposite is true. All day, all night the body intervenes; blunts or sharpens, colours or discolours, turns to wax in the warmth of June, hardens to tallow in the murk of February. The creature within can only gaze through the pane—smudged or rosy; it cannot separate off from the body like the sheath of a knife or the pod of a pea for a single instant; it must go through the whole unending procession of changes, heat and cold, comfort and discomfort, hunger and satisfaction, health and illness, until there comes the inevitable catastrophe; the body smashes itself to smithereens, and the soul (it is said) escapes. But of all this daily drama of the body there is no record. People write always of the doings of the mind; the thoughts that come to it; its noble plans; how the mind has civilised the universe. They show it ignoring the body in the philosopher's turret; or kicking the body, like an old leather football, across leagues of snow and desert in the pursuit of conquest or discovery. Those great wars which the body wages with the mind a slave to it, in the solitude of the bedroom against the assault of fever or the oncome of melancholia, are neglected. Nor is the reason far to seek. To look these things squarely in the face would need the courage of a lion tamer; a robust philosophy; a reason rooted in the bowels of the earth. Short of these, this monster, the body, this miracle, its pain, will soon make us taper into mysticism, or rise, with rapid beats of the wings, into the raptures of transcendentalism.

Source: Woolf, Virginia. 2003. *On Being Ill.* Ashfield, MA: Paris Press. Originally published 1930. Reprinted by permission of the Society of Authors as the literary representative of the estate of Virginia Woolf.

▣ Erich Maria Remarque, from *The Road Back* (1931)

Another source of the solidarity of disabled veterans has been their persistent difficulties in dealing with the state in its capacity as a provider of assistance and benefits. Impersonal and insensitive administration of programs, declining commitment to fund programs during periods of fiscal stringency, and ignorance of specific disabling conditions have consistently plagued relations between disabled veterans and government. These difficulties are exacerbated under circumstances of defeat, in which governments have to contend with demoralization as well as economic collapse. In this selection, from a novel written by the most significant German interpreter of the World War I experience, the desperate situation of German disabled veterans after World War I is captured, as is the terrible toll of war upon the bodies of the veterans involved in the ghostly protest demonstration that Remarque describes.

Demonstrations in the streets have been called for this afternoon. Prices have been soaring everywhere for months past, and the poverty is greater even than it was during the war. Wages are insufficient to buy the bare necessities of life, and even though one may have the money it is often impossible to buy anything with it. But ever more and more gin palaces and dance halls go up, and ever more and more blatant is the profiteering and swindling.

Scattered groups of workers on strike march through the streets. Now and again there is a disturbance. A rumor is going about that troops have been concentrated at the barracks. But there is no sign of it as yet.

Here and there one hears cries and counter-cries. Somebody is haranguing at a street corner. Then suddenly everywhere is silence.

A procession of men in the faded uniforms of the frontline trenches is moving slowly toward us. It is

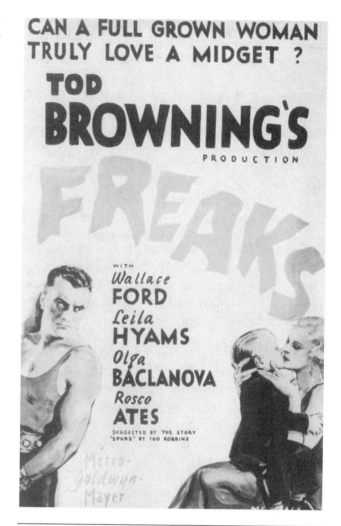

In Freaks, *a community of circus "freaks" takes revenge on a female trapeze artist and her strong-man lover after she has married Hans, a short-statured performer, for his fortune. The director, Tod Browning, cast in key parts disabled actors, including Harry Earles, Daisy Earles, Daisy and Violet Hilton, Johnny Eck, Randion, and others. The film became deeply controversial in its day, largely because of the fact that living disabled people were employed in key roles. In the 1960s, the film experienced a revival as a cult classic as an insightful social allegory about intolerance.*

Source: *Freaks* (1932), directed by Tod Browning. B&W, 60 minutes.

formed up by sections, marching in fours. But white placards are carried before: *Where is the Fatherland's gratitude?—The War Cripples are starving.*

The men with one arm are carrying the placards, and they look around continually to see if the procession is still coming along properly behind them, for they are the fastest.

These are followed by men with sheep dogs on short, leather leads. The animals have the red cross of the blind at their collars. Watchfully they walk along beside their masters. If the procession halts they sit down, and then the blind men stop. Sometimes dogs off the street will rush in among the column, barking and wagging their tails, wanting to romp and play with them. But these merely turn their heads and take no notice of all the sniffing and yapping. Yet their ears are erect, pricked and alert, and their eyes are alive; but they walk as if they no longer wished to run and to jump, as if they understood for what they are there. They have separated themselves from their fellows, as Sisters of Mercy separate themselves from jolly shop girls. Nor do the other dogs persist long; after a few minutes they give up and make off in such haste that it looks almost as if they were flying from something. Only a powerful mastiff stands still, and with front legs widely straddling, barks slowly, deep and hollow, till the procession is past.

It is strange how a face without eyes alters—how in the upper half it becomes extinct, smooth and dead; and how odd the mouth is in comparison, when it speaks! Only the lower half of the face lives. All these have been shot blind; and so they behave differently from men born blind. They are more violent, and at the same time more cautious, in their gestures that have not yet gained the sureness of many years of darkness. The memory of colors, of sky, earth and twilight still lives with them. They move still as if they had eyes; involuntarily they lift and turn their heads to see who it is that speaks to them. Some have black patches or bandages over their eyes, but most go without them, as if by that means they would stand nearer to colors and the light. Their eyelids are withered and closed: only the narrow strip of the lower lid still protrudes a little, blotched, wet and red like a dim, cheerless dawn. Many of them are healthy, powerful fellows with strong limbs that would like well to move freely and have play. The pale sunset of the March sky gleams behind their bowed heads. In shop windows the first lamps are being lighted. But they hardly feel the mild, sweet air of evening on their brow. In their heavy boots they move slowly through the everlasting darkness that stretches about them like a cloud; and troubled and persistent, their thoughts clamber up and down the meager scale of figures that would mean bread and comfort and life to them, and yet cannot be. Hunger and penury stir idly in the darkened rooms of their mind. Helpless and full of dull fear, they sense their nearness; yet they cannot see them nor do aught against them but to walk slowly in their numbers through the streets, lifting up their dead

faces from the darkness toward the light, in dumb appeal to others, who can still see.

Behind the blind come the men with one eye, the tattered faces of men with head wounds: wry, bulbous mouths, faces without noses and without lower jaws, entire faces one great red scar with a couple of holes where formerly were a mouth and a nose. But above this desolation, quiet, questioning, sad human eyes.

On these follow the long lines of men with legs amputated. Some already have artificial limbs that spring forward obliquely as they walk and strike clanking on the pavement, as if the whole man were artificial, made up of iron and hinges. Others have their trouser legs looped up and made fast with safety pins. These go on crutches or sticks with black rubber pads.

Then come the shakers, the shell-shocked. Their hands, their heads, their clothes, their bodies quake as though they still shuddered with horror. They no longer have control of themselves; the will has been extinguished, the muscles and nerves have revolted against the brain, the eyes become void and impotent.

One-eyed and one-armed men are pushing along wicker carriages with oilcloth covers, wherein are other men so badly wounded that they can now only live in wheeled chairs. Among them a few men come trailing a flat handcart, such as carpenters use to transport bedsteads or coffins. On it there sits a torso. The legs are gone from the hips. It is the upper half of a powerful man, nothing more. He has broad, stalwart shoulders and a big, brave face with a heavy moustache. On his head he wears a peaked cap. It may be that he was formerly a furniture mover. Beside him is a placard with wobbly lettering that he has, no doubt, painted himself—I should like to walk too, mate. With solemn face he sits there; now and then, supporting himself on his arms, he will swing a little farther up the wagon so as to change his seat.

A young, pale fellow without arms, and legs amputated at the knees, follows after him. The knees stand in thick, leather wrappings like great hooves. It appears so odd that one involuntarily looks under the wagon, as if the legs must surely carry on there beneath it. In his arm stumps he carries a placard: Many thousands of us are still lying in the hospitals.

The procession drags slowly along the streets. Wherever it passes, all is still. Once, at the corner of Hook Street, it has to wait a long time. A new dance palace is being erected there, and the street is blocked with heaps of sand, cement mixers and girders. Between the struts over the entrance is the name in illuminated letters: "Astoria Dance-Palace and Wine Saloon." The trolley with the torso stands directly beneath it, waiting until some iron girders have been shifted. The dull glow of the lighted sign floods over him, coloring the silent face to an awful red, as if it were swelling with some terrible fury and must suddenly burst into a hideous cry.

But then the column moves on, and again it is just the face of the furniture mover, pallid from the hospital in pale evening, and smiling gratefully as a comrade puts a cigarette between his lips.

Quietly the groups pass on through the streets, without cries, without indignation, resigned—a complaint, not an accusation. They know that those who can shoot no more need not expect over-much help. They will go on to the Town Hall and stand there a while; some secretary or other will say something to them, then they will break up and return singly to their rooms, their narrow dwellings, their pale children and their awful misery, without much hope, prisoners of the destiny that others made for them.

Source: Remarque, Erich Maria. 1931. Wheen, A. W., trans. Pp. 266–271 in *The Road Back*. Boston: Little, Brown, and Co. Copyright © 1931 by A.G. Ullstein; copyright renewed © 1958 by Erich Maria Remarque.

⊡ Ernest Hemingway, from "A Way You'll Never Be" (1933)

Here Hemingway plays with the stream-of-consciousness technique used by modernist writers, the style of writing by association, to represent Nick Adams's shell-shocked state of mind. This story is one of Hemingway's most successful experiments with how to picture the cognitive breakdown of a protagonist.

"I am a veteran of the Eritrea campaign," said the adjutant stiffly. "I fought in Tripoli."

"It's quite something to have met you," Nick put out his hand. "Those must have been trying days. I noticed the ribbons. Were you, by any chance, on the Carso?"

"I have just been called up for this war. My class was too old."

"At one time I was under the age limit," Nick said. "But now I am reformed out of the war."

"But why are you here now?"

"I am demonstrating the American uniform," Nick said. "Don't you think it is very significant? It is a little tight in the collar but soon you will see untold millions wearing this uniform swarming like locusts. The grasshopper, you know, what we call the grasshopper in America, is really a locust. The true grasshopper is small and green and comparatively feeble. You must not, however, make a confusion with the seven-year locust or cicada which emits a peculiar sustained sound which at the moment I cannot recall. I try to recall it but I cannot. I can almost hear it and then it is quite gone. You will pardon me if I break off our conversation?"

"See if you can find the major," the adjutant said to one of the two runners. "I can see you have been wounded," he said to Nick.

"In various places," Nick said. "If you are interested in scars I can show you some very interesting ones but I would rather talk about grasshoppers. What we call grasshoppers, that is, and what are, really, locusts. These insects at one time played a very important part in my life. It might interest you and you can look at the uniform while I am talking."

Source: Hemingway, Ernest. 1987. "A Way You'll Never Be." In *The Complete Short Stories of Ernest Hemingway*. New York: Charles Scribner's Sons. Copyright 1933 by Charles Scribner's Sons. Copyright renewed © 1961 by Mary Hemingway. Reprinted with permission of Scribner, an imprint of Simon and Schuster Adult Publishing Group.

⊡ Nathanael West, *Miss Lonelyhearts* (1933)

The medium of film creates and reinforces a series of socially horrific predicaments that are seen as simply generated by an obscene body. These are largely located around disfigurement and around those bodies that have been deemed to be repulsive in a field of vision. Many novelists of the twentieth century, including Elizabeth Bowen in Death of the Heart, *Harper Lee in* To Kill a Mockingbird, *and Manuel Puig in* The Kiss of the Spider Woman, *wrestled with the implications of film as a burgeoning and influential mode of storytelling. Because film operates as a more visual narrative medium than printed text, film stories have tended to emphasize physical appearance as a social value. Similarly, film mobilizes audiences around the suspense and shock value that can be precipitated in a simple narrative premise: the placing of visually different bodies on exhibition.*

Hence, the crafting of narratives around repulsive bodies and the development of film as a craft have occurred hand in hand. In the history of film production, one finds an entire genre of horror films developing within the visually sophisticated era of silent cinema and remaining heavily influential into the 1930s. For example, during the eugenics era in Germany, influential films developed at Babelsburg studios made the new "horror" genre a principal part of their repertoire. In the United States, subsequent to a break with Edison's efforts to control production, an alliance among Hollywood studios became the central source of filmed story products. The excerpt below is from Nathanael West's Miss Lonelyhearts. *West was among the authors who wrote about the culture and effects of classic or "golden"-era Hollywood.*

In his novels, West, like the cinema of which he writes, explored the implications of a predominantly visual medium upon those it casts as visually repulsive. This excerpt is also significant because it appears as a preface to Erving Goffman's influential, and contemporaneous, study entitled Stigma: Notes on the Management of Spoiled Identity. *Most important, primary sources on film narrative and disability are significant because a central strand of disability studies involves a critique of the misrepresentations of cinema in its presentation of disability as a horror and a personal tragedy.*

Dear Miss Lonelyhearts—

I am sixteen years old now and I don't know what to do and would appreciate it if you could tell me what to do. When I was a little girl it was not so bad because I got used to the kids on the block makeing fun of me, but now I would like to have boy friends like the other girls and go out on Saturday nites, but no boy will take me because I was born without a nose—although I am a good dancer and have a nice shape and my father buys me pretty clothes.

I sit and look at myself all day and cry. I have a big hole in the middle of my face that scares people even myself so I cant blame the boys for not wanting to take me out. My mother loves me, but she crys terrible when she looks at me.

What did I do to deserve such a terrible bad fate? Even if I did do some bad things I didn't do any before I was a year old and I was born this way. I asked Pape and he says he doesnt know, but that maybe I did something in the other world before I was born or that maybe I was being punished for his sins. I dont believe that because he is a very nice man. Ought I commit suicide?

Sincerely yours,
Desperate

Source: West, Nathanael. 1933. *Miss Lonelyhearts.* New York: James Loughlin.

◉ Kye Yong Muk, from "Adada the Idiot" [*Paegch'i Adada*] (1935)

"Adada the Idiot" depicts Adada, a disabled woman with speech and cognitive impairment. This short story has been interpreted as offering a critique of the increasing materialism of Korean society by depicting that society as morally disabled. The story was made into films in 1956 and 1987.

Adada was a mute. When she tried to talk the only sounds she could make were a stuttering "a-da-da" over and over. Sometimes however, when she really tried, the words would come out one at a time fairly well, but this was so only with simple words.

So people ridiculed her and even though her real name was Hwak-sil, everyone called her "Adada." Naturally the name stuck, with even her father and mother coming to call her that. And for her part, whenever anyone called "Adada" she responded as though it were her real name.

"I'm getting gray hair because of you, bitch," her mother spat. "Either go on back to your husband or get the hell out of here and go somewhere and die. Bitch! Bitch! Bitch!" . . .

As if to say, "I'll do as you wish," Adada shook her head sadly and filled with fright, uncertain as to what she should do, dragged herself outside the gate.

Once outside, she still had no idea where she could go. . . .

The realization that she had no place to go made her feel a deep longing for her husband's home of five years ago, which was now useless except for the solace of tears. In those days her mother- and father-in-law had treated her well. They were concerned lest she be cold or warm, whether the work was too hard for her or whether she was tired. How eagerly they had humored her. And at night her husband had held her close to his bosom, melting her weariness. Ah, how well her husband and his parents had treated her!

And it was true. For the first five years of her marriage she had been loved by the whole family. Not that the idea of marrying a mute had been particularly appealing, but otherwise he never could have married without actually buying a wife. At 28 and still single he was finding it difficult enough to fill his own gullet. . . .

On top of that, Adada was a good worker. She docilely did whatever she was told and had never complained in the least. So it was that this family whose poverty had kept them at each other's throats with sullen looks and unpleasant words suddenly became wreathed in smiles of harmony, like a garden blessed with spring showers.

Of course, Adada was not normal and she did make mistakes, but [the] in-laws, who were being supported by her, did not look upon her with disgust, but rather made every effort to console her and to cover up her faults.

It was there that Adada felt human happiness for the first time in her life. She felt bitter whenever she thought of how her own parents had not even considered her as a human being because she was a "worthless child," or more to the point that she was a "wicked child" who was disgracing the family's good name. . . .

The years have passed and the one somjigi of paddy field which had been the foundation of their existence gradually brought them to a comfortable life. And with several hundred yen in savings, this man who was her husband began to hate his mute wife for no reason. . . .

"Bitch," he would say, "I'm sick of looking at you. Go back to your parents." And that would be followed by a beating. Still, Adada suffered patiently and did her duty as a wife and as a daughter-in-law. All of this endeared Adada even more to her in-laws. Finally the son, sensing that the daughter-in-law could not be pried away from the father and feeling domestic frustration, sold off the entire year's harvest and left home. In his quest for emotional solace he squandered all his money on sex and drink, lived a worthless life and then, joining up with some friends, crossed over the river into Antung in Manchuria.

Immersing himself in the life of this speculative city he managed, by dint of physical labor, to get together some capital, and with a few good speculative investments his dream of wealth began miraculously to come true, and almost inadvertently he managed to accumulate close to 20,000 yen. With this small fortune he picked, from the vast number of women who had been following his money, a true love for this perfect wife and took her home with him.

Then dreaming of a completely new way of life, he built another house, and his cruelty toward Adada became even worse than before. [On] top of this, his father was much taken with the intelligent, gracious new daughter-in-law whom they had no reason to be ashamed of.

No longer in favor with her in-laws, with no one to take her side, and unable to bear the beatings of her insensitive husband, she was finally driven out. . . .

But where to go? As she turned the problem over in her mind she came to the conclusion that the only one in this world she could turn to was Surong.

A bachelor, now over thirty, Surong had no parents, no brothers or sisters, no cousins. . . .

Surong had been playing up to Adada for the past year. Even though she was a mute and had been driven from her husband's home, she was nevertheless Kim Ch'o-si's daughter, so he was self-effacing, and taking care not to act too boldly, he trained his sights on her and watched carefully to determine her feelings toward him. . . .

[The] two of them exchanged wedding vows without a formal ceremony and at daybreak left the village and slipped away to an island called Simmi-do to settle down to a peaceful life. . . .

"Look," he said. "It doesn't look like a lot but there's 1,500 ryang here—that's 150 in yen. At today's prices we can easily buy 2,000 p'yŏng of land." Adada did not answer. A definite tinge of sadness flashed across her face. . . . Adada simply shook her head without speaking. . . . As a matter of fact, even when he said he had money, Adada never imagined it was so much, and when she heard Surong say he was going to buy land with all that money she could feel all the happiness she had dreamed of slipping away from her. . . .

Adada put down the basket on the sand and removed the roll of money from the waist of her trousers. With a twirl she loosened the piece of rag which had been wrapped around the money in who knows how many layers. Adada stood there staring vacantly, waiting, wishing that they would quickly either sink beneath the water of float out to sea. . . .

Adada felt exhilarated beyond description. When she thought how those countless pieces of money which were being pulled down into the water were taking all of her own misfortunes with them into the great boundless sea from which there would be no return, Adada was so happy she could have danced. . . .

"Ya, ya. Adada! The money! Did you take the money? The money, the money . . . !" he shouted. His voice a shattering bolt from the blue. . . .

Little by little the sweep and flow of the waves quickened their pace. The bills flowed to and fro, playing a game of hide and seek with him, as if trying to lure him into the deep waters. . . .

Surong realized that the money was gone now, but he could not lift his eyes from the water and stood there like a man bereft of his senses staring dumbfoundedly. Then like a shot, he became running to the small hill by the water's edge where Adada stood trembling and, without saying a word, kicked her viciously in the midsection. The sound of a grunt pierced the air at almost the same time the muck splattered in all directions as Adada slid down head first into the slime of the edge of the sea. And then a scream. . . .

Surong, his fist still clenched, stands there like a statue peering into the heaving waves. . . .

Above, flocks of seagulls wheel about and glide in circles looking for their mates, oblivious to the grim human tragedy which has taken place. They screech noisily and with the sound of their wings beating in great flaps they grace the seaside panorama with a joyful dance.

Source: Kye Yong Muk. 1974. Clippinger, Morgan E., trans. "Adada the Idiot." *Korea Journal* (April):45–52, 67. Originally published 1935; reprinted by permission of the *Korea Journal*.

◉ The League of the Physically Handicapped (1935)

In 1935, at the height of the Great Depression, a group of disabled people joined together as the League of the Physically Handicapped to protest job discrimination. Bureaucratic rules and individual prejudices kept many disabled people from benefiting from the government employment supports provided by President Roosevelt's New Deal programs. This excerpt includes the League's assessment of the problem and their demands for change.

The fliers handed out by members of the League of the Physically Handicapped, explained that people with handicaps "cannot get regular jobs as teachers or librarians in New York State. . . . Even a typist must pass a physical examination. . . . In private business the Physically Handicapped invariably are discriminated

against. They work harder for less wages. [Given this disability-based employment bias,] our League demands that handicapped people receive a just share of the millions of jobs being given out by the government. . . . The Handicapped still are discriminated against by Private Industry. It is because of this discrimination that we demand the government recognize its obligation to make adequate provisions for handicapped people in the Works Relief Program."

Source: Blumberg, Barbara. 1979. P. 49 in *The New Deal and the Unemployed: The View from New York City*. Lewisburg, PA: Bucknell University Press. Blumberg & Brown: Reprinted by permission of the Associated University Presses.

◉ Kang Kyong-Ae, from *The Underground Village* [*Jihachon*] (1936)

Kang Kyong-Ae, a feminist novelist, focused on depicting people in the lower classes and women's lives in colonial Korea in a form of critical realism. The Underground Village is a novella portraying the impoverished countryside life of a man with partially paralyzed limbs, Ch'il-sŏng; his love interest, the blind woman K'ŭnnyon; and his mother and siblings. The excerpts include Ch'il-sŏng's encounters with another man with a physical disability from a work injury as well as the end of the story.

The sun was burning upon the western hill. Ch'il-sŏng, as usual, staggered past this village with his beggar's sack slung over his shoulder. He kept pulling down his crownless straw hat, but the sun continued broiling his forehead, and drops of sweat rolled down. Dust rose up from the parched road like smoke and made it difficult for him to breathe.

"There he comes again!"

"Come on!"

The little urchins at play by the roadside shouted and ran toward him. Ch'il-sŏng swore to himself and hurried his steps, but the children soon overtook him and pulled at his clothes.

"Cry, lad! Cry!" One of the urchins blocked Ch'il-sŏng's way and laughed. The children surrounded him in a circle.

"Hey, kid, how old are you?"

"Show us what you earned today."

One of the urchins snatched at the beggar's sack, and all the others clapped their hands. Ch'il-sŏng stood immobile and glared at the biggest of the group. He knew that if he tried to advance or swore at them they would pester him still more vigorously.

"Oh, he looks like a gentleman today."

One bristly-haired urchin brandished a stick before him with a bit of cowdung at the tip. The children all giggled and made as if to smear cowdung on Ch'il-sŏng with their sticks. Ch'il-sŏng could not stand it, so he ran as fast as he could. . . .

It was not the first time that he had been chased away by a dog; and countless times he had been abused and persecuted by men, too.

But somehow he felt an uncontainable fury today.

"Why are you standing there like that?"

He looked back in surprise to find that he was standing before a small building which was a water-mill. The man who was looking at him with out-stretched neck seemed between forty and fifty, and Ch'il-sŏng could instantly tell that he was a cripple and a beggar like himself. The man grinned. He did not feel like going in, but entered after some hesitation. With a strong smell of rice husks came also the stink of horse droppings.

"Come to this side . . . Oh, your clothes are all wet."

The man stood on his crutches, spread the straw mat he had been sitting on, and sat down on one corner of it. Ch'il-sŏng quickly noted the man's gray hair and beard. He feared that the man might try to take away his earnings.

"You must be cold because of those wet clothes. You put on my old clothes and take them off and dry them." The man searched his bundle and said, "Here it is. Come here."

Ch'il-sŏng looked back. It was a dark western jacket patched in several places. He envied him such a good garment and looked directly in his smiling eyes. He did not look like a man who would try to snatch away other beggars earnings. Ch'il-sŏng dropped his glance and looked at the water dripping from his sleeves. The man walked toward him, leaning on his crutch.

"Why are you standing there like that? Put this on."

"Oh, no." Ch'il-sŏng stepped back one step and looked at the western jacket. His heart throbbed before a garment the like of which he had never worn in his life.

"Oh, aren't you a stubborn fellow! Then come here and sit on this mat." The man led him by the hand and made him sit on the straw mat. The man pretended not to notice Ch'il-sŏng's twisted legs. . . .

"Are you a born cripple?" the man suddenly asked. Ch'il-sŏng bowed his head and, after much hesitation, answered, "No."

"Then it was because of an illness. Did you get any treatment?"

Ch'il-sŏng looked long at his legs again, hesitating. At last he muttered: "No. None at all."

"Ugh, in this world sound legs get broken. It's no surprise not to get treatment for sicknesses."

The man laughed into void. The laughter made Ch'il-sŏng shudder. He glanced at the man. As he looked out at the road with fiercely dilated eyes, blue veins stood out on the man's forehead and his lips were tightly shut.

"Oh, I curse myself to think how stupid I was! I should have fought till death! What a damned stupid fool I was." . . .

"Listen fellow. I was head of a family once. I was a model worker in a factory, too. A first-rate engineer . . . After my leg was broken I was fired from the factory, and my woman ran away and the kids cried from hunger. . . . My parents died of sorrow. Oh, there's no use telling it."

The man stared at Ch'il-sŏng. Ch'il-sŏng's heart throbbed for some reason and he could not face the man's glance, so he looked at his broken leg, and at the mute bovine earth beneath that leg. . . .

"Oh, ours will all be swept away now! Our field can't escape being flooded when K'ŏnnyon's field got swept away. . . . Oh, K'ŏnnyon's lucky she doesn't have to live through this. She got married yesterday."

"What?" Ch'il-sŏng screamed. The precious material stored in his bosom struck his skin like a rock. His mother, startled, looked at her son.

"Mom, look at that!" Ch'il-un jumped up and groaned. They all looked. The cloth wrapped round the baby's head was about half torn off and maggots big as rice grains were crawling out of it.

"Oh, God! What has happened? What has happened!" His mother went over to the baby and snatched away the cloth. The rat skin came away at that, and from it dropped hordes of maggots bathed in blood.

"Baby! My baby! Wake up! Oh, wake up!" Hearing his mother's scream, Ch'il-sŏng ran outside frantically. The rain poured down fiercely and the gale blew like mad, and the sky, torn mercilessly by the lightning, wailed with thunder. Ch'il-sŏng glared at the sky.

Source: Kang Kyong-Ae. 1983. Suh Ji-moon, trans. "The Underground Village" [Jihachon]. In *The Rainy Spell and Other Korean Stories.* London: Onyx Press. Originally published 1936; reprinted by permission of the *Korea Journal.*

◉ National Socialist Propaganda, *Volk und Rasse* (1936)

The National Socialist propaganda machine got up to speed in the 1930s as the German population was infiltrated with eugenic ideology. The German people were supposed to consider their family planning and reproduction as entirely in the service of creating a healthy, national body. The following is an example from the monthly newsletter, Volk und Rasse *["Nation and Race"].*

"Healthy marriage is a national duty."

"The nation has the duty to return consecration to the institution of marriage, which is appointed the task of conceiving images of God and not freaks between man and ape."

Source: *Volk und Rasse: Illustrierte Monatsschrift für das deutsche Volkstum: Zeitschrift des Reichsausschusses für Volksgesundheitsdienst und der Deutschen Gesellschaft für Rassenhygiene.* 1936. Berlin, Germany: H8, title page. [*Volk and Race: Illustrated Monthly Magazine for the German Volk: Magazine of the Reich's Commission for the Medical Service of the Volk and the German Society for Race Hygiene.* Vogt, Sara, trans.].

◉ Japanese Schools for the Physically and Mentally Handicapped (1937)

The following excerpt about the history of schools for students with physical and sensory disabilities is taken from a book written in 1937 about the educational history of Japan. The discussion demonstrates the country's commitment to schooling disabled children but also the common practice of educating them in separate facilities. The discussion ends with a critique of nonsystematic education for students with cognitive disabilities.

The Imperial Ordinance relating to schools for the blind, deaf and dumb makes it compulsory for each prefecture and the Hokkaido to establish at least one school of each class of the afflicted. Further, permission is given to cities, towns and villages, or to private persons, to found schools for the blind, deaf and dumb. At the present time in Japan there are two government institutions of this type, one the Tokyo School for the Blind and the other the Tokyo School for the Deaf and Dumb. Both are under the immediate control of the Department of Education. In addition, there are twenty-nine public schools for such afflicted persons, and forty-two private schools. The discrepancy between the number of public schools is explained by the fact that the government rules permit prefectures to adopt schools established by private individuals or by cities or towns as prefectural schools, and advantage has been taken of this regulation by a number of prefectures.

Schools of this type generally consist of two departments, the elementary and the middle grade, although in some schools permission is granted to dispense with either department. To be admitted to the elementary department of any school for the blind, or the deaf and dumb, candidates must be over six years of age. For admission to the middle grade department they must have completed the elementary training or give proof of an equivalent standard.

In the schools for the blind the curriculum in general emphasizes such subjects as music, acupuncture and massage. Teaching by the Braille method is not so advanced as in the West. But there is a system adapted by a Japanese teacher, and based on the Braille, by which the blind are taught to read. For the most part, however, blind Japanese students are taught by ear and memory-training. Throughout the whole period of Japanese history, massage, which plays so large a part in the therapeutics of the country, has been looked upon as an art particularly suited to the blind. This traditional attitude is still maintained, so that the schools for the blind offer a first-class training in massage.

The annual number of applicants for admission to the Tokyo School for the Blind is about 125, of whom approximately 60 are admitted. The subsequent careers of the graduates from this school, to take a typical year, are as follows:

Teachers	14
Engaged in acupuncture and massage	6
Hospital workers	2
Further study	10
Others	2

The schools for the deaf and dumb are similarly divided into two departments, providing an elementary and a middle course. The ordinary curriculum is confined very largely to drawing, sewing and the industrial arts. Some success has been achieved in teaching articulation and lip-reading, for which purpose the most modern Western methods have been introduced into a few schools, which have thereby trained instructors for other schools.

The Tokyo School for Deaf-mutes has in the neighbourhood of 130 applicants each year, but of these only about 90 are admitted.

Unfortunately, there is as yet in Japan no well-arranged system of training mentally defectives. Their education in separate classes is carried on experimentally in a few schools, thanks to the initiative of the local authorities. There is, however, no properly organized public system designed to provide the care and training that could so well be utilized by this unfortunate type, which for the most part are left to the care, or otherwise, of their families.

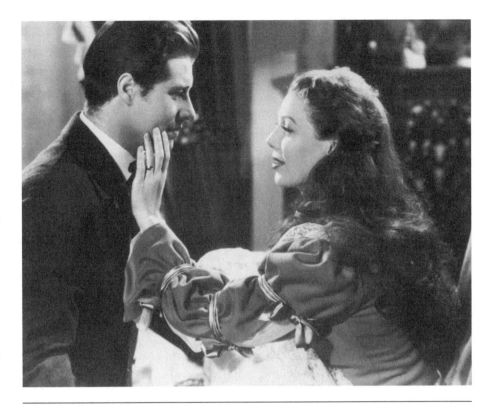

In The Story of Alexander Graham Bell, *the inventor of the telephone, whose mother is deaf, marries a woman who is deaf as well. The film depicts Bell as heroic in his efforts to assist individuals with hearing and speech impairments to communicate.*

Source: *The Story of Alexander Graham Bell* (1939), directed by Irving Cummings. B&W, 105 minutes. Reprinted by permission of Paul Darke.

Source: Keenleyside, Hugh, and A. F. Thomas. 1937. Pp. 259–261 in *History of Japanese Education and Present Educational System*. Tokyo, Japan: Hokuseido Press. Reprinted by permission of Hokuseido Press.

▣ John Steinbeck, from *Of Mice and Men* (1937)

Steinbeck plays with the stereotype of the well-meaning but dangerous idiot. Lennie is attracted to beautiful things but destroys them, turning the world against him and his brother, George. George is his brother's keeper, but the job seems too hard to bear when that brother is mentally disabled.

Lennie went behind the tree and brought out a litter of dried leaves and twigs. He threw them in a heap on the old ash pile and went back for more and more. It was almost night now. A dove's wings whistled over the water. George walked to the fire pile and lighted the dry leaves. The flame cracked up among the twigs and fell to work. George undid his bindle and brought out three cans of beans. He stood them about the fire, close in against the blaze, but not quite touching the flame.

"There's enough beans for four men," George said.

Lennie watched him from over the fire. He said patiently, "I like 'em with ketchup."

"Well, we ain't got any," George exploded. "Whatever we aint' got, that's what you want. God a'mighty, if I was alone I could live so easy. I could go get a job an' work, an' no trouble. No mess at all, and when the end of the month come I could take my fifty bucks and go into town and get whatever I want. Why, I could stay in a cat house all night. I could eat any place I want, hotel or any place, and order any damn thing I could think of. An' I could do all that every damn month. Get a gallon of whisky, or set in a pool room and play cards or shoot pool." Lennie knelt and looked over the fire at the angry George. And Lennie's face was drawn with terror. "An' whatta I got," George went on furiously. "I got you! You can't keep a job and you lose me ever' job I get. Jus' keep me shovin' all over the country all the time. An' that ain't the worst. You get in trouble. You do bad things and I got to get you out." His voice rose nearly to a shout. "You crazy son-of-a-bitch. You keep me in hot water all the time." He took on the elaborate manner of little girls when they are mimicking one another. "Jus' wanted to feel that girl's dress—jus' wanted to pet it like it was a mouse—Well, how the hell did she know you jus' wanted to feel her dress? She jerks back and you hold on like it was a mouse. She yells and we got to hide in a irrigation ditch all day with guys lookin' for us, and we got to sneak out in the dark and get outta the country. All the time somethin' like that—all the time. I wisht I could put you in a cage with about a million mice an' let you have fun." His anger left him suddenly. He looked across the fire at Lennie's anguished face, and then he looked ashamedly at the flames.

It was quite dark now, but the fire lighted the trunks of the trees and the curving branches overhead. Lennie crawled slowly and cautiously around the fire until he was close to George. He sat back on his heels. George turned the bean cans so that another side faced the fire. He pretended to be unaware of Lennie so close beside him.

"George," very softly. No answer. "George!"

"Whatta you want?"

"I was only foolin,' George. I don't want no ketchup. I wouldn't eat no ketchup if it was right here beside me."

"If it was here, you could have some."

"But I wouldn't eat none. George. I'd leave it all for you. You could cover the beans with it and I wouldn't touch none of it."

George still stared morosely at the fire. "When I think of the swell time I could have without you, I go nuts. I never get no peace."

Lennie still knelt. He looked off into the darkness across the river. "George, you want I should go away and leave you alone?"

"Where the hell could you go?"

"Well, I could. I could go off in the hills there. Some place I'd find a cave."

Source: Steinbeck, John. 1993. *Of Mice and Men*. New York: Penguin. Copyright 1937 renewed © 1965 by John Steinbeck. Used by permission of Viking Penguin, a division of Penguin Group (USA) Inc.

◉ Social Security Report on Disability Insurance (1938)

The report demonstrates the degree of U.S. government resistance to efforts to adjust the Social Security Act in order to include permanent disability within its provisions.

The Board recognizes that the administrative problems involved are difficult, although it does not believe them insuperable. It also recognizes that provision for permanent total disability would increase the cost of the system both now and in the future. For these reasons it is not making any positive recommendations on this matter at this time.

Source: Proposed Changes in the Social Security Act, Report of the Social Security Board to the President and to the Congress of the United States, 30 Dec. 1938, H.R. 110, 76th Cong., 1st sess. (1939).

◉ Public Speech by the Bishop of Munster (1941)

This sermon, delivered August 3, 1941, by Cardinal August Count von Galen, Bishop of Munster, came as a bombshell. Thousands of copies were printed and circulated. Nazi leaders were furious but helpless to prohibit the critique without fueling public opposition.

Fellow Christians! In the pastoral letter of the German Bishops of 26 June 1941, which was read out in all the Catholic churches in Germany on 6 July, 1941, it states among other things: It is true that there are definite commandments in Catholic moral doctrine which are no longer applicable if their fulfillment involves too many difficulties. However, there are sacred obligations of conscience from which no one has the power to release us and which we must fulfill even if it costs us our lives. Never under any circumstances may a human being kill an innocent person apart from war and legitimate self-defence. On 6 July, I already had cause to add to the pastoral letter the following explanation: for some months we have been hearing reports that, on the orders of Berlin, patients from mental asylums who have been ill for a long time and may appear incurable, are being compulsorily removed. Then, after a short time, the relatives are regularly informed that the corpse has been burnt and the ashes can be delivered. There is a general suspicion verging on certainty, that these numerous unexpected deaths of mentally ill people do not occur of themselves but are deliberately brought about, that the doctrine is being followed, according to which one may destroy so-called 'worthless life' that is kill innocent people if one considers that their lives are of no further value to the nation and the state.

I am reliably informed that lists are also being drawn up in the asylums of the province of Westphalia as well of those patients who are to be taken away as so called 'unproductive national comrades' and shortly to be killed. The first transport left the Marienthal institution near Munster during this past week.

German men and women §211 of the Reich Penal Code is still valid. It states: 'he who deliberately kills another person will be punished by death for murder if the killing is premeditated.'

Those patients who are destined to be killed are transported away from home to a distant asylum presumably in order to protect those who deliberately kill those poor people, members of our families, from this legal punishment. Some illnesses are then given the cause of death. Since the corpse has been burnt straight away the relatives and also the criminal police are unable to establish whether the illness really occurred and what the cause of death was. However, I have been assured that the Reich Interior Ministry and the office of the Reich Doctor's Leader, Dr. Conti, make no bones about the fact that in reality a large number of mentally ill people in Germany have been deliberately killed and more will be killed in the future.

The Penal Code lays down in §139: 'he who receives credible information concerning the intention to commit a crime against life and neglects to alert authorities or the person who is threatened in time will be punished.' When I learnt of the intention to transport patients from Marienthal in order to kill them, I brought a formal charge at the State Court in Munster and with the Police President in Munster by means of

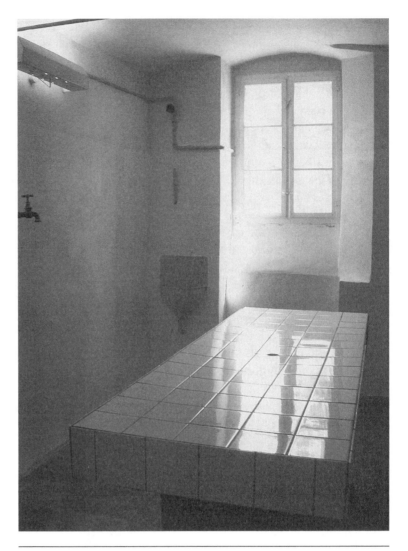

Autopsy area where murdered disabled inmates with gold teeth or "unusual" anatomies were studied after the gassing. The autopsy table itself continued to be used into the 1970s by occupational and physical therapists for stretching exercises into the 1970s. Today the site exists as memorial to the victims of National Socialist medical violence during World War II.

Source: Photo by Sharon Snyder.

a registered letter which reads as follows: 'According to information which I have received, in the course of this week a large number of patients from the Marienthal Provincial Asylum near Munster are to be transported to the Eighberg asylum so-called "unproductive national comrades" and will then be soon deliberately killed, as is generally believed has occurred with such transports from other asylums. Since such an action is not only contrary to the moral laws of God and Nature but is also punishable by death as murder under §211 of the Penal Code, I hereby bring a charge in accordance with my duty under §139 of the Penal Code, and request you to provide immediate protection for national comrades threatened in this way by taking action against those agencies who are intending the removal and murder, and that you inform me of the steps that have been taken.' I have received no news concerning intervention by the Prosecutor's Office or by the police. . . .

Thus we must assume that the poor helpless patients will soon be killed. For what reason? Not because they have committed a crime worthy of death. Not because they attacked their nurses or orderlies so that the latter had no other choice but to use legitimate force to defend their lives against their attackers. Those are cases where, in addition to the killing of an armed enemy in a just war, the use of force to the point of killing is allowed and is often required. No, it is not for such reasons that these unfortunate patients must die but rather because, in the opinion of some department, or the testimony of some commission, they have become 'worthless life' because according to this testimony they are 'unproductive national comrades.' The argument goes: they can no longer produce commodities, they are like an old machine which no longer works, they are like an old horse which has become incurably lame, they are like a cow which no longer gives milk. What does one do with such an old machine? It is thrown on the scrap heap. What does one do with a lame horse, with such an unproductive cow? No, I do not want to continue the comparison until the end—however fearful the justification for it and the symbolic force of it are. We are not dealing with machines, horses and cows whose only function is to serve mankind, to produce goods for man. One may smash them, one may slaughter them as soon as they no longer fulfill this function. No, we are dealing with human beings, our fellow human beings, our brothers and sisters. With poor people, sick people, if you like unproductive people. But have they for that reason forfeited the right to life? Have you, have I the right to live only so long as we are productive, so long as we are recognised by others as productive? If you establish and apply the principle that you can kill 'unproductive' fellow human beings then woe betide us all when we become old and frail! If one is allowed to kill the 'unproductive' people then woe betide the invalids who have used up, sacrificed and lost their health and strength in the productive process. If one is allowed forcibly to remove one's unproductive fellow human beings then woe betide loyal soldiers who return to the homeland seriously disabled, as cripples, as invalids. If it is once accepted that people have

the right to kill 'unproductive' fellow humans—and even initially if it only affects the poor defenceless mentally ill—then as a *matter of principle* murder is permitted for all unproductive people, in other words for the incurably sick, the people who have become invalids through labor and war, for us all when we become old, frail, and therefore unproductive.

Then, it is only necessary for some secret edict in order that the method developed for the mentally ill should be extended to other 'unproductive' people, that it should be applied to those suffering from incurable lung disease, to the elderly who are frail or invalids, to the severely disabled soldiers. Then none of our lives will be safe any more. Some commission can put us on the list of the 'unproductive,' who in their opinion have become worthless life. And no police force will protect us and no court will investigate our murder and give the murderer the punishment he deserves. Who will be able to trust his doctor any more? He may report the patient as 'unproductive' and receive instructions to kill him. It is impossible to imagine the degree of moral depravity, of general mistrust that would then spread even through families if this dreadful doctrine is tolerated, accepted, and followed. Woe to mankind, woe to our German nation if God's holy commandment 'Thou shalt not kill,' which God proclaimed on Mount Sinai amidst thunder and lightning, which God our Creator inscribed in the conscience of mankind from the very beginning, is not only broken, but if this transgression is actually tolerated and permitted to go unpunished.

I'll give you an example of what is going on. In Marienthal there was a man of about 55, a peasant from a rural parish in the Munster area—I could give you his name—who for some years had been suffering from mental disturbance and who had therefore been put in the care of the Marienthal asylum. He was not really mentally ill, he could receive visitors and was very pleased whenever his relatives came to see him. Only a fortnight ago, he received a visit from his wife and from one of his sons who is a soldier at the front and had home leave. So the farewell was a sad one: who knows if the soldier will return, will see his father again, for after all he may die in the struggle on behalf of his national comrades. The son, the soldier, will almost certainly never see his father again here on earth because since then he has been put on the list of the 'unproductive.' A relative who wanted to visit the father in Marienthal last week was turned away with the news that the patient has been transported away from here on the orders of the Ministerial Council for the Defence of the Reich. Nobody could say where to: the relatives would be informed in a few days time. What will the news be? Will it be the same as in other cases? That the person had died, that the corpse had been burnt, that the ashes can be delivered after payment of a fee? In that case, the soldier who is at the front risking his life for his German national comrades, will not see his father again here on earth because German national comrades at home have killed him . . .

Source: Noakes, J., and G. Pridham, eds. 1988. Pp. 1036–1039 in *Nazism: A History in Documents and Eyewitness Accounts, 1919–1945*, Volume 3, *Foreign Policy, War and Racial Extermination. A Documentary Reader.* Published with permission of the University of Exeter Press.

▣ Katharine Butler Hathaway, from *The Little Locksmith* (1943)

The Little Locksmith is an extraordinary autobiography written by a woman who spent 10 years of her life strapped to a board in an unsuccessful attempt to prevent curvature of the back from a spinal tumor. The first excerpt included here discusses her transition from a carefree childhood to a "bedridden" and contemplative existence. During the course of the story, she changes from a child repulsed by the hunchbacked figure of a local locksmith to one who longs to find a house best fitted to her life as a disabled woman.

This is the story of such transformations, both large and small, and now in the beginning I will tell the nature of the predicament which first made this kind of magic dear to me—the predicament and the magic together which made necessary and possible at last my visit to the almond-shaped island which lay in the palm of my right hand. For of course, without a predicament, there is no need of magic.

When I was five years old I was changed from a rushing, laughing child into a bedridden, meditative one. As the years passed, my mother explained to me just what had happened, and why I had to be so still. She told me how lucky I was that my parents were able to have me taken care of by a famous doctor. Because, without the treatment I was having, I would have had to grow up into a—well, I would have had to be, when I grew up, like the little locksmith who used to come to our house once in a while to fix locks.

I knew the little locksmith, and after this, when he came, I stared at him with a very strange intimate feeling. He never looked back at me. His eyes were always down at what he was doing, and he apparently did not want to talk with or look at anybody. He was very fascinating indeed. He was not big enough to be considered a man, yet he was not a child. In the back his coat hung down from an enormous sort of peak, where the cloth was worn and shiny, between his shoulders, and he walked with a sort of bobbing motion. In front his chin was almost down on his chest, his hands were long, narrow, and delicate, and his fingers were much cleverer than most people's fingers. There was something about him, something that was indescribably alluring to a child. Because he was more like a gnome than a human being he naturally seemed to belong to our world more than to the grown-up world. Yet he seemed to refuse to belong to our world or anybody else's. He acted as if he lived all alone in a very private world of his own.

Somehow I knew that there was a special word that the grownups called a person shaped like the little locksmith, and I knew that to ordinary healthy grownups it was a terrible word. And the strange thing was that I, Katharine, the Butlers' darling little girl, had barely escaped that uncanny shape and that terrible word. Because I was being taken care of by a famous doctor nobody would ever guess, when I grew up, that I might have been just like the little locksmith.

Staring wonderingly at him, I knew it. I knew that compared with him I was wonderfully lucky and safe. Yet deep within me I had a feeling that underneath my luck and safeness the real truth was that I really belonged with him, even if it was never going to show. I was secretly linked with him, and I felt a strong, childish, amorous pity and desire toward him, so that there was even a queer erotic charm for me about his gray shabby clothes, the strange awful peak in his back, and his cross, unapproachable sadness which made him not look at other people, not even at me lying on my bed and staring sideways at him. (Pp. 14–15)

A house such as I was dreaming of would be only another example, I thought, of the easy magic of transformation by which one thing becomes its opposite. All that was needed, I thought, was a person bold and independent enough to undertake it. That person would need to be very bold indeed, because the process of transformation was so entirely a matter of faith and magic and simplicity that nobody would believe that it could be done until after it had been done. I thought for several reasons that I might be the bold person.

Sometimes a worm will sew a stitch in a young leaf, and even though the leaf may partly unfold, and partly grow and live, it will always be a crumpled and imperfect leaf. My body, like the leaf, represented that mysterious element of imperfection in Nature, which allows the worm to maim the leaf; I represented the flaw which exists side by side with a design which appears to be flawless. Because the worm had sewed a stitch in me and made me forever crumpled, I belonged to the fantastic company of the queer, the maimed, the unfit. It was understood that I could not play a part in the ordained dance of love, in obedience to the design. I was obliged, therefore, in a certain sense, to skip in my own life all the years and all the force and strength which other women gave to love and to the bearing of children. I was obliged to skip the years of sexual activity and become, while I was still young and joyous, the equivalent of an old woman, a detached, sexless, meditative observer. But I was too sympathetic and ardent to be a passive observer. I had to act in some way. I had to participate, myself, in the ritual of love and experience. With my belief in the magic of transformation and my belief in my own power to exert it, I suddenly knew that I was the suitable bold person, the little, old, young crumpled person who could accomplish, if anyone could, this amazing project. I saw myself as the potent little figure, not old and not young, conspicuously lacking in size and in beauty, who appears and reappears in all folk tales as the good godmother, the talismangiver, the magic-bringer, who inevitably comes to the rescue of young people who are much bigger and more beautiful than she is, yet who get themselves entangled in their life-size and more than life-size human troubles and are weak and helpless until that familiar little nonhuman figure arrives on the scene. I knew that my destiny would reach its mark if I could work this unheard-of transformation and make my house the place of refuge and solace I had been dreaming of. I sat on my doorstep in Castine in the still autumn sunlight, and I began to be quite astonished and a little appalled by the things that I found myself thinking. But I did not let that scare me. For my third wish I wrote in my imagination across the panel under the mantelpiece in the square room behind me the last two lines of Shelley's Epipsychidion. "Come, leave the crowd which errs and which reproves, And come and be my guest, for I am Love's."

I wrote them only in my imagination, but in my imagination they were always there, as long as the house belonged to me—the invitation which I wanted to give to all the people in the world who needed it. I might have written beside it, "Unto the pure all things are pure; but unto them that are defiled and unbelieving is nothing pure"; but it seemed to me it came to the same thing.

I wanted my house, then, to be a safe refuge for three kinds of people, who are all alike in being at a particular disadvantage in the outside world because they all possess and are guided by the mystic's innocence toward life, the fearless innocence which is not afraid of facing everything, and, facing everything, dares to believe, as Blake says, that all that is, is holy. My feeling of affinity toward that fundamental kind of innocence was the basis of each of my three wishes concerning the future of the house. It was the essential attitude which I wanted my house to prove possible and to defend. (Pp. 199–201)

Source: Hathaway, Katharine Butler. 2000. Excerpts from *The Little Locksmith: A Memoir*. Copyright 1942, 1943 by Coward-McCann, Inc., renewed © 1974 by Warren H. Butler. Reprinted with permission of The Feminist Press at the City University of New York, www.feministpress.org.

▣ "N–P": The Case of Neuropsychiatric Disability (1944)

The program of aggressive normalization remained in force throughout the twentieth century and was improved and expanded on in numerous ways, especially as new understandings of disability and new conditions of war demanded. One particularly significant area of transformation was in the provision of psychological services, especially to those sustaining neuropsychiatric disabilities, which were as old as warfare itself, but largely misunderstood until the twentieth century as evidence of cowardice and malingering. Through preinduction testing, some armed forces tried to weed out men unlikely to have the emotional stability to serve under wartime conditions, but the greater the manpower needs, the more such standards were relaxed, and the more the armed services needed to be able to provide psychological treatment.

Every month thousands of men return home from preinduction examinations or from the U.S. Army with N-P stamped on their medical records. N-P (neuropsychiatric) sometimes means insane but usually means psychoneurotic. What psychoneurotic means, few laymen know. Most psychoneurotics do not know either. Many of them think they are insane or soon will be. So do family and neighbors who look askance, and employers who sometimes refuse jobs. (Last week the Army changed its N-P stamp to read "Unsuited for military service.") Because few N-Ps discuss their plight, few people realize how many there are.

But last week 2,000 psychiatrists at the 100th meeting of the American Psychiatric Association heard some startling figures from the Army's Colonel William Clare Menninger (brother of famed Psychiatrist Karl Menninger). Since Pearl Harbor the Army has turned down 1,340,000 men for neuropsychiatric causes, has discharged 216,000. These figures would be even higher if the men in Army neuropsychiatric wards were included.

Most practical report on the N-P problem was made to the meeting by New York Hospital's white-haired, 40-year-old Dr. Thomas Alexander Cumming Rennie. Dr. Rennie realized that discharged and deflected N-Ps need psychiatric care, without it might develop real mental illness. He also realized that there was no place where they could get such help. So last August he started a psychiatric clinic at the hospital, manned one night a week by twelve psychiatrists, a psychologist, seven social workers. The clinic gives psychiatric interviews, group treatment, occupational therapy, arranges social gatherings, dates, helps men get jobs.

Dr. Rennie told last week's meeting that the clinic has definitely proved its value to N-Ps. Of its 200 patients (about one-third from the Army, only 14 actual combat veterans) 104 are improved (some became perfectly well after only one one-hour psychiatric interview), many are still under treatment: a very few had to be sent to mental hospitals. (Some of these have since been discharged, now hold jobs.)

New York City already has six such psychiatric clinics; Boston has four, and there are a few others. But Dr. Rennie will not be satisfied until all available psychiatrists are helping in such clinics. Even so most of the cases would go untended—the U.S. has only about 3,000 psychiatrists altogether, of whom 800 are at war.

Source: "N-P." 1944. *Time* (May 29):44–45. © TIME Inc. Reprinted by permission.

▣ Gwendolyn Brooks, from *A Street in Bronzeville* (1945)

This poem provides reflections on heaven from the perspective of a physically disabled African American girl. The poem focuses on locating a "straight" environment that will better accommodate and accept the speaker's differences.

hunchback girl: she thinks of heaven

My Father, it is surely a blue place
And straight. Right. Regular. Where I shall find
No need for scholarly nonchalance or looks
A little to the left or guards upon the
Heart to halt love that runs without crookedness
Along its crooked corridors. My Father,
It is a planned place surely. Out of coils,
Unscrewed, released, no more to be marvelous,
I shall walk straightly through most proper halls
Proper myself, princess of properness.

Source: Brooks, Gwendolyn. 1999. *Selected Poems.* New York: Harper Perennial. Originally published 1945. Reprinted by consent of Brooks Permissions.

Frida Kahlo (1907–1954)

Frida Kahlo constructed images of a disabled female body out of seemingly disparate pieces. Her work interweaves traditional Mexican votive painting, technical images of the body that emerged from modern medical science (x-rays, surgical implements, hospital experience), and Christian iconography of redemption through physical suffering. In this way, she rendered an entirely new view of personal experience. Kahlo is among the first, and perhaps the most daring, to render a portrait of transparent, explicit, literalized bodily trauma. Prior to her work, pain was shown through the gestures of agony (e.g., scenes of crucifixion or martyrdom, as in the work of Käthe Kollwitz or Picasso's *Guernica*) or explicit gore (e.g., battle scenes, beheadings by Salome or Judith, any number of mythological illustrations).

Kahlo's work is particularly of interest to disability studies not only for the autobiographical renditions of her injuries, illnesses, and surgeries, but also because of the nature of the body she invents. Often the interior of the body is visible and continuous with the exterior in a kind of psychic Möbius strip. In works such as *The Broken Column, The Two Fridas, Roots, The Tree of Hope,* and *Without Hopes,* there is no clear division between inner reality and outer appearance, and thus the unsharable nature of individual pain becomes explicit. By the 1930s, x-ray technology had been in public use for some time, ending the concept of the opaque body, and public hospitals had also been established as places of collective community experience. Kahlo demolishes the idea of the body in pain as a shameful or hidden object. Her body is offered up in many contexts, but her pain imagery is never separate from her life at large, and her pain is never represented as a different sphere of experience

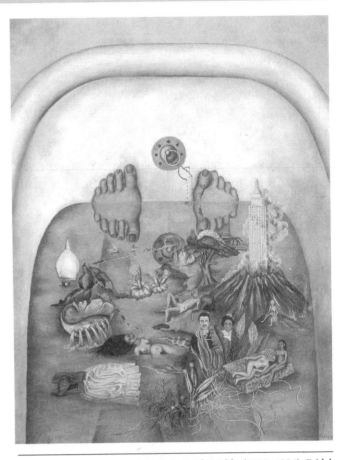

What the Water Gave Me (1938), by Frida Kahlo (1907–1954). Frida's body is both intimately present and hidden, while the water of her private bathtub transforms into the river of life. She contemplates the flow of her history as images of her family, her European and Mexican heritage, and intense love relationships emerge from the reflecting pool of the self.
Source: Art Resource, New York.

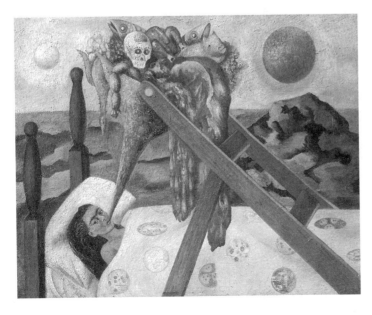

Without Hopes (1945), by Frida Kahlo (1907–1954). The painting depicts a postsurgery Frida vomiting her insides into a harsh, Aztec landscape. Fears of internal decay, the seeds of death, and the rotten remains of still-life objects erupt and seem to be a truer representation of her body than the hidden form under the infected blanket.
Source: Art Resource, New York.

in kind or degree. Her illnesses are fully in context of the rest of her life. The examinations of marriage, sexuality, cultural patrimony, and family are in the same visual iconographies as those of disability.

Her paintings must also be seen in the context of the traditional image of the female body as a mysterious, irrational, and secretive vessel. The baring of her body inside and out is more transgressive than a simple nude self-portrait. Her body is small and doll-like. It appears as a toy in the thrall of immense forces, not as a mythic goddess-like being. In embedding the matter-of-fact details of her medical experiences within a highly emotional language, she both demystifies disability and presents it outside of the context of the casebook (again, she may be the first to do this). To open oneself to a Kahlo painting is to feel the vulnerability of one's own body and to immediately experience its transcendence through art.

Another aspect of disability is the mutability of her body (a factor of chronic but unpredictable illness), symbolized in her portrayals of her body in partial transmutation with animals, partners, or the natural world in general. One could view her deep pairing with monkeys, with Diego, with the Little Deer, and with her doubled self as a reflection of the way

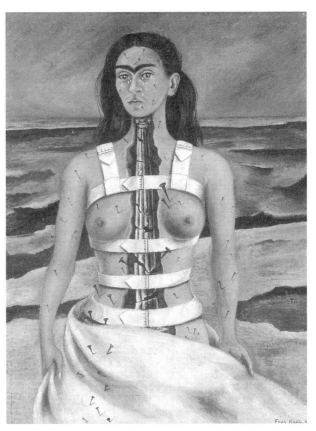

The Broken Column *(1944), by Frida Kahlo (1907–1954). The most explicit image in her canon of work, this painting fully exposes the nature of Kahlo's injury and gives no hint of the possibility of relief inside or outside her body. It is a brilliant rendering of the way in which illness can cause the entire world to seem bleak and hostile to the body in pain.*
Source: Art Resource, New York.

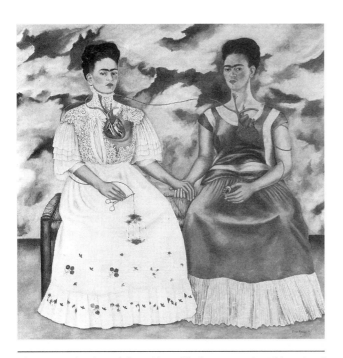

The Two Fridas *(1939), by Frida Kahlo (1907–1954). Kahlo painted this immediately after her divorce from Diego Rivera. Reminiscent of a wedding portrait, one Frida (in traditional Mexican Tehuna dress) comforts an injured and bleeding Frida (in Victorian gown). In nurturing her discarded self, she also seems to marry her disabled self, equating the states of emotional and physical pain.*
Source: Art Resource, New York.

that disabled people must often render all control or custody over their bodies. A kind of permeability arises, a thinning of boundaries that enables her to see herself as an amalgam of parts. History, love, and culture build her self-portraits. She depicts herself or others in isolation only when in a state of deep emotional pain and despair (*Self-Portrait with Cropped Hair, Suicide of Dorothy Hale*).

Disability is often imagined as a state of weakness and withdrawal. Frida Kahlo gives us a world in which pain becomes a fire in the machine, a state of wild ferocity, a disrobing to reveal a body in full communion.

—Riva Lehrer

Further Reading

Herrera, Hayden. 1983. *Frida: A Biography of Frida Kahlo.* New York: Harper & Row.

Part Three

Culture and Resistance

◉ 1946–present

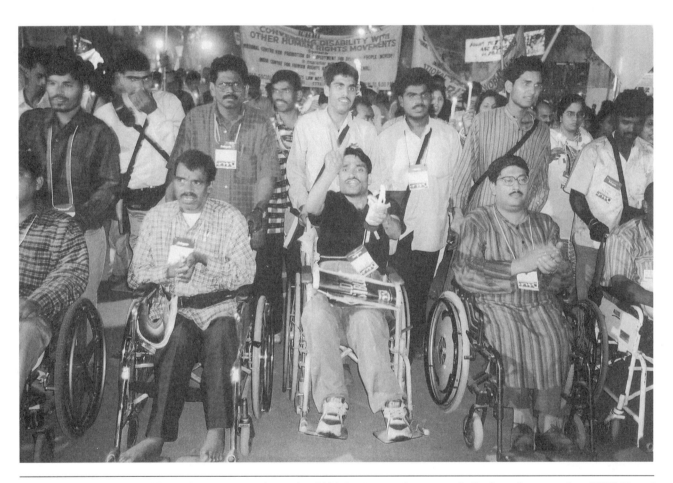

Disability protest at the World Social Forum in Mumbai, India, 2004. Participants from across India shout slogans such as "WSF Shame! Shame!" and "WSF Inaccessible, Inaccessible!"

Source: National Centre for Promotion of Employment for Disabled People, New Delhi, India.

Culture and Resistance
1946–Present

▣ William Carlos Williams, from *Paterson* (1946)

The American imagist poet-physician William Carlos Williams quotes from a lengthy newspaper account of a visit to "a natural curiosity" as a metaphor for humanity as a monstrous exhibit.

A gentleman of the Revolutionary Army, after describing the Falls, thus describes another natural curiosity then existing in the community: "In the afternoon we were invited to visit another curiosity then existing in the neighborhood. This is a monster in human form, he is twenty-seven years old, his face from the upper part of his forehead to the end of his chin, measures *twenty-seven inches,* and around the upper part of his head is twenty-one inches: his eyes and nose are remarkably large and prominent, chin long and pointed. His features are coarse, irregular and disgusting, his voice rough and sonorous. His body is twenty-seven inches in length, his limbs are small and much deformed, and he has the use of one hand only. He has never been able to sit up, as he cannot support the enormous weight of his head; but he is constantly in a large cradle, with his head supported in pillows. He is visited by great numbers of people, and is peculiarly fond of the company of clergymen, always inquiring for them among his visitors, and taking great pleasure in receiving religious instruction. General Washington made him a visit, and asked 'whether he was a Whig or a Tory.' He replied that he had never taken an *active* part on either side."

Source: Williams, William Carlos. 1946. *Paterson.* New York: New Direction. Copyright © 1946, 1948, 1949, 1951, 1958 by William Carlos Williams. Reprinted by permission of New Directions Publishing Corporation.

▣ Ann Petry, from *The Street* (1946)

One of the great works of African American literature, Ann Petry's The Street *documents the corrupt systems of economic inequity and food distribution that undermine the community's health and well-being. In the second excerpt, the story describes the physically massive and largely immobile body of Mrs. Hedges, who functions in the novel as a moral center.*

She thought about the stores again. All of them—the butcher shops, the notion stores, the vegetable stands—all of them sold leavings, the sweepings, the impossible unsalable merchandise, the dregs and dross that were reserved especially for Harlem.

Yet the people went on living and reproducing in spite of the bad food. Most of the children had straight bones, strong white teeth. But it couldn't go on like that. Even the strongest heritage would one day run out. Bub was healthy, sturdy, strong, but he couldn't remain that way living here. (P. 153)

In the middle of the block there was a sudden thrust of raw, brilliant light where the unshaded bulbs in the big poolroom reached out and pushed back the darkness. A group of men stood outside its windows watching the games going on inside. Their heads were silhouetted against the light.

Lutie, walking quickly through the block, glanced at them and then at the women coming toward her from Eighth Avenue. The women moved slowly. Their shoulders sagged from the weight of the heavy shopping bags they carried. And she thought, That's what's wrong. We don't have time enough or money enough to live like other people because the women have to work until they become drudges and the men stand by idle.

She made an impatient movement of her shoulders. She had no way of knowing that at fifty she wouldn't be misshapen, walking on the sides of her shoes because her feet hurt so badly; getting dressed up for church on Sunday and spending the rest of the week slaving in somebody's kitchen.

It could happen. Only she was going to stake out a piece of life for herself. She had come this far poor and black and shut out as though a door had been slammed in her face. Well, she would shove it open; she would beat and bang on it and push against it and use a chisel in order to get it open. (Pp. 185–186)

Lutie's mouth closed. She had never seen Mrs. Hedges outside of her apartment and looked at closely she was awe-inspiring. She was almost as tall as the Super, but where he was thin, gaunt, she was all hard, firm flesh—a mountain of a woman.

She was wearing a long-sleeved, high-necked flannelette nightgown. It was so snowy white that her skin showed up intensely black by contrast. She was barefooted. Her hands, her feet, and what could be seen of her legs were a mass of scars—terrible scars. The flesh was drawn and shiny where it had apparently tightened in the process of healing.

The big white nightgown was so amply cut that, despite the bulk of her body, it had a balloon-like quality, for it billowed about her as she stood panting slightly from her exertion, her hands on her hips, her hard, baleful eyes fixed on the Super. The gaudy bandanna was even now tied around her head in firm, tight knots so that no vestige of hair showed. And watching the wide, full nightgown as it moved gently from the draft in the hall, Lutie thought Mrs. Hedges had the appearance of a creature that had strayed from some other planet.

Her rich, pleasant voice filled the hallway, and at the sound of it the dog slunk away, his tail between his legs. 'You done lived in basements so long you ain't human no more. You got mould growin' on you,' she said to Jones.

Lutie walked away from them, intent on getting up the stairs as quickly as possible. Her legs refused to carry her and she sat down suddenly on the bottom step. The long taffeta skirt dragged on the tiled floor. Bits of tobacco, the fine grit from the street, puffed out from under it. She made no effort to pick it up. She put her head on her knees, wondering how she was going to get the strength to climb the stairs.

'Ever you even look at that girl again, I'll have you locked up. You oughtta be locked up, anyway,' Mrs. Hedges said.

She scowled at him ferociously and turned away to touch Lutie on the shoulder and help her to her feet. 'You come sit in my apartment for a while till you get yourself back together again, dearie.'

She thrust the door of her apartment open with a powerful hand, put Lutie in a chair in the kitchen. 'I'll be right back. You just set here and I'll make you a cup of tea. You'll feel better.'

The Super was about to go into his apartment when Mrs. Hedges returned to the hall. 'I just wanted to tell you for your own good, dearie, that it's Mr. Junto who's interested in Mis' Johnson. And I ain't goin' to tell you again to keep your hands off,' she said.

'Ah, shit!' he said vehemently.

Her eyes narrowed. 'You'd look awful nice cut down to a shorter size, dearie. And there's folks that's willin' to take on the job when anybody crosses up they plans.'

She stalked away from him and went into her own apartment, where she closed the door firmly behind her. In the kitchen she put a copper teakettle on the stove, placed cups and saucers on the table, and then carefully measured tea into a large brown teapot. Lutie, watching her as she walked barefooted across the bright-colored linoleum, thought that instead of tea she should have been concocting some witch's brew.

The tea was scalding hot and fragrant. As Lutie sipped it, she could feel some of the shuddering fear go out of her.

'You want another cup, dearie?'

'Yes, thank you.'

Lutie was well on the way to finishing the second cup before she became aware of how intently Mrs. Hedges was studying her, staring at the long evening skirt, the short coat. Again and again Mrs. Hedges' eyes would stray to the curls on top of Lutie's head. She should feel grateful to Mrs. Hedges. And she did. But her eyes were like stones that had been polished. There was no emotion, no feeling in them, nothing visible but shiny, smooth surface. It would never be possible to develop any real liking for her.

'You been to a dance, dearie?'

'Yes. At the Casino.'

Mrs. Hedges put her teacup down gently. 'Young folks has to dance,' she said. 'Listen, dearie,' she went on. 'About tonight'—she indicated the hall outside with a backward motion of her head. 'You don't have to worry none about the Super bothering you no more. He ain't even going to look at you again.'

'How do you know?'

'Because I scared him so he's going to jump from his own shadow from now on.' Her voice had a purring quality.

Lutie thought, You're right, he won't bother me any more. Because tomorrow night she was going to find out from Boots what her salary would be and then she would move out of this house.

'He ain't really responsible,' Mrs. Hedges continued. 'He's lived in cellars so long he's kind of cellar crazy.'

'Other people have lived in cellars and it didn't set them crazy.'

'Folks differs, dearie. They differs a lot. Some can stand things that others can't. There's never no way of knowin' how much they can stand.'

Lutie put the teacup down on the table. Her legs felt stronger and she stood up. She could get up the stairs all right now. She put her hand on Mrs. Hedges' shoulder. The flesh under the flannel of the gown was hard. The muscles bulged. And she took her hand away, repelled by the contact.

'Thanks for the tea,' she said. 'And I don't know what I would have done if you hadn't come out in the hall—' Her voice faltered at the thought of being pulled down the cellar stairs, down to the furnace room—

'It's all right, dearie.' Mrs. Hedges stared at her, her eyes unwinking. 'Don't forget what I told you about the white gentleman. Any time you want to earn a little extra money.'

Lutie turned away. 'Good night,' she said. She climbed the stairs slowly, holding on to the railing. Once she stopped and leaned against the wall, filled with a sick loathing of herself, wondering if there was something about her that subtly suggested to the Super that she would welcome his love-making, wondering if the same thing had led Mrs. Hedges to believe that she would leap at the opportunity to make money sleeping with white men, remembering the women at the Chandlers' who had looked at her and assumed she wanted their husbands. It took her a long time to reach the top floor.

Mrs. Hedges remained seated at her kitchen table, staring at the scars on her hands and thinking about Lutie Johnson. It had been a long time since she thought about the fire. But tonight, being so close to that girl for so long, studying her as she drank the hot tea and seeing the way her hair went softly up from her forehead, looking at her smooth, unscarred skin, and then watching her walk out through the door with the long skirt gently flowing in back of her, had made her think about it again—the smoke, the flame, the heat. (Pp. 237–241)

Source: Petry, Ann. 1992. *The Street*. Boston: Beacon Press. Copyright 1946, renewed 1974 by Ann Petry. Reprinted by permission of Houghton Mifflin Company. All rights reserved.

Murrogh De Burgh Nesbitt, from *The Road to Avalon* (1949)

In 1944, after 40 years of energetic life with physical disability, and having experience of counseling many South Africans with serious impairments, Murrogh Nesbitt sketched his dream of a rehabilitation center run by disabled people in a mountain setting that would enhance the self-healing process. Focusing initially on servicemen disabled in World War II, Nesbitt believed they needed more than surgical and medical interventions, more than aids and gadgets. They needed a time and context in which their spirits could heal. They needed the comradeship of active disabled people to prepare for the challenges ahead.

Disabled men do not want to be coddled. They must never be allowed to think that they have lost any of their potential manhood because of their disabilities.

I know that the real battle for the disabled men will begin when they face the world and have to earn their own living. The medical men and the surgeon have their place in the scheme when these men have to be treated for their wounds. The psychiatrist and psychologist have their places, but surely there is also room in rehabilitation schemes for the services of disabled men who have conquered all difficulties and have lived normal lives.

Disabled men have told me that I have changed their mental outlook. They have told me that when they have seen what I can do the urge comes to them to do likewise. They know that I have trekked out of the valley of shadows, that I have climbed mountains. I am not saying these things in a spirit of egoism. These are facts, and facts are worth all your tons of theory.

Source: Nesbitt, Murrogh De Burgh. 1949. P. 218 in *The Road to Avalon*. London: Hodder & Stoughton.

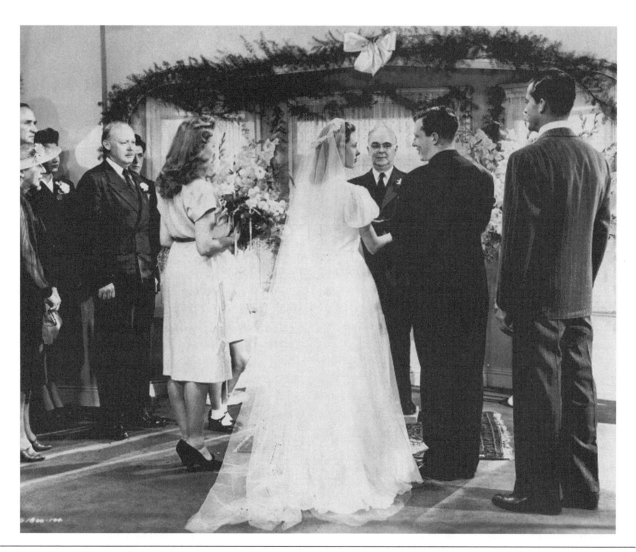

In the 1946 film The Best Years of Our Lives, *three men return from World War II to a small town in middle America and have varying degrees of success adjusting to postwar civilian life. The part of Homer Parrish, a Navy veteran who has lost both his hands, is played by nonprofessional actor Harold Russell. While serving as a demolitions instructor at a military base in North Carolina in 1944, Russell's hands were blown off in an accident involving a defective fuse. Ten days after his accident, he was transferred from the base hospital to the amputees' ward at Walter Reed General Hospital for advanced medical care. There, he was fitted for prosthetic replacements for his hands and given instruction in how to use them. His proficiency in their use was profiled in an army documentary,* Diary of a Sergeant. *For his role as Homer Parish, Russell received two Oscars: one for Best Supporting Actor and one for "bringing aid and comfort to disabled veterans." The film also received the Academy Award for Best Picture.*

Russell became an advocate for veterans and people with disabilities. He helped organize the World Veterans Federation and served as vice president of its World Veterans Fund, served three terms as the National Commander of the AMVETS, and was appointed chair of the President's Committee on Hiring the Handicapped by President Lyndon Johnson. He wrote two autobiographies, Victory in My Hands *(1949, with Victor Rosen) and* The Best Years of My Life *(1981, with Dan Ferullo). Russell died in 2002 at the age of 88.*

▣ Anzia Yezierska, from Red Ribbon on a White Horse (1950)

One of 10 children who immigrated at age 15 from Russian Poland to New York City's Lower East Side, Yezierska's writing spoke eloquently to the plight of Yiddish immigrants, the poor, and aged. Yezierska had a significant visual impairment, and her daughter *hired transcribers to allow her to continue writing after she became blind. This excerpt from her fictionalized autobiography details her childhood friendship with a disabled man.*

Always whenever I saw Zalmon Shlomoh I would feel that I too was a cripple. It leaped out of my eyes like the guilt of secret sin, that devouring hunger in me. People ran away from it as from a deformity. Only Zalmon Shlomoh, the hunchback, could feel and see the wild wolves of that hunger and not be frightened away.

I wondered, as I recalled the days when Zalmon was my only friend, whether he was still alive. If I could reach him, would he be glad to see me? Dared I look him up, to find out? But I knew he could never forgive my becoming one of the bloody rich. I never would look him up.

I thought of the time Zalmon had come to see me with a newspaper package under his arm. In the secondhand shop he had picked up, for a dime, an old record of Beethoven's "Moonlight Sonata." Instead of talking, he turned on the record again and again, filling the small room with the melancholy tenderness of all the unspoken love in the world.

One night he had taken me to hear Caruso in Pagliacci. The grief of the clown reached up to us in the gallery. That glorious voice cried out the ache of our own unlived lives.

Even while we sat together, cousins in sorrow, I was affronted by Zalmon's fish smells. In his new suit he looked as incongruous as a dog in a praying shawl. His charm was great enough to make me forget the dwarfed deformity of his body, but his fish smells drove me away. I could smell them even now.

Source: Yezierska, Anzia. 1950. *Red Ribbon on a White Horse.* New York: Scribner.

▣ Josephine Miles, Poems (20th c.)

Josephine Miles (1911–1985), an award-winning poet who taught at the University of California at Berkeley during the mid-twentieth century, was the first woman ever to be tenured in the English Department there. Miles lived with severe rheumatoid arthritis and, in the absence of elevators and wheelchair-accessible entrances, had to be carried across campus and up stairs by male assistants.

Reason (1955)

Said, Pull her up a bit will you, Mac, I want to
    unload there.
Said, Pull her up my rear end, first come first serve.
Said, Give her the gun, But, he needs a taste of his
    own bumper.
Then the usher came out and got into the act.

Said, Pull her up, pull her up a bit, we need this
    space, sir.
Said, For God's sake, is this still a free country or what?
You go back and take care of Gary Cooper's horse
And leave me handle my own car.
Saw them unloading the lame old lady,
Ducked out under the wheel and gave her an elbow,
Said, all you needed to do was just explain;
Reason, Reason is my middle name.

Doll (1979)

Through the willows bent down to shelter us where
    we played
House in the sandy acres, though our dolls,
Especially Lillian, weathered all the action,
I kept getting so much earlier home to rest
That medical consultation led to cast
From head to toe. It was a surprise for my parents
And so for me also, and I railed
Flat out in the back seat on the long trip home
In which three tires blew on our trusty Mitchell.
Home, in a slight roughhouse of my brothers,
It turned out Lillian had been knocked to the floor
    and broken
Across the face. Good, said my mother
In her John Deweyan constructive way,
Now you and Lillian can be mended together.
We made a special trip to the doll hospital
To pick her up. But, They can't fix her after all, my
    father said,
You'll just have to tend her with her broken cheek.
I was very willing. We opened the box, and she lay
In shards mixed among tissue paper. Only her eyes
Set loose on a metal stick so they would open
And close, opened and closed, and I grew seasick.
A friend of the family sent me a kewpie doll.
Later Miss Babcox the sitter,
After many repetitious card games,
Said, We must talk about bad things.
Let me tell you
Some of the bad things I have known in my life.
She did not ask me mine, I could not have told her.
Among the bad things in my life, she said.
Have been many good people, good but without
    troubles;
Her various stories tended
To end with transmigrations of one sort or another,
Dishonest riches to honest poverty; kings and queens
To Indians over an adequate space and time.

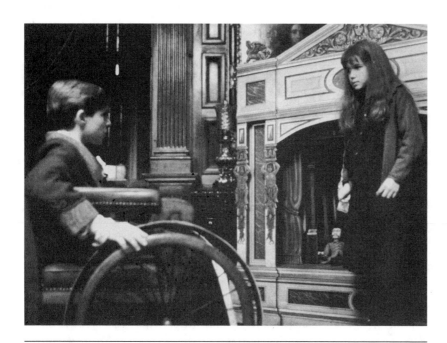

In The Secret Garden, *an adaptation of Frances Hodgson Burnett's classic story, Margaret O'Brien stars as the orphan who transforms the lives of her embittered uncle and his bedridden son when she starts tending a garden on the grounds of their country mansion. The sobriety of black and white gives way to a blast of Technicolor.*

Source: *The Secret Garden* (1949), directed by Fred M. Wilcox. United Kingdom. B&W/color, 92 minutes. Reprinted by permission of Paul Darke.

Take this cat coming along here, she said,
A glossy black cat whom she fed her wages in
    salmon,
He is a wise one, about to become a person.
Come to think of it, possibly Lillian
Is about to become a cat.
She will have different eyes then, I said.
Obviously. Slanted, and what is more
Able to see in the dark.

Source: Miles, Josephine. 1983. *Collected Poems, 1930–1983.* Urbana: University of Illinois Press. Copyright © 1983 by Josephine Miles. Used with permission of the University of Illinois Press.

▣ Hah Keun-Chan, from "Ill-fated Father and Son" [*Sunan I'dae*] (1957)

The title "Ill-fated Father and Son" can also be translated as "The Sufferings of Two Generations." In the story, the father, Man-do, who lost his arm in World War II during his conscripted labor in the South

Pacific, greets his son, Chin-su, who is returning from the Korean War with one leg. Hah Keun-Chan's works mostly deal with national tragedy such as war experience and the lives of the lower class.

Chin-su comes back alive; there is the lingering sad news that some have died in the war and some haven't heard whether or not their sons were killed! Oh my son Chin-su is still alive, he's coming back.

Thinking of it has made Mr. Pak Man-do climb to the top of Yongmaru hill in one breath; usually he would sit and rest once or twice in order to climb the hill. . . .

It was not hard to climb down the hill. As Man-do's only arm, his right, swung back and forth, his pace naturally began to quicken. The sleeve of his left arm was carelessly stuck in the pocket of his vest. My only son to be shot dead in the war was unimaginable! Of course he had to come back alive! But since he's coming back from a hospital, he must have been wounded slightly. But surely not like I was.

Man-do looked down at the sleeve stuck in the pocket of his vest. Nothing in it. It was merely a cloth cylinder without any left arm. The sleeve was always stuck in the pocket of his vest; it hung and swung from the left shoulder. Perhaps a bullet only slightly grazed Chin-su's calf or buttocks. If he was wounded so badly as to lose an arm like me, that cry baby surely couldn't put up with the pain. Inwardly worried about his son, Man-do muttered to himself. . . .

Squatting down at the edge of the brook, Man-do untied his belt, passed water, and felt better. Bubbles formed due to the urine on the mirror surface of the water, and a school of fishes swam up. There were some fish as big as your thumb.

I sure wish I could have a drink and some of those raw fish dipped in red pepper sauce. His mouth watered at the sight of the fish as he thought about a drink. But he blew his nose noisily and began to cross the log bridge carefully. . . .

He lit a cigarette. He never sat on a bench in the waiting room of the station without recalling a memory which always struck terror into his heart. His lost arm with fingers turned black and blue like a moss-clad log, seemed to lie heavily on his mind.

At that time there had been a crowd of over a hundred people in this station. Among them had been Man-do. Waiting for a train to carry them away, none of them had known their destination. They had been draftees pressed into service by the Japanese government-general; none of them had any choice but to get on the train; all of them like puppets had been manipulated by order of the Japanese.

Some of them had been told they would be sent to the coal-mines in Hokkaido and others had asserted that the islands of Southeast Asia would be their destination. There had been some people who said even Manchuria would be alright for them. Man-do, thinking that any place would be alright for him, [had] puffed out his cigarette smoke through the nostrils of his turned-up nose. . . .

When he had heard the train enter the vicinity, its sad warning whistle merged into his deep vast grief, . . . Man-do felt his eyes misty with tears. But as the train pulled away from the station, his sad feeling began to fade from his mind. Man-do, then, found himself somewhat inwardly pleased. . . .

On the day of the accident they were, as usual, preparing a hole in which to set dynamite in the crack of a rock. When everything was ready all but one would get out of the tunnel. . . . Man-do was almost out of the entrance when he heard a bomb-shell blast with a gust of wind. He nearly went crazy. It was bombs from a plane flying directly over the entrance. Backing and falling, he saw another plane swooping down from the mountain ridge, and dashed back. As soon as he plunged inside, the tremendous explosion of the dynamite swept the inside of the tunnel. Man-do felt his consciousness dimmed in a flash. . . .

He found himself on a soft mattress of a hospital, after regaining consciousness. He felt the terrible pain making a sudden attack on his ill-fated shoulder. They had already operated on his disfigured shoulder.

The sudden whistle of a train from the bend of the mountain awoke him, drenched in the mournful memory. Jumping up from the bench, he gripped the bunch of mackerel beside him. His heart throbbed more quickly as the whistle became closer and louder. . . .

In the wave of people moving toward the exit, he saw a wounded soldier limping on crutches; he did not pay any attention. It seemed there were no more people getting off at this stop. A few people who had not yet gotten aboard were only walking up and down along the platform to get on the train.

I think he wouldn't lie about this coming in his letter to me. . . . Feeling his heart somewhat troubled, Man-do muttered to himself.

"Father!"

A voice from behind him came to him. He started and turned his head in a great hurry. At the moment he looked back, he became pop-eyed and opened his mouth wide. The man standing on his crutches was surely his son, but utterly unlike before. A trouser leg of his pants was flapping in the wind!

Astounded by Chin-su's disfigurement, Man-do found himself falling into despair. At last, his eyes began to water with tears.

"Oh, my goodness!"

They were the first words that came from Man-do, in a tone trembling with excitement. He doubled up his fist firmly, holding the bunch of mackerel.

"God, what on earth is the matter with you?"

"Father!"

"Oh, you poor boy!"

Man-do's [turned]-up nose was running snivel. Tears were flowing down Chin-su's cheeks. "Come on, let's go!" said Man-do bluntly as he began to walk briskly ahead of Chin-su with the grim look that the unexpected misfortune was entirely due to Chin-su himself. Chin-su, licking the salty tears that ran down over his upper lip, limped after his father.

Man-do, never turning his head toward his son, went on walking, averting his eyes. Looking down at the ground like a man with a heavy load on his back, Man-do went on walking without a pause. Chin-su, supported by crutches, couldn't by any means keep up with the pace of a healthy man, and to make him more miserable, Man-do was quickening his steps. At last the distance between the two became so great that the low voice hardly reached Man-do. . . .

Then both father and son came out of the wine house and walked along a footpath between the rice-fields.

This time, unlike before, Chin-su walked ahead of his father. From behind, looking at his son who was limping on his crutches, Man-do followed him at a snail's pace, dangling the mackerel from his one arm. Man-do felt uneasy in his stomach, and staggered. He drank too much, he thought. He began to lose his senses. But it didn't matter, he felt.

"Hey, Chin-su!"

"Yes."

"What happened to your leg?"

"I was hit by a grenade fragment."

"By a grenade fragment?"

"Yes."

"Um . . ."

"The whole leg turned bad so they had to cut it off at the hospital."

There was a brief silence.

"Father."

"What?"

"I'm afraid I can't live like this!"

"What do you mean? Until they die, everyone struggles to live. Don't be so stupid!"

Again the silence.

"Look, son! I live well enough with only one arm, don't I? Of course, it doesn't look too good, but that doesn't have anything to do with living."

"I wish I were you. Walking on this one leg is killing me."

"Oh, boy, you're wrong. What's the use of walking? You can do any work you want with two good hands."

"Really?"

"Sure. In fact, we can share the work between us; you can do the indoor housework sitting down, while I take care of the heavy work outside. We'll have no problems at all."

"I guess not."

Chin-su, sighing slightly, looked back at his father. Man-do smiled gently, turning his face toward him. The alcohol had passed through his system quickly and Man-do's bladder was bursting.

Man-do squatted by the roadside and tried to grasp the string binding the mackerel with his teeth. Seeing this, Chin-su said, "Let me hold the fish, father."

Until his father finished urinating, Chin-su with his crutches in one hand and the fish in the other waited in the road. After finishing, Man-do promptly took the bunch of fish from his son.

At last, they arrived at the brook with the narrow log bridge across it. Chin-su saw that he was going to have a problem getting across. The sandy stream-bed didn't seem firm enough to support him on his crutches, though the water was shallow enough. What's more, it was absolutely impossible for him to cross the narrow log bridge. The only thing, he believed, left to him was to roll up his trousers after all, and so flopping on the bank, he began to do so.

"That's alright, just ride on my back, son."

Man-do looked down at Chin-su a little vacantly.

"All you have to do is climb on my back and we can both get across. Come on. Take the fish."

He thrust out the bunch of mackerel toward Chin-su.

With a look of embarrassment, Chin-su hesitatingly took it. With his back to his son, Man-do stretched out his only arm and said,

"Climb on, son."

Chin-su rode gently on the back of his father, holding his crutches in one hand and the mackerel in the other. With his single arm stretched behind, Man-do clutched Chin-su's leg firmly, and told him, "You'd better hold on to my neck tightly."

Clutching the fish and crutches as he hugged his father with both arms, Chin-su's eyes began to fill and his face tightened with emotion. Man-do, straining his stomach muscles, stood up slowly. His knees were shaking slightly under the weight, but he thought he could make it.

Stepping out on the narrow log bridge, Man-do began muttering to himself: How pitiful for this strong young body to be disfigured! Chin-su, you have met a sad lot in this misguided world. Damn it! Your whole future is hopelessly doomed. Hopeless!

While these thoughts were running through Man-do's mind, Chin-su, clinging to his father's back with his face shrouded in despair, groaned inwardly: Now I have been cursed too. My father has no luck at all. It'd have been better if I'd . . . died. . . .

Still swayed by the wine and weighted down by his son, Man-do stepped carefully on the bridge.

The Yongmaru hill standing tall before them looked down silently on this ill-fated father and son.

Source: Hah Keun-Chan. 1972, August 1. Choi, W. S., trans. "Ill-fated Father and Son" [*Sunan I'dae*]. *Korea Journal*: 7–12. (Originally published 1957) Reprinted by permission of the *Korea Journal*.

◨ German Movement of Mentally Disabled People (1958)

The Bundesvereinigung Lebenshilfe für Menschen mit geistiger Behinderung (Federal Association of Assisted Living for People with Cognitive Disabilities) is one of the most successful and largest disability self-help organizations in Germany. It was founded in 1958 as Lebenshilfe für das geistige behinderte Kind

(Assisted Living for the Mentally Handicapped Child) by a small group of experts and parents of cognitively disabled children. Its foundation was a reaction to the crimes perpetrated against disabled people during the National Socialist era. Thanks to the Bundesvereinigung, the Federal Republic of Germany was able to connect with the standard of education for cognitively disabled children and youth in other Western countries and in Northern European countries.

Letter of Invitation to the First Meeting, being held in Marburg/Lahn, November 13, 1958

Re: Preliminary discussion towards the foundation of a German organization of parents and friends of the mentally handicapped.

On the 23rd of November at 1:30 p.m., a meeting will take place in the educational counseling center in Marburg/Lahn regarding the possibility of founding a German national organization of parents and friends of the mentally handicapped as well as the goals and purposes of such an organization.

You are cordially invited to this meeting.

Organizations of this type already exist in many countries. The largest and so far most successful of such is the "National Association for Retarded Children" in the United States. . . .

The fact that the general public in Germany has to date done so relatively little for the general welfare of the mentally handicapped, has for many affected families needlessly increased the difficulties with their problem children in such a way that not seldom they become hardly bearable burdens.

As we know from the U.S., England, Holland, and a few other countries, institutions such as remedial kindergartens, schools for children that are only on the motor level trainable (imbeciles), schools for mongoloid children, training schools [*Anlernwerkstätten*], sheltered workshops, short-stay homes, summer camps, night schools, and evening clubs for the mentally handicapped, can highly contribute to limiting this problem to its narrowest borders.

The suggestion to call into being such institutions in this country as well will have to come from an influential parent organization, which will not grow weary in fighting again and again, wherever necessary for the welfare and happiness of its charges. With the help of the collective experiences from parent organizations in other countries, it should be possible in the foreseeable future to achieve a fundamental expansion of facilities for the mentally handicapped here as well. Also, the present period of economic prosperity should undoubtedly favor the success of such efforts. . . .

1958–Protocol of the Inaugural Meeting from November 23, 1958, Marburg

. . . After greeting those individuals present, the Summoner of the meeting, Mr. Tom Mutters, gave an overview of parental organizations for mentally handicapped children in other countries and underlined . . . the goals and purposes of a similar organization in Germany. . . . There was agreement, above all, on the following individual items:

- Contact should be made with all neighboring institutions that have similar objectives.
- The new organization should fight for, above all, a reform of home care; in particular, it should aim at supporting the institutions to stay in contact with the families.
- For the time being, the reform movement will emphasize the promotion of 'sheltered workshops and remedial kindergartens.' . . .

There was also a warning given to the new organization of following too strongly the course of already existing umbrella organizations of a denominational or solicitous sort, and it was unanimously pleaded for the creation of an independent organization that is fundamentally led by parents of disabled children.

The main task of the association was defined as fostering exemplary helping institutions, not however, to establish or maintain such institutions itself. The planned assistance should benefit all mentally handicapped (not only mongoloids and not only children). However, out of psychological grounds it seems opportune to anchor the expression, "Help for Children" in the association's description.

After a thorough discussion of the various possibilities, the group reached an agreement on the following description: "Lebenshilfe für das geistig behinderte Kind e.V." [Assisted Living for the Mentally Handicapped Child, a Registered Organization].

Source: Möckel, Andreas, Heidemarie Adam, and Gottfried Adam, eds. 1999. Pp. 154–157 in *Quellen zur Erziehung von Kindern mit geistiger Behinderung.* Würzburg, Germany: Bentheim. [*Sources on the Education of Children with Cognitive Disabilities: Vol. 2. 20th Century.* Vogt, Sara, trans.]

▣ Harper Lee, from To Kill a Mockingbird (1960)

Harper Lee's classic novel about growing up in the racially segregated U.S. South hinges on a variety of disability-based revelations. The falsely accused African American character, Tom Robinson, is proven innocent by Atticus Finch on the basis of an impairment he received when his arm was caught in a cotton gin. Nevertheless, the all-white jury finds him guilty of the crime of raping a lower-class white woman, Mayella Ewell. Additionally, a cognitively disabled character, Boo Radley, ultimately saves the children from a violent attack by Mayella's father, who is enraged by their father's willingness to defend a black man. In this excerpt, the children (Jem, Scout, and Dill) create horror stories about Boo's disability and incarceration within his family home.

Jem gulped down his second glassful and slapped his chest. "I know what we are going to play," he announced. "Something new, something different."

"What?" asked Dill.

"Boo Radley."

Jem's head at times was transparent: he had thought that up to make me understand he wasn't afraid of Radleys in any shape or form, to contrast his own fearless heroism with my cowardice.

"Boo Radley? How?" asked Dill.

Jem said, "Scout, you can be Mrs. Radley—"

"I declare if I will. I don't think—"

"Smatter?" said Dill. "Still scared?"

"He can get out at night when we're all asleep . . ." I said.

Jem hissed. "Scout, how's he gonna know what we're doin'? Besides, I don't think he's still there. He died years ago and they stuffed him up the chimney."

Dill said "Jem, you and me can play and Scout can watch if she's scared."

I was fairly sure Boo Radley was inside that house, but I couldn't prove it, and felt it best to keep my mouth shut or I would be accused of believing in Hot Steams, phenomena I was immune to in the daytime.

Jem parceled out our roles: I was Mrs. Radley, and all I had to do was come out and sweep the porch. Dill was old Mr. Radley: he walked up and down the sidewalk and coughed when Jem spoke to him. Jem, naturally, was Boo: he went under the front steps and shrieked and howled from time to time.

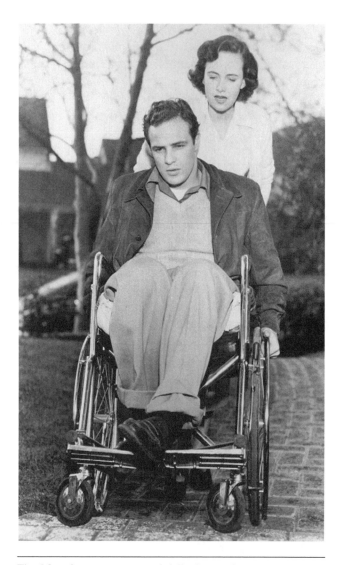

The Men *focuses on a ward full of paraplegic war veterans, including Marlon Brando as a wheelchair user, who struggle to come to terms with their altered bodies and a hostile social world beyond the rehabilitation unit.*

Source: *The Men* (1950), directed by Fred Zinnemann. United States. B&W, 85 minutes. Reprinted by permission of Paul Darke.

As the summer progressed, so did our game. We polished and perfected it, added dialogue and plot until we had manufactured a small play upon which we ran changes every day.

Dill was a villain's villain: he could get into any character part assigned him, and appear tall if height was part of the devilry required. He was as good as his worst performance; his worst performance was Gothic. I reluctantly played assorted ladies who entered the script. I never thought it was as much fun as Tarzan, and I played that summer with more than vague anxiety despite Jem's assurances that Boo

Radley was dead and nothing would get me, with him and Calpurnia there in the daytime and Atticus home at night.

Jem was a born hero.

It was a melancholy little drama, woven from bits and scraps of gossip and neighborhood legend: Mrs. Radley had been beautiful until she married Mr. Radley and lost all her money. She lost most of her teeth, her hair, and her right forefinger (Dill's contribution. Boo bit it off one night when he couldn't find any cats or squirrels to eat.); she sat in the living room and cried most of the time, while Boo slowly whittled away at all the furniture in the house. The three of us were the boys who got into trouble; I was the probate judge, for a change; Dill led Jem away and crammed [him] beneath the steps, poking him with the brush broom. Jem would reappear as needed in the shapes of the sheriff, assorted townsfolk, and Miss Stephanie Crawford, who had more to say about the Radleys than anybody in Maycomb.

When it was time to play Boo's big scene, Jem would sneak into the house, steal the scissors from the sewing machine drawer when Calpurnia's back was turned, then sit in the swing and cut up newspapers. Dill would walk by, cough at Jem, and Jem would fake a plunge into Dill's thigh. From where I stood it looked real.

When Mr. Nathan Radley passed on his daily trip to town, we would stand still and silent until he was out of sight, then wonder what he would do to us if he suspected. Our activities halted when any of the neighbors appeared, and once I saw Miss Maudie Atkinson staring across the street at us, her hedge clippers in mid-air.

One day we were busily playing Chapter XXV, Book II of One Man's Family, we did not see Atticus standing on the sidewalk looking at us, slapping a rolled magazine against his knee. The sun said twelve noon.

"What are you all playing?" he asked.

"Nothing," said Jim.

Jem's evasion told me our game was a secret, so I kept quiet.

"What are you doing with the scissors, then? Why are you tearing up that newspaper? If its today's I'll tan you."

"Nothing."

"Nothing what?" said Atticus.

"Nothing sir."

"Give me those scissors," Atticus said. "They're nothing to play with. Does this, by any chance have anything to do with the Radleys?"

"No sir," said Jem, reddening.

"I hope it doesn't," he said shortly, and went inside the house.

"Jem-m . . .."

"Shut up! He's gone into the living room, he can hear us in there."

Safely in the yard, Dill asked Jem if we could play anymore.

"I don't know. Atticus didn't say we couldn't—"

"Jem," I said, "I think Atticus knows it anyway."

I was not so sure, but Jem told me I was being a girl, that girls always imagine things, that's why other people hated them so, and if I started behaving like one I could just go off and find some to play with.

"All right, you just keep it up then," I said. "You'll find out."

Atticus's arrival was the second reason I wanted to quit the game. The first reason happened the day I rolled into the Radley front yard. Through all the head-shaking, quelling of nausea and Jem-yelling, I heard another sound, so low I could not have heard it from the sidewalk. Someone inside the house was laughing.

Source: Lee, Harper. 1960. Pp. 38–41 in *To Kill a Mockingbird*. New York: Warner. Copyright © 1960 by Harper Lee, renewed 1988 by Harper Lee, foreword © 1993 by Harper Lee. Reprinted by permission of HarperCollins Publishers.

Erving Goffman, from *Asylums: Essays on the Social Situation of Mental Patients and Other Inmates* (1961)

Many psychiatric survivors credit Erving Goffman's work as significant in revealing how a dependency on long-term institutionalization creates an inherently disempowering system of psychiatric care.

Like the neophytes in many of these total institutions, the new inpatient finds himself cleanly stripped of many of his accustomed affirmations, satisfactions, and defenses, and is subjected to a rather full set of mortifying experiences: restriction of free movement, communal living, diffuse authority of a whole echelon of people, and so on. Here one begins to learn about the limited extent to which a conception of oneself can be sustained when the usual setting of supports for it are suddenly removed. . . . While undergoing these humbling moral experiences, the inpatient learns to orient himself in terms of the "ward system." (P. 148)

. . . Once lodged on a given ward, the patient is firmly instructed that the restrictions and deprivations he encounters are not due to such blind forces as tradition or economy—and hence dissociable from self—but are intentional parts of his treatment, part of his need at the time, and therefore an expression of the state that his self has fallen to. Having every reason to initiate requests for better conditions, he is told that when the staff feel he is "able to manage" or will be "comfortable with" a higher ward level, then appropriate action will be taken. In short, assignment to a given ward is presented not as a reward or punishment, but as an expression of his general level of social functioning, his status as a person. (P. 149)

Source: Goffman, Erving. 1961. *Asylums: Essays on the Social Situation of Mental Patients and Other Inmates.* New York: Doubleday.

The Korean Child Welfare Committee, from *Handicapped Children's Survey Report* (1961)

These excerpts are from the first nationwide disability census in Korea, which has unique categories of disability different from later statistics. For example, children of mixed races were classified as socially handicapped, but this classification disappears from the disability category in later statistics. The survey was funded by various international social welfare foundations, the U.S. Army, and Korean governmental and church-related organizations. The report was published in Korean and English. The report includes the history of welfare services for handicapped children, case studies, essays by professionals on social issues and concerns of each category, and statistical descriptions of the results.

Foreword

Soon Yung Kwon

The Korea Child Welfare Committee has contributed to the promotion of child welfare in Korea in many ways for the past ten years, and this survey of children with physical, mental or social handicaps was one of its largest undertakings to date.

The Children's Survey Sub-committee, organized in September 1960 prepared for the nation-wide survey that was effectively carried out as of 10 April 1961. The Committee received financial assistance from both Korean and international voluntary agencies and individuals, administrative and technical participation of the Ministry of Health and Social Affairs, and those of provincial and local government.

Based on the decision of the Committee to use as interviewers, the Tong or Dong chiefs of villages who have little knowledge in handicaps of people, the survey had to be limited to such severe handicaps as a layman could plainly identify. Therefore, the children with slight handicaps and the children who are suffering from sicknesses or diseases that might cause handicaps in the future were not included in the Survey.

Some socially handicapped children such as juvenile delinquents; orphans; children born outside marriage, children of leper parents, and children of widows were not included in this survey. . . .

Healthy children of leper parents find themselves rejected by and ostracized from society. However, the survey did not include the group because of technical difficulties in the method of survey that was employed. An article on the subject was included in this report. Loss of husbands and fathers during the Korean War produced many widows and orphans. Widows living with their dependent children often find it difficult to get married again in this society and feel that they are a complicated social problem.

As the result of this survey many facts have been discovered. Handicapped boys are 27.2% more in number than the girls, as the total 77,903 handicapped children include 49,560 boys and 28,343 girls. The largest in number of handicaps is "paralytic or palsied" with 31,475 children with paralytic handicaps (38.7% is the total). The four Provinces that have the largest number of handicapped children are in order of Cheju-do, Cholla Namdo, Kyongsang Namdo and Cholla Pukdo. Seoul City has the smallest. 46,563 handicapped children or 82.6% are the children of low income families whose tax assessment is under category number 5. 58,947 handicapped children or 65.9% of the total indicated their desire for medical care.

Introduction

In Korea, many national crises and rapid social changes during the past twenty years have spawned serious problems contributing to human suffering in all walks of life. A large number of these problems are related directly to the welfare of children, such as care of orphans, prevention of and guidance for steadily increasing juvenile delinquents, rehabilitation of children with physical or mental handicaps, as well as protection of children placed under social discrimination. There is a growing awareness of the need for better provision of educational opportunities for the less fortunate, attention for child health, cultivation of recreational activities and other programs and services promoting general welfare of children.

Faced with the tremendous task of meeting so many needs on every side with little experience and resources, both government and voluntary agencies have been placed under pressure to develop adequate welfare services based on systemic assessment of needs and resources through a social survey. The need to fill this gap in the development of social welfare services was well demonstrated by the fact that there was extremely meager statistical information available on the nation's children when this committee began the collection of preliminary statistics.

This survey on handicapped children was the first such experiment on a nation-wide scale in the social welfare field, undertaken with scientific approach in an effort to introduce facts which we hope will be used for planning and implementation of needed services. It has been duly recognized by the committee that the problems of handicapped children are only a small portion of those related to the total family and child welfare needs in Korea. (P. 14)

The Mixed Racial Child, by Anne M. Davison

Most of the mixed racial children in Korea are illegitimate because mothers are casual or regular prostitutes of foreign servicemen. Of course the girl does not want to remain in that category, and she hopes constantly that he will marry her and take her away. If he is a white serviceman, he is the most [desirable]. If

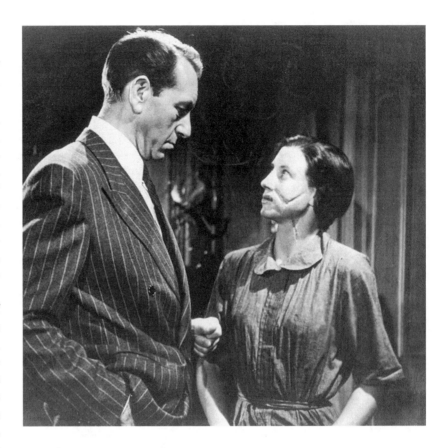

In A Stolen Face, *a plastic surgeon attempts to transform the face of a female convict into that of a lost lover.*

Source: *A Stolen Face* (1952), directed by Terrence Fisher. United Kingdom. B&W, 80 minutes. Reprinted by permission of Paul Darke.

she lives with him and has his child, the baby may be used as a lever to try to press him into marriage. In the marriage of an oriental and an occidental, the marriage custom of one or the other or both may be followed. If a western marriage is registered, the Korean community accepts it, but if the eastern custom is followed in a mixed marriage, the western country may not recognise it legally. When there is a marriage by Korean custom, as long as her "husband" remains in Korea, she is a respectable member of society, but when her "husband" leaves and returns to his own country, leaving her behind, everyone feels that he is a deserter. She is then thrust back into the community as an outcast and joins the group of cast-off wives, and other rejected people. Her chances of rehabilitation become very small.

There are girls as well as men who use the present social situation for their own ends. Sometimes the girl leads the man on, with no intention of leaving her way of life. She promises to marry and emigrate. Their marriage is made a legal one. If he must leave early, then she may refuse to follow him. She blames legal offices, friends and welfare worker, as excuses for her own indecision. The husband on the other side of the world feels that her delays in joining him are caused by outside attitudes of prejudice against his oriental wife because he does not really understand her basic problem.

What happens to the children in all these situations? They follow along and share the insecurity that their parents have made for them. They share the hope of the mother, that the father will return and marry her and take them all away, or marry the mother for debts, living expenses, and school fees. Such hopes keep the child's life uncertain and constantly insecure. Sometime the father says, "Send my son, even if my wife won't come." Very often another foreign man will feel that this girl has been badly treated, and pity may drive him to marry her and adopt her illegitimate children as well.

The decision to release a child for foreign adoption abroad is reached in various ways.

1. It may be complete economic inability to support that is the deciding factor. Having a child is costly, and the mother has probably become deeply indebted to the brothel keeper. Legally she cannot be made to meet debts of this nature, but she knows that she has a social obligation, that will weigh heavily on her until it is met.

2. A release for adoption may be given by a girl who has reached the end of her hope that the father will return as he promised he would do. By this time the child may be ten years old.

3. She may release her baby because he hampers her movement, is costly, and may remind her of a man who is no longer around. An oriental girl finds it hard to accept the fact that a foreign man is not interested in what happens to his child, especially if the child is a boy, and she constantly wants to have the father consulted about plans for their child. This may delay an adoption for years.

4. Some girls realise that foreign adoption in the long view will give more opportunity to the child, than anything they can give, and unselfishly they face the separation and make plans together with the adoption agency for his emigration.

Girls who make a success of prostitution financially are in a position where they can hire an older woman or a friend to care for the child. The mother can then write directly to the father, ask for support, or better still, from her point of view, beg him to divorce his wife and come back and marry her. The children are being held for blackmail purposes, and not loved by the mother or given the security of a home environment. These are the children that suffer the most and the longest. They are usually living in the middle of a prostitute community, and they must face each day the fact that they are consequences that have made no one happy, and often no one wants. Girls who move to some sections of an urban community, and who thus lose their identity somewhat, may find themselves and their children accepted more readily in the new community. This is so especially if the school teacher's attitude is one of acceptance and understanding. Of course children tease each other unmercifully, but if the teacher and the mother understand, and are a strength to a child, an adjustment may by made. However, when that point is reached, often the child may be behind in his school grade. It may mean that if the mother has no money for school fees, the child may have to leave school altogether, even though he is getting along well. As most of the prostitutes have very little education themselves, few of them having completed primary school, and have lost their self for an education for their children as other parents in the community.

The social and psychological handicaps of these children may be complicated by the addition of the physical or mental ones as well, such as polio, tuberculosis, feeble-mindedness etc.

Until the channel is opened to change a child's surname legally, there is not likely to be extensive adoption of mixed racial children in Korea. There needs to be a great deal more publicity and supervised assistance before families will be able to accept the challenge and do anything as radical as this. However, the government has taken the stand that a child should not be penalised for any misbehaviour of the parents. They have made . . . provisions for legal birth registrations for *all* [children]. As mixed racial marriage are increasing, there are growing numbers of mixed racial legitimate children in the community.

Foreign adoption is only a partial solution for the problems of mixed racial children's problems. There has not been enough time yet to evaluate the results of placing oriental children in western homes. For the present, plans should be made for the best possible solution to each situation may be found, either here in Korea or aboard. (Pp. 71–74)

Source: The Korean Child Welfare Committee. 1961. *Handicapped Children's Survey Report.* Seoul, South Korea: Korean Child Welfare Committee. Reprinted by permission of the Korean Department of Social Welfare.

▣ Thomas S. Szasz, from *The Myth of Mental Illness* (1961)

Thomas S. Szasz's popular work remains controversial. Recommended by psychiatric survivor/user advocates who are also affiliated with the antipsychiatry movement, many credit Szasz's ideas as providing instrumental theoretical support during the movement's early years.

It is customary to define psychiatry as a medical specialty concerned with the study, diagnosis, and treatment of mental illnesses. This is a worthless and misleading definition. Mental illness is a myth. Psychiatrists are not concerned with mental illnesses and their treatments. In actual practice they deal with personal, social, and ethical problems in living.

Source: Szasz, Thomas S. 1961. P. 262 in *The Myth of Mental Illness: Foundations of a Theory of Personal Conduct.* New York: Harper & Row. Copyright 1961 by Paul B. Hoeber, Inc. © 1974 by Thomas S. Szasz, M.D. Reprinted by permission of HarperCollins Publishers Inc.

▣ Michel Foucault, from *The Birth of the Clinic* (1963)

In The Birth of the Clinic, *Foucault analyzes the objectifying rhetoric of diagnosis applied by clinical medicine to its human objects. The work, along with his* Madness and Civilization, *furthers his anatomy of institutions as disciplinary spaces. Collectively, the two works demonstrate Foucault's lifelong critique of pathology as a distancing formula of empiricism that empties subjects of their humanity.*

From the Preface

Commentary questions discourse as to what it says and intended to say; it tries to uncover that deeper meaning of speech that enables it to achieve an identity with itself, supposedly nearer to its essential truth; in other words, in stating what has been said, one has to re-state what has never been said. In this activity known as commentary which tries to transmit an old, unyielding discourse seemingly silent to itself, into another, more prolix discourse that is both more archaic and more contemporary—is concealed a strange attitude toward language: to comment is to admit by definition an excess of the signified over the signifier; a necessary, unformulated remainder of thought that language has left in the shade—a remainder that is the very essence of thought, driven outside its secret—but to comment also presupposes that this unspoken element slumbers within speech (*parole*), and that, by a superabundance proper to the signifier, one may, in questioning it, give voice to a content that was not explicitly signified. . . . Is it not possible to make a structural analysis of discourses that would evade the fate of commentary by supposing no remainder, nothing in excess of what has been said, but only the facts of its historical appearance?

From Chapter One: Spaces and Classes

In order to know the truth of the pathological fact the doctor must abstract the patient . . . paradoxically, in relation to that which he is suffering from, the patient is only an external fact; the medical reading must take him into account only to place him in parentheses. . . .

Medical perception must be directed neither to series nor to groups; it must be structured as a look through a magnifying glass, which, when applied to different parts of an object, makes one notice other parts that one would not otherwise perceive, thus initiating the endless task of understanding the individual. . . .

In fact, no hostile disease is a pure disease. . . .

From Chapter Two: A Political Consciousness

Being a collective phenomenon, it [an epidemic] requires a multiple gaze; a unique process, it must be described in terms of its special, accidental, unexpected qualities. The event must be described in detail but it must also be described in accordance with the coherence implied by multi-perception: being an imprecise form of knowledge, insecurely based while ever partial, incapable of acceding of itself to the essential or fundamental, it finds its own range only in the cross-checking of viewpoints, in repeated, corrected information, which finally circumscribes,

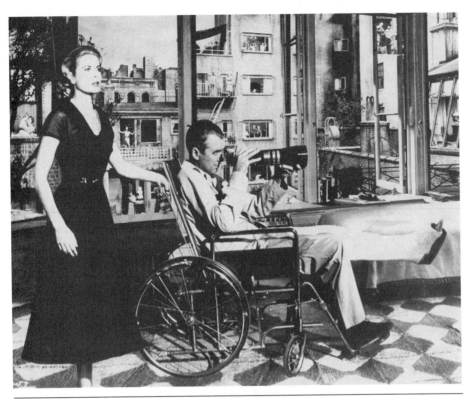

In Rear Window, *a news photographer, confined to his room by a broken leg, believes that he has seen a murder committed in an apartment on the other side of the courtyard. The film employs physical mobility as a metaphor for masculine oedipal conflicts with women.*

Source: *Rear Window* (1954), directed by Alfred Hitchcock. United States. Color, 110 minutes. Reprinted by permission of Paul Darke.

compassion; in this way, the poor would find "in companions of their own kind naturally sympathetic creatures who are not necessarily strangers to them." Thus disease would everywhere find its natural, or almost natural, locale, where it would be free to follow its own course and to abolish itself in its truth. . . .

The hospital is an anachronistic solution that does not respond to the real needs of the poor and that stigmatizes the sick in a state of penury. . . .

From Chapter Four: The Old Age of the Clinic

The clinic, on the other hand, was thought to be the element of its positive accumulation: it was this constant gaze upon the patient, this age-old, yet ever renewed attention that enabled medicine not to disappear entirely with each new speculation, but to preserve itself, to assume little by little the figure of the truth that is definitive, if not completed, in short, to develop, below the level of the noisy episodes of its history, in a continuous historicity. In the non-variable of the clinic, medicine, it was thought, had bound truth and time together. . . .

From Chapter Five: The Lesson of the Hospitals

What allows man to resume contact with childhood and to rediscover the permanent birth of truth is this bright, distant, open naivety of the gaze. . . .

Once the criteria of competence had been laid down, a selection could be made of those to whom the lives of citizens might be safely entrusted; medicine would then become a closed profession. . . .

A structure had to be found for the preservation of both the hospitals and the privileges of medicine, that was compatible with the principles of liberalism

where gazes meet, the individual, unique nucleus of these collective phenomena. At the end of the eighteenth century this form of experience was being institutionalized. . . .

A medicine of epidemics could exist only if supplemented by a police. . . .

The myth of a nationalized medical profession, organized like the clergy, and invested, at the level of man's bodily health, with power similar to those exercised by the clergy over men's souls; in the myth of a total disappearance of disease in an untroubled, dispassionate society restored to its original state of health. . . .

Medicine will also embrace a knowledge of *healthy man* that is a study of *nonsick-man* and a definition of the model man. . . .

From Chapter Three: The Free Field

For these, "communal houses for the sick" must be set up that would function as family substitutes and spread, in the form of reciprocity, the gaze of and the need for social protection—the latter understood somewhat ambiguously as the protection of the poor by the rich and the protection of the rich against the poor. . . .

But to look in order to know, to show in order to teach, is not this a tacit form of violence, all the more abusive for its silence, upon a sick body that demands to be comforted, not displayed? . . .

And in accordance with a structure of reciprocity, there emerges for the rich man the utility of offering help to the hospitalized poor: by paying for them to be treated, he is, by the same token, making possible a greater knowledge of the illnesses with which he himself may be affected; what is benevolence towards the poor is transformed into knowledge that is applicable to the rich. . . .

From Chapter Six: Signs and Cases

The symptom—hence its uniquely privileged position—is the form in which the disease is presented: of all that is visible, it is closest to the essential; it is the first transcription of the inaccessible nature of the disease. . . .

The sign announces: the prognostic sign, what will happen; the anamnestic sign, what has happened; the diagnostic sign, what is now taking place. . . . Through the invisible, the sign indicates that which is further away, below, later. It concerns the outcome, life and death, time, not that immobile truth, that given, hidden truth that the symptoms restore to their transparency as phenomena. . . .

Individual variations are spontaneously effaced by integration. In the medicine of species, this effacement of particular modifications was assured only by a positive operation: in order to accede to the purity of essence, it was first necessary to possess it, and then to use it to obliterate the excessively rich content of experience; it was necessary, by a prior choice, "to distinguish what is constant from what is variable in it, the essential from the purely accidental." . . .

From Chapter Seven: Seeing and Knowing

The glance, on the other hand, does not scan a field: it strikes at one point, which is central or decisive; the gaze is endlessly modulated, the glance goes straight to its object. . . .

From Chapter Eight: Open up a Few Corpses

A fine transmutation of the corpse had taken place: gloomy respect had condemned it to putrefaction, to the dark work of destruction; in the boldness of the gesture that violated only to reveal, to bring to the light of day, the corpse became the brightest moment in the figures of truth. . . .

Anatomy could become pathological only insofar as the pathological spontaneously anatomizes. Disease is an autopsy in the darkness of the body, dissection alive. . . .

From Chapter Nine: The Visible Invisible

Life, with its finite, defined margins of variation, was to play the same role in pathological anatomy as the broad notion of nature played in nosology: it was the inexhaustible, but closed basis in which disease finds the ordered resources of its disorders. . . .

Death is disease made possible in life . . . deviation in life is of the order of life but of a life that moves towards death. . . .

Source: Foucault, Michel. 1975. Sheridan, Alan, trans. *The Birth of the Clinic: An Archaeology of Medical Perception.* New York: Vintage. Copyright © 1975 Alan Sheridan. Originally published in French as *Naissance de la Clinique—Une archeologie du regard medical,* copyright © 1963 by Editions Gallimard, reprinted by permission of Georges Borchardt, Inc. for Editions Gallimard.

Thomas Pynchon, from *The Crying of Lot 49* (1966)

This excerpt from the American postmodern writer's first novel provides an important example of disability as a marker of social ostracism. However, rather than foregrounding physical difference as undesirable, the passages employ disability as that which identifies the existence of alternative political communities outside of a stultifying mainstream.

Out at the airport Oedipa, feeling invisible, eavesdropped on a poker game whose steady loser entered each loss neat and conscientious in a little balance-book decorated inside with scrawled post horns. "I'm averaging a 99.37 percent return, fellas," she heard him say. The others, strangers, looked at him, some blank, some annoyed. "That's averaging it out, over 23 years," he went on, trying a smile. "Always just that little percent on the wrong side of breaking even. Twenty-three years. I'll never get ahead of it. Why don't I quit?" Nobody answering.

In one of the latrines was an advertisement by ACDC, standing for Alameda County Death Cult, along with a box number and post horn. Once a month they were to choose some victim from among the innocent, the virtuous, the socially integrated and well-adjusted, using him sexually, then sacrificing him. Oedipa did not copy the number.

Catching a TWA flight to Miami was an uncoordinated boy who planned to slip at night into aquariums and open negotiations with the dolphins, who would succeed man. He was kissing his mother passionately goodbye, using his tongue. "I'll write, ma," he kept saying. "Write by WASTE," she said, "remember. The government will open it if you use the other. The dolphins will be mad." "I love you, ma," he said. "Love the dolphins," she advised him. "Write by WASTE."

So it went. Oedipa played the voyeur and listener. Among her other encounters were a racially-deformed welder, who cherished his ugliness, a child roaming the night who missed the death before birth as certain outcasts do the dear lulling blankness of the community; a Negro woman with an intricately-marbled scar along the baby-fat of one cheek who kept going through rituals of miscarriage each for a different reason, deliberately as others might the ritual of birth, dedicated not to continuity but to some kind of interregnum; an aging night-watchman, nibbling at a bar of Ivory Soap, who had trained his virtuoso stomach to accept also lotions, air-fresheners, fabrics, tobaccoes and waxes in a hopeless attempt to assimilate it all, all the promise, productivity, betrayal, ulcers, before it was too late; and even another voyeur, who hung outside one of the city's still-lighted windows, searching for who knew what specific image. Decorating each alienation, each species of withdrawal, as cufflink, decal, aimless doodling, there was somehow always the post horn. She grew so to expect it that perhaps she did not see it quite as often as she later was to remember seeing it. A couple-three times would really have been enough. Or too much.

She busrode and walked on into the lightening morning, giving herself up to a fatalism rare for her. Where was the Oedipa who'd driven so bravely up here from San Narciso? That optimistic baby had come on so like the private eye in any long-ago radio drama, believing all you needed was grit, resourcefulness, exemption from hidebound cops' rules, to solve any great mystery.

But the private eye sooner or later has to get beat up on. This night's profusion of post horns, this malignant,

deliberate replication, was their way of beating up. They knew her pressure points, and the ganglia of her optimism, and one by one, pinch by precision pinch, they were immobilizing her.

From the Social Security Act of 1967, Section 223 (d)(3) (United States)

The U.S. Social Security Act presented a variety of iterations of the definition of disability over the course of its development and implementation. In the 1967 version, disability was narrowed to a category of incapacity to work.

An individual . . . shall be determined to be under a disability only if his physical or mental impairment or impairments are of such severity that he is not only unable to do his previous work but cannot, considering his age, education, and work experience, engage in any kind of substantial gainful work which exists in the national economy, regardless of whether such work exists in the immediate area in which he lives, or whether a specific job vacancy exists for him, or whether he would be hired if he applied for work.

R. D. Laing, from *The Politics of Experience* (1968)

R. D. Laing, a psychiatrist who came to be known as the father of the antipsychiatry movement, stressed that our modern sense of "normality" creates and then camouflages deep intrinsic loss. The antipsychiatry movement is often associated with the psychiatric survivor/user movement.

What we call "normal" is a product of repression, denial, splitting, projection, introjection and other forms of destructive action on experience. . . . It is radically estranged from the structure of being.

The more one sees this, the more senseless it is to continue with generalized descriptions of supposedly specifically schizoid, schizophrenic, hysterical "mechanisms."

There are forms of alienation that are relatively strange to statistically "normal" forms of alienation. The "normally" alienated person, by reason of the fact that he acts more or less like everyone else, is taken to be sane. Other forms of alienation that are out of step with the prevailing state of alienation are those that are labeled by the "normal" majority as bad or mad.

The condition of alienation, of being asleep, of being unconscious, of being out of one's mind, is the condition of normal man.

Source: Laing, R. D. 1968. Pp. 27–28 in *The Politics of Experience.* New York: Ballantine Books. Copyright © R. D. Laing, 1967.

▣ From the Rehabilitation Act of 1973 (United States)

The Rehabilitation Act of 1973 was one of the earliest efforts to formalize legislation in the United States that guaranteed disabled people protection from discrimination under the law. The Vocational Rehabilitation Act of 1920 had marked the first major legislation establishing public rehabilitation programs for persons with disabilities in the United States. Funds were provided for vocational guidance, training, occupational adjustment, prosthetics, and placement services. Amendments during subsequent decades expanded the scope of federal programs. The Rehabilitation Act of 1973, which changed the name of the legislation from the Vocational Rehabilitation Act to the Rehabilitation Act, man dated a priority to serve persons with severe disabilities and affirmative action programs were established in Title V, Sections 501, 502, 503, and 504.

The Rehabilitation Act of 1973 was the predecessor of the 1990 Americans with Disabilities Act and promoted equal access throughout all segments of society. This excerpt is from the act as it was amended in 1998 by the Workforce Investment Act.

Section 2 (a): Findings

Congress finds that—

(1) millions of Americans have one or more physical or mental disabilities and the number of Americans with such disabilities is increasing;

(2) individuals with disabilities constitute one of the most disadvantaged groups in society;

(3) disability is a natural part of the human experience and in no way diminishes the right of individuals to—

   (A) live independently;
   (B) enjoy self-determination;
   (C) make choices;
   (D) contribute to society;
   (E) pursue meaningful careers; and
   (F) enjoy full inclusion and integration in the economic, political, social, cultural, and educational mainstream of American society;

(4) increased employment of individuals with disabilities can be achieved through implementation of statewide workforce investment systems under title I of the Workforce Investment Act of 1998 that provide meaningful and effective participation for individuals with disabilities in workforce investment activities and activities carried out under the vocational rehabilitation program established under title I, and through the provision of independent living services, support services, and meaningful opportunities for employment in integrated work settings through the provision of reasonable accommodations;

(5) individuals with disabilities continually encounter various forms of discrimination in such critical areas as employment, housing, public accommodations, education, transportation, communication, recreation, institutionalization, health services, voting, and public services; and

(6) the goals of the Nation properly include the goal of providing individuals with disabilities with the tools necessary to—

(A) make informed choices and decisions; and

(B) achieve equality of opportunity, full inclusion and integration in society, employment, independent living, and economic and social self-sufficiency, for such individuals.

(b) Purpose

The purposes of this Act are—

(1) to empower individuals with disabilities to maximize employment, economic self-sufficiency, independence, and inclusion and integration into society, through—

(A) statewide workforce investment systems implemented in accordance with title I of the Workforce Investment Act of 1998 that include, as integral components, comprehensive and coordinated state-of-the-art programs of vocational rehabilitation;

(B) independent living centers and services;

(C) research;

(D) training;

(E) demonstration projects; and

(F) the guarantee of equal opportunity; and

(2) to ensure that the Federal Government plays a leadership role in promoting the employment of individuals with disabilities, especially individuals with significant disabilities, and in assisting States and providers of services in fulfilling the aspirations of such individuals with disabilities for meaningful and gainful employment and independent living.

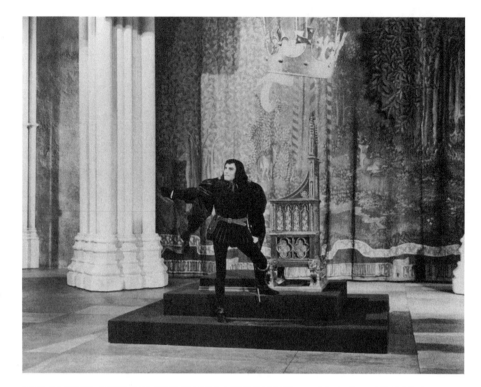

Laurence Olivier directs and stars in Richard III, *a triple Bafta-winning adaptation of Shakespeare's "hump-backed" king turned power-mongering usurper of the British throne.*

Source: *Richard III* (1955), directed by Laurence Olivier. United Kingdom. Color, 158 minutes. Reprinted by permission of Paul Darke.

(c) Policy

It is the policy of the United States that all programs, projects, and activities receiving assistance under this Act shall be carried out in a manner consistent with the principles of—

(1) respect for individual dignity, personal responsibility, self-determination, and pursuit of meaningful careers, based on informed choice, of individuals with disabilities;

(2) respect for the privacy, rights, and equal access (including the use of accessible formats), of the individuals;

(3) inclusion, integration, and full participation of the individuals;

(4) support for the involvement of an individual's representative if an individual with a disability requests, desires, or needs such support; and

(5) support for individual and systemic advocacy and community involvement.

Section 7: Definitions

(20) Individual with a disability
(A) In general
Except as otherwise provided in subparagraph (B), the term "individual with a disability" means any individual who—

(i) has a physical or mental impairment which for such individual constitutes or results in a substantial impediment to employment; and

(ii) can benefit in terms of an employment outcome from vocational rehabilitation services provided pursuant to title I, III, or VI.

(21) Individuals with a significant disability
(A) In general
Except as otherwise provided in subparagraph (B), the term "individual with a significant disability" means an individual with a disability—

(i) who has a severe physical or mental impairment which seriously limits one or more functional capacities (such as mobility, communication, self-care, self-direction, interpersonal skills, work tolerance, or work skills) in terms of an employment outcome;

(ii) whose vocational rehabilitation can be expected to require multiple vocational rehabilitation services over an extended period of time; and

(iii) who has one or more physical or mental disabilities resulting from amputation, arthritis, autism, blindness, burn injury, cancer, cerebral palsy, cystic fibrosis, deafness, head injury, heart disease, hemiplegia, hemophilia, respiratory or pulmonary dysfunction, mental retardation, mental illness, multiple sclerosis, muscular dystrophy, musculo-skeletal disorders, neurological disorders (including stroke and epilepsy), paraplegia, quadriplegia, and other spinal cord conditions, sickle cell anemia, specific learning disability, end-stage renal disease, or another disability or combination of disabilities determined on the basis of an assessment for determining eligibility and vocational rehabilitation needs described in subparagraphs (A) and (B) of paragraph (2) to cause comparable substantial functional limitation.

(B) Independent living services and centers for independent living

For purposes of title VII, the term "individual with a significant disability" means an individual with a severe physical or mental impairment whose ability to function independently in the family or community or whose ability to obtain, maintain, or advance in employment is substantially limited and for whom the delivery of independent living services will improve the ability to function, continue functioning, or move towards functioning independently in the family or community or to continue in employment, respectively.

(C) Research and training

For purposes of title II, the term "individual with a significant disability" includes an individual described in subparagraph (A) or (B).

(D) Individuals with significant disabilities

The term "individuals with significant disabilities" means more than one individual with a significant disability.

(E) Individual with a most significant disability

(i) In general

The term "individual with a most significant disability," used with respect to an individual in a State, means an individual with a significant disability who meets criteria established by the State under section 101(a)(5)(C).

(ii) Individuals with the most significant disabilities

The term "individuals with the most significant disabilities" means more than one individual with a most significant disability.

(22) Individual's representative; applicant's representative

The terms "individual's representative" and "applicant's representative" mean a parent, a family member, a guardian, an advocate, or an authorized representative of an individual or applicant, respectively.

(23) Institution of higher education

The term "institution of higher education" has the meaning given the term in section 1201(a) of the Higher Education Act of 1965 (20 U.S.C. 1141(a)).

(24) Local agency

The term "local agency" means an agency of a unit of general local government or of an Indian tribe (or combination of such units or tribes) which has an agreement with the designated State agency to conduct a vocational rehabilitation program under the supervision of such State agency in accordance with the State plan approved under section 101. Nothing in the preceding sentence of this paragraph or in section 101 shall be construed to prevent the local agency from arranging to utilize another local public or nonprofit agency to provide vocational rehabilitation services if such an arrangement is made part of the agreement specified in this paragraph.

(25) Local workforce investment board

The term "local workforce investment board" means a local workforce investment board established under section 117 of the Workforce Investment Act of 1998.

(26) Nonprofit

The term "nonprofit," when used with respect to a community rehabilitation program, means a community rehabilitation program carried out by a corporation or association, no part of the net earnings of which inures, or may lawfully inure, to the benefit of any private shareholder or individual and the income of which is exempt from taxation under section 501(c)(3) of the Internal Revenue Code of 1986.

(27) Ongoing support services

The term "ongoing support services" means services—

(A) provided to individuals with the most significant disabilities;

(B) provided, at a minimum, twice monthly—

(i) to make an assessment, regarding the employment situation, at the worksite of each such individual in supported employment, or, under special circumstances, especially at the request of the client, off site; and

(ii) based on the assessment, to provide for the coordination or provision of specific intensive services, at or away from the worksite, that are needed to maintain employment stability; and

(C) consisting of—

(i) a particularized assessment supplementary to the comprehensive assessment described in paragraph (2)(B);

(ii) the provision of skilled job trainers who accompany the individual for intensive job skill training at the worksite;

(iii) job development, job retention, and placement services;

(iv) social skills training;

(v) regular observation or supervision of the individual;

(vi) followup services such as regular contact with the employers, the individuals, the individuals' representatives, and other appropriate individuals, in order to reinforce and stabilize the job placement;

(vii) facilitation of natural supports at the worksite;

(viii) any other service identified in section 103; or

(ix) a service similar to another service described in this subparagraph.

(28) Personal assistance services

The term "personal assistance services" means a range of services, provided by one or more persons, designed to assist an individual with a disability to perform daily living activities on or off the job that the individual would typically perform if the individual did not have a disability. Such services shall be designed to increase the individual's control in life and ability to perform everyday activities on or off the job.

(29) Public or nonprofit

The term "public or nonprofit," used with respect to an agency or organization, includes an Indian tribe.

(30) Rehabilitation technology

The term "rehabilitation technology" means the systematic application of technologies, engineering methodologies, or scientific principles to meet the needs of and address the barriers confronted by individuals with disabilities in areas which include education, rehabilitation, employment, transportation, independent living, and recreation. The term includes rehabilitation engineering, assistive technology devices, and assistive technology services.

Source: The complete text of the Rehabilitation Act (29 U.S.C. 701 et seq.) is available at http://204.245.133.32/law/rehabact.htm

▣ Toni Morrison, from *The Bluest Eye* (1970)

In this novel, Morrison employs disability as a constitutive feature of several of her most memorable characters. In the excerpt here, Polly's identity forms around a limp that she develops after stepping on a rusty nail in childhood. The work's key argument explores concepts of racial beauty as "the most destructive idea in western culture."

Polly

The easiest thing to do would be to build a case out of her foot. That is what she herself did. But to find out the truth about how dreams die, one should never take the word of a dreamer. The end of her lovely beginning was probably the cavity in one of her front teeth. She preferred, however, to think always of her foot. Although she was the ninth of eleven children and lived on a ridge of red Alabama clay seven miles from the nearest road, the complete indifference with which a rusty nail was met when it punched clear through her foot during her second year of life saved Pauline Williams from total anonymity. The wound left her with a crooked archless foot that flopped when she walked—not a limp that would have eventually twisted her spine, but a way of lifting the bad foot as though she were extracting it from little whirlpools that threatened to pull it under. Slight as it was, this deformity explained for her many things that would have been otherwise incomprehensible: why she alone of all the children had no nickname; why there were no funny jokes and anecdotes about funny things she had done; why no one ever remarked on her food preferences—no saving of the wing or neck for her—no cooking of the peas in a separate pot without rice because did not like rice; why nobody teased her; why she never felt at home anywhere, or that she belonged anyplace. Her general feeling of separateness and unworthiness she blamed on her foot. Restricted as a child, to this cocoon of her family's spinning, she cultivated quiet and private pleasures. She liked, most of all, to arrange things. To line things up in rows—jars on shelves at canning, peach pits on the step, sticks, stones, leaves—and the members of her family let these arrangements be. When by some accident somebody scattered her rows, they always stopped to retrieve them for her, and she was never angry, for it gave her a chance to rearrange them again. Whatever portable plurality she found, she organized into neat lines, according to their size, shape or gradations of color. Just as she would never align a pine needle with the leaf of a cottonwood tree, she would never put the jars of tomatoes next to the green beans. During all of her four years of going to school, she was enchanted by numbers and depressed by words. She missed—without knowing she missed—paints and crayons. . . . When the war ended and the twins were ten years old, they too left school to work. Pauline was fifteen, still keeping house, but with less enthusiasm. Fantasies about men and love and touching were drawing her mind and hands away from her work. Changes in weather began to affect her, as did certain sights and sounds. These feelings translated themselves into extreme melancholy. She thought of the death of newborn things, lonely roads, and strangers who appear out of nowhere simply to hold one's hand, woods in which the sun was always setting. In church especially did these dreams grow. The songs caressed her, and while she tried to hold her mind on the wages of sin, her body trembled for redemption, salvation, a mysterious rebirth that would simply happen, with no effort on her part. In none of her fantasies was she ever aggressive; she was usually idling by the river bank, or gathering berries in a field when a someone appeared, with gentle and penetrating eyes, who—with no exchange of words—understood; and before whose glance her foot straightened and her eyes dropped. The someone had no face, no form, no voice, no odor. He was a simple Presence, an all-embracing tenderness with strength and a promise of rest. It did not matter that she had no idea of what to do or say to the Presence—after the wordless knowing and the soundless touching, her dreams disintegrated. But the Presence would know what to do. She had only to lay her head on his chest and he would lead her away to the sea, to the city, to the woods . . . forever. . . . Thus it was that when the Stranger, the someone, did appear out of nowhere, Pauline was grateful but not surprised. He came, strutting right out of a Kentucky sun on the hottest day of the year. He came big, he came strong, he came with yellow eyes, flaring nostrils, and he came with his own music.

Pauline was leaning idly on the fence, her arms resting on the crossrail between the pickets. She had just put down some biscuit dough and was cleaning the flour from under her nails. Behind her at some distance she heard whistling. One of these rapid, high-note riffs that black boys make up while sweeping, shoveling. Or just walking along. A kind of city-street music where laughter belies anxiety, and joy is as short

and straight as the blade of a pocketknife. She listened carefully to the music and let it pull her lips into a smile. The whistling got louder, and still she did not turn around, for she wanted it to last. While smiling to herself and holding fast to the break in somber thoughts, she felt something tickling her foot. She laughed aloud and turned to see. The whistler was bending down tickling her broken foot and kissing her leg. She could not stop her laughter—not until he looked up at her and she saw the Kentucky sun drenching the yellow, heavy-lidded eyes of Cholly Breedlove.

◉ Toni Morrison, from *Sula* (1973)

In this novel, African American novelist Toni Morrison explores disability as a source of individual authority rather than a disqualification. In this scene, her protagonist, Eva Peace, presides over her neighborhood while communal memory grows dim about her previous life as a nondisabled woman. For Morrison, Eva's power becomes increasingly the subject of her mythical qualities as a communal storyteller.

1921

The creator and sovereign of this enormous house with the four sickle-pear trees in the front yard and the single Elm in the back yard was Eva Peace, who sat in a wagon on the third floor directing the lives of her children, friends, strays, and a constant stream of boarders. Fewer than nine people in the town remembered when Eva had two legs, and her oldest child, Hannah was not one of them. Unless Eva introduced the subject, no one ever spoke of her disability; they pretended to ignore it, unless, in some mood of fancy, she began some fearful story about it—generally to entertain children. How the leg got up by itself one day and walked on off. How she hobbled after it but it ran too fast. Or how she had a corn on her toe and it just grew and grew and grew until her whole foot was a corn and then it traveled on up her leg and wouldn't stop growing until she put a red rag at the top but by that time it was already at her knee.

Somebody said Eva stuck it under a train and made them pay off. Another said she sold it to a hospital for

$10,000—at which Mr. Reed opened his eyes and asked, "Nigger gal legs goin' for $10,000 *a piece?*" as though he could understand $10,000 *a pair*—but for *one?*

Whatever the fate of her lost leg, the remaining one was magnificent. It was stockinged and shod at all times and in all weather. Once in a while she got a felt slipper for Christmas or her birthday, but they soon disappeared, for Eva always wore a black laced-up shoe that came well above her ankle. Nor did she wear overlong dresses to disguise the empty place on her left side. Her dresses were mid-calf so that her one glamorous leg was always in view as well as the long fall of space below her left thigh. One of her men friends had fashioned a kind of wheelchair for her: a rocking-chair top fitted to a large child's wagon. In this contraption she wheeled around the room, from bedside to dresser to the balcony that opened out the north side of her room or to the window that looked out on the back yard. The wagon was so low that children who spoke to her standing up were eye-level with her, and adults, standing or sitting, had to look down at her. But they didn't know it. They all had the impression that they were looking up at her, up into the open distances of her eyes, up into the soft black of her nostrils and up at the crest of her chin.

Source: Morrison, Toni. 1973. Pp. 30–31 in *Sula.* New York: Plume. Reprinted by permission of International Creative Management, Inc. Copyright © Toni Morrison.

◙ Union of the Physically Impaired Against Segregation, from *Aims* (1974)

This reading is excerpted from a policy statement created by British disability protestors as a critique against social obstacles to their full equality. The group was started by disabled activist Paul Hunt when he wrote an open letter to a local newspaper, The Guardian, and invited other disabled people to join him in his protest. Hunt spent a number of years as a resident of an institution and actively sought to expose the lack of control allowed to disabled people. The Union of the Physically Impaired Against Segregation also engaged in key struggles for the rights to integrated education, accessible housing, as well as meaningful employment. The organization disbanded in 1990 but still serves as one of the earliest examples of organizing against socially created obstacles to disabled peoples' integration.

The Union aims to have all segregated facilities for physically impaired people replaced by arrangements for us to participate fully in society. These arrangements must include the necessary financial, medical, technical, educational and other help required from the State to enable us to gain the maximum possible independence in daily living activities, to achieve mobility, to undertake productive work, and to live where and how we choose with full control over our lives.

Policy Statement

1. *Disability and Segregation.* Britain today has the necessary knowledge and the advanced technology to bring physically impaired people into the mainstream of life and enable us to contribute fully to society. But instead of the Country's resources being concentrated on basic human problems like ours, they are frequently misspent, for example, on making sophisticated weapons of destruction, and on projects like Concorde and Centre Point. So despite the creation today of such an enormous capacity, which could help overcome disability, the way this capacity is misdirected means that many physically impaired people are still unnecessarily barred from full participation in society. We find ourselves isolated and excluded by such things as flights of steps, inadequate public and personal transport, unsuitable housing, rigid work routines in factories and offices, and a lack of up-to-date aids and equipment.

2. There are a few individual examples of severely impaired people being able to overcome many of these barriers by the use of sufficient resources in the right way. They prove that integration is possible. But as a group we are still often forced to put up with segregated and inferior facilities. We get sent to special schools, colleges or training centres. We are systematically channelled into segregated factories, centres, Homes, hostels and clubs. If we do manage to become mobile, it is often in antiquated tricycles or specially labelled transport. All these segregated forms of help represented progress in years past. But since the means for integration now undoubtedly exists, our confinement to segregated facilities is increasingly oppressive and dehumanising. . . .

5. *Low Bargaining-Power.* When we do succeed in getting employment, our comparatively low productivity means that we have low bargaining-power when it comes to negotiating decent treatment and facilities. Our position is similar to that of many people who are middle-aged or elderly, who have had break-downs,

or are mentally handicapped, black, ex-prisoners, unskilled workers, etc. We are usually among the first to lose our jobs and be cast on the scrap-heap when it suits the needs of the economy. If we are lucky we may be drawn in again, to do the worst paid work, when business starts to boom once more. If we are unlucky, then we could face a lifetime on the degrading, means-tested poverty line. If we are very unlucky we may be consigned to a soul-destroying institution.

6. *Institutions—The Ultimate Human Scrap-Heaps.* The union of the Physically Impaired believes that the reality of our position as an oppressed group can be seen most clearly in segregated residential institutions, the ultimate human scrap-heaps of this society. Thousands of people, whose only crime is being physically impaired, are sentenced to these prisons for life— which may these days be a long one. For the vast majority there is still no alternative, no appeal, no remission of sentence for good behaviour, no escape except the escape from life itself.

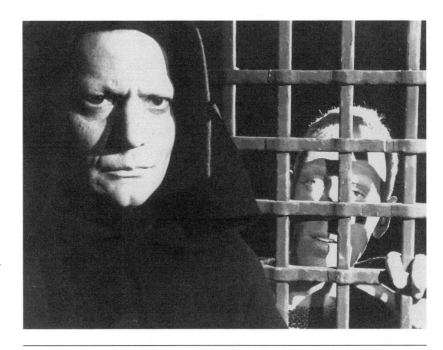

The Seventh Seal *is a doom-laden allegory set in medieval times when plague is raging through the land. A knight is challenged to a game of chess by Death, and the knight attempts to reveal the goodness of humankind in order to stave off his own encroaching mortality.*

Source: *The Seventh Seal* (1957), directed by Ingmar Bergman. Sweden. B&W, 100 minutes. Reprinted by permission of Paul Darke.

7. The cruelty, petty humiliation, and physical and mental deprivation suffered in residential institutions, where isolation and segregation have been carried to extremes, lays bare the essentially oppressive relations of this society with its physically impaired members. As in most similar places, such as special schools, there are some staff and volunteers doing their best to help the residents. But their efforts are systematically overwhelmed by the basic function of segregated institutions, which is to look after batches of disabled people— and in the process convince them that they cannot realistically expect to participate fully in society and earn a good living. This function was generally appropriate when special residential institutions first came into being, since in the competitive conditions of the time many physically impaired people could not even survive without their help. But now it has become increasingly possible for severely impaired people not just to survive, but also to work and become fully integrated, the need for segregated institutions no longer exists in the way it did. They have become seriously out of step with the changed social and technological conditions of Britain today. . . .

12. *Disablement Outside Institutions.* Our Union maintains that the present existence of segregated institutions and facilities is of direct relevance even for less severely impaired people who may expect to avoid having to use them. Those of us who live outside institutions can fully understand the meaning of disability in this society only when we take account of what happens to the people who come at the bottom of our particular group. Their existence and their struggles are an essential part of the reality of disability and to ignore them is like assessing the condition of elderly people in this society without considering the existence of geriatric wards.

13. It is also true that the kind of prejudiced attitudes we all experience (other people being asked if we take sugar in our tea is the usual example) are related to the continued unnecessary existence of sheltered institutions. Those who [do this] are indicating that they think we are not capable of participating fully and making our own decisions. They are harking back to the time when disabled people had to be sheltered much more, and they imply that really we ought to be back in our rightful place—that is, a special school, club, hospital unit, Home or workshop. Physically impaired people will never be fully accepted in ordinary

society while segregated institutions continue to exist, if only because their unnecessary survival today reinforces out of date attitudes and prejudices.

14. *Medical Tradition.* Both inside and outside institutions, the traditional way of dealing with disabled people has been for doctors and other professionals to decide what is best for us. It is of course a fact that we sometimes require skilled medical help to treat our physical impairments—operations, drugs and nursing care. We may also need therapists to help restore or maintain physical function, and to advise us on aids to independence and mobility. But the imposition of medical authority, and of a medical definition of our problems of living in society, have to be resisted strongly. First and foremost we are people, not "patients," "cases," "spastics," the "deaf," "the blind," "wheelchairs," or "the sick." Our Union rejects entirely any idea of medical or other experts having the right to tell us how we should live, or withholding information from us, or [making] decisions behind our backs.

15. We reject also the whole idea of "experts" and professionals holding forth on how we should accept our disabilities, or giving learned lectures about the "psychology" of disablement. We already know what it feels like to be poor, isolated, segregated, done good to, stared at, and talked down to—far better than any able-bodied expert. We as a Union are not interested in descriptions of how awful it is to be disabled. What we are interested in, are ways of changing our conditions of life, and thus overcoming the disabilities which are imposed on top our physical impairments by the way this society is organised to exclude us. In our view, it is only the actual impairment which we must accept; the additional and totally unnecessary problems caused by the way we are treated are essentially to be overcome and not accepted. We look forward to the day when the army of "experts" on our social and psychological problems can find more productive work.

Source: Union of the Physically Impaired Against Segregation. 1974. *Union of the Physically Impaired Against Segregation: Aims.* Available at: www.leeds.ac.uk/disability-studies/archiveuk/ UPIAS/UPIAS.pdf. Reprinted by permission of Paul Hunt.

▣ Alice Walker, from *Meridian* (1976)

Following in a long tradition of stories about children raised without parents in nature (such as Itard's writings on Victor of Aveyron, for instance, described in Fernald's excerpt in Part Two), Walker's chapter extends the analogy to dehumanizing beliefs about African Americans during the civil rights era. In order to "tame" the wild child's renegade nature, she is captured by administrators at an all-black university for women. However, the do-gooders tragically decide that she is incapable of living alongside other educated individuals and attempt to find a school for "special children" in which to house her.

The Wild Child

The Wild Child was a young girl who had managed to live without parents, relatives or friends for all of her 13 years. It was assumed she was thirteen, though no one knew for sure. She did not know herself, and even if she had known, she was not capable of telling. Wile Chile, as the people in the neighborhood called her (saying it slowly, musically, so that it became a kind of lewd, suggestive song), had appeared one day in the slum that surrounded Saxon College when she was already five or six years old. At that time there were two of them, Wile Chile and a smaller boy. The boy soon disappeared. It was rumored that he was stolen by the local hospital for use in experiments, but this was never looked into. In any case, Wile Chile was seen going through garbage cans and dragging off pieces of discarded furniture, her ashy black arms straining at the task. When a neighbor came out of her house to speak to her, Wile Chile bolted, not to be seen again for several weeks. This was the pattern she followed for years. She would be seen scavenging for food in the garbage cans, and when called to, she would run.

In the summer she wore whatever was available in castoff shorts and cotton tops. Or she would wear a pair of large rayon panties, pulled up under her arms, and nothing else. In winter she put together a collection of wearable junk and topped it with a mangy fur jacket that came nearly to the ground. By the age of eight (by the neighbors' reckoning) she had began to smoke, and, as she dug about in the debris, kicking objects this way and that (cursing, the only language she knew), she puffed on cigarette butts with a mature and practiced hand.

It was four or five winters after they first spotted her that the neighbors noticed Wile Chile was pregnant. They were critical of the "low-down dirty dog" who had done the impregnating, but could not imagine what to do. Wile Chile rummaged about as before, eating rancid food, dressing herself in castoffs, cursing and bolting, and smoking her brown cigarettes.

It was while she was canvassing voters in the neighborhood that Meridian first heard of the Wild Child. The neighbors had by then tried to capture her: A home for her lying-in had been offered. They failed to catch her, however. As one neighbor explained it, Wile Chile was slippier than a greased pig, and unfortunately the comparison did not end there. Her odor was said to be formidable. The day Meridian saw the Wild Child she withdrew to her room in the honors house for a long time. When the other students looked into her room they were surprised to see her lying like a corpse on the floor beside her bed, eyes closed and hands limp at her sides. While lying there she did not respond to anything; not the call to lunch, not the phone, nothing. On the second morning the other students were anxious, but on that morning she was up.

With bits of cake and colored beads and unblemished cigarettes she tempted Wile Chile and finally captured her. She brought her onto the campus with a catgut string around her arm; when Wile Chile tried to run Meridian pulled her back. Into a tub went Wile Chile, whose body was caked with mud and rust, whose hair was matted with dust, and whose loud obscenities mocked Meridian's soothing voice. Wile Chile shouted words that were never uttered in the honors house. Meridian, splattered with soap and mud, broke down and laughed.

At dinner Wile Chile upset her tablemates with the uncouthness of her manners. Ignoring their horrified stares she drank from the tea pitcher and put cigarette ashes in her cup. She farted, as if to music, raising a thigh.

The housemother, called upon in desperation by the other honor students, attempted to persuade Meridian that the Wild Child was not her responsibility.

"She must not stay here," she said gravely. "Think of the influence. This is a school for young ladies." The housemother's marcel waves shone like real sea waves, and her light-brown skin was pearly under a mask of powder. Wile Chile trembled to see her and stood cowering in a corner.

The next morning, while Meridian phoned schools for special children and then homes for unwed mothers—only to find there were none that would accept Wile Chile—The Wild Child escaped. Running heavily across a street, her stomach the largest part of her, she was hit by a speeder and killed.

Source: Walker, Alice. 1976. Pp. 35–37 in *Meridian*. New York: Pocket Books. Copyright © 1976 by Alice Walker, reprinted by permission of Harcourt, Inc.

John Gliedman and William Roth, from "The Grand Illusion" (1976)

In the fall of 1976, the organizers of the 1977 White House Conference on Handicapped Individuals invited John Gliedman and William Roth to submit an "Awareness Paper" on the communications disabilities. Deciding to run with the topic, they responded with "The Grand Illusion," a 37-page Goliath of an essay, typeset on an IBM Selectric Composer to conserve space, that contained large chunks of the 1976 working draft of their book The Unexpected Minority *(1980). Although "The Grand Illusion" was not the first work to highlight the analogies between the disabled and other stigmatized minorities, the essay's relentless emphasis on the degree to which disability is a social construction was unusual for the times. The authors developed their analysis further in* The Unexpected Minority, *where they presented the first comprehensive critique of traditional lay and expert views of disability and embedded the need for legal and political action within a perspective that integrated the minority group model with what today is variously called the postmodern or "disability as human variation" model. Perhaps because of its laser-like focus on developing the minority group model of disability, "The Grand Illusion" had its intended effect of shaking people up. "The Grand Illusion" was distributed to all who attended the White House conference, but it was not included in the volume of Awareness Papers that the organizers subsequently published, an omission that the authors have always considered a signal bureaucratic honor.*

The individual's communication options are generated by the nature of the setting. Is the individual among friends? Is he among strangers who respect him for what he is rather than see him as a handicap? And to an equally remarkable extent, the social possibilities of any normal setting are in turn partly determined by an individual's earlier social experience. Has he had a good education? Has he had sexual experience? Has he been able to travel? What was (or is) the individual's childhood like? The answers to these questions are as decisive as the answers to the medical questions. Indeed, in a certain sense, they are far more decisive because they determine the ultimate significance of the medical answers in the individual's life.

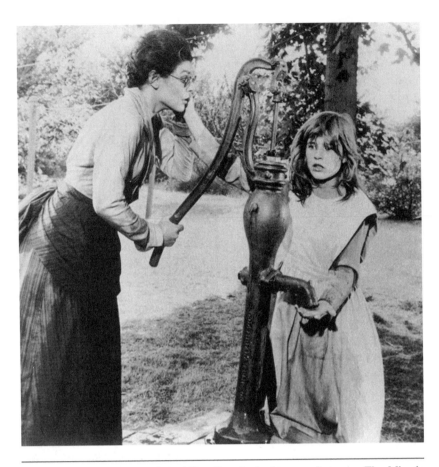

One of the most recognized disability films in the history of cinema, The Miracle Worker *tells the story of Annie Sullivan's struggles to teach the deaf and blind Helen Keller how to communicate in sign language.*
Source: *The Miracle Worker* (1962), directed by Arthur Penn. United States. B&W, 106 minutes.
Reprinted by permission of Paul Darke.

In recent years there has been much talk about the emphasis upon meaningless academic credentials in American life. [In] a cruel and largely unperceived way, the able-bodied world practices a parallel kind of credentialing on the disabled. All too often the child or the newly disabled adult learns that the prerequisite for being in social settings where a simple cry by a person with CP, a touch by a blind person, or a nod or grimace of joy is exactly right—and communicates far more than mere words—is a normal body. As much as anything our emphasis on the most mechanical aspects of communication reflects (or at least is congruent with) an important fact about cultural attitudes toward disability. To focus so exclusively on the sensory and motor obstacles to the message—and to overlook the sociological medium upon which all communication depends—is, in effect, to ratify the systematic exclusion of large numbers of disabled individuals from situations of genuine intimacy. It is to ratify their exile to the impoverished setting of the classroom, the doctor's office, the hospital ward, and the family bedroom which visitors are not shown. All too often we wind up helping the severely communication-disabled communicate as *patients* not as self-sufficient adults.

But to even mention in passing the importance of a rich and varied life experience to successful communication—however communication be defined—is to touch upon one of the great tragedies of handicap. Characteristically we make every effort to help the disabled individual compensate for his reduced ability to transmit or receive messages by teaching him how to be more explicit. In the process what is often forgotten—especially in the education of the handicapped child—is the positive functions of ellipsis for the able-bodied. Nowhere is this clearer than in the most meaningful and intimate situations of life—the touch of two lovers, the telegraphic speech of two old friends on the same wavelength, the poetry of silence. Here again the severely communication disabled individual often possesses more than enough biological capacity for effective communication. What is often lacking is not the biological potential but the social potential—i.e., a life in which intimacy is possible with anyone.

In sum, even if we restrict ourselves to the considerations of the classically defined communications disabilities, much of what the individual experiences as the most limiting and destructive aspect of his communications disability is the result of an ultimately social and ultimately arbitrary set of decisions, not an inevitable consequence of his biological deficit. Society not biology decrees that individuals crippled by severe CP are denied access to the mainstream of life. Society not biology decrees that the deaf must use cumbersome visual devices or speech instead of sign language to communicate with the hearing.

If most communications disabilities contain a sociological component of no mean importance, what of other kinds of handicaps? Might their not inconsiderable sociological component also produce significant obstacles to communication—obstacles whose ultimate origins are to be found not in the bodies of the disabled but in the minds of the able-bodied?

To broach these questions requires a significant expansion of the definition of communication common in the specialized literature which treats [of] communication disorders. It requires that we explore all kinds of communication, verbal and nonverbal. It requires that we recognize that each of us speaks many "languages" besides English—languages which communicate our self image to the other, our state of mind, our character, our social status, and our feelings about the other; language which communicates to the other whether we think he has a future and whether we have a future, in our private life and in professional life; language which passes judgment on the quality of the interaction between self and other, whether we might be compatible acquaintances, business associates, friends or lovers. And it is to recognize that each of us broadcasts this information on many "wavelengths" simultaneously, only one of these wavelengths being captured by a summary of what was actually said. We broadcast by means of our oral speech style, our grammar, our choice of words, our wit, and our accent. We broadcast by means of our tone of voice, our intonation, our clarity of articulation; by the way we pause between phrases and words: by our pitch, and our timber. We broadcast by means of the gestures we consciously or unconsciously make with our arms and legs, and if our arms and legs are paralyzed that very fact broadcasts a message. We broadcast by means of our facial expressions. We do so even if we are blind and do not control what the other reads into our face. We broadcast by our posture, our motor control, and by the overall way we look; an atrophied limb broadcasts a message; so does a wheel chair or an iron lung. We broadcast information by means of each of these channels, and what is communicated on one channel affects what is communicated on the other channels. Indeed, even our interpretation of the literal meaning of spoken speech is far more dependent upon what is broadcast on other "wavelengths." As anyone who has puzzled his way through transcripts of taped conversations knows, much that is self-evident face-to-face becomes unclear and ambiguous when we do not know what gestures, and tones of voice were used—or, even, upon occasions, the physical context in which the words were uttered, or the speaker's job, status, or sex.

But to adopt a definition of communication which is more in consonance with current linguistic, anthropological, and sociological practice, is to see that the communication problems of the disabled represent one side of what is perhaps the root problem of handicap in America—a problem which might aptly be called "The Other American Dilemma." The problem of handicap is multitudinous in its complexity. It involves medicine, rehabilitation, education, psychiatry. But first and foremost it is a problem of the able-bodied. By accident or by design, the world which the able-bodied have built interposes all manner of physical and social obstacles to the achievement of an adult identity for the disabled. For the individual with a relatively minor disability, these obstacles exert at the very least a severe psychic toll in unnecessarily low self-esteem, anxiety, demoralization, and diminished communication possibilities and abilities. For the more severely handicapped, biologically imposed limitations loom larger, but the really insuperable obstacles remain those imposed upon the individual by an able-bodied world which all too often returns his efforts for self-realization and communication with stigma, indifference, ignorance, and even, upon occasion, systematic efforts to persuade him to adjust to a life of needless dependency.

In the pages which follow we shall pursue a path which arches back and forth between these two faces of "The Other American Dilemma." In sections II and III, by means of analysis and copious example we explore some of the more important sociological obstacles experienced by most handicapped individuals. First appearing in the very act by which an able-bodied person sees a handicapped person, they are rooted in deep-seated cultural definitions of the meaning of disability. These definitions impede communication on many levels. After exploring some of these levels, we briefly examine some of the strategies the handicapped adopt to overcome these sociological obstacles—strategies which also often exact a terrible human cost. In sections IV and V we turn to a consideration of possible ways of improving the sociological situation of handicap. As we will see, one of the best ways may lie through the handicapped, as a social group, seeking to emulate the strategy which has proven so successful for the members of other stigmatized minority groups in the last generation. An important precondition for pursuing this course is the elimination of the many environmental barriers to the mobility of disabled individuals—e.g., buildings without ramps or adequate rest rooms, public telephones, and elevators not coded in Braille, and automobiles and public transportation systems which often are virtually unusable. Besides sharply curtailing the exercise of fundamental civil liberties, these physical barriers also represent a major obstacle to interpersonal communication on their own account. Next we briefly examine some of the other obstacles to communication, self-realization, and the achievement of an adult identity that that society puts in the way of the handicapped child and adult. These obstacles range from the way in which our helping services treat an individuals handicap and not the needs of the whole person, to the way society structurally discriminates against the handicapped as independent producers and consumers. We shall see that the effects of these institutional obstacles parallel the effects of environmental barriers to mobility: both represent concrete social precipitates of our underlying cultural definition of handicap. Finally, in the Appendix, we attempt systematically to catalogue some of the main ways in which break downs in communication between able-bodied and handicapped individuals can occur.

* * *

Before we can perceive a biological difference as a handicap, we must know—or have reason to believe—that it is chronic. Because this knowledge is not unambiguously transmitted by the rays of light which are focused into an image on the retina, the fact that we seem to instantaneously see that the man is handicapped reflects an interpretation of what our retina receives. To be sure, knowledge that a biological deficit is chronic is, in the everyday sense of the word, a reasonably objective matter. One consults a doctor, a textbook, or one's own experience. There is nothing subjective about knowing that a man with a spinal cord injury will not be able to use his legs again unless there is a breakthrough in treating his kind of spinal block. But suppose that in addition to such facts, other, less impeccable and less objective pieces of knowledge intervene between the image of the handicapped man on our retina and our seeing him, suppose that beliefs with little or no basis in reality intervene and govern what we see?

In her biography of Moshe Dayan, the general's daughter writes that after he lost his right eye in battle, her father was mystified by the fascination which his injury seemed to hold for many women. Dayan's disability is one of the few which change dramatically in character as one moves from childhood to adulthood. The nature of this change tells us something important about what we have to assume before we perceive something as a handicap.

A thought experiment. Conjure up in your mind a military man with an eye-patch. Now examine your feelings. Is there not something romantic and heroic about the injury? Doesn't it suggest a dark and complex past, a will of uncommon strength, perhaps a capability for just enough brutality to add an agreeable trace of sinister and virile unpredictability to the man? Depending on one's politics, it can suggest a resourceful ally or a dangerous enemy. Mustn't one be very tough and very competent indeed, to escape so lightly from a brush with death? No doubt these reactions explain why the only time Madison Avenue used a disability to enhance the glamour (and salability) of a commodity was in the Hathaway shirt ads of the 1960's.

Now replace the image of the Hathaway man with an eye-patch with the image of a young child with an eye-patch. For most people, something strange happens. The romance and mystery of the disability disappear. What we see is a handicapped child. There is something sad and even pitiful about him. Looking at his face we fear for his future and worry about his present. We think: this poor kid is going to have a hard time growing up and making it in this world. Where the presence of an eye-patch made the Israeli leader seem even more of a general (an adult role), the presence of an eye-patch on a child is a sign of damage, a cause for pity, an indication that this is a child whose ability to fit into some adult role in the future is in serious jeopardy.

Similar shifts in valence as a function of age or sex occur with a host of minor disfigurements or cosmetic blemishes—with scars and with certain kinds of ugliness which seem quite terrible in a child or a woman and seem sexy or virile in an adult male. Such shifts also appear to occur with certain kinds of limps requiring the use of a cane, as an acquaintance of ours learned to his astonishment when, after a hiking accident which left him hobbling about for several weeks, he was told by a number of friends that he looked very distinguished using a cane and should consider always using one. Needless to say, this is not something which anyone ever says to a young child who is forced to use a cane.

But General Dayan's eye-patch also points to something else. It points to a class of fairly serious physical disabilities which shuttle back and forth between being perceived as handicaps, or as enhancers, the direction of the shuttle being a function of one's adult role. (All of them, let us add at once, are perceived as handicaps when they appear in women and children.) In Jean Renoir's "La Grand Illusion," Erich von Stroheim plays the part of a man with a brace under his chin, a lame leg, a body scarred by burns, and a back injury which requires that he wear a steel corset. While the enumeration of these disabilities suggests a rather severely disabled man, we do not perceived the commandant as handicapped when we watch the film.

There are at least three possible explanations for this, and each suggests a cluster of special adult roles which are able to assimilate certain kinds of major handicaps more readily than most adult roles.

First, the movie is set during wartime. During war, our tacit definitions of handicap are relaxed. We adopt—if that be the word—a more sane approach, what counts is not so much how a man looks (within limits) but whether he can still function. And while von Stroheim is no longer fit for combat duty, he is perfectly capable of running a prisoner of war camp, and controlling the lives of hundreds of able-bodied people.

The second explanation involves the kind of character von Stroheim plays. An old Prussian aristocrat with a Spartan sense of morality and honor which elicits respect, he quite literally refuses to cease being an adult. And because society gives him the means—a war, a position of responsibility behind the lines and an aristocratic identity—he carries it off.

The final explanation is, we believe, generic. It is easier to integrate (and therefore to defuse) a disability into one's adult identity if one is cast as a villain. Villains are supposed to be scary. They are also supposed to be cunning, resourceful, and capable of outwitting death. A disability or two serves to indicate these characteristics—hence the false arm of Dr. No in the James Bond thriller, *The Island of Dr. No,* or in Bond's *From Russia With Love,* the thug with the hook on his arm which can cut through metal and glass. Hence the cluster of disabilities which afflict Dr. Strangelove, in Stanley Kubrick's "Dr. Strangelove," but which do not always succeed in causing us to view him as handicapped—the arm which is not fully under his control, the partial paralysis which results in his being pushed about in a wheelchair and wearing braces on his legs.

Closely related to these implicit rules about when a physical imperfection is perceived as a disability or a handicap, is the phenomenon of anthropomorphicization.

All of us remember childhood stories about four-footed creatures of the plains and forests—horses running wild and free, lion cubs overcoming the dangers of the veldt and becoming hunters, deer and bear living out their lives in the green solitude of the forest. When we heard these stories as children—and when we retell them to our own children—there seems nothing strange or unnatural to ascribing a full range

of (juvenile and adult) human characteristics to creatures who hunt with their claws or live by grazing on grass and shrubbery. One thinks of *Winnie-The-Pooh,* of *Bambi,* of *Lassie,* or Jack London's *The Call of the Wild,* of *Black Beauty,* of *Born Free,* of a multitude of other stories about animals in which a perfect equation is made between human child and animal child, human adult and animal adult.

But now perform the following thought experiment. Replace the animal figures in one of these stories with human beings who possess exactly the same range of functional capacities as the animals in question. For a deer who can run swiftly but can only manipulate objects with his mouth and tongue, substitute the image of a man paralyzed from the neck down who is as mobile as a deer in his electric wheelchair, and who can also manipulate objects with his mouth and tongue. Or instead of a family of lions, imagine a family of severely retarded individuals with intact bodies. Here, too, there is a perceptual "snap." Our willingness to expand the category of human to include juvenile and adult forms other than our own dissolves when we try to make it embrace severely handicapped people as well. Indeed, the very idea seems a contradiction in terms, an exercise in sick humor, and certainly something that we are not about to expose our children to.

Yet reflect a moment. Why is it a contradiction in terms to ascribe human characteristics to a man in an electric wheelchair or to a profoundly retarded person? Is it not because, bound up in our perception of animals, is the belief that on their own terms, they are complete, whole, and either adult or in the process of growing up to become adult, whereas it is precisely this quality of adultness (future or present) which is absent in our perception of these people we perceive as handicapped?

Source: Gliedman, John, and William Roth. 1977. "The Grand Illusion: Stigma, Role Expectations, and Communication: A Sociological Overview of the Problem of Handicap." In *The White House Conference on Handicapped Individuals Delegate Workbook.* New York: The Carnegie Corporation.

▣ Judi Chamberlin, from *On Our Own: Patient-Controlled Alternatives to the Mental Health System* (1978)

Described by many in the antipsychiatric movement as a landmark work, On Our Own *represents one of the earliest writings by a self-proclaimed psychiatric survivor.*

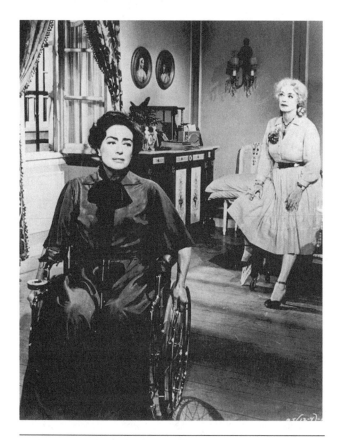

In Whatever Happened to Baby Jane? *two former movie stars live in their gloomy Hollywood mansion; one is in a wheelchair, and the other is mentally ill. The plot revolves around the responsibility for the accident that confined the matinee star to a wheelchair.*

Source: *Whatever Happened to Baby Jane?* (1962), directed by Robert Aldrich. United States. B&W, 130 minutes. Reprinted by permission of Paul Darke.

This excerpt, from the chapter entitled "Consciousness Raising," discusses the importance of raising the consciousness of both mental patients and others.

Consciousness raising is an ongoing process. Negative stereotypes of the "mentally ill" are everywhere and are difficult not to internalize, no matter how sensitive one becomes. This stereotyping has been termed "sane chauvinism" or "mentalism" by mental patients' liberation groups. Like sexism, mentalism is built into the language—*sick* and *crazy* are widely used to refer to behavior of which the speaker disapproves. The struggle against mentalism is one of the long-range activities of mental patients' liberation. . . . My feelings began to change when I discovered the existence of the Mental Patients' Liberation Project in New York, one of the earliest mental patients' liberation groups. We talked about our experiences and discovered how similar they were. Whether we had been in grim state

hospitals or expensive private ones, whether we were there voluntarily or involuntarily, whether we had been called schizophrenic, manic-depressive, or whatever, our histories had been extraordinarily similar. We had experienced depersonalization, the stupefying effects of drugs, the contempt of those who supposedly "cared" for us. Out of this growing awareness came a deeper understanding of the true purpose of the mental health system. It is primarily social control.

Source: Chamberlin, Judi. 1978. Pp. 66–67 in *On Our Own: Patient-Controlled Alternatives to the Mental Health System*. New York: McGraw-Hill. Printed with permission from Slack, Inc.

Sherwood Hall, from *With Stethoscope in Asia: Korea* (1978)

Sherwood Hall was the son of Dr. Rosetta S. Hall and Dr. William Hall, American missionaries and physicians in Korea. Dr. Rosetta Hall established modern special education in Korea in 1894. Sherwood Hall wrote a book based on his mother's diary. This excerpt shows the Western Christian perspective on disabled people in traditional Korea and the missionaries' roles.

Dr. [William?] Hall's first Christian convert in Pyong Yang was Mr. O Syok Hyong (who was among those cast into prison and later released during the recent persecutions). Mr. O had a little daughter who was blind. Mrs. Hall had encountered blind and deaf-mute patients in her medical work and longed to be able to do something to help them. However, the condition of both the blind and deaf-mutes in Korea at that time, Mrs. Hall discovered, was indeed pitiable. The deaf-mutes were considered imbeciles who survived by their animal instincts and the blind became fortune tellers or sorcerers (*mudongs*) if their parents were rich enough to have them thus trained. Otherwise, they were neglected and ignored, often poorly fed and clothed and allowed to sit in a corner until eventually they lost even the ability to walk.

Although Mrs. Hall had wanted to do something to help blind children, she had been cautioned that the Koreans might not understand her purpose. In time of any disturbances, they might point to the blind students as proof of the false tale that circulated during the Baby Riots of 1888 that doctors were taking out the children's eyes to make medicine.

When Mrs. Hall observed that Mr. O's eldest daughter was blind, she thought, "Here's my chance to begin. Her father is a Christian, and will not misinterpret my motive." . . .

Pongnai responded so eagerly and with such intelligence, that Mrs. Hall felt that she could be helped to learn to read if only Mrs. Hall had knowledge of the proper technique for teaching the blind. She resolved to learn more about it, for it could be a means of combating the superstition which prevented the blind from enjoying a life of usefulness. . . .

After moving to Pyong Yang, my mother had started working again with Mr. O's blind daughter, Pongnai. Teaching Pongnai with these new resources was at first slow and tedious work, but once she had mastered the alphabet and the syllabary, it was plain sailing. In a year, Pongnai could read all that my mother had been able to prepare and she learned to write in point and to make her own lessons from dictation. My mother also taught her to knit.

Patients, seeing Pongnai so happy and industrious, would ask my mother if other blind girls they knew might join her. Thus began the first school for the blind in Korea, and after the Pyong Yang Girls' School was built, a classroom for blind girls was added. My mother's belief was that the blind girls should be taught together with the seeing girls and should participate in their games. All that was necessary was to add a special teacher to the school staff for the beginners. Pongnai eventually became such a teacher as the work for the blind and deaf expanded.

Source: Hall, Sherwood. 1978. *With Stethoscope in Asia: Korea.* McLean, VA: MCL Associates. Copyright © 1978. Reprinted by permission.

▣ Leslie Fiedler, from *Freaks, Myths and Images of the Secret Self* (1978)

In one of the earliest analyses of freak shows as a social forum for producing difference, Fiedler adopts his characteristic psychoanalytic framework from which to read freak relations in the sideshow context. For Fiedler, the freak show provided audiences with opportunities to more directly encounter the Other of embodiment. One gazed at freaks while experiencing an internal catharsis that ultimately confirmed one's own membership in the ranks of the normal.

Even the ritualized murder of Freaks, however, seemed in ancient times to verge on sacrilege, and its incidence, therefore, was much lower than we might suppose. Sometimes, indeed, they were preserved and worshipped, as was clearly the case of a hideously distorted shamanka (female medicine woman) found in an underground cave in Czechoslovakia in the midst of ritual splendor 25,000 years after her interment. And even the Emperor Augustus, convinced that all freaks, especially Midgets, possessed the Evil Eye, nonetheless had created for his court a gold statue with diamond eyes representing his pet Dwarf, Lucius.

So there never was in earlier times any total genocidal onslaught against Freaks like that launched by Hitler against Dwarfs in the name of modern "eugenics." And it is even likely that fewer monsters were denied a chance to live in "priest-ridden" societies than in an AMA-controlled age like our own, in which "therapeutic abortions" are available to mothers expecting monstrous births, and infanticide is practiced under the name of "removal of life-supports from non-viable major terata."

At any rate, the word "monster" retains much of the awe once felt in the presence of newborn malformations, and the word, therefore, along with its variant form, "monstrosity," has never disappeared from the working vocabulary of carnivals and side shows. Indeed, I can still play in my head a spiel of a "freak show talker," familiar to me since childhood. Jo-Jo, the dog-faced boy, that ghost of a voice keeps saying, the greatest an-thro-po-log-i-cal-mon-ster-os-i-ty in captivity Brought back at great expense from the jungles of Bary-zil. Walks like a boy. Barks like a dog. Crawls on his belly like a snake. And at the drawled five syllables of mon-ster-os-i-ty, I feel my spine tingle and my heart leap as I relive the wonder of seeing for the first time my own most private nightmares on public display out there.

Why have I not used the word "monster," then, to describe those "unnatural creatures" whose natural history I am trying to write? In 1930, C. J. S. Thompson called a similar study, *The Mystery and Lore of Monsters.* But over the more than four decades since its appearance, the term "monster," has been preempted to describe creations of artistic fantasy like *Dracula, Mr. Hyde,* the *Wolf Man, King Kong,* and the nameless metahuman of Mary Shelley's *Frankenstein.* . . .

To be sure, monsters have a mythological dimension like Freaks, and in this respect they are unlike the category of unfortunates whom early French teratologists called mutiles: the blind, deaf, dumb, crippled, perhaps even hunchbacks and harelips, though these are marginal; along with amputees, paraplegics, and other victims of natural or man-made disaster. Children who are born legless or armless, their limbs amputated by a tangled umbilical cord, are sometimes hard to tell from true phocomelics, or seal children, with vestigial hands and feet attached directly to the torso. But once identified, they are primarily felt as objects not of awe but of pity.

Source: Fiedler, Leslie. 1978. Pp. 21–23 in *Freaks, Myths and Images of the Secret Self.* New York: Simon and Schuster. Reprinted by permission.

◙ Self-Advocacy in Australia (1981)

The Code of Rights of REINFORCE, the Victorian Association for Intellectually Disadvantaged Citizens, was drawn up in August 1981 at the Fifth Strand, an international conference of people labeled as mentally retarded. The Fifth Strand was an alternative conference that ran parallel with a "professional" conference on mental retardation.

Code of Rights

We want more training for jobs outside.

We want to see more people out of institutions.

We want better transport and lower fares and better services.

We are humans first and disadvantaged second.

All theatres to have concessions for each session.

We need more access to community facilities.

Everybody living in institutions has the right to community living, to be trained for jobs and to education.

We want more group homes to be built and more half-way houses.

Each pension should be above the poverty line and increase quarterly.

We want the right to have our own choice of medical insurance and our own doctor.

We have the right to have our rights protected, to be protected from violence and crime.

We have the right to information about marriage and relationships.

We have the right to live in our own home.

We have the right to spend our own money.

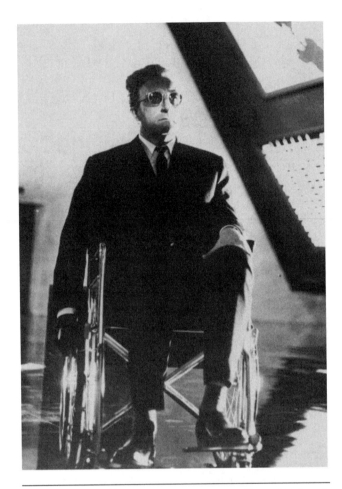

Kubrick's cool cynicism and screenwriter Terry Southern's caustic humor are perfectly wedded in Dr. Strangelove, *a vision of nuclear apocalypse brought about by a mad U.S. general's paranoia about women and Commies. Peter Sellers excels as a black-gloved, wheelchair-using, Kissinger-esque president.*

Source: *Dr. Strangelove* (1964), directed by Stanley Kubrick. United Kingdom. B&W, 93 minutes. Reprinted by permission of Paul Darke.

We demand all discrimination to cease.

We have the right to live with whom we want.

We have the right to know where our money is going.

Intellectually disadvantaged citizens should have access to low-rent flats and houses in the community.

We demand the closing of institutions for intellectually disadvantaged people.

We have the right to education.

We have the right to privacy.

We have the right to private ownership.

We have the right to equal day's pay for a fair day's work.

We have the right to worker's compensation.

Images of Disability on Stamps

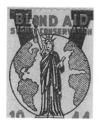

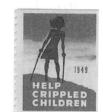

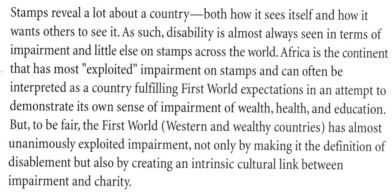

Stamps reveal a lot about a country—both how it sees itself and how it wants others to see it. As such, disability is almost always seen in terms of impairment and little else on stamps across the world. Africa is the continent that has most "exploited" impairment on stamps and can often be interpreted as a country fulfilling First World expectations in an attempt to demonstrate its own sense of impairment of wealth, health, and education. But, to be fair, the First World (Western and wealthy countries) has almost unanimously exploited impairment, not only by making it the definition of disablement but also by creating an intrinsic cultural link between impairment and charity.

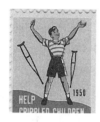

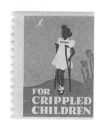

Charity and education about the prevention of impairment are givens and are seen as a wholly "good" thing. Thus, some images of impairment on stamps are so gloriously non-PC that they seem almost a joy in their celebration of otherness. Though a massive explosion of postal images of disability and impairment took place after the United Nations' 1981 International Year of the Disabled, prior to that, postal images of disability had appeared consistently in relation to wars (veterans), charity, immunization programs (polio in particular), and health education programs.

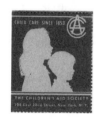

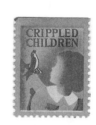

As with any stamp-collecting theme, there are always many more examples of the theme than one would ever hope for, be it images of disabled people; of particular impairments; or of wheelchairs, crutches, hearing aids, and the like. Stamps have been—and still are—advertisements for a (usually dubious) collective ideology of disablement; thus, we see the current increase in representations of disability on stamps linked to current issues such as stem cell research or HIV issues. But, like disability itself, disability and impairment are now and will continue to be on stamps in virtually every country in the world. (See www.outside-centre.com for listing and images.)

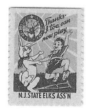

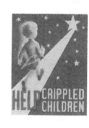

Paul Darke

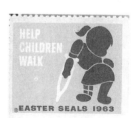

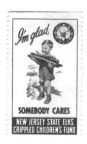

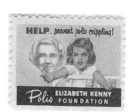

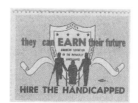

▣ Tetsuko Kuroyanagi, from *Totto-chan: The Little Girl at the Window* (1981)

This excerpt is from Totto-chan: The Little Girl at the Window, *a best-selling memoir by Japanese television talk show host and author Tetsuko Kuroyanagi. The book recalls her year as a first grader at Tomoe Academy, a progressive school created and run by Sosaku Kobayashi. (The school was destroyed in 1945 when the United States bombed Tokyo.) Kuroyanagi appreciated Headmaster Kobayashi's philosophy of "leveling the playing field" for all children, a very unusual approach to education in Japan before the surrender and occupation. The title of the book draws on a Japanese expression: people who were "over by the window" were marginalized, not part of the larger group (a similar Western expression would be to say that someone at work was "moved to a corner office" and thus taken out of the mainstream—though of course this expression conveys a positive separation). There isn't much mention of physical disability in this context in the book, but the epilogue refers to one particular classmate of the author's, Akira Takahashi. The reference to Sports Day is to a day when everyone in a school (and sometimes the parents as well) takes part in a festival of track and field events. Normally, a person of short stature would stand little chance at such events; however, the Headmaster had arranged for first-grade events that would actually be simpler for a person of short stature than for a child of average height. "Lunchtime speeches" at Tomoe referred to the Headmaster having children get up during lunch and make short speeches about almost anything, in order to help them develop self-confidence. At least in the first grade at Tomoe, swimming was "clothing optional"; the Headmaster thought that the children would get over any "morbid curiosity" about their bodies, especially with someone like Akira Takahashi in the class.*

The Swimming Pool

That was a red-letter day for Totto-chan. It was the first time she had ever swum in a pool. And without a stitch on!

It happened in the morning. The headmaster said to them all, "It's become quite hot all of a sudden, so I think I'll fill the pool."

"Wow!" everybody cried, jumping up and down. Totto-chan and the first grade children cried "Wow" too, and jumped up and down with even greater excitement than the older students. The pool at Tomoe was not rectangular like most pools, as one end was narrower than the other. It was shaped pretty much like a boat. The lay of the land probably had something to do with it. But nonetheless, the pool was a large and splendid one. It was situated between the classrooms and the Assembly Hall.

All during their lessons, Totto-chan and the others kept stealing glances out of the window at the pool. When empty it had been littered with fallen leaves just like the playground. But now that it was clean and beginning to fill up, it started to look like a real swimming pool.

Lunchtime finally arrived, and when the children were all gathered around the pool, the headmaster said, "We'll do some exercises and then have a swim."

"Don't I need a swimsuit to go swimming?" thought Totto-chan. When she went to Kamakura with Mother and Daddy, she took a swimsuit, a rubber ring, and all sorts of things. She tried to remember if the teacher had asked them to bring swimsuits.

Then, just as if he had read her thoughts, the headmaster said, "Don't worry about swimsuits. Go and look in the Assembly Hall."

When Totto-chan and the other first graders got to the Assembly Hall the bigger children were taking off their clothes with shrieks of delight as if they were going to have a bath. They ran out, one after the other, stark naked, onto the school grounds. Totto-chan and her friends hurriedly followed them. In the warm breeze it felt wonderful not to have any clothes on. When they got to the top of the steps outside the Assembly Hall they found the others already doing warm-up exercises. Totto-chan and her classmates ran down the steps in their bare feet.

The swimming instructor was Miyo-chan's elder brother—the headmaster's son and an expert in gymnastics. He wasn't a teacher at Tomoe but he was on the swimming team of a university. His name was the same as the school's—Tomoe. Tomoe-san wore swimming trunks.

After their exercises, the children let out screams as cold water was poured over them, and then they jumped into the pool. Totto-chan didn't go in until she had watched some of the others and satisfied herself they could stand. It wasn't hot, like a bath, but it was lovely and big, and as far as you could stretch your arms there was nothing but water.

Thin children, plump children, boys, girls—they were all laughing and shouting and splashing in their birthday suits.

What fun, thought Totto-chan, and what a lovely feeling! She was only sorry [her dog] Rocky couldn't come to school. She was sure that if he knew he could go in without a swimsuit he'd be in the pool, too.

You might wonder why the headmaster allowed the children to swim naked. There were no rules about it. If you brought your suit and wanted to wear it, that was perfectly all right. On the other hand, like today, when you suddenly decided to go in and hadn't a suit, that was perfectly all right, too. And why did he let them swim in the nude? Because he thought it wasn't right for boys and girls to be morbidly curious about the differences in their bodies, and he thought it was unnatural for people to take such pains to hide their bodies from each other.

He wanted to teach the children that all bodies are beautiful. Among the pupils at Tomoe were some who had had polio, like Yasuaki-chan, or were very small, or otherwise handicapped, and he felt if they bared their bodies and played together it would rid them of feelings of shame and help to prevent them developing an inferiority complex. As it turned out, while the handicapped children were shy at first, they soon began to enjoy themselves, and finally they got over their shyness completely.

Some parents were worried about the idea and provided their offspring with swimsuits which they insisted should always be worn. Little did they know how seldom the suits were used. Observing children like Totto-chan—who right from the start decided swimming naked was best—and those who said they had forgotten to bring their suits and went in anyway, most of them became convinced it was much more fun swimming naked like the others, so all they did was make sure they took wet swimsuits home! Consequently, almost all the children at Tomoe became as brown as berries all over, and there were hardly any with white swimsuit marks. (Pp. 66–69)

Takahashi

One morning, when they were all running about the school grounds, the headmaster said, "Here's a new friend for you. His last name is Takahashi. He'll be joining the first grade train."

The children, including Totto-chan, looked at Takahashi. He took off his hat and bowed, and said shyly, "How do you do?"

Totto-chan and her classmates were still quite small, being only in the first grade, but Takahashi, although he was a boy, was much smaller still, with short arms and legs. His hands, in which he held his hat, were small, too. But he had broad shoulders. He stood there looking forlorn.

"Let's talk to him," said Totto-chan to Miyo-chan and Sakko-chan. They went over to Takahashi. As they approached him he smiled affably, and they smiled back. He had big round eyes and looked as if he wanted to say something.

"Would you like to see the classroom in the train?" Totto-chan offered.

"Mm!" replied Takahashi, putting his hat back on his head.

Totto-chan was in a great hurry to show him the classroom and bounded over to the train, calling to him from the door, "Hurry up."

Takahashi seemed to be walking fast but was still a long way off.

"I'm coming," he said as he toddled along trying to run.

Totto-chan realized that while Takahashi didn't drag his leg like Yasuaki-chan, who had had polio, he was taking the same amount of time to get to the train. She quietly waited for him. Takahashi was running as fast as he could and there was no need to say, "Hurry," for he *was* hurrying. His legs were very short and he was bow-legged. The teachers and grown-ups knew that he had stopped growing. When he saw that Totto-chan was watching him, he tried to hurry faster, swinging his arms, and when he got to the door, he said, "You do run fast." Then he said, "I'm from Osaka."

"Osaka?" cried Totto-chan excitedly. Osaka was a dream city she had never seen. Mother's younger brother—her uncle—was a university student, and whenever he came to the house he used to take her head in both his hands and lift her up as high as he could, saying, "I'll show you Osaka. Can you see Osaka?"

It was just a game grown-ups used to play with children, but Totto-chan believed him. It stretched the skin of her face horribly and pulled her eyes out of shape and hurt her ears, but she would frantically look into the distance to try and see Osaka. But she never could. She always believed, however, that one day she would be able to see it, so whenever her uncle came, she would ask, "Show me Osaka." So Osaka had become the city of her dreams. And Takahashi came from there!

"Tell me about Osaka," she said to Takahashi.

"About Osaka?" he asked, smiling happily. His voice was clear and mature. Just then the bell rang for the first class.

"What a pity," said Totto-chan. Takahashi went in gaily, swinging the little body that was almost hidden by his bag, and sat down in the front row. Totto-chan hurriedly sat down next to him. She was glad you could sit anywhere you liked. She didn't want to leave him. Thus, Takahashi became one of her friends, too. (Pp. 90–100)

Sports Day

Tomoe's Sports Day was held every year on the third of November. The headmaster had decided on that day after a lot of research, in which he found out that the third of November was the autumn day on which it had rained the fewest times. Perhaps it was due to his skill in collecting weather data, or perhaps it was just that the sun and clouds heeded his desire— that no rain should mar the Sports Day so anticipated by the children, who had decorated the school grounds the day before and made all sorts of preparations. Whatever it was, it was almost uncanny the way it never rained on that day.

As all kinds of things were done differently at Tomoe, its Sports Day, too, was unique. The only sports events that were the same as at other elementary schools were the Tug of War and the Three-Legged Race. All the rest had been invented by the headmaster. Requiring no special or elaborate equipment, they made use of familiar everyday school things.

For instance, there was the Carp Race. Large tubular cloth streamers, shaped and painted like carp—the kind that are flown from poles in May for the Boys' Day Festival—were laid in the middle of the school grounds. At the signal, the children had to start running toward the carp streamers and crawl through them from the mouth end to the tail end and then run back to the starting point. There were only three carp—one red and two blue—so three children raced at a time. The race looked easy but was quite difficult. It was dark inside, and the carp were long, so you could easily lose your sense of direction. Some children, including Totto-chan, kept coming out of the mouth, only to realize their mistake and hurriedly burrow inside again. It was terribly funny to watch

because the children crawling backward and forward inside made the carp wriggle as if they were alive.

There was another event called Find-A-Mother Race. At the signal the children had to run toward a wooden ladder propped up on its side, crawl through it between the rungs, take an envelope from a basket, open it, and if the paper inside said, for instance, "Sakko-chan's mother," they would have to find her in the crowd of spectators, take her hand, and return together to the finishing line. One had to ease oneself through the ladder with catlike grace or one's bottom could get stuck. Besides that, a child might know well enough who Sakko-chan's mother was, but if the paper read "Miss Oku's sister," or "Mr. Tsue's mother," or "Mrs. Kuninori's son," whom one had never met, one had to go to the spectators' section and call in a loud voice, "Miss Oku's sister!" It took courage. Children who were lucky and picked their own mothers would jump and down shouting, "Mother! Mother! Hurry!" The spectators, too, had to be alert for this event. There was no telling when their names might be called, and they would have to be ready to get up from the bench or from the mat where they were sitting, excuse themselves, and wend their way out as fast as they could to where someone's child was waiting, take his or her hand, and go running off. So when a child arrived and stopped in front of the grown-ups, even the fathers held their breath, wondering who was going to be called. There was little time for idle chit-chat or nibbling food. The grown-ups had to take part in events almost as much as the children.

The headmaster and other teachers joined the children in the two teams for the Tug of War, pulling and shouting, "Heave-ho, heave-ho!" while handicapped children, like Yasuaki-chan, who couldn't pull, had the task of keeping their eyes on the handkerchief tied to the center of the rope to see who was winning.

The final Relay Race involving the whole school was also different at Tomoe. No one had to run very far. All one had to do was run up and down the semicircular flight of concrete steps leading to the Assembly Hall. At first glance it looked absurdly easy, but the steps were unusually shallow and close together, and as no one was allowed to take more than one step at a time, it was quite difficult if you were tall or had large feet. The familiar steps, bounded up each day at lunchtime, took on a fresh, fun aspect on Sports Day, and the children hurried up and down them shrieking gaily. To anyone watching from afar, the scene would have looked like a beautiful kaleidoscope. Counting the top one there were eight steps in all.

The first Sports Day for Totto-chan and her classmates was a fine day just as the headmaster had hoped. The decorations of paper chains and gold stars made by the children the day before and the phonograph records of rousing marches made it seem like a festival.

Totto-chan wore navy blue shorts and a white blouse, although she would have preferred to wear athletic bloomers. She longed to wear them. One day after school the headmaster had been giving a class in eurythmics to some kindergarten teachers, and Totto-chan was very taken with the bloomers some of the women were wearing. What she liked about them was that when the women stamped their feet on the ground, their lower thighs showing beneath the bloomers rippled in such a lovely grown-up way. She ran home and got out her shorts and put them on and stamped on the floor. But her thin, childish thighs didn't ripple at all. After trying several times, she came to the conclusion it was because of what those ladies had been wearing. She asked what they were and Mother explained they were athletic bloomers. She told Mother she definitely wanted to wear bloomers on Sports Day, but they couldn't find any in a small size. That was why Totto-chan had to make do with shorts, which didn't produce any ripples, alas.

Something amazing happened on Sports Day. Takahashi, who had the shortest arms and legs and was the smallest in the school, came first in everything. It was unbelievable. While the others were still creeping around inside the carp, Takahashi was through it in a flash, and while the others only had their heads through the ladder, he was already out of it and running several yards ahead. As for the Relay Race up the Assembly Hall steps, while the others were clumsily negotiating them a step at a time, Takahashi—his short legs moving like pistons—was up them in one spurt and down again like a speeded-up movie.

"We've got to try and beat Takahashi," they all said.

Determined to beat him, the children did their utmost, but try as they might, Takahashi won every time. Totto-chan tried hard, too, but she never managed to beat Takahashi. They could outrun him on the straight stretches, but lost to him over the difficult bits.

Takahashi went up to collect his prizes, looking happy and as proud as Punch. He was first in everything so he collected prize after prize. Everyone watched enviously.

"I'll beat Takahashi next year!" said each child to himself. But every year it was Takahashi who turned out to be the star athlete.

Now the prizes, too, were typical of the headmaster. First Prize might be a giant radish; Second Prize, two burdock roots; Third Prize, a bundle of spinach. Things like that. Until she was much older Totto-chan thought all schools gave vegetables for Sports Day prizes.

In those days, most schools gave notebooks, pencils, and erasers for prizes. The Tomoe children didn't know that, but they weren't happy about the vegetables. Totto-chan, for instance, who got some burdock roots and some onions, was embarrassed about having to carry them on the train. Additional prizes were given for various things, so at the end of Sports Day all the children at Tomoe had some sort of vegetable. Now, why should children be embarrassed about going home from school with vegetables? No one minded being sent to buy vegetables by his mother, but they apparently felt it would look odd carrying vegetables home from school.

A fat boy who won a cabbage didn't know what to do with it.

"I don't want to be seen carrying this," he said. "I think I'll throw it away."

The headmaster must have heard about their complaints for he went over to the children with their carrots and radishes and things.

"What's the matter? Don't you want them?" he asked. Then he went on, "Get your mothers to cook them for dinner tonight. They're vegetables you earned yourselves. You have provided food for your families by your own efforts. How's that? I'll bet it tastes good!"

Of course, he was right. It was the first time in her life, for instance, that Totto-chan had ever provided anything for dinner.

"I'll get Mother to make spicy burdock!" she told the headmistress. "I haven't decided yet what to ask her to make with the onions."

Whereupon the others all began thinking up menus, too, describing them to the headmaster.

"Good! So now you've got the idea," he said, smiling so happily his cheeks became quite flushed. He was probably thinking how nice it would be if the children and their families ate the vegetables while talking over the Sports Day events.

No doubt he was thinking especially of Takahashi—whose dinner table would be overflowing with First Prizes—and hoping the boy would remember his pride and happiness at winning those First Prizes before developing an inferiority complex about his size and the fact he would never grow. And maybe, who knows, the headmaster had thought up those singularly Tomoe-type events just so Takahashi would come first in them. (Pp. 109–114)

From the Epilogue

What are they doing now, those friends of mine who "traveled" together with me on the same classroom "train?"

Akira Takahashi

Takahashi, who won all the prizes on Sports Day, never grew any taller, but entered, with flying colors, a high school famous in Japan for its rugby team. He went on to Meiji University and a degree in electronic engineering.

He is now personnel manager of a large electronics company near Lake Hamana in central Japan. He is responsible for harmony in the work force and he listens to complaints and troubles and settles disputes. Having suffered much himself, he can readily understand other people's problems, and his sunny disposition and attractive personality must be a great help, too. As a technical specialist, he also trains the younger men in the use of the large machines with integrated circuitry.

I went to Hamamatsu to see Takahashi and his wife—a kindly woman who understands him perfectly and has heard so much about Tomoe she says it is almost as if she had gone there herself. She assured me Takahashi has no complexes whatever about his dwarfism. I am quite sure she is right. Complexes would have made life very difficult for him at the prestigious high school and university he attended, and would hardly enable him to work as he does in a personnel department.

Describing his first day at Tomoe, Takahashi said he immediately felt at ease when he saw there were others with physical handicaps. From that moment he suffered no qualms and enjoyed each day so much he never even once wanted to stay home. He told me he was embarrassed at first about swimming naked in the pool, but as he took off his clothes one by one, so he shed his shyness and sense of shame bit by bit. He even got so he did not mind standing up in front of the others to make his lunchtime speeches.

He told me how Mr. Kobayashi had encouraged him to jump over vaulting-horses higher than he was, always assuring him he could do it, although he suspects now that Mr. Kobayashi probably helped him over them—but

not until the very last moment, letting him think he had done it all by himself. Mr. Kobayashi gave him confidence and enabled him to know the indescribable joy of successful achievement. Whenever he tried to hide in the background, the headmaster invariably brought him forward so he had to develop a positive attitude to life willy-nilly. He still remembers the elation he felt at winning all those prizes. Bright-eyed and sensible as ever, he reminisced happily about Tomoe.

A good home environment must have contributed, too, to Takahashi's developing into such a fine person. Nevertheless, there is no doubt about the fact that Mr. Kobayashi dealt with us all in a very far-sighted way. Like his constantly saying to me, "You're really a good girl, you know," the encouraging way he kept saying to Takahashi, "You can do it!" was a decisive factor in shaping his life.

As I was leaving Hamamatsu, Takahashi told me something I had completely forgotten. He said he was often teased and bullied by children from other schools on his way to Tomoe and would arrive there crestfallen, whereupon I would quickly ask him what children had done it and was out of the gate in a flash. After a while I would come running back and assure him it was all right now and wouldn't happen again.

"You made me so happy then," he said when we parted. I had forgotten. Thank you, Takahashi, for remembering. (Pp. 193–195)

◙ Stanley Elkin, from *The Magic Kingdom* (1985)

Elkin's novel exposes the absurdities lurking beneath charity efforts to treat terminally ill children to fantasy vacations in order to lessen their "suffering." Instead, the trip descends into sentimental nightmare that benefits no one other than the resort owners. In this excerpt, the group's aptly named personal assistant, Colin Bible, uses the Disneyland parade as an opportunity for a lesson about human variation across body types.

"Come, children," Colin said.

"We already seen that parade," said Benny Maxine.

"I want you to see it again."

"Where are you taking them?" Nedra Carp asked.

"You needn't come, Miss Carp, if you don't wish to."

"Oh, I couldn't let you go by yourself. Who'd push the girl's wheelchair?"

"I'll push it. Benny can handle Mudd-Gaddis's."

Maxine looked at the nurse.

"Anyway, I don't see what the rush is. The parade don't start for nearly an hour yet."

There were frequent parades in the Magic Kingdom. Mr. Moorhead had given them permission to stay up one night to watch the Main Street Electrical Parade, a procession of floats outlined in lights like the lights strung across the cables, piers, spans, and towers of suspension bridges. There were daily "character" parades in which the heroes and heroines of various Disney films posed on floats, Alice perched on her mushroom like the stem on fruit; Pinocchio in his avatar as a boy, his strings fallen

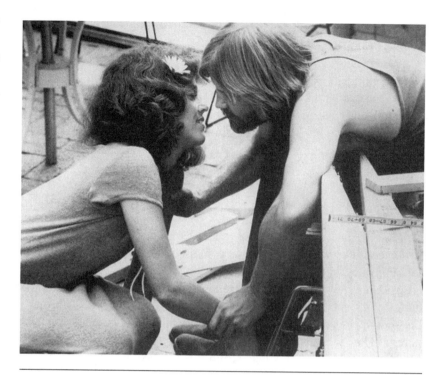

In Coming Home, *Jane Fonda portrays a woman who is married to a man fighting in Vietnam. After volunteering to work at a local veteran's hospital, she falls in love with a paralyzed veteran who becomes an active antiwar protester.*

Source: *Coming Home* (1978), directed by Hal Ashby. United States. Color, 126 minutes. Reprinted by permission of Paul Darke.

away, absent as shed cocoon; Snow White flanked by her dwarfs; Donald Duck, his sailor-suited, nautical nephews. They'd seen this one, too. There'd been high school marching bands, drum majors, majorettes, pom-pom girls, drill teams like a Swiss Guard. Tall, rube-looking bears worked the crowd like advance men, parade marshals. Some carried balloons in the form of Mickey Mouse's trefoil-shaped head, vaguely like the club on a playing card. (Pluto marched by, a Mickey Mouse pennant over his right shoulder like a rifle. "Dog soldier!" Benny Maxine had shouted through his cupped hands. The mutt turned its head and, in spite of its look of pleased, wide-eyed, and fixed astonishment, had seemed to glare at him.) Everywhere there were Mickey Mouse banners, guerdons, pennants, flags, color pikes, devices, and standards, the flash heraldics of all blazoned envoy livery. Music blared from the floats, from the high-stepping tootlers: Disney's greatest hits, bouncy and martial as anthems. It could almost have been a triumph, the bears, ducks, dogs, and dwarfs like slaves, like already convert captives from exotic far-flung lands and battlefields. The Mouse stood like a Caesar in raised and

isolate imperiality on a bandbox like a decorated cake. He was got up like a bandmaster in his bright red jacket with its thick gold braid, his white, red-striped trousers. His white gloves were held stiff and high as a downbeat against his tall, white-and-red shako. His subjects cheered as he passed. (You wouldn't have guessed that Minnie was his concubine. In her polka dot dress that looked almost like homespun, and riding along on a lower level of a lesser float, she could have been another pom-pom girl.)

It was toward this parade they thought they were headed.

But Main Street was practically deserted.

"What was the rush?" Nedra Carp asked.

"Yeah, where's the fire?" said Benny Maxine.

"Hang on," Colin Bible told them. "You'll see."

"It's another half hour yet," Lydia Conscience said.

"Are we just going to stand around?" Janet Order asked from her wheelchair.

"We could be back in our rooms resting," Rena Morgan said.

"We can sit over there," Colin said. He pointed across Main Street to the tiny commons.

Old-fashioned wood benches were placed outside a low iron railing that ran about a fenced green.

"We sit here we won't see a thing once it starts," Noah Cloth said.

"He's right," Tony Word said. "People will line up along the curb and block out just everything."

"Hang on," Colin Bible said. "You'll see."

About twenty minutes before the parade was scheduled to start, a few people began to take up positions along the parade route.

"Look there," Colin said.

"Where, Colin?" Janet said.

"There," he said, "the young berk crossing the street, coming toward us." He was pointing to an odd-looking man with a wide thin mustache, macho and curved along his lip like a ring around a bathtub. His dark thick sideburns came down to a level just below his mouth. "They're dyed, you know," Colin whispered. "They're polished with bootblack."

"How would you know that, Colin?" Noah asked.

"Well, not to blind you with science, I'm a nurse, aren't I? And 'haven't a nurse eyes, 'haven't a nurse 'air? When you see stuff so inky? There ain't such darkness collected together in all the dark holes."

"All the dark holes," Benny Maxine repeated, pretending to swoon.

"Look alive, mate," Colin scolded, "we're on a field trip, a scientifical investigation."

"We're only waiting for the parade to begin," Lydia said.

"A parade we already seen."

"Two times."

"By day and by night."

"M-I-C-K-E-Y M-O-U-S-E."

"Can't we give the parade a pass?"

"*This,*" Colin hissed, "*This* is the parade! This is the parade and you've *never* seen it! All you seen is the cuddlies, all you seen is the front runner, excellent dolls, happy as Larry and streets ahead of life."

"Really, Mister Bible," Nedra Carp said, "such slangy language!"

"Lie doggo, dearie, please. Keep your breath to cool your porridge, Miss Carp."

"I don't think this is distinguished, Mister Bible," Miss Carp said.

"Jack it in," he told her sharply. "Distinguished? *Distinguished?* I'm showing them the popsies; I'm showing them the puppets. I'm displaying the nits and flourishing the nut cases. The bleeders and bloods, the yobbos and stooges. I'm furnishing them mokes and bringing them muggings. All the mutton dressed as lamb. No one has yet, God knows, so old Joe Soap will must."

"Why?"

"Ask me another," he said.

"Why?"

"They've got to find out how many beans make five, don't they? It's only your ordinary level pegging, merely keeping abreast. There's a ton of niff in this world, you know. There's just lashings and lashings of death. Hark!" He broke off. "*Watch what you think you're going to miss.* Hush! Squint!" The man in the mustache and sideburns was passing in front of them.

And now you couldn't have dragged them away. You couldn't have rolled Janet Order's or Mudd-Gaddis's wheelchair downhill.

"Uh-oh," Colin Bible said, "we've been sold a pup."

"Snookered!" said one of the children.

"Skinned!" said another.

"Socked!"

"Some mothers have 'em," Benny Maxine said.

Because they saw that Colin had been wrong.

The man was not young, after all. He could have been in his fifties. He wore cowboy boots, the cheap imitation leather not so much worn as peeling, chipped as paint and mealy and rotten as spoiled fruit. His high raised heels were of a cloudy translucent plastic. Flecks of gold-colored foil were embedded in them like sparks painted on a loud tie. Up close he had the queer, pale, lone, and fragile look of men who cut themselves shaving. Of short-order cooks, of men wakened in drunk tanks or beaten in fights. A bolo tie, like undone laces, hung about a bright pink rayon shirt that fit over a discrete paunch tight and heavy as muscle. A chain that ran through a wallet in the back pocket of his pants was attached to his belt.

Nor were his broad sideburns dyed. They were tattooed along his ears and down his cheeks. His mustache was tattooed. The actual gloss and sheen tattooed too—like highlights in a landscape. Everything only indelible, deep driven inks among the raised scars of his illustrious whiskers.

They were gathering, coming together quickly now, lining up along the curbs, building a crowd, rapidly taking up the best vantage points like people filling a theater. "See 'em? They look like fans at the all-in wrestling," Colin said wickedly. And they did. Something not so much supportive as impatient and partisan about them. Apple Annies of style, Typhoid Marys of spirit, the men as well as the women, they could have been carriers, not of disease but of vague, pandemic strains on the psyche, on tastes not depleted but somehow made to accommodate to the surrender terms of their lives and conditions. As though they'd survived their dreams, even their lives, only to find a need to be at a parade of cartoon characters at Disney World.

It was different with the children, their parents. Oddly in the minority, Colin barely made mention of them, as though most lives came with a grace period, thirty or thirty-five years, say, some fifty-thousand-mile guarantee of the agreeable and routine. It was the widows traveling together he pointed out, the senior citizens up from Miami or down from such places as Detroit or Cleveland on package tours. It was the retirees, the couples unescorted by kids. They were casually dressed, the women in pants suits or sometimes in shorts—it was a mild fall day—the men in Bermudas, in slacks the color of artificial fruit flavors, in white shoes, in billed caps with fishermen's patches. (Cinderella Castle, towering above them in the background, made them seem even more like subjects than ever, reasonably content, well off, even, but with a whiff of the indentured about them, of an obligated loyalty.)

"Look there!" Colin Bible said. "And *there*. Look at those over there!"

There was a couple with the lined, bloated, and satisfied heads of midgets. Wens were sprinkled across their faces like a kind of loose change of flesh.

There was a potbellied, slack-breasted man, his wife with bad skin, wrinkled, scarred, pitted as scrotum. They had smooth, fat fingers, and their hands were balled into the ineffectual, hairless fists of babies.

"Look, look there, how ugly!" Colin said.

An angry woman with long dark hair, her back to the street, stood near the couple with the wens. Her hair, tied beneath her chin, looked like a babushka. She stared back at Colin and the children, her black, thick eyebrows exactly the color and shape of leeches above eyes set so deep in her skull they seemed separated from her face, hidden as eyes behind a mask or holes cut from portraits in horror films. A set of tiny lips, Kewpie-doll, bow-shaped, red and glossy as wet paint, and superimposed, grafted onto her real lips like a botched bookkeeping or clumsy work in a child's coloring book, tinted an additional ferocity into her scrutiny.

"It breaks your heart," Colin said. "Imperfection everywhere, everywhere. Not like in nature. What, you think stars show their age? Oceans, the sky? No fear! Only in man, only in woman. Trees never look a

day older. The mountains are better off for each million years. Everywhere, everywhere. Bodies mismanaged, malfeasance, gone off. Like styles, like fashions gone off. It's this piecemeal surrender to time, kids. You can't hold on to your baby teeth. Scissors cut paper, paper covers rock, rock smashes scissors. A bite of candy causes tooth decay, and jaw lines that were once firm slip off like shoreline lost to the sea. Noses balloon, amok as a cancer. Bellies swell up and muscles go down. Hips and thighs widen like jodhpurs. My God, children, we look like we're dressed for the horseback! (And everywhere, everywhere, there's this clumsy imbalance. You see these old, sluggish bodies on thin-looking legs, like folks carrying packages piled too high. Or like birds puffed out, skewed, out of sorts with their foundations.) And hair. Hair thins, recedes, is gone. Bodies fall away from true. I don't know. It's as if we've been nickel-and-dimed by the elements: by erosion, by wind and water, by the pull of gravity and the oxidation of the very air. Look! Look there!"

A middle-aged woman in a print dress waited in house slippers for the parade to begin. She was crying. Tears pushed over the ledges of her eyes. A clear mucus filled a corner of one nostril.

A dowager's hump draped a pretty young woman's shoulders and back like a shawl.

They saw the details of a man's face, the stubble, lines, cleft, dimples, and pores, sharp and clarified as close-ups in black-and-white photographs.

Sunglasses in the form of swans, masks, butterflies, or random as the form of costume jewelry. Odd-shaped wigs and hairdos sat on people's heads like a queer gardening, a strange botany. And, everywhere, penciled eyebrows, painted lips, like so many prostheses of the cosmetic.

It had begun now, the parade. A well-dressed man in a business suit stood at attention as the floats passed by. He held his hat over his heart. (And sanity, sanity too, marred, scuffed as a shoe, wrinkled as laundry.) It had begun now, but the children weren't watching. They couldn't take their eyes off the crowd. ("*This, this* is the parade!") They stared at the special area the park had provided for guests in wheelchairs, at the old men and women who sat in them, bundled against some internal chill on even this warm day, wrapped in blankets that tucked over their feet, in sweaters, in scarves, in wool gloves and mittens, covered by hats, by caps, Mickey Mouse's eared beanies, dark as *yarmulkes,* on top of their other headgear; at, among them, an ancient woman in a rubber Frankenstein mask for warmth; at her nurse, feeding her cigarettes, venting her smoke through a gap in the monster's wired jaws. At other women, depleted, tired, who sat on benches, their dresses hiked well above their knees, their legs (in heavy stockings the color of miscegenetic, coffee-creamed flesh) not so much spread as forgotten, separated, guided by the collapsing, melted lines of their thighs. At their husbands (or maybe just the men they lived with, for convenience, for company, for making the welfare checks go farther), their hands in their laps, incurious as people who have just folded in poker. (And *everywhere* those dark glasses. "It ain't for the glare," Colin told them, "it's for the warmth!") At grown men and women wearing the souvenirs of the Magic Kingdom: sweat shirts, T-shirts, with Eeyore, with Mickey Mouse, with Jiminy Cricket, Alice-in-Wonderland pinafores, Minnie Mouse dresses, carryalls with Dumbo and Tigger and Tramp. At a woman in her sixties, inexplicably wearing a boa, a turban, a veil of wide, loose black mesh; at hands and arms and shoulders blotched by liver spots; at a man in baggy pants suspiciously, unscrupulously bulging. At a man in shorts, the enlarged veins on his legs like wax dripping down Chianti bottles in Italian restaurants.

At a woman with oily skin and pores like a sort of goose-flesh, visible as the apertures of chickens where their pinfeathers had been plucked. At a still handsome woman with bare, shapely, but hairy legs (hair even on the tops of her feet), carefully trimmed as sideburns or rolled as stockings two inches below her knee; at a powerfully built man in his sixties whose chest hair, visible through his sheer tank top, had been as lovingly, patiently groomed as a high school boy's. (Everywhere, everywhere hair—the strange feeling they had that they were among birds, the wigs, the boa, the babushka of hair beneath the woman's chin, the piled hairdos, the thinning hair, the penciled eyebrows, the tattooed mustache and sideburns of the strange Westerner. Mudd-Gaddis's own baldness and the chemotherapeutic fuzz of several of the children. Because everything has a reasonable explanation, and almost all had heard that hair didn't stop growing after you died. Because everything has a reasonable explanation and hair was the gnawed, tenuous rope by which they hung on to immortality.)

Everywhere there were peculiar couples. A boy and a girl who couldn't have been more than twelve but looked in their runt intimacy as if they could have been married. The boy held his arm protectively about the girl's shoulder, his free hand in the pocket of his three-quarter-length trench coat as though he fondled a gun. He wore a jacket, a shirt, and a tie. His floods, honed as a knife along their permanent crease, rose above sharp, snazzy shoes. The girl, shorter than her small boyfriend, in a decent wool coat that looked as if it had been bought at a back-to-school sale, smiled wanly. Her black full hair showed signs of gray and she seemed a little nervous, wary, even long-suffering, beneath the arm of her protector, as if she knew his faults, perhaps, his diseases—which weren't diseases in her book—his excessive drinking, his compulsive gambling, his quick fists and rude abuse.

And stared openly at the mismatched couples: at the big, powerful girls next to undersized men and the men large as football players beside bloodless, scrawny women, at the couples widely discrepant in age in open attitudes of love and regard, handholding or clutching butts, the men's fingers casually resting along breasts as if they lolled in water. Or their arms thrown abruptly across each other's shoulders. Sending the smug signals of secret satisfactions, like the wealthy, perhaps, like people in drag.

And at a closely supervised group of the retarded, oddly ageless, the males in overalls, the females in loose, shapeless dresses and rolled stockings, clutching one another with their short fat fingers, their strange, pleased eyes fixed in their happy Smile Faces like raisins in cakes, beaming above their neglected teeth, beaming, beaming beneath their close-cropped hair on their broad, short skulls.

(Yet most were not defective, merely aging or old, or anyway beyond that thirty- or thirty-five-year grace period that seemed to come with most lives.)

Not even needing Colin now to direct their attention, to point things out. In it themselves now, raising their voices, like people outbidding each other in some hot contest, not even listening; or, if listening, then listening for the break in the other's discourse, for that opportune moment when they could have their say, get in their licks; or, if listening, then listening not just for the other to finish but for some generalized cue, some more or less specific tag on which they could build, add, like players of dominoes, say, or card games that followed strict suit. But generally too excited even for that. Only half listening, really, less, fractionally, marginally, seeing how it was with them and concentrating only on the essence, pith, and gist of what they would say, thinking in a sort of deliberate and polite headlines but settling finally into a kind of conversation and still using the language of that other kingdom, the one they'd come from to get to this one.

"Lord love a duck!" said Janet Order. "Just clap eyes on these gaffers."

"My word, Janet! They're for it, I'd say so," Rena Morgan agreed.

"Lamb turning to mutton." Janet sighed.

"Fright fish."

"Blood puddles."

"Lawks!" said Benny Maxine. "Look at the bint with the healthy arse. I'm gone dead nuts on that fanny."

"Ooh, it's walloping big, ain't it?" Tony Word said.

"If it ever let off it wouldn't 'alf make a pongy pooh," Benny asserted.

"Like Billy-O!" Tony said.

"Good gracious me!" said Lydia Conscience. "Say what you will, my heart goes out to the old biddy what looks like someone put her in the pudding club."

"Yar, ain't she dishy? There's one in every village."

Tony Ward considered. "No," he said. "She's just put on the nose bag. It's simply a case of your lumping, right grotty greedguts."

"Only loads of grub then, you think?" Lydia asked.

"Oh, yes," said Tony. "Oodles of inner man. Tub and tuck."

"Jesus weeps!" said illiterate Noah Cloth, looking about, his gaze settling on the little group of the retarded. "He weeps for all the potty, pig-ignorant prats off their chumps, for all the slow-coach clots and dead-from-the-neck-up dimbos, and wonky, puddle coots and gits, goofs and goons, for all his chuckle-headed, loopy muggings and passengers past praying for."

"Put a sock in it, old man," Benny Maxine said softly.

"For all the nanas," Noah said, crying now. "For all the bright specimens."

"Many's the nosh-up gone down that cake hole," Tony Ward said, his eyes fixed on the fat woman Lydia Conscience had thought pregnant. "Many's the porky pots of tram-stopper scoff and thundering stodge through that podge's gob," he said without appetite.

"She's chesty," Rena Morgan said, weeping, of a woman who coughed. "She should put by the gaspers."

"She's had her day," said Janet Order.

"Coo! Who ain't?" Rena, sobbing, wanted to know. "Which of us, hey? Which of them?"

"Are they all on the dream holiday then?" Charles Mudd-Gaddis asked.

"All, old son, and no mistake," Lydia Conscience said wearily.

"A shame," he said. "Letting themselves go like that. And them with their whole lives in front of them."

And, at last, just rudely pointing. (They could have been mutes waving at entrées, aiming at desserts in a cafeteria line.) Whirling, indiscriminate, flailing about in some random *"J'accuse"* of the spontaneous. Whining, wailing, whimpering, weeping.

Because everything has a reasonable explanation. They lived in England's cold climate. They came from a place where clothes made their men and their women. They were unaccustomed to sportswear, to shorts and the casual lightweights and washables of the near tropics. They were unaccustomed, that is, to the actual shapes of people and simply did not know that what they saw was just the ordinary let-hung-out wear and tear of years, of meals, of good times and comforts and all the body's thoughtless kindnesses to itself. So that when Colin said what he said they believed him.

"I tell you," he told them, "that's you in a few years, never mind those three-score-and-ten you thought was your birthright. All that soured flesh, all those bitched and bollixed bodies. You see? You see what you thought you were missing?"

"Bodies," Nedra Carp said. "Don't tell me about bodies. I *know* about bodies."

Source: Elkin, Stanley. 2000. Pp. 218–229 in *The Magic Kingdom*. Normal, IL: Dalkey Archive Press. Copyright © 1985 by Stanley Elkin. Reprinted by permission of Georges Borchardt, Inc.

Australian Disability Advocacy (1980s)

The Disability Services Act of 1986 shapes funding for disability services in Australia. It marks a shift away from charitable, segregated services and toward community-based services aimed at community integration and participation, increased workforce participation, independence, and promoting positive images of persons with disabilities. The entry of "advocacy services" into the program represented a significant triumph for activist groups in the Australian disability scene, which had increased voice after the International Year for Disabled Persons in 1981.

From Disability Services Act of 1986 Part II, Divisions 1 and 7

Advocacy services means:

(a) self advocacy services, namely, services to assist persons with disabilities to develop or maintain

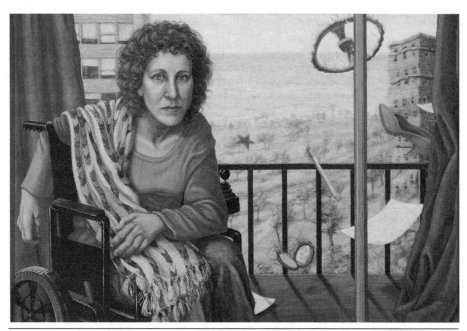

"Circle Story #3: Susan Nussbaum," *by Riva Lehrer. 1998. Acrylic on panel. 16" by 26." Susan Nussbaum is a playwright, actress, director, and disability rights activist. She has starred in, written and/or directed productions at the Goodman, Victory Gardens, and Blue Rider theaters, and other major venues. Her play Mishuganismo is included in Staring Back, and her latest play, No One As Nasty, opened at Chicago's Victory Gardens Theater in 2000. She also teaches pla writing at the Mark Taper Forum in Los Angeles. Nussbaum was injured in a car accident twenty years ago, and she has examined the disability experience with an unsparing, critical wit.*

the personal skills and self confidence necessary to enable them to represent their own interests in the community;

(b) citizen-advocacy services, namely, services to facilitate persons in the community to assist:

(i) persons with disabilities; or

(ii) the families of, and other persons who provide care or assistance, to persons with disabilities; to represent their interests in the community; or group-advocacy services, namely, services to facilitate community organisations to represent the interests of groups of persons with disabilities.

Commentary

Australian disability activist groups were influenced by two main streams of analysis. Physical disability activists, shaped by the disability rights movement emerging from the United Kingdom and the United States, adopted a "social model" of disability. This analysis was taken up by some individuals with intellectual impairment, arguing that with skills and training individuals previously judged incompetent could speak up for themselves. This stream is characterized as

the empowerment model of advocacy.

The other stream emerged from the Syracuse University Training Institute for Human Service Planning, Leadership and Change Agentry. The theory of social devaluation was taken into the model for citizen advocacy. It also influenced many parents, especially those with family members with intellectual or multiple impairments. This stream can be characterized as the social role valorization model. It was this stream that gave the advocacy services section of the Disability Services Act of 1986 its name and configuration—thereby providing great opportunities as well as opening up continuing debates.

The two streams have many points of confluence, especially the centrality of the demand for community life and the dissolution of institutional and congregate services and for the defense of certain rights. However, many contested issues continue to reflect their divergence: the clash between a collectivist rights movement and the incipient individualism of social valorization.

But this can never be the full story. Such a division is too crude. Disability advocacy in Australia has taken on a new spirit of cooperation, building on contributions from community development, enriched by understandings of new social movements. Activists and scholars are expanding the social model of disability with wisdom about relationality, the learnings of seeking normalization, and the critical insights of postmodern thought.

The quest remains—to hold faith with the streams of this history while developing creative theory and practice that can deal with the challenges still faced by many people with impairments.

Source: Disability Services Act of 1986 (Australia). Available at: http://www.comlaw.gov.au/comlaw/Legislation/ActCompilation1 .nsf/0/A92AC1C00AC724E0CA256F71004CD94F/$file/Disability Services1986.pdf

▣ Cheryl Marie Wade, "I Am Not One of The" (1987)

In this work, disabled U.S. poet and performance artist Cheryl Marie Wade celebrates the differences across disabilities that normative culture rejects. In doing so, the poem creates an alternative value system that turns socially imposed "deviance" into a revelation about the persistence of human variation.

I am not one of the physically challenged

I'm a sock in the eye with gnarled fist

I'm a French kiss with cleft tongue

I'm orthopedic shoes sewn on a last of your fears

I am not one of the differently abled

I'm an epitaph for a million imperfect babies left untreated

I'm an ikon carved from bones in a mass grave at Tiergarten, Germany

I'm withered legs hidden with a blanket

I am not one of the able disabled

I'm a black panther with green eyes and scars like a picket fence

I'm pink lace panties teasing a stub of milk white thigh

I'm the Evil Eye

I'm the first cell divided

I'm mud that talks

I'm Eve I'm Kali

I'm The Mountain That Never Moves

I've been forever I'll be here forever

I'm the Gimp

I'm the Cripple

I'm the Crazy Lady

I'm The Woman With Juice

Source: Wade, Cheryl Marie. 1987. "I Am Not One of The." Available at: http://www.disabledandproud.com/prideart.htm. Reprinted by permission.

▣ Sally Zinman, Howie T. Harp, and Su Budd, from *Reaching Across: Mental Health Clients Helping Each Other* (1987)

In this excerpt from this groundbreaking self-help manual for psychiatric survivors, Su Budd explains why client-centered, peer-driven support is a keystone of the psychiatric survivor/user movement.

In a mutual support group, we can develop our own power base. As we reach out horizontally to each other, recipients become providers and vice versa. We can feel a certain independence or distance from the mental health system that empowers us to discern the differences between available services more clearly, and to choose only those services provided by that system, which we find to be beneficial to us. This makes the mental health system more accountable to us and holds it responsible to answer our needs as we define them. Since we are not part of the mental health system, we do not keep medically oriented records, which dehumanize people. We do not need records to provide each other with good support. We do not have to wonder what is being written into our "charts" by others, and we do not have to deal with the feelings that come up with being diagnosed.

Source: Zinman, Sally, Howie T. Harp, and Su Budd, eds. 1987. Ch. 5 in *Reaching Across: Mental Health Clients Helping Each Other.* Sacramento, CA: California Network of Mental Health Clients. Reprinted by permission.

▣ "Position of the Students, Faculty and Staff of Gallaudet University" (1988)

In March 1988, students at Gallaudet University protested the selection of a hearing president out of three candidates—the other two were deaf. The excerpt below lays out the demands of the protestors, which successfully resulted in the hiring of the deaf university's first deaf president.

The appointment of the new president of Gallaudet University has resulted in an OVERWHELMING vote of NO CONFIDENCE in the Board of Trustees!

DEMANDS

1) We demand that the Board of Trustees appoint one of the two deaf finalists as President, Gallaudet University . . . NOW!

2) We demand that Jane Basset Spilman resign from the Board immediately and that a deaf Board Member be elected as chairperson.

3) We demand that the Board [initiate] the process of changing its By-Laws to conform with the C.O.E.D.'s [recommendations] to Congress of a 51% deaf member representation on the Board of Trustees.

4) We demand that no student, staff or faculty member of Gallaudet University be subject to any reprisals as a result of their standing on this matter.

11:30 am, March 7, 1988

Source: President's Council on Deafness. 1988. "Position of the Students, Faculty and Staff of Gallaudet University." Available at: http://pr.gallaudet.edu/dpn/issues/pcddemands.html. Copyright © 1995–2003 Gallaudet University.

▣ Audre Lorde, "A Burst of Light: Living with Cancer" (1988)

Born in New York in 1934 to West Indian parents, Audre Lorde went on to be a teacher and international lecturer. Her book The Cancer Journals *details her efforts to survive breast cancer while also combating the sexism, racism, and able-ism of the medical industry. She refused to separate the struggle for dignity in the wake of her diagnosis from other civil rights agendas, and her writing insightfully dovetails with these political concerns to form a new alignment for collective action.*

If I am to put this all down in a way that is useful, I should start with the beginning of the story.

Sizable tumor in the right lobe of the liver, that's what the doctors said. Lots of blood vessels in it means it's most likely malignant. Let's cut you open right now and see what we can do about it. Wait a minute, I said. I need to feel this thing and see what's going on inside myself first, I said, needing some time to absorb the shock, time to assay the situation and not act out of panic. Not one of them said, I can respect that, but don't take too long about it.

Instead, that simple claim to my body's own process elicited such an attack from a reputable Specialist in Liver Tumors that my deepest—if not necessarily most useful—suspicions were totally aroused.

What a doctor could have said to me that I would have heard was, 'You have a serious condition going on in your body and whatever you do about it you must not ignore it or delay deciding how you are going to deal with it because it will not go away no matter what you think it is.' Acknowledging my own responsibility for my own body. Instead, what he said to me was, 'if you do not do exactly what I tell you to do right now without questions you are going to die a horrible death.' In exactly those words.

I felt the battle lines Danny being drawn up within my own body.

I saw this specialist in liver tumors at a leading cancer hospital in New York City, where I had been referred to as an outpatient by my own doctor.

The first people who interviewed me in white coats from behind a computer were only interested in my health care benefits and proposed method of payment. Those crucial facts determined what kind of plastic ID card I would be given, and without a plastic ID card, no one at all was allowed upstairs to see any doctor, as I was told by the uniformed, pistoled guards at all the stairwells.

From the moment I was ushered into the doctor's office and he saw my x-rays, he proceeded to infantilize me with an obviously well practiced technique. When I told him I was having second thoughts about a liver biopsy, he glanced at my chart. Racism and Sexism joined hands across the table as he saw I taught at a university. 'Well, you look like an *intelligent* girl,' he said, staring at my one breast all the time he was speaking. 'Not to have this biopsy immediately is like sticking your head in the sand.' Then he went on to say that he would not be responsible when I wound up screaming in agony one day in the corner of his office!

I asked this specialist in liver tumors about the dangers of a liver biopsy spreading an existing malignancy, or even encouraging it in a borderline tumor. He dismissed my concerns with a wave of his hand, saying, instead of answering, that I really did not have any other sensible choice.

I would like to think that this doctor was sincerely motivated by a desire to me to seek what he truly believed to be the only remedy for my sickening body, but my faith in that scenario is considerably diminished by his $250 consultation fee and his subsequent report to my own doctor containing numerous supposedly clinical observations of remaining pendulous breast.

In any event, I can thank him for the fierce shard lancing through my terror that shrieked there must be some other way, this doesn't feel right to me. If this is cancer and they cut me open to find out, what is stopping that intrusive action from spreading the cancer, or turning a questionable mass into an active malignancy? All I was asking for was the reassurance of a realistic [answer] to my real questions, and that was not forthcoming. I made up my mind that if I was going to die in agony on someone's office floor, it certainly wasn't going to be his! I needed information, and pored over books on the liver in Barnes & Noble Medical Textbook Section on Fifth Avenue for hours. I learned, among other things, that the liver is the largest, most complex, and most generous organ in the human body. But that did not help me very much.

In this period of physical weakness and psychic turmoil, I found myself going through an intricate inventory of rage. First of all at my breast surgeon—had he perhaps done something wrong? How could such a small breast tumor have metastasized? Hadn't he assured me he'd gotten it all, and what was this now anyway about micro-metastases? Could this tumor in my liver have been seeded at the same time as my breast cancer? There were so many unanswered questions, and too much that I just did not understand.

But my worst rage was the rage at myself. For a brief time I felt like a total failure. What had I been busting my ass doing these past six years if it wasn't living and loving and working to my utmost potential? And wasn't that all a guarantee supposed to keep exactly this kind of thing from ever happening again. So what had I done wrong and what was I going to have pay for it? Why Me?

But finally a little voice inside me said sharply 'Now really, is there any other way you would have preferred living the past six years that would have been any more satisfying? And be that as it may, *should* or *shouldn't* isn't even the question. How do you want to live the rest of your life from now on and what are you going to do about it?' Time's awasting!

Gradually, in those hours in the stacks of Barnes & Noble, I felt myself shifting into another gear. My resolve strengthened as my panic lessened. Deep breathing regularly. I'm not going to let them cut into body again until I'm convinced that there's no other alternative. And this time, the burden of proof rests with the doctors because their record of success with liver cancer is not so good that it would make me jump at a surgical solution. And scare tactics are not going to work. I have been scared for six years and that hasn't stopped me. I've given myself

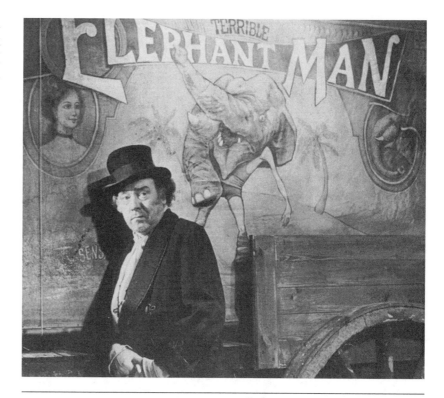

Elephant Man *tells the extraordinarily moving tale of the unfortunate Joseph Merrick, born with a rare disease, who was taken from the world of the freak show to the pinnacle of Victorian society.*

Source: *Elephant Man* (1980), directed by David Lynch. United Kingdom. B&W, 124 minutes. Reprinted by permission of Paul Darke.

plenty of practice in doing whatever I need to do, scared or not, so scare tactics are just not going to work. Or I hoped they were not going to work. At any rate, thank the goodness, they were not working yet. One step at a time.

But some of my nightmares were pure hell, and I started having trouble sleeping.

In writing this I have discovered how important some things are that I thought were unimportant. I discovered this by the high price they exact for scrutiny. At first I did not want to look again at how slowly I came to terms with my own mortality on a deeper level than before. Medical textbooks on the liver were fine, but there were appointments to be kept, and bills to pay, and decisions about the upcoming trip to Europe to be made. And what do I say to my children. Honesty has always been the bottom line between us, but did I really need them going through this with me during their final, difficult years at college? On the other hand, how could I shut them out of the most important decision of my life?

I made a visit to my breast surgeon, a doctor with whom I have always been able to talk frankly, and it was

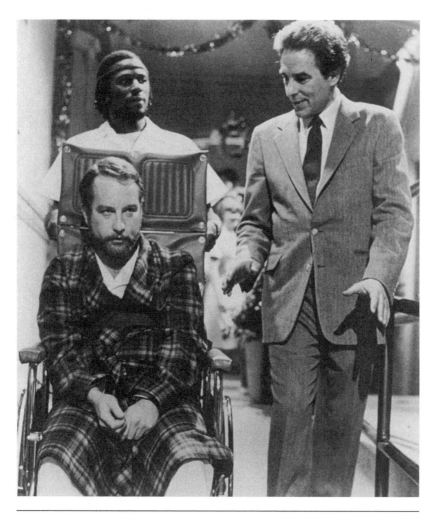

In Whose Life Is It Anyway?, *a wisecracking sculptor, paralyzed from the neck down after a car crash, struggles for his right to die.*

Source: *Whose Life Is It Anyway?* (1981), directed by John Badham. United States. Color, 118 minutes. Reprinted by permission of Paul Darke.

from him that I got my first trustworthy and objective sense of timing. It was from him that I learned that the conventional forms of treatment for liver metastases made little more than one year's difference in the survival rate. I heard my old friend Clem's voice coming back to me through the dimness of thirty years: 'I see you coming here trying to make sense where there is no sense. Just try living in it. Respond, alter, see what happens.' I thought of the African way of perceiving life, as experience to be lived rather than as problem to be solved.

Homeopathic medicine calls cancer the cold disease. I understand that down to my bones that quake sometimes in their need for heat, for the sun, even for just a hot bath. Part of the way in which I am saving my own life is to refuse to submit my body to cold whenever possible.

In general, I fight hard to keep my treatment scene together in some coherent and serviceable way, integrated into my daily living and absolute. Forgetting is no excuse. It's as simple as one missed shot could make the difference between a quiescent malignancy and one that is growing again. This not only keeps me in an intimate, positive relationship to my own health, but it also underlies the responsibility for attending to my own health. I cannot simply hand over that responsibility to anyone else.

Which does not mean I give into the belief, arrogant or naïve, that I know everything I need to know in order to make informed decisions about my body. But attending to my own health, gaining enough information to help me understand and participate in the decisions made about my body by people who know more medicine than do I, are all crucial strategies in my battle for living. They also provide me with important prototypes for doing battle in all other areas of my life.

Battling racism and battling sexism and battling apartheid share the same urgency inside me as battling cancer. None of these struggles are ever easy, and even the smallest victory is never to be taken for granted. Each victory must be applauded, because it is so easy not to battle at all, to just accept and call that acceptance inevitable.

And all power is relative. Recognizing the existence as well as the limitations of my own power, and accepting the responsibility for using it in my own behalf, involve me in direct and daily actions that preclude denial as a possible refuge. Simone de Beauvoir's words echo in my head: 'It is in the recognition of the genuine conditions of our lives that we gain the strength to act and our motivation for change.'

Source: Lorde, Audre. 1999. "A Burst of Light: Living with Cancer." In Price, Janet, and Margaret Shildrick, eds. *Feminism and the Body.* New York: Routledge. (Originally published 1988)

Michelle Cliff, "If I Could Write This in Fire, I Would Write This in Fire" (1988)

In this passage, the Jamaican American writer Michelle Cliff describes how race and disability conjoin in the minds of English and American missionaries during a girl's experience of a grand mal seizure.

Some of the girls were out-and-out-white (English and American), the rest us were colored—only a few were dark. Our uniforms were blood-red Gabardine, heavy and hot in buildings meant to re-create England; damp with stone floors, facing onto a cloister, or quad as they called it. We began each day with the headmistress leading us in English hymns. The entire school stood for an hour in the zinc-roofed Gymnasium.

Occasionally a girl fainted, or threw up. Once, a girl had a grand mal seizure. To any such disturbance the response was always "keep singing." While she flailed on the stone floor, I wondered what the mistress would do. We sang "Faith of our Fathers," and watched our classmate as her eyes rolled back in her head. I thought of people swallowing their tongues. This student was dark—here on a scholarship—and the only woman who came forward to help her was the gamesmistress, the only dark teacher. She kneeled beside the girl and slid the white webbed belt from her tennis shorts, clamping it between the girl's teeth. When the seizure was over, she carried the girl to a tumbling mat in a corner of the gym and covered her so she wouldn't get chilled.

Were the other women unable to touch the girl because of her darkness? I think that now. Her darkness and her scholarship. She lived on Windward Road with her grandmother; her mother was a maid. But darkness is usually enough for women like those to hold back. Then, we usually excused that kind of behavior by saying they were "ladies" (we were constantly being told that we should be ladies also. One teacher went so far as to tell us many people thought Jamaicans lived in trees and we had to show these people they were mistaken). In short, we felt insufficient to judge the behavior of these women. The English ones (who had the corner on power in the school) had come all this way to teach us. Shouldn't we treat them as missionaries they were certain they were?

The Creole Jamaicans had a different role; they were passing on those of us who were light-skinned the Creole heritage of collaboration, assimilation, loyalty to our betters. We were expected to be willing subjects in this outpost of civilization.

The girl left school that day and never returned.

Source: Cliff, Michelle. 1988. "If I Could Write This in Fire, I Would Write This in Fire." Pp. 66–67 in Simonson, Richard, and Scott Walker, eds. *Multicultural Literacy.* St. Paul, MN: Greywolf.

Katherine Dunn, from *Geek Love* (1989)

In these excerpts from Dunn's fantasy novel, the bald, albino, hunchbacked, female narrator, Olympia, describes her status in a disabled family that purposefully breeds "human oddities" for their freak show exhibition. The second passage details the loss of anonymity often experienced by disabled people in public settings.

I was born three years after my sisters. My father spared no expense in these experiments. My mother had been liberally dosed with cocaine, amphetamines, and arsenic during her ovulation and throughout her pregnancy with me. It was a disappointment when I emerged with such commonplace deformities. My albinism is the regular pink-eyed variety and my hump, though pronounced, is not remarkable in size or shape as humps go. My situation was far too humdrum to be marketable on the same scale as my brother's and sisters.' Still, my parents noted that I had a strong voice and decided I might be an appropriate shill and talker for the business. A bald albino hunchback seemed the right enticement toward the esoteric talents of the rest of the family. The dwarfism, which was very apparent by my third birthday, came as a pleasant surprise to the patient pair and increased my value. From the beginning I slept in the built-in cupboard beneath the sink in the family living van, and had a collection of exotic sunglasses to shield my sensitive eyes. (P. 8)

She talks. People talk easily to me. They think a bald albino hunchback dwarf can't hide anything. My worst is all out in the open. It makes it necessary for people to tell you about themselves. They begin out of simple courtesy. Just being visible is my biggest confession, so they try to set me at ease by revealing our equality, by dragging out their own less-apparent deformities. That's how it starts. But I am like a stranger on the bus and they get hooked on having a listener. They go too far because I am one listener who is in no position to judge or find fault. They stretch out their dampest secrets because a creature like me has no virtues or morals. If I am "good" (and they assume that I am), it's obviously for lack of opportunity to be otherwise. And I listen. I listen eagerly, warmly, because I care. They tell me everything eventually. (P. 156)

My tall stool was cutting off blood to my legs and I squirmed and craned my neck. Arty was turned away from me, watching McGurk, who slumped down and sat on the bed. "I'll show you the lubrication and drainage system, but . . ." He hiked at his trousers until both knees were bare, white and hairless. The shoes came up his shins and turned into grey socks. "But I guess you want my credentials," McGurk said. He reached up his right pant leg. There was a snap and the shoe toppled over with the plastic shin and knee sticking out of it. A dim gleam came from the dark fold of the empty trouser leg. He slid his hand up the other trouser leg and both legs lay on the floor with steel shining out of the hollow tops of the knees. He pulled his pant legs up his thighs and showed the steel caps on the stumps. There were a groove, a few grip protrusions, and a number of electrical contact points protruding from each unit. He looked up, calmly waiting. (P. 169)

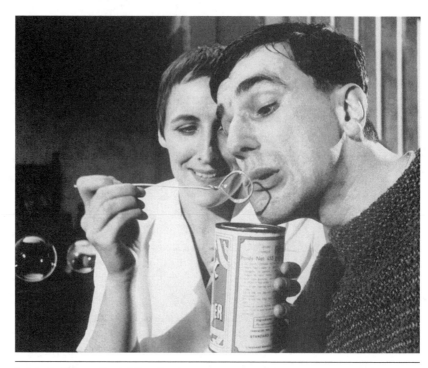

In My Left Foot, *Daniel Day-Lewis re-creates the Irish painter/writer Christy Brown with extraordinarily matter-of-fact detail and precision. Brown emerges not just as a victim of cerebral palsy but as a complex and often vexing character.*
Source: *My Left Foot* (1989), directed by Jim Sheridan. United Kingdom. Color, 103 minutes. Reprinted by permission of Paul Darke.

Source: Dunn, Katherine. 1989. *Geek Love.* New York: Knopf. Copyright © 1989 by Katherine Dunn. Used by permission of Alfred A. Knopf, a division of Random House, Inc.

▣ From the Americans with Disabilities Act of 1990 (United States)

Building on the landmark protections established in Section 504 of the Rehabilitation Act (see entry above), the Americans with Disabilities Act codified the definition of disability beneath three sweeping categories: (a) incapacity in at least one major life function, (b) an established history of such an impairment, or (c) a belief that one has such an impairment. While the first two designations continued a long tradition of medical pathology as a key qualifying category, the third definition established the social basis of disability. The Act further established disability as involving a class of individuals protected under the law against discrimination in employment, education, public access, and so forth. Most legal analysts are in agreement that, since its passage, its protections have been significantly eroded by conservative U.S. judiciary forces that have ruled in favor of businesses and other public institutions seeking to protect their monetary interests.

Sec. 2. Findings and Purposes

(a) Findings.—The Congress finds that—

(1) some 43,000,000 Americans have one or more physical or mental disabilities, and this number is increasing as the population as a whole is growing older;

(2) historically, society has tended to isolate and segregate individuals with disabilities, and, despite some improvements, such forms of discrimination against

individuals with disabilities continue to be a serious and pervasive social problem;

(3) discrimination against individuals with disabilities persists in such critical areas as employment, housing, public accommodations, education, transportation, communication, recreation, institutionalization, health services, voting, and access to public services;

(4) unlike individuals who have experienced discrimination on the basis of race, color, sex, national origin, religion, or age, individuals who have experienced discrimination on the basis of disability have often had no legal recourse to redress such discrimination;

(5) individuals with disabilities continually encounter various forms of discrimination, including outright intentional exclusion, the discriminatory effects of architectural, transportation, and communication barriers, overprotective rules and policies, failure to make modifications to existing facilities and practices, exclusionary qualification standards and criteria, segregation, and relegation to lesser services, programs, activities, benefits, jobs, or other opportunities;

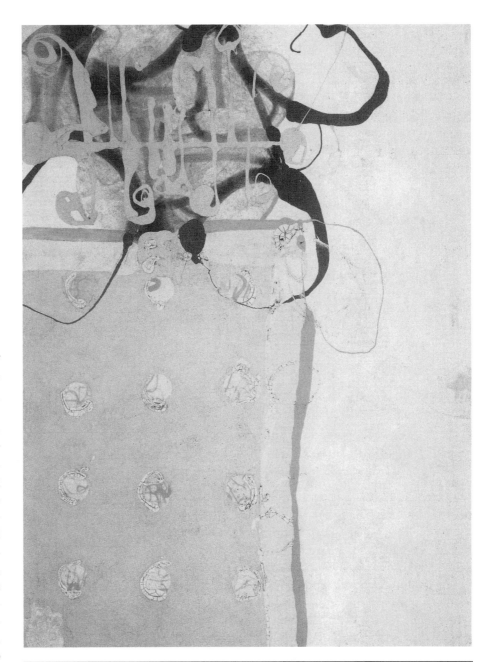

"Fidelity," by Katherine Sherwood. 2000. Mixed media on paper. An artist with a visual impairment, Sherwood works with abstract imagery that comments on ways of seeing and perceiving the world.

(6) census data, national polls, and other studies have documented that people with disabilities, as a group, occupy an inferior status in our society, and are severely disadvantaged socially, vocationally, economically, and educationally;

(7) individuals with disabilities are a discrete and insular minority who have been faced with restrictions and limitations, subjected to a history of purposeful unequal treatment, and relegated to a position of political powerlessness in our society, based on characteristics that are beyond the control of such individuals and resulting from stereotypic assumptions not truly indicative of the individual ability of such individuals to participate in, and contribute to, society;

(8) the Nation's proper goals regarding individuals with disabilities are to assure equality of opportunity, full participation, independent living, and economic self-sufficiency for such individuals; and

(9) the continuing existence of unfair and unnecessary discrimination and prejudice denies people with disabilities the opportunity to compete on an equal basis and to pursue those opportunities for which our free society is justifiably famous, and costs the United States billions of dollars in unnecessary expenses resulting from dependency and nonproductivity.

(b) Purpose.—It is the purpose of this Act—

(1) to provide a clear and comprehensive national mandate for the elimination of discrimination against individuals with disabilities;

(2) to provide clear, strong, consistent, enforceable standards addressing discrimination against individuals with disabilities;

(3) to ensure that the Federal Government plays a central role in enforcing the standards established in this Act on behalf of individuals with disabilities; and

(4) to invoke the sweep of congressional authority, including the power to enforce the fourteenth amendment and to regulate commerce, in order to address the major areas of discrimination faced day-to-day by people with disabilities.

Sec. 3. Definitions

As used in this Act:

(1) Auxiliary aids and services.—The term "auxiliary aids and services" includes—

(A) qualified interpreters or other effective methods of making aurally delivered materials available to individuals with hearing impairments;

(B) qualified readers, taped texts, or other effective methods of making visually delivered materials available to individuals with visual impairments;

(C) acquisition or modification of equipment or devices; and

(D) other similar services and actions.

(2) Disability.—The term "disability" means, with respect to an individual—

(A) a physical or mental impairment that substantially limits one or more of the major life activities of such individual;

(B) a record of such an impairment; or

(C) being regarded as having such an impairment.

(3) State.—The term "State" means each of the several States, the District of Columbia, the Commonwealth of Puerto Rico, Guam, American Samoa, the Virgin Islands, the Trust Territory of the Pacific Islands, and the Commonwealth of the Northern Mariana Islands.

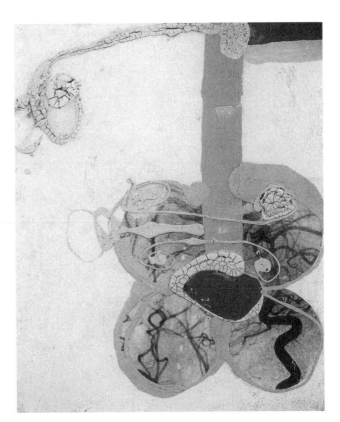

"Fidelity II," by Katherine Sherwood. 2000. Mixed media on canvas. An artist with a visual impairment, Sherwood works with abstract imagery that comments on ways of seeing and perceiving the world.

▣ Law on the Protection of Disabled Persons of 1990 (China)

The Law of the People's Republic of China on the Protection of Disabled Persons was passed at the 17th Meeting of the Standing Committee of the Seventh National People's Congress on December 28, 1990, and was implemented on May 15, 1991. This is a significant and landmark legal document, because it is the first disability law to safeguard the legal rights and interests of disabled people since the founding of the People's Republic of China. Although many terms in the law are too general to implement in practice, it does mark the beginning of a recognition of basic human rights of this much-neglected group of people in China.

Article 1 [Purpose and Basis]

This Law is formulated in accordance with the Constitution for the purpose of protecting the lawful rights and interests of, and developing undertakings for disabled persons, and ensuring their equal and full

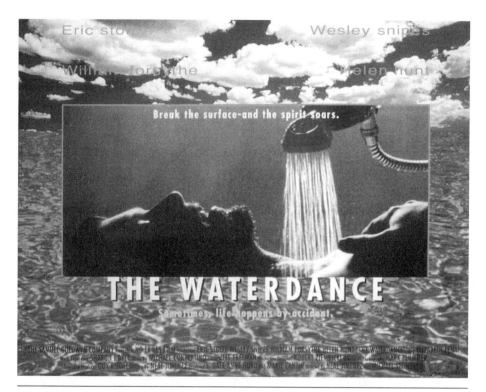

The Waterdance *is an important film about author Joel Garcia's efforts to adjust to his paralysis after a hiking accident. The story delves into the hassles and humiliations of life in a rehabilitation center, including the tensions that erupt between disabled residents.*

Source: *The Waterdance* (1992), directed by Neil Jimenez and Michael Steinberg. United States. Color, 106 minutes. Reprinted by permission of Paul Darke.

participation in social life and their share of the material and cultural wealth of society.

Article 2 [Definition, Categories and Criteria]

A disabled person refers to one who suffers from abnormalities or loss of a certain organ or function, psychologically or physiologically, or in anatomical structure and has lost wholly or in part the ability to perform an activity in the way considered normal.

The term "disabled persons" refers to those with visual, hearing, speech or physical disabilities, mental retardation, mental disorder, multiple disabilities and/or other disabilities.

The criteria for classification of disabilities shall be established by the State Council.

Article 3 [Protection of Rights]

Disabled persons shall enjoy equal rights with other citizens in political, economic, cultural and social fields, in family life and other aspects. The citizen's rights and personal dignity of disabled persons shall be protected by law.

Discrimination against, insult of and infringement upon disabled persons shall be prohibited.

Article 4 [Special Assistance]

The state shall provide disabled persons with special assistance by adopting supplementary methods and supportive measures with a view to alleviating or eliminating the effects of their disabilities and external barriers and ensuring the realization of their rights.

Article 5 [Special Assurance]

The state and society shall provide special assurance, preferential treatment and pension for wounded or disabled servicemen and persons disabled while on duty or for protecting the interests of the state and people.

Article 6 [Responsibilities of Government]

The people's governments at all levels shall incorporate undertakings for disabled persons into plans for economic and social development through budget arrangement, overall planning and coordination and other measures under strengthened leadership with a view to ensuring that undertakings for disabled persons develop in coordination with economic and social progress.

The State Council and the people's governments of provinces, autonomous regions and municipalities directly under the Central Government shall adopt organizational measures to coordinate departments concerned in the work for people with disabilities. The establishment of specific institutions shall be decided upon by the State Council and/or the people's governments of provinces, autonomous regions and municipalities directly under the Central Government.

Departments concerned under the people's governments at various levels shall keep in close contact with disabled persons, solicit their opinions and fulfill respectively their own duties in the work for disabled persons.

Article 7 [Responsibilities of the Society]

The whole society should display socialist humanitarianism, understand, respect, care for and assist people with disabilities and support the work for disabled persons.

State organs, non-governmental organizations, enterprises, institutions and urban and rural organizations at grassroots level should do their work for disabled persons well, as is within their responsibility.

State functionaries and other personnel engaged in the work for disabled persons should work hard to fulfill their lofty duties in serving disabled people.

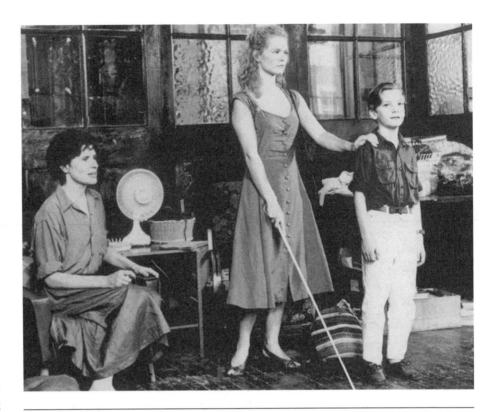

In Afraid of the Dark, *an 11-year-old boy with a blind mother worries about the identity of the psychopath who is attacking blind women and begins to suspect those around him.*

Source: *Afraid of the Dark* (1992), directed by Mark Peploe. United Kingdom/France. Color, 91 minutes. Reprinted by permission of Paul Darke.

Article 8 [Responsibilities of Disabled Persons' Federation]

China Disabled Persons' Federation (CDPF) and its local branches shall represent the common interests of disabled persons, protect their lawful rights and interests, unite, educate disabled persons, and provide service for disabled persons.

CDPF shall undertake tasks entrusted by the government, conduct work for disabled persons and mobilize social forces in developing undertakings for disabled persons.

Article 9 [Responsibilities of Fosterer, Guardian and Family Member]

Legal fosterers of disabled persons must fulfill their duties towards their charges.

Guardians of disabled persons must fulfill their duties of guardianship and protect the lawful rights and interests of their charges.

Family members and guardians of disabled persons should encourage and assist disabled persons to enhance their capability of self-reliance.

Maltreatment and abandoning of disabled persons shall be prohibited.

Article 10 [Obligations of Disabled Persons]

Disabled persons must abide by laws, carry out their due obligations, observe public order and respect social morality.

Disabled persons should display an optimistic, and enterprising spirit, have a sense of self-respect, self-confidence, self-strength and self-reliance, and make contributions to the socialist construction.

Article 11 [Prevention of Disabilities]

The state shall undertake, in a planned way, the work of disability prevention, strengthen leadership in this regard, publicize and popularize knowledge of good pre-natal and post-natal care as well as disability prevention, formulate laws and regulations dealing with disability causing factors such heredity, diseases, medical poisoning, accidents, calamity and environmental pollution and adopt measures to prevent the occurrence and aggravation of disabilities by organizing and mobilizing social forces.

Article 12 [Award]

Governments and departments concerned shall award those disabled persons who have made notable achievements in socialist construction and those units or individuals who have made remarkable contributions to safeguarding the lawful rights and interests of disabled people, promoting undertakings and providing service for disabled persons.

Source: Law of the People's Republic of China on the Protection of Disabled Persons. 1990. Available at: http://www.apcdproject .org/trainings/web-based/pant_homepages/jiang/laws.html

▣ Walt Stromer on the Functional Brutality of Military Medicine (1990)

Dealing with large numbers of often desperately injured or chronically ill men and believing in the program of aggressive normalization, military doctors were known to spare few feelings in informing men that their disabilities were permanent and that they needed to begin to adjust to them immediately, without self-pity or self-deception. While this often caused great resentment, it also served for many as a stimulus to make the necessary adjustments to new circumstances. Walt Stromer, long a member of the Blinded Veterans Association, went on to become a Professor of Speech at Cornell College in Iowa, where he was on the faculty for 32 years before retiring.

The View From Here

Editor's Note: Walt Stromer, guest columnist for this issue, lives in Mt. Vernon, Iowa. He is retired from Cornell College, where he taught speech for 32 years. Now he reaches adult education classes in other subjects he likes, and goes to the library a lot.

A Letter Too Late
By Walt Stromer

It was March 1945, and we were headed home on the Queen Mary. We sailed at 23 knots, zigzagging for fear of torpedoes. There were more than three thousand survivors aboard, wounded and disabled of the great crusade. Going home to cold drinks, hot dogs and assorted miracles.

A month later at Dibble General Hospital in California, no one had talked to me about miracles, so I made an appointment to see Lt. Fritchie, the ward officer. At ten the next morning, I knocked on his door. He opened it saying, "There's a chair straight ahead of you—sit down." He rustled through papers for a few seconds. Then he said, "I've looked through your files. I guess you know your case is hopeless. You'll never see again. Any questions?" After a few seconds, I said, "No." He said, "All right," and opened the door.

I walked out and closed the door. I didn't slam it. Lying back in my bunk, I don't remember all the thoughts, but suicide did come to mind. In about fifteen minutes, someone yelled, "Chow," which changed my thinking for the moment.

Before that morning I had just disliked Lt. Fritchie. After that I hated him. But a strange thing happened. I began to think about it from his position. He had to give that same terrible news to several hundred young men . . . news that could tear a man apart. Also some of us needed to be told to stop wishing and dreaming and to get on with living and the business of rehabilitation.

Five years later, I wrote to the Lieutenant to tell him I understood why he had been so brusque. His wife wrote back to say he had died two years earlier of cancer.

Sorry, sir.

Source: Stromer, Walt. 1990. "A Letter Too Late." *The BVA Bulletin* 45(July–August):8. Printed with permission of the Blinded Veterans Association.

▣ World Federation of Psychiatric Users, Minutes of the First Committee Meeting (1991)

The first organizational committee meeting for the World Federation of Psychiatric Users was held in Mexico City on August 23, 1991. Representatives included those from the United States, Mexico, Japan, Netherlands, and New Zealand.

Mexico City, 23 August 1991

Present: Jan Dirk van Abshoven (Netherlands), Paolo del Vecchio (USA), Bob Long (USA)—replacing Esperanza Isaac, Mary O'Hagan (New Zealand), Pauline Hinds (New Zealand), Natosughi (Japan), Masaji Koganezawa (Japan) Adriana Lopez (Mexico)

Agenda

1. Meeting rules
2. Name for organisation
3. Priority tasks
4. Who will do what and when

1. Meeting Style and Voting Rules

Mary began by stating the need for cooperation. She said the meeting would run by consensus but there will be a vote for some agenda items. There will be no formal 'rules of order.' Each country represented will have one vote.

2. Name

There was some discussion about what term to call ourselves by. Survivor, client, inmate, psychiatrically labelled, purchaser and ex-patient were rejected. Opinion was divided between "user" and "consumer." The USA favoured "consumer." Mexico, New Zealand, Japan and the Netherlands favoured "user."

The following suggestions for the name of the organisation were put to the vote.

- World Federation of Mental Health Users Holland
- World Federation of Psychiatric Users Mexico, NZ
- International Federation of Psychiatric Survivors
- Worldwide Congress of MH Consumers
- Worldwide Network of Psych Users Japan
- World Union of Mental Health Consumers USA

The name of the organisation is:
World Federation of Psychiatric Users

3. Prioritising Tasks for the Next Two Years

The following tasks were developed before the meeting. Each country voted on what they thought should be the top three priorities for the next two years.

1. Network and inform users and user groups of the WFPU and increase membership. Produce and distribute a newsletter.
2. Hold international teleconferences

3. Produce and distribute discussion papers to users, professionals etc on the following issues:

- ECT
- Neuroleptics
- third world issues
- self-help / self-advocacy
- psychiatric labelling
- international bill of rights

4. Unified and coordinated response to any major rights violations that occur
5. Administrative tasks:

- fundraising
- yearly lists and censuses
- information storage
- coordination of tasks
- development of rules
- correspondence
- logo / letterhead
- committee meetings
- pamphlets

6. Continue user contact with WFMH and encourage users to go to Tokyo and to organise a user only conference before or after the World Congress for Mental Health, in Tokyo in 1993.

All countries voted for 1, 5 and 6 as priorities for the next two years.

- Newsletter / Networking / Membership
- Administrative tasks
- Contact with WFMH / Users to Tokyo

The non-priority tasks could still be done if there was time and energy for it.

4. Details on Priority Tasks

Many of the details decided on about the priority tasks are in the WFPU Plan (enclosed) which allocates who will do what and by when. Discussion not included in the Plan follows.

Newsletter

The newsletter will be free. It will be published every 6 months.

Membership

Membership shall be US $5.00 but users will have the option of paying no fee if they cannot afford it.

Administration

New Zealand will provide the office and administrative tasks for WFPU for the next two years.

Funding

There was a wide ranging discussion on ways to get funding. People felt it would be unethical to get sponsorship from drug companies. Funding will be needed for a pamphlet on WFPU. The Japanese could be approached for funding for user travel/conference to Tokyo. Fifty percent of funding should go to groups in originating country once WFPU is well-established.
MEETING ENDS

Source: World Federation of Psychiatric Users. 1991. *First Committee Meeting*. Available at: http://www.wnusp.org/wnusp%20evas/Dokumenter/mexico1991.html. Reprinted by permission.

▣ Robert Brown and Hope Schutte, from *Our Fight: A Battle against Darkness* (1991)

A wealthy nation, fortunate to have never suffered the humiliation of total defeat, surrender, and occupation, the United States nonetheless has seen many of the same general problems in administering benefits and programs of assistance for disabled veterans that we see in defeated nations, such as Germany after the world wars. The history of American disabled veterans' organizations, especially at the level of the national office, has often been a struggle against bureaucratic lethargy, incompetence, and insensitivity. As this selection makes clear, the Blinded Veterans Association, which was founded by 100 blinded veterans of World War II then undertaking mobility and orientation training at an Army facility in Connecticut, has a long history of representing a wide variety of visually impaired veterans in their struggles with the bureaucracies in charge of overseeing programs relevant to its members' interests.

There is a special room on the first floor of the Blinded Veterans Association national headquarters building in Washington, D.C. It's where we keep our files, the records of all the men and women who, over nearly the past 46 years, have come to us for help.

Well, it isn't really a room—just an area walled off by an arrangement of room dividers, room dividers obscured by long rows of gray, brown, and green filing cabinets. Many of the cabinets are quite old and beat up. Yet they contain the names and experiences of men and women, thousands of blinded veterans who have been a part of BVA.

They tell stories, true stories, of the individual struggles of veterans blinded in combat, or though accident or disease, to regain their dignity and independence—stories of sacrifice and courage, of suffering and damaged lives and disappointment. Theirs is an accounting, a history of the desperation, and the hopes and dreams of thousands of American veterans who lost their sight.

And the file cabinets contain the story of the early days of the Blinded Veterans Association, the joyous successes and disappointing failures, the work accomplished and the work left undone by our early founders—a group of dedicated, determined young blinded veterans pulling together to do all they could to help their comrades so that they, too, might reclaim the basic rights of any human—dignity and independence.

One evening after all the other office staff had left for home, and feeling somewhat tired after a day of "working the phones," I stopped by the file room. I had some time to spend until I could get a ride home so I started opening some of the older cabinets and thumbing through the files I found there.

The file folders themselves are all different sizes and colors. Some, dating back to BVA's beginnings in the mid-1940s, are yellowed with age and have that dusty, old paper odor. Yet whether from World War II or the present time, each folder contains the personal history of a blinded veteran who has asked BVA for help.

Most of them contain letters, frequently laboriously hand written by the blinded servicemen themselves. These are quite difficult to read. Others are typewritten and frequently full of typing errors made by veterans struggling to communicate the best they could.

Usually, there are also military service records, medical records, and letters from doctors chronicling what had happened to the veteran, i.e., explaining the source of his blindness and other injuries, if he has them. There are copies of applications to the Veterans Administration for whatever benefits were needed and available copies of completed forms for compensation of injuries, educational and vocational training programs, and prosthetic equipment; and copies of job applications and resumes. The records of the men and women in the files come from every branch of service. Folder after folder, the lives of the blinded veterans who have come to BVA for help.

I continued pulling files and reviewing the old records, although with some hesitation, with a feeling that I was unearthing old troubles and sufferings long laid to rest and, probably, best left as they were. With a sense that there might be more in the old folders than I wanted to know about right then, because I had worked on veterans cases all that day and some of the blinded veterans who come to BVA asking for help have problems so daunting, so intractable that each and every one of us here has questioned our own ability and competence. We frequently wonder and worry: Did we do enough? Could we have done more? Perhaps done a better job? Did we try hard enough?

But my curiosity overcame my hesitation and I continued looking back in the early days, in 1946 and 1947, just after World War II had ended and just after BVA was organized, our headquarters office was located in New York City. We didn't have much to offer then—no Field Service Program, no Service Officers, no board of Veterans Appeals Claims Representative. Not much but togetherness.

Still, it was obvious that the early BVA staff did an excellent job. And the value of blinded veterans helping other blinded veterans was also apparent because our early workers took a realistic, down-to-earth approach, accepting the fact of their blindness and building upon what was left. They were good advice to their fellow blinded veterans; and they were tough, pushing and prodding much needed changes through the frequently unyielding Veterans Administration bureaucracy.

In many ways, these files are almost a chronology of America's wars in the Twentieth Century: World War II; Korea; Vietnam; and even the "cold war" in Europe, the Mid-East and the Pacific. There are even folders on blinded veterans from World War I, the folders of blinded servicemen who came to BVA for help after we were formed.

The files showed me that the injuries of the men blinded in Korea were much the same as those of the men blinded in World War II: bullet wounds to the head, grenade fragments in the eyes, artillery bursts, land mines, burns, airplane crashes. All the horrible aspects of war.

A large number of files show an initial date of contact with the BVA as the late 1960s and early 1970s. The awful consequences of the Vietnam War: men and women, most in their forties now, many of whom are still struggling to build a life for themselves. Soldiers, marines and airmen whose eyes were blasted or burned away by rocket propelled grenades, or

"RPGs" as the men called them; or by AK-47s; or in the fires of downed airplanes or helicopters. And land mines, land mines, land mines—dirt and stones and metal fragments blasted into faces and eyes. Records on men and women blinded in exploding ammunition dumps; blinded in vehicle crashes; blinded by artillery malfunctions. And although we haven't reached as many of these veterans as we'd like to, or been able to do all that we know needs doing, we at BVA are still trying to help them as much as we possibly can.

Then, there are folders with more recent dates, too, because each year a substantial number of servicemen go blind whether or not there is a war in progress: servicemen who are blinded in accidents or by disease while on active duty; those who go blind after leaving service; or servicemen manifesting age-related diseases which cause blindness. In fact, many of the files dated 1980 and up belong to veterans of World War II, Korea, and the long years of the cold war and show a real change in the origins of blindness—Diabetes, Glaucoma, Macular Degeneration, Retinitis Pigmentosa, Multiple Sclerosis, Optic Atrophy—diseases with strange names that usually do not strike until later in life, yet with devastating impact. They all destroy precious sight.

To me, on that late night, I realized that the files at BVA speak not only of war, of suffering, but of bravery and courage and sacrifice, of the meaning of service and the price of freedom. And I believe they also speak of fellowship. Because we at BVA are all blinded veterans—whether we served during war or peacetime; were blinded in combat or in an accident; lost our sight to disease while in service or many years later. And we are all bound together by our love of country and our desire for a peaceful world. We do our best to serve and help one another without regard to race, creed, sex, religion or political affiliation.

To receive our assistance, you need only be a veteran and be "legally blind." Currently, the standard definition of legal blindness is: "best corrected vision in the better eye of no more than 20/200 or a visual field of no more than 20 percent in the better eye."

Since World War II, America's blinded veterans have encountered many frustrations in their dealings with the Veterans Administration. Continual turnover in Veterans Administration Regional Office . . . staff; lack of training about the special needs of blinded veterans; indifference caused by heavy workloads; difficulties with communicating and implementing updated benefit rulings; and a pervasive ignorance about the causes of blindness and its actual—as opposed to imagined—limitations have all resulted in inequities in the VA's treatment of blinded soldiers. Unfortunately, many of these inequities are still prevalent today. For example, up until 1972 blinded veterans who had suffered anatomical loss of both eyes usually received much larger VA disability compensation awards than those veterans who were equally sightless but whose eyes had not been enucleated.

And because one of the most serious problems facing nearly all blinded veterans is not having enough money to meet even the most basic of their living expenses, the matter of compensation or pensions has become an overriding issue.

It is, in fact, along with our personal advocacy of blind rehabilitation for nearly all blinded veterans, the most prevalent issue involved with the blinded veterans we try to help and, therefore, occupies a great deal of our time.

The issue is a complex one. Originally disability compensation was awarded for injuries sustained during battle. It was conceived as unrelated to economic need: the Military Service or the Veterans Administration was simply "compensating" the veteran for his blindness or other injuries incurred in combat as a means for insuring that his future standard of living would not be affected by his diminished earning capacity. The amount, or rate, of service-connected compensation was to be proportionately related to the severity of his disability or loss. Basically, this is the system still in effect today.

Therefore, in most cases, veterans blinded while on active duty through either disease or injury, and through no fault of their own, are subsequently compensated for their loss. Additionally, veterans whose "aggravation" of blindness can be proven—that is, if a veteran has a certain disease affecting vision, for example Multiple Sclerosis, which manifests itself following active duty and, if the disease follows an abnormally rapid progression which can be presumed to be a consequence of the stresses of military service—may also be certified as service connected, and thus become eligible to receive all corresponding service-connected compensation. Today, these benefits now also include medical care, educational and vocational training benefits, housing grants, automobile grants and dependent benefits.

Pension, on the other hand, was established as recompense or recognition for services rendered to the nation. It was a means of assisting veterans in living out their days with the dignity that comes from having one's basic needs met and was, therefore, intended for any veteran in temporary or permanent need of financial assistance due to non-service-connected illness or disability, or old age. Current criteria for being awarded a VA pension generally include: total disability; service during a wartime period; and low-income status. Today's VA pensions also entitle the veteran to medical care and several other benefits as well.

Determining amounts for either compensation or pension awards is a complex process based upon an elaborate and highly detailed rating system. Compensation and pension amounts are also frequently revised upward to reflect increases in cost of living.

When a veteran contacts BVA, we immediately try to determine whether or not the veteran may be eligible for either service-connected or non-service-connected benefits. If so, we assist him or her in preparing claims applications and monitor the application as it works its way through the VA process, solving whatever problems arise and helping track down whatever additional information is needed to insure that the compensation or pension award received is an equitable one.

Our experiences over the years have taught us the sad truth that fairness and equity on the part of the VA, as well as other service agencies, simply cannot be assumed. For some reason, VA rating officials sometimes seem to take an almost whimsical approach to blinded veterans, denying their legitimate compensation claims and insisting on injury ratings far below those allowed by regulation. Part of the problem seems to lie in the misreading of medical evaluations; and part of it from medical evaluations that were performed poorly to begin with, resulting in inadequate measures and descriptions of the nature and extent of veterans' blindness. Strange as it may sound, despite the high level of technology that exists in medical science today, many doctors remain incredulously ignorant of blindness—of its sources and of its attendant problems.

Consequently, much of our work on behalf of blinded veterans becomes very technical. In response, we have established, and maintain, a high level of technical expertise that enables us to challenge the bureaucracy when such mistakes are made.

Naturally, wherever and whenever possible we try to get the blinded veteran "service connected." As need dictates, we search for old records and documents from military service years that may show a service-related cause for the blindness. We review old claims and claim denials to see if errors have been made. And when we feel that a veteran's claim has been unfairly turned down at the VA Regional Office level, we represent the veteran's case at the next level of appeal, the Board of Veterans Appeals.

Indeed, many, if not most, of the benefits blinded veterans receive today stem from BVA's efforts over the years, and the work continues. Through often bitter experience we have learned that the VA, like many other federal agencies, simply cannot be trusted to look after us. The present system of blind rehabilitation centers and clinics and of Visual Impairment Service Teams . . . and many other services now available to all veterans will persist only as long as BVA and its sister veterans organizations remain vigilant.

We at BVA are here to help all blinded veterans, both individually and collectively. We, sometimes alone, sometimes in conjunction with our sister veterans service organizations, present legislative initiatives and frequently attend hearings on veteran's legislation. Our officers, directors, national office and field staff all represent blinded veterans before departments and agencies at the state, regional, and national levels, including the U.S. Congress, the Department of Veterans Affairs, the President's Committee on Employment of People with Disabilities, the Small Business Administration, the U.S. Office of Personnel Management, the U.S. Department of Labor, the Department of Health and Human Services and the Department of Education—as we have since our formation in 1945.

We also testify on behalf of blinded veterans at hearings of the House and Senate Committees on Veterans Affairs, on problems related to blind rehabilitation, veterans' access to health care, improved prosthetic services, and on the budget for the Department of Veterans Affairs.

Over the years BVA has taken on a lot. But we know that many pressing needs of blinded veterans remain unmet. And it is our sincere hope that one day, funds and continuing strong leadership providing, we will be given the opportunity to grapple with these issues, too, in order to more completely fulfill our mission to provide mutual support and assistance to all blinded veterans.

Source: Brown, Robert, and Hope Schutte. 1991. Pp. 26–33 in *Our Fight: A Battle against Darkness.* Washington, DC: Blinded Veterans Association. Printed with permission of the Blinded Veterans Association.

▣ From *Dendron News* (1992)

This excerpt, which appeared on the back page of Dendron News, *provides a brief explanation of the name chosen for one of the first "Psychiatric Survivors & Allies Independent Media."*

What is "Dendron" anyway?

Your brain has billions of cells called *neurons*. Information flows between neurons through the branches of DENDRITES, which comes from the Greek word for *tree,* DENDRON. This paper is printed on recycled paper from dendrons (post-consumer). Brains look like ancient, wild forests. Psychiatry is like modern forestry—clearcutting brains to prop up the current failing, dominating system. So connect your liberating thoughts with others globally through DENDRON.

Source: *Dendron News* (27–29). 1992, May 1. Eugene, OR: Clearinghouse on Human Rights & Psychiatry. Reprinted with permission of Mindfreedom International (www.mindfreedom .org), formerly known as *Dendron News.*

▣ Disability Discrimination Act of 1992 (Australia)

The Australian Disability Discrimination Act (DDA) 1992 was enacted at a time in Australia's history when there was a concerted effort to address the social exclusion of disability people. The Australian Disability Discrimination Act 1992 reflected many of the principles enshrined in the Americans with Disabilities Act 1990 and included coverage for work, education, accommodation, sport and recreation.

While the initial proposal for the enactment of the legislation appeared as an unprecedented move by government to redress discrimination on the grounds of disability, increasingly, the limitations of the DDA are being revealed. The national legislative framework pursued a policy of restrained social recognition of equality before the law. Reforming social institutions for the collective good of disabled people has been constrained by the legislation's "complaints framework," as the onus of reporting experiences of discrimination is placed on disabled individuals. Further, organizations and social institutions can be absolved of legal accountability and compliance with the DDA if they can prove "unjustifiable hardship" on economic grounds. Other constraining factors consist of the Australian Government's National Competition Policy. In Australia, national legislation is reviewed to ensure that it does not impede the competitive capacity of the economy, in line with competitive market ideology. During 2003 and 2004, the DDA underwent extensive review with national public consultations. There was overwhelming public support to strengthen the DDA, particularly in the area of employment. However, many of the recommendations and the current government's commitment to National Competition Policy do not appear to redress discrimination on the grounds of disability.

Section I–This Act may be cited as the Disability Discrimination Act 1992

Objects

The objects of this Act are:

(a) to eliminate, as far as possible, discrimination against persons on the ground of disability in the areas of

(i) work, accommodation, education, access to premises, clubs and sport; and

(ii) the provision of goods, facilities, services and land; and

(iii) existing laws; and

(iv) the administration of Commonwealth laws and programs; and

(b) to ensure, as far as practicable, that persons with disabilities have the same rights to equality before the law as the rest of the community; and

(c) to promote recognition and acceptance within the community of the principle that persons with disabilities have the same fundamental rights as the rest of the community.

Disability discrimination

(1) For the purposes of this Act, a person (*discriminator*) discriminates against another person (*aggrieved person*) on the ground of a disability of the aggrieved person if, because of the aggrieved person's disability, the discriminator treats or proposes to treat the aggrieved person less favourably than, in circumstances that are the same or are not materially different, the discriminator

treats or would treat a person without the disability.

(2) For the purposes of subsection (1), circumstances in which a person treats or would treat another person with a disability are not materially different because of the fact that different accommodation or services may be required by the person with a disability.

Indirect disability discrimination

For the purposes of this Act, a person (*discriminator*) discriminates against another person (*aggrieved person*) on the ground of a disability of the aggrieved person if the discriminator requires the aggrieved person to comply with a requirement or condition:

(a) with which a substantially higher proportion of persons without the disability comply or are able to comply; and (b) which is not reasonable having regard to the circumstances of the case; and (c) with which the aggrieved person does not or is not able to comply.

Disability discrimination–interpreters, readers and assistants

For the purposes of this Act, a person (*discriminator*) discriminates against another person with a disability (*aggrieved person*) if the discriminator treats the aggrieved person less favourably because of the fact that the aggrieved person is accompanied by:

(a) an interpreter; or (b) a reader; or (c) an assistant; or (d) a carer; who provides interpretive, reading or other services to the aggrieved person because of the disability, or because of any matter related to that fact, whether or not it is the discriminator's practice to treat less favourably any person who is accompanied by: (e) an interpreter; or (f) a reader; or (g) an assistant; or (h) a carer.

Disability discrimination–guide dogs, hearing assistance dogs and trained animals

(1) For the purposes of this Act, a person (*discriminator*) discriminates against a person with: (a) a visual disability; or (b) a hearing disability; or (c) any other disability; (*aggrieved person*) if the discriminator treats the aggrieved person less favourably because of the fact that the aggrieved person possesses, or is accompanied by: (d) a guide dog; or (e) a dog trained to ssist the aggrieved person in activities where hearing is required, or because of any matter related to hat fact; or (f) any other animal

trained to assist the aggrieved person to alleviate the effect of the disability, or because of any matter related to that fact; whether or not it is the discriminator's practice to treat less favourably any person who possesses, or is accompanied by, a dog or any other animal.

(2) Subsection (1) does not affect the liability of a person with a disability for damage to property caused by a dog or other animal trained to assist the person to alleviate the effect of the disability or because of any matter related to that fact.

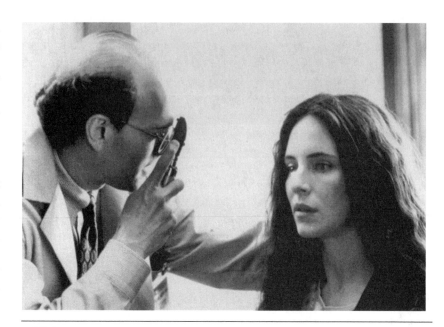

In Blink, *a musician recovers her sight after 20 years and believes that she has witnessed a murder. A detective decides to trust her account and protects her from danger.*

Source: *Blink* (1994), directed by Michael Apted. United States. Color, 102 minutes. Reprinted by permission of Paul Darke.

Act done because of disability and for other reason

If: (a) an act is done for 2 or more reasons; and (b) one of the reasons is the disability of a person (whether or not it is the dominant or a substantial reason for doing the act); then, for the purposes of this Act, the act is taken to be done for that reason.

Unjustifiable hardship

For the purposes of this Act, in determining what constitutes unjustifiable hardship, all relevant circumstances of the particular case are to be taken into account including: (a) the nature of the benefit or detriment likely to accrue or be suffered by any persons concerned; and (b) the effect of the disability of a person concerned; and (c) the financial circumstances and the estimated amount of expenditure required to be made by the person claiming unjustifiable hardship; and (d) in the case of the provision of services, or the making available of facilities—an action plan given to the Commission under section 64.

Discrimination in employment

(1) It is unlawful for an employer or a person acting or purporting to act on behalf of an employer to discriminate against a person on the ground of the other person's disability or a disability of any of that other person's associates: (a) in the arrangements made for the purpose of determining who should be offered employment; or (b) in determining who should be offered employment; or (c) in the terms or conditions on which employment is offered.

(2) It is unlawful for an employer or a person acting or purporting to act on behalf of an employer to discriminate against an employee on the ground of the employee's disability or a disability of any of that employee's associates: (a) in the terms or conditions of employment that the employer affords the employee; or (b) by denying the employee access, or limiting the employee's access, to opportunities for promotion, transfer or training, or to any other benefits associated with employment; or (c) by dismissing the employee; or (d) by subjecting the employee to any other detriment.

(3) Neither paragraph (1)(a) nor (b) renders it unlawful for a person to discriminate against another person, on the ground of the other person's disability, in connection with employment to perform domestic duties on the premises on which the first-mentioned person resides.

(4) Neither paragraph (1)(b) nor (2)(c) renders unlawful discrimination by an employer against a person on the ground of the person's disability, if taking into account the person's past training, qualifications and experience relevant to the particular employment

and, if the person is already employed by the employer, the person's performance as an employee, and all other relevant factors that it is reasonable to take into account, the person because of his or her disability: (a) would be unable to carry out the inherent requirements of the particular employment; or (b) would, in order to carry out those requirements, require services or facilities that are not required by persons without the disability and the provision of which would impose an unjustifiable hardship on the employer.

Accommodation

(1) It is unlawful for a person, whether as principal or agent, to discriminate against another person on the ground of the other person's disability or a disability of any of that other person's associates: (a) by refusing the other person's application for accommodation; or (b) in the terms or conditions on which the accommodation is offered to the other person; or (c) by deferring the other person's application for accommodation or according to the other person a lower order of precedence in any list of applicants for that accommodation.

(2) It is unlawful for a person, whether as principal or agent, to discriminate against another person on the ground of the other person's disability or a disability of any of the other person's associates: (a) by denying the other person access, or limiting the other person's access, to any benefit associated with accommodation occupied by the other person; or (b) by evicting the other person from accommodation occupied by the other person; or (c) by subjecting the other person to any other detriment in relation to accommodation occupied by the other person; or (d) by refusing to permit the other person to make reasonable alterations to accommodation occupied by that person if:

(i) that person has undertaken to restore the accommodation to its condition before alteration on leaving the accommodation; and

(ii) in all the circumstances it is likely that the person will perform the undertaking; and

(iii) in all the circumstances, the action required to restore the accommodation to its condition before alteration is reasonably practicable; and

(iv) the alteration does not involve alteration of the premises of any other occupier; and

(v) the alteration is at that other person's own expense.

(3) This section does not apply to or in respect of:
(a) the provision of accommodation in premises if:

(i) the person who provides or proposes to provide the accommodation or a near relative of that person resides, and intends to continue to reside on those premises; and

(ii) the accommodation provided in those premises is for no more than 3 persons other than a person referred to in subparagraph (a)(i) or near relatives of such a person; or

(b) the accommodation is provided by a charitable or other voluntary body solely for persons who have a particular disability and the person discriminated against does not have that particular disability; or

(c) the provision of accommodation in premises where special services or facilities would be required by the person with a disability and the provision of such special services or facilities would impose unjustifiable hardship on the person providing or proposing to provide the accommodation whether as principal or agent.

▣ National Empowerment Center's Mission Statement (1992)

The National Empowerment Center was founded in 1992 through a grant from the Center for Mental Health Services, Substance Abuse and Mental Health Services Administration, U.S. Department of Health and Human Services, to act as a consumer-run National Technical Assistance Center. Located in Lawrence, Massachusetts, it remains a significant component of the psychiatric survivor/user movement. The group's website is at http://www.power2u.org.

Our Mission

The mission of the National Empowerment Center Inc. is to carry a message of recovery, empowerment, hope and healing to people who have been diagnosed with mental illness. We carry that message with authority because we are a consumer/survivor/expatient-run organization and each of us is living a personal journey of recovery and empowerment. We are convinced that recovery and empowerment are not the privilege of a few exceptional leaders, but rather are possible for each person who has been diagnosed with mental illness. Whether on the back ward of a state mental institution or working as an executive in a corporation, we want people who are mental health consumers/ survivors/ex-patients to know there is a place to turn to in order to receive the information they might need in order to regain control over their lives and the resources that affect their lives. That place is the National Empowerment Center.

Source: National Empowerment Center. 1992. *Mission Statement.* Available at: http://www.power2u.org/what.html. Reprinted by permission.

▣ Richard Powers, from *Operation Wandering Soul* (1993)

Powers's dystopic novel takes place on a pediatric ward for disabled children in Los Angeles. Rather than passively submitting to their destiny as wards of the state, medical guinea pigs, or sentimentalized charity objects, the children begin to do research in order to re-create a more meaningful history of disability and adult neglect for themselves. Specifically, they spend each evening having their nurse, Linda, read tales about other disabled children from around the world from whom they might better learn to navigate their own stigmatized lives. In this excerpt, they listen to a version of the ancient Japanese myth of Hiruko, the Leech Child, who is abandoned by his parents to die because of his disabilities but ends up sailing around the world in search of comradeship (see an excerpt from the original version of this story in Part One).

(Night 57, Japan)

This is how the world begins. At first, the All was no more than a blurry egg, full of seeds and shaken together. After a time beyond telling, the heavier parts began to sink down and the lighter floated upon them, forming the plain of high heaven. On this plain, three gods were born of no one, lived out an eternity, and then vanished back into nothing.

How you gonna be born of no one? Everybody got . . .

Shh. Come on. It's a makeup; that's how it opens. Next there came about, on their own, a few pairs of gods who lived in the drifting middle of nowhere. The youngest couple among them were called Izanami and Izanagi, or She-the-Inviter and He-the-Inviter. She

and He were ordered by their elders to collect a solid world from out of the shapeless, muddy waters that flowed beneath the high plain of heaven. They stood on the bridge of the sky and dipped a jeweled spear into the sandy broth below them, stirring it slowly. They pulled their spear out of the waters. A drop of brine sticking to the shaft fell off to form Onogoro, the first island.

She-the-Inviter and He-the-Inviter climbed down onto the island and began exploring it. They circled slowly around one another at the pillar at the center of the solid world. Slowly, they discovered each other, and learned that they wanted one another.

Uh-oh. They in trouble now. When my daddy found my big brother and me . . .

No, sweetheart; it wasn't like that. Remember, these two gods had no parents. Slowly, by experiment and chance, She-the-Inviter and He-the-Inviter learned how to make a baby. But their first child was born with something wrong with it. Because She did not yet know the rules of courtship she accidentally broke them. So the first infant who laid eyes on the world was born deformed.

Heh. Like me, you mean?

Yes, Chuck, my man. A little like you. She and He named their boy Hiruko, the Leech Child. They didn't know what they were supposed to do with him, so they built him a boat of reeds and set the boy adrift on the open sea. So you see, the very first child *ever* was abandoned. As soon as the Leech Child drifted out of sight, his parents began making other babies, more deities to cover every walk of creation.

Among their new children were the eight main islands of the world. She-the-Inviter was burned to death while giving birth to her last child, Fire. Gods spilled out of her dying body. Other gods arose from the tears of her husband's eyes. In a rage, He-the-Inviter swung his great blade and cut off the head of Fire, his son. From out of the bleeding neck of Fire there sprang Thunder, with several more gods.

The soul of She-the-Inviter went down into Yomi, the land of darkness, where He-the-Inviter madly followed. He wanted to find her and bring her back to life. But his wife had already eaten food cooked in the land of darkness, so she could not come back. The dead She warned her husband not to look upon her. But he disobeyed her command. He looked at her face, and saw something horrible. His wife was rotting. Maggots covered her. Shh! Yes, like the ones in old garbage. He-the-Inviter ran back up into the world in terror. She was hurt and angry, and She sent a pack of Furies to chase after her husband.

When He reached the surface once again, He sealed up the entrance to the land of darkness with an enormous rock. His wife became furious. She threatened to kill a thousand of their children every day that He kept her trapped. But He just sneered at her. He said that he would father fifteen hundred new children for every thousand that She killed. She and He knew they had come to an end.

To purify himself, He bathed in the waters. As He washed, more gods sprang from him. From the water sprinkling from his left eye was born the Sun, and from his right the Moon. Out of his nose there came Susanoo, the God of the Wind and Storm.

His nose? Gross. But what about the boy in the boat? The Leech?

It doesn't say. He must have floated for a long, long time. Reeds can be very watertight in these stories. But the ocean can be pretty big too. The Leech Child probably drifted in the current for years, farther and farther away, into places where land was completely unheard of.

Maybe the boat was held together by little metal clasps. That's it; I once read something like this. He pulled one of these metal strands loose and fashioned a bit of tinsel from it, which he dangled in the water just to amuse himself, because it looked pretty. And that's how, by accident, he learned that fish will bite at a hook. And he figured out that by eating fish, he could live pretty much as long as he needed.

Yeah? Well, all right. It's possible. Read us another one.

(Night 139, central Italy. Twin infant sons of a vestal virgin and the God of War are sentenced by the king to be drowned in the Tiber. Miraculously, the cask they are put in floats. They are found and suckled by a wolf more loving than human parents. The foundlings grow up to invent the West.)

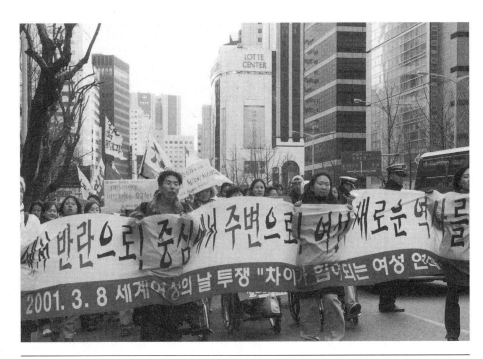

Korean Protest of Socially Marginalized Peoples: Intersexed. Lesbian, Disabled, Prostitutes, Seoul, Korea, 2003.

Go on. We want more.

(Night 21, the Near East. Another terrified tyrant orders all the male offspring of a certain tribe to be drowned to death. The mother makes a little reed ark for the boy, and lays him in the rushes on the riverbank. The tyrant's daughter finds the infant, and hires the boy's own mother to nurse him. The boy grows up to bring God's law to . . .)

Why drowning? Why water all the time? Why little boats?

Yes, that's odd, isn't it? Happens all over the place. Look at this: Night 308, the Mississippi. Night 145, Norway. Night 98, Kashmir. Night 114, Zimbabwe.

(Across the planet, attempted drownings, tiny bound bodies thrown deliberately back into the sea. All through the time line, vanishing into the current, carried along by the undertow. Every other story in any anthology—children sealed up, locked in casks, keelhauled, strapped on rafts, sucked down by the departing tide. A few miraculously saved, for future purposes.)

And some mom and dad always want to kill them.

Yes, true! Notice how the stories always blame some evil step-something, or foster fathers, or kings? Guilty conscience, I'll bet you anything. These cats have something to hide, I'm here to tell you. If they're not putting the kids out to drown in chests, then they're leaving them on church steps or by a roadside out of town. Or here, look: dropped off deep in the woods, bricked up into cornerstones, rolled over on in the parents' shared bed . . .

(. . . swaddled too tightly, delivered with a club to the skull or butterfly slit in the trachea, wrung with a bit of old cloth, or, for maximum efficiency—Night 3, Greece—eaten.)

Awesome. Any that stuff really happen?

(Night Before Last, Pacific Islands: two thirds of offspring. West Africa: any twins. Sarawak: boys strung from trees. China: daughters given instant turnaround chance to return as sons. Germany, Italy, France: 1.8 "live birth" males to one female. SE England: "Three drowned in pond, two in well, five buried, two suffocated by pillow, two left in ditch, one thrown on dung heap, one slammed against bedpost, two twisted necks . . . Chicago; Houston; Portland, OR: discreet suburban fatalities, malign neglect, everyday police roundups dribbling out of radio speakers in the dark, on all-night talk stations turned down low, between choruses of that old folk tune, *I am no stranger to your town.*)

Why?

(Tales 101 and 343: postpartum birth control.)

Source: Powers, Richard. 1993. Pp. 80–89 in *Operation Wandering Soul.* New York: William Morrow. Reprinted by permission.

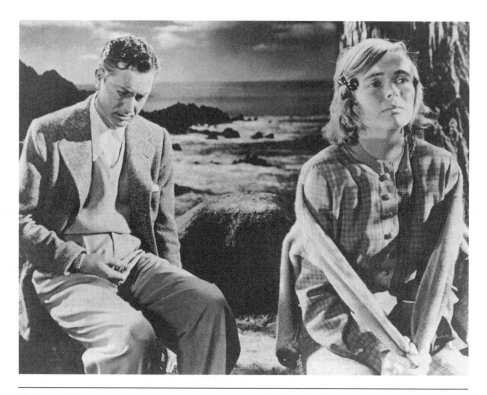

Enchanted Cottage is a queasily sentimental tale in which a blind pianist persuades a disfigured war veteran and a homely woman that they are, in fact, beautiful.

Source: *Enchanted Cottage* (1994), directed by John Cromwell. United States. B&W, 90 minutes. Reprinted by permission of Paul Darke.

undertaken in the 1990s by disability studies faculty at Hunter College in New York City. The following is an excerpt from the rationale offered to allow disability to serve as fulfillment of the multicultural studies requirement. Although the proposal ultimately failed, the effort sparked other efforts to adopt similar requirements at U.S. universities and colleges across the country.

▣ The Hunter College Disability Studies Project, "Definition of Disability Studies" (1990s)

One effort at the university level to gain recognition of disability as a multicultural experience was

Hunter College of the City University of New York
    Simi Linton
    Susan Mello
    John O'Neill

The Disability Studies Project
    Hunter College
    Department of Educational Foundations and
    Counselling Programs
    695 Park Avenue
    New York, NY 10021

Disability Studies

Disability Studies reframes the topic of disability by focusing on disability as a social phenomenon, as a social construct, as a metaphor and in fact as a culture. It does this by examining myths and ideas related to disability in all forms of cultural representations and throughout history. This focus shifts the emphasis away from examining the characteristics of impairments and their prevention, treatment and remediation to the study of disability as a social/cultural/political phenomenon. This shift does not indicate a denial of the presence of impairments and physical limitations, nor a rejection of the utility of intervention and treatment. Rather, the examination of disability as a socially constructed category is conducted in order to disentangle those impairments and limitations from the myth, ideology and stigma that influence social interaction and social policy. This analysis challenges the idea that the economic and social status and the assigned roles of people with disabilities are an inevitable outcome of their impairments, an idea similar to the argument that women's roles and status are biologically determined.

It is useful to disentangle the social construction from the physical realities of disability. One can begin to understand the breadth and depth of discrimination, marginalization, alienation and oppression of people with disabilities. In addition, Disability Studies is a prism through which we can gain a broader understanding of society and human experience, and the significance of human variation. Just as looking at American Studies from an African-American perspective provides a more comprehensive view of America's history, Disability Studies provides a more complex view [of] many critical social issues: competence, wholeness, independence/dependence, autonomy, health, physical appearance, aesthetics, and community, which pervade every aspect of the civic and pedagogical culture. Scholarship in this field addresses such fundamental ideas as who is considered a burden and who is a resource, who is expendable and who is esteemed, who should engage in the activities that might lead to reproduction and who should not, and if reproduction is not the aim, who can engage in erotic pleasures and who should not. Disability Studies examines the eugenics ideology that informs the discourse on abortion, pre-natal screening, birth control, euthanasia and medical ethics. And as Longmore (1992) points out, it also deepens the "historical comprehension of a broad range of subjects, for instance the history of values and beliefs regarding human

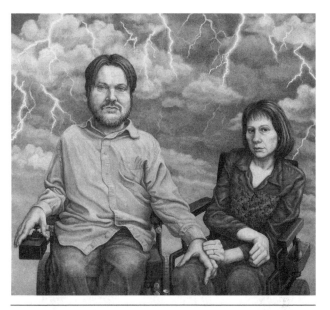

Circle Story #5: Mike Ervin and Anna Stonem, *by Riva Lehrer. 1998. Mixed media on paper, 22" by 21." Mike Ervin, journalist, writer and playwright, and Anna Stonum, poet, and visual artist, are shown in a double portrait. Ervin and Stonum were both dedicated disability rights activists and traveled the country to participate in political actions. They had been married for a decade before Anna Stonum's sudden death of heart failure in February 1999. Ervin's disability is Duchenne's muscular dystrophy, and Stonum's was Friedreich's ataxia.*

nature, gender and sexuality; American notions of individualism and equality, and the social and legal definitions of what constitutes a minority group."

The field of Disability Studies is multidisciplinary, includes both theory and research and has relevance to both liberal arts and applied fields. It draws on paradigms and constructs from anthropology, literature, sociology, history, political science, education and others. Incorporated into the liberal arts curriculum, it has the potential to organize and critique the existing representations of disability and ability in the culture. This process can expose ways that disability has been socially constructed and reveal the consequences of that construction for the pedagogic and civic cultures.

The myths and ideologies about disability entrenched in the curriculum parallel those that wield influence in the civic culture. The present curriculum supports the social organization and practices within the civic culture whose institutions often maintain an inequitable distribution of power and opportunity based on perceptions of competence and value. Therefore, a goal of Scholars in Disability Studies is to expose, deconstruct, and analyze fallacies and inconsistencies and examine their implications for social interaction. When incorporated into the curriculum, Disability Studies has the potential to redress the inadequacies in the structure and content of the curriculum by approaching disability as a phenomenon that organizes social, political and intellectual experience.

◉ Mike Ervin, *The History of Bowling* (1999)

The History of Bowling is the story of Chuck, a 32-year-old quadriplegic college freshman who, after 15 years of watching TV in his mother's attic, has gathered the courage to return to college. As he begins to relish coming out of the disability closet, he finds love in, of all places, PE class. His paramour, Lou, is a senior with an invisible disability (epilepsy) who has spent her life trying to hide her condition. When an insensitive coach forces the two to collaborate on a project, love blossoms and lovers' quarrels ensue, comically spurred on by Chuck's seductive roommate, Cornelius, who is deaf and blind, as well as a cad and a con. The playwright, Mike Ervin, is a well-known Chicago writer and disability rights activist. He coordinates the Victory Gardens Access Project, a program that uses technology to make live theater accessible for persons with disabilities.

Act I : Scene I: Lou and Chuck
are in opposite corners of the stage.

LOU (to audience): I finally broke down and got a doctor's note. I hated to do it but I had to. It was the only way I could get out of that stupid mandatory PE credit. I had the doctor at the student infirmary write me a note saying it was unsafe for me to take PE because it could set off a seizure if I got hit in the head with a ball. Of course it was bull shit. But the doctors at the student infirmary are like retired podiatrists. They don't know any better. I felt cheap and sleazy after I did it. Not because it was a lie, but because I played the cripple game. I only played the cripple game once before in my whole life. I could have played it a thousand times. But the only time I ever did, I stood up and said, "Well, your honor, sir, it's just that I have epilepsy. And if I were to have a seizure in the jury box . . ."

CHUCK (to audience): I, on the other hand, am the king of the doctor's notes. I could fill [the] gymnasium

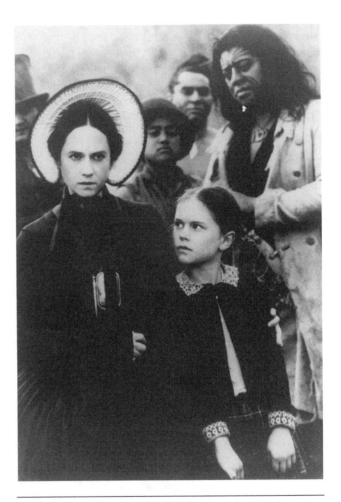

In The Piano, *a mute Scottish woman travels with her young daughter for an arranged marriage to a landowner in New Zealand. She is forced to leave her most treasured possession, her piano, on the beach, but she enters into a bizarrely erotic relationship with the half-Maori who purchases it.*

Source: *The Piano* (1994), directed by Jane Campion. Australia. Color, 120 minutes. Reprinted by permission of Paul Darke.

with all the doctor's notes I've had to get. When I got the license plates with the little wheelchair hieroglyphic, I had to get a doctor's note. When I got this wheelchair, doctor's note. When I applied to this university, doctor's note again. One time I was in a shoe store and the manager rushed up and he said that before he would let any of his sales people touch my feet, I would have to bring a doctor's note.

LOU (to audience): I know, I know, I should have stood up and said, "I have epilepsy, your honor, but it will in no way interfere with my ability to do the job!" But I didn't have time for jury duty.

CHUCK (to audience): The shoe store manager was so uptight. He said, "I'm sorry sir, but I don't want them to be responsible if something should happen." I said, "What, you had a cripple come in here once and his feet exploded?" And he said, "It's not that I don't have empathy for your situation." That really made me laugh. I said, "How can YOU feel sorry for ME? You manage a shoe store!"

LOU (to audience): My mother would hate it if she knew I got a doctor's note. The one thing she has no patience for is "those people who use their handicap as a weapon."

CHUCK (to audience): Beggars on the street are like that too. They try to hit up everyone who comes by, but never me. It's an insult. They're wearing shoes they found in the dumpster, but they think they're better off than me. I wish I could afford to flash 500 bucks at one of them! I'd show them boy!

LOU (to audience): I should have known it wouldn't be that easy. I delivered my doctor's note to Mr. Barnes, the PE teacher. I tried to act like I was really broken up about not being able to take PE.

(Enter BARNES, perusing a note. He's the devil wearing gym teacher's clothes with a whistle around his neck.)

BARNES: Oh dear. Epilepsy, huh?

LOU: Yes. And I really can't [take] the risk.

BARNES: Oh, mercy no. Most certainly not.

LOU: I'm really sorry. I'll have to get an exemption, I guess.

BARNES: We'll have to put you in the special section.

LOU: What!

BARNES: Oh yes. The special section. For the people with handicaps. Maybe you can't literally participate in athletic activities, but you surely can write term papers about them. You and your partner.

LOU: Partner?

BARNES: But of course. Another handicapped person.

LOU: You mean, someone who's blind, or in a wheelchair?

BARNES: Could be a hemophiliac. (Laughs a diabolical laugh.)

(Barnes exits.)

CHUCK (to audience): The street preachers are the worst. I try my best to ignore them, until they start with that, "Pray to Jesus and he'll make you walk!" One day I passed that one who's always in front of the drug store with the bullhorn shouting, "Jesus! Jesus! Jesus!" And he says to me, "You better get right with Jesus, or he ain't never gonna make you walk!"

LOU (to audience): Oh God! A partner! My mother would say, "Serves you right! You can either use your handicap to make excuses or you can stand on your own two feet!"

CHUCK (to audience): "You better get right with Jesus or he ain't never gonna make you walk!" Who the hell does he think he is? So I turned to him and I said, "You better get right with Jesus, or he ain't never gonna make you white!"

LOU (to audience): I had to meet my partner at the cafeteria. Two o'clock Tuesday. All I knew was his name was Chuck. That's all I knew. Oh God! I don't belong here!

CHUCK (to audience): He told me don't think my wheelchair will keep me from going to hell! I said I hope not. One time I made airplane reservations and they told me before I could board I'd have to have a doctor's note. I just bet you if I did go to hell, Satan would hit me up for a doctor's note.

LOU (to audience): There was this black boy named Terry. His face was hideously burned. It was like his face was made of wax and big wax tears dripped down and solidified. His face was smeared, like someone tried to put it back in place with a putty knife.

(Lou walks toward Chuck and sees him sitting at a cafeteria table.)

LOU: Chuck?

CHUCK: Yeah.

LOU: I'm Lou.

CHUCK: My partner?

LOU: Yes.

CHUCK: What are you? Hemophiliac?

LOU: Epilepsy.

CHUCK: Epilepsy people can't take PE?

LOU: There's been a mistake. I was supposed to get an exemption.

CHUCK (Laughing): An exemption from Barnes? That sadistic bastard? They say he wouldn't let his dead grandma off the hook for P.E. We're lucky he's not making us run laps.

LOU: I wish he was.

CHUCK: Thanks.

LOU: I didn't mean it like that.

CHUCK: Right.

LOU: I didn't.

(Pause.)

CHUCK: You a freshman?

LOU: No. A senior. It's my last semester.

CHUCK: A senior? And just taking PE now?

LOU: I put it off until the last minute. And now I can't avoid it anymore. What are you?

CHUCK: A freshman.

LOU: How old are you?

CHUCK: Thirty two.

LOU: And you're a freshman?

CHUCK: It's a long story.

(*Pause.*)

LOU: I didn't mean anything by what I said. It's just that I hate writing term papers. And especially about sports. I don't know anything about sports. I hate sports. I have no idea what to write about.

CHUCK: Yeah well that's OK. I know a lot about sports. That's all I did for the last fucking 15 years. Watch sports on cable. Stock car racing, water polo, the world table tennis championships. But I was about to tell Barnes he could shove his busy work. Then I got to thinking about it and pretty soon I got real excited. So don't worry. I know exactly what we're gonna write about!

LOU: Oh good. What?

CHUCK (*bitterly*): Bowling!

LOU: Bowling?

CHUCK: Bowling.

LOU: I hate bowling.

CHUCK: So do I.

LOU: I don't know anything about bowling. I've never set foot in a bowling alley.

CHUCK: That's all right. I know all about bowling. I did it enough times.

LOU: You? Bowling?

CHUCK: Yep. Bowling Buddies. Crippled kids bowling club. Every third Saturday. The bastards! I think they were Christian kids. Real clean rah-rah types. I think maybe we were extra credit. They'd close down Rainbow Lanes for the afternoon and bring the cripples in. Sons of bitches!

LOU: My God.

CHUCK: I know. And bowling buddies motto was "anybody can bowl a strike." They had this ramp. It looked like a miniature playground slide. They'd put the ball on top and you'd push it and would roll down the ramp and head down the lane. Anybody could do it. There was this kid with no arms. He pushed the ball with his head.

LOU: Please. I don't want to hear anymore

CHUCK: He was a maniac. He'd get a running start and butt heads with the bowling ball. They made him wear a leather helmet. We called him kamikaze. And in bowling buddies, no one ever threw a gutter ball. You know why?

LOU: Don't tell me.

CHUCK: Because the Christians ran along side the lane and if the ball headed for the gutter, they'd kick it back on course.

LOU: All right! All right! We'll do bowling!

CHUCK: It's all true. Every word.

LOU (*to audience*): He made me feel how I felt when my friend Amy told me about the bastard she was married to who beat her up for years. The Amy I knew was the head of an agency, served on several boards. She was an activist. If any man tried that with the Amy I knew, she'd break his neck. Same way with Chuck. I couldn't believe he let them do that to him. Somewhere along the line, he'd completely transformed.

(*Lou approaches Chuck.*)

CHUCK: Still exists, bowling buddies. Chapters all over the country.

(*Lou crawls up onto his lap and kisses him long and hard. Barnes runs out frantically blowing his whistle and he throws a penalty flag.*)

Scene II: The cafeteria. Lou and Chuck sit at a table with food trays on it. Lou has a pen and writing pad.

CHUCK: OK. Read that back.

LOU: Again?

CHUCK: Yes. Again. Got to get it right. You know what a fucker Barnes is.

LOU: All right, all right! (*reading*). The history of bowling.

CHUCK: Not from the top. Start from the part about Old Lady McDonald.

LOU (Reading): Bowling buddies was founded in 1962 by Mrs. Roger McDonald as a monument to her late husband. She wanted to combine his two great passions in life: service to the less fortunate and bowling.

CHUCK: Ok. Great. Now skip down to the part about the blind kids.

LOU: This is depressing.

CHUCK: I know. Keep reading.

LOU: Blind kids . . . blind kids. . . . Ok: (*Reading*) The blind kids were the worst bowlers in the world. Everybody ran for cover. But even the blind kids never threw a gutter ball. No one ever threw a gutter ball in bowling buddies. That was another one of our proud mottoes. But why not? What's wrong with throwing a gutter ball? What were they afraid of? And we all accepted it. No one questioned it. Not one of us ever demanded our inalienable right to throw a gutter ball!

CHUCK: OK. Good. Now add, "In life, there's gutter balls. It's a fact. Better learn how to deal with it."

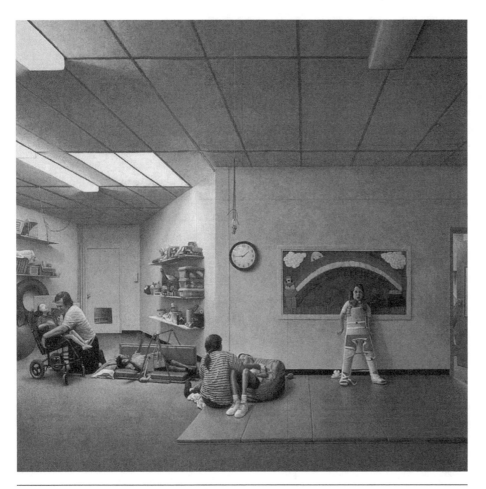

Big Picture, *by Tim Lowly. 1997. Tempera on panel. 120" by 120," In this work, Lowly captures the students and teachers interacting in a special education class in Seoul, Korea.*

LOU: That's sick!

CHUCK: I know. I told you he's a sadist. That's how he gets his jollies. Him and the jocks. But we're gonna get the last laugh.

LOU: Oh God! Why did I try to get an exemption!

CHUCK: Oral presentation's a tough job. Takes a tough woman. So see. I have respect for you.

LOU: No way! Why don't you do it?

CHUCK: Oh don't worry. I'll be there. I just haven't figured out in what capacity.

LOU: No way am I doing any oral presentations!

CHUCK: We need to finish this.

LOU: I'm serious.

CHUCK: We'll discuss it later. Now what did I say before? Life is full of gutter balls.

(Lou reluctantly picks up the pad.)

LOU: Oh screw it. I don't care. Write about whatever you want. I just want to get this over with so I can graduate.

CHUCK: Good. Ok so write that down about gutter balls.

LOU: The minute I get out of here, I've already decided what I'm gonna do. You know what I'm gonna do?

CHUCK: I'd love to hear every detail. Really I would. But let's do the gutter balls first.

LOU: I'm gonna hop a boxcar. I don't care which one. Just pick one and go. I did it once before. All by myself. Rode all the way across Indiana. Changed my life. I know it's hard to believe riding across Indiana could change your life. But it's the boxcar. It's magic. The moonlight.

CHUCK: Even Indiana.

LOU: Yes! Even Indiana! Exactly. That's the beauty of it. I'm glad I wasn't in West Virginia or some place that really is beautiful or I wouldn't have got the full impact. It was the only time I rode. It scares me when I think back. Not because I was alone.

LOU: This is bull shit. You don't have any respect for me. We're supposed to be partners! I'm just a fucking secretary!

CHUCK: No. I just think better out loud.

LOU: And this whole paper is all about you.

CHUCK: No way. It's more about you than me. It's your worst nightmare.

LOU: What the hell is that supposed to mean?

CHUCK: They're gonna kidnap you and make you a bowling buddy!

LOU: Write your own fucking paper!

CHUCK (*mocking Lou*): Help! Help! Zombies! Hey, you think I don't have respect for you? You get the toughest job of all. You get to do the oral presentation.

LOU: Presentation? To whom?

CHUCK: To Barnes. He didn't tell you that part?

LOU: No!

CHUCK: Oh yeah. Oral presentation. To the whole gym class. It's our final. At the end of the semester he parades all the cripples into the gym and they present their papers to all the jocks.

I'm glad I was alone. I wouldn't have got the full impact if I wasn't alone. But when I think back, I'm lucky I didn't kill myself when I jumped off. I could've broken both legs. Then what? In the middle of a prairie. I could've died out there. I could've been eaten by wolves. People hop moving boxcars and they get sucked under the train and killed. That's the thing. I was so depressed and I did it all with such a sudden rush of abandon—almost suicidal. Not completely suicidal. It wasn't guaranteed death like jumping off a cliff. There was just a chance. But I didn't care. But I trust my motivations now. They're positive. I'm doing it to reward myself. And I'll wait until the train is stopped from now on before I hop on and off. But God, it's so amazing out in a box car. I was howling at the moon like a coyote.

CHUCK: Yeah well I wouldn't know. I don't do boxcars.

LOU: Oh. Sorry. Where were we?

CHUCK: Gutter balls. Ever since the dawn of time there have been gutter balls.

LOU: I want to tell you something.

CHUCK (*irritated*): Can we write that down first?

LOU: I want to tell you now before we go any further.

CHUCK: OK! What!

LOU: Because it may make a difference.

CHUCK: In what?

LOU: In general.

CHUCK: It won't. What?

LOU: This is my third college.

CHUCK: Uh huh?

LOU: And I'm only 22.

CHUCK: OK?

LOU: I started college when I just turned 17. I was double promoted twice. I was honor society.

CHUCK: Congratulations.

LOU: So I dropped out of two colleges in two years. I was running from lovers.

CHUCK: So?

LOU: So the second one was a woman.

CHUCK: Was it fun?

LOU: Fun? I don't know. I guess. Mostly. Until the end.

CHUCK: Well good. Can we finish with the gutter balls?

LOU: Will you pose for me?

CHUCK: What?

LOU: I'm a photographer too. I want you pose for me. Please?

CHUCK: OK sure. Now please—

LOU: Nude.

(*Pause.*)

CHUCK: You're kidding, right?

LOU: No. It's an on-going series I'm doing. People I know. I don't ask everybody I know to pose. Very few, actually. They have to have a certain charisma. Not really charisma. More like audacity. Audacity and a certain playfulness. The audacity to be playful. But I guess that's charisma. I've only asked four or five of my friends. And my aunt.

CHUCK: You took naked pictures of your aunt?

LOU: She's not like most aunts. She's real cool. What I do is I take their picture in their natural habitat—doing something they do every day, except nude. And they do it like they don't even realize they're nude. Just go about their business. Except nude. Like the one I took of my aunt, she was vacuuming. And my friend Gordon, the thing he does every day is wait for the stupid subway. So we went down to the subway late at night when no one was around. And he stood there naked waiting for the train. So with you, I'd probably do it in your dorm room working on your bowling paper. Except nude. It's the juxtaposition of the mundane and the extraordinary. A statement about freedom. So will you do it?

CHUCK: I don't know.

LOU: Why not? Can't you handle it?

CHUCK: I can handle it!

LOU: Then you'll do it?

CHUCK: Maybe.

Source: Ervin, Mike. 2005. *The History of Bowling.* In Lewis, Victoria Ann, ed. *Beyond Victims and Villains: Contemporary Plays by Disabled Playwrights.* Minneapolis, MN: Consortium Books. (Originally performed 1999)

▣ Steven Brown, *Institute on Disability Culture Manifesto* (1999)

This manifesto documents the long list of disability activist complaints against media spectacles such as Jerry Lewis's Labor Day Telethon for Muscular Dystrophy. In his cyber newsletter, author Steven Brown galvanizes public opposition to the telethon by explaining why charity activities do more harm than good for disabled populations. In this excerpt, he brings together some of his previous publications in his cyber newsletter.

August 1999, Number Six

IT'S TELETHON TIME–AGAIN

Labor Day will be here before we know it—and once again Jerry Lewis and hopefully Jerry's Orphans, the protest group developed to oppose the MDA telethon, will be in the spotlight. Telethons have the ability to bring about some of the most vituperative arguments about disability issues. Here's what I've written about telethons in the past:

THE TRUTH ABOUT TELETHONS

"Recently, I chanced upon an article in DISABLED USA describing the efforts of a person with Multiple Sclerosis first to retain her well-paying job, then to find a new one that matched her abilities and expectations. She failed. Or, more properly, her society failed her. She unnerved prospective employers who were afraid her dreaded disease would frighten both co-workers and the public, not to mention render her unfit to be a productive, and compatible, employee. After several years of searching for appropriate employment she has determined that her best route to continued success and continued productivity is through free-lance photography and other artistic endeavors. Her disability did not force her out of the employment mainstream. Society's handicapping barriers did.

For several years now, I've been receiving the GAUCHER'S DISEASE REGISTRY NEWSLETTER. I've even published articles in it addressing the importance of the disability movement. I was pleased to note that the Newsletter's editor was starting to refer to "people with disabilities" and to include articles about disability rights and advocacy. But two issues ago, I was horrified to read two articles concerning a young Englishwoman with Gaucher's Disease. She was constantly being described, and describing herself, as being victimized by this disease. Now I'm not going to maintain that Gaucher's Disease is a welcome guest that should be greeted with a fervor of hospitality. I'm much too familiar with its broken bones, heartaches, and physical pain. But I'm also unwilling to be labeled a victim who has survived its ravages. You see, "victim" has an ugly connotation that offends—no, enrages—me. Being told, or believing,

I'm a victim places all the responsibility for the results of the disease in the disease itself. Now I ask you, does a disease feel; is it cognizant, does it manipulate? As far as I know, disease does none of these things, but people do. I resent being called a victim because that implies that I have no control over the way I react to my disease, to my disability. But the fact is, I do have control. I can decide whether to succumb to my pain or to adapt myself to it. I can decide whether I want to grind my bones into pieces or to use a wheelchair for mobility. I can decide whether to risk passing this inherited disease onto my own natural children or to remain childless. I can decide. I am a victim only when I let my disease rule me. I am a person with a disability when I choose how to react to the characteristics of my disease. Anyone can choose to be a victim of anything. And anyone can choose not to be.

You're probably wondering, if you've been tenacious enough to read this far, what these thoughts have to do with telethons. Two things. First, I chose that title to grab your attention, just like telethons are supposed to do. Second, it has occurred to me that the way the majority of us think and feel about disability has been shaped by telethons, by what we might call "the telethon mentality." When I think about Multiple Sclerosis, the first phrase that comes to me is "killer of young adults." When I think about Muscular Dystrophy, it is "Jerry's Kids." Telethons may do some good. They may expose some people to disability. They may raise money for research and charity. They may give attention to people who need it. But they also isolate people with disabilities as victims, as subjects of charity, as a "thing" to be considered annually when their group's time comes to appear on TV. While disability advocates continue to insist that we want to be integrated into a society organized to allow us access to all its avenues, telethons continue to segregate us as a population to be pitied, to be identified as distinct, and to be helped. The truth about telethons is that they are mechanisms of segregation. The truth about accessibility is that it is a mechanism of integration.

The long-winded point of this essay is that it is time for us to stop being victims. It is time for us to stop being ruled by our diseases, our impairments, our limitations. It is time for us to stop being ruled by our disabilities. It is time for us to control our lives, our environments, ourselves. It is time for us to control our disabilities. It is time for us to make telethons and "the telethon mentality" a thing of the past. It is time."

(From Volume VII, Summer/Fall 1985 OKLAHOMA COALITION OF CITIZENS WITH DISABILITIES NEWSLETTER, 4–5)

"Telethons have generated great controversy for the past decade or so. Entertainer Jerry Lewis has become the focal point of this conflict. Best known for his comedy routines and slapstick movie roles, Lewis has been identified with the Muscular Dystrophy Association (MDA) for many years. The MDA has sponsored an annual telethon during the Labor Day weekend since 1981. Each year Lewis takes the opportunity to write an article about MDA in PARADE magazine which is distributed with many Sunday papers. Lewis' articles have tended to bemoan the plight of children who have Muscular Dystrophy and to include pleas to support "his children," some of whom are almost as old as he is.

Several years ago Lewis spent some time in a wheelchair to see what it was like. He wrote about his experiences in PARADE. His comments were so disparaging that two advocates with Muscular Dystrophy formed a group called, "Jerry's Orphans," to sponsor annual Labor Day weekend demonstrations to protest Lewis' demeaning approach to disability.

The two combatants have waged a public battle, which led to a 1993 article in VANITY FAIR magazine characterizing Lewis' personality and the substance of the issues involved. In the article, Paul Longmore, a historian with a disability known for his studies of the media and telethons, described the impact of telethons on the American public.

> Four major telethons—Easter Seals, the Arthritis Foundation, United Cerebral Palsy, and the M.D.A.— are the single most powerful cultural mechanism defining the public identities of people with disabilities in our society today, mainly because they reach so many people. . . . The telethon sponsors claim that, collectively, they have a combined audience of 250 million people.
>
> That's the equivalent of the population of this country. The message of telethons is that whatever condition people with disabilities have, that condition has essentially spoiled their lives, and the only way to correct that is to cure them. The message of the disability-rights movement is that it's possible to be a whole person with a disability.

The final two sentences of Longmore's analysis form a precise description of the models of charity and celebration of disability that have emerged in the late twentieth century. The most comprehensive assessment of the charity mentality comes from an English photographer with a disability, David Hevey. In his 1992 book, THE CREATURES TIME FORGOT, Hevey exposes charities as the most visible appendage of what he calls the "disability industry." Hevey contends that charities have created a hegemony, an almost complete dominance, of what the public perceives as the one voice of people with disabilities. But in reality, disabled people wait at the end of the line of the disability industry's priorities.

Foremost among any charity's goals are survival and ensuring that those individuals who contribute to the agency's success feel good about themselves. This can be accomplished by attaining the dual objectives of raising money for the organization and determining how to distribute it to the organization's needy clientele.

One result of this model [is] that the needs of the charity, or disability industry, must come before all other concerns. A more invidious consequence is that the only way charities and their ilk can continue to exist and to feel good about their selfless contributions to those less fortunate than themselves is to have a perpetual supply of victims of disability's tragic ravages." . . .

In 1999, the biggest problem I have with telethons of any kind continues to be that they promote segregation, not integration. It is long beyond time to be rid of telethons. Since they are not going away, I can only suggest the next best thing: do whatever you can to oppose them, including not sending money to any of them! If you want to make a charitable donation, find another way to do it. Let's give telethons a simple message: GO AWAY.

Source: Brown, Steven. 1999. *Institute on Disability Culture Manifesto.* Available at: http://www.dimenet.com/disculture/archive.php?mode=A&id=18

▣ Emma Morgan, "Attention Deficit Disorder" (1996)

In this ironically entitled poem, the disabled poet Emma Morgan demonstrates how attention deficit disorder (ADD) proves a reasonable response to the chaotic backdrop of world events in the mid-1990s. Rather than portraying her own mental state and tendency to shift from activity to activity as a liability, the poem helps readers recognize ADD as a viable mode of attention that allows the narrator to sift through seemingly insignificant details in order to highlight their overlooked importance.

In my world of mental anarchy
The task "to clean the house"
Breaks into ten
And ten again
Like a seven breaking into two and five
One and six then three and four
Each another sum of parts
So that I might wash a dish
Dust three shelves
Read one page
And return a phone call
Before I finally settle
Into sweeping half the stairs
Or scouring one sink
With a ferocity of purpose.

When you speak to me
of Russian borders rearranging—
your hair-do
the glimmer of your nail polish
the dream I had last night
and one pattern on the wallpaper

at your back
vie for my attention
like a class of eager children
sliding off their seats
with the sheer potency of right answers
Your world of global puzzles
Loses me in a grand collage of universes
Each the size of the pen cap
Held between your teeth
But give me just your shoe
Or one braided lace
To you a detail—
To me a world of six strands
Each a set of threads
The tension of the weave precise
And I can see what isn't visible to you

You couldn't stand to pay attention
In that small world
Snaking through the eyelets of your shoe

I dismiss the boundaries

Of minute, hour, day
Until there's only task—
Task so focused it becomes world

My mind a sheet of paper
Folded in on itself
And again
Until it becomes a crane
A Moor on horseback
Or a hummingbird
Poised on the lip of a blossom
Balanced on a stillness
Built of motion

Source: Morgan, Emma. 1996. "Attention Deficit Disorder." Available at: http://www.realityengineering.org/poetrycastle/viewthread.php?fid=143&tid=1826&action=printable

Michael Bérubé, from *Life as We Know It: A Father, a Family, and an Exceptional Child* (1996)

This essay on the birth of the author's son, Jamie, with Down syndrome reinterprets the meaning of a pathologized genetic condition as valued difference. Employing arguments from evolutionary biology, civil rights politics, and science fiction film, Bérubé rejects a pitying or patronizing attitude in order to reclaim the social context for almost a half million people in the United States.

There has never been a better time to be born with Down syndrome—and that's really saying something, since Down syndrome appears to have been with us for ten million years or more. How do we know? Because in the 1970s, Down syndrome was reported in gorillas and chimpanzees. Since there's no chance that we humans "gave" Down syndrome to other primate species, it would seem that trisomy 21 has been an integral part of being "human" ever since our evolutionary tree split off from that of apes. Cro-Magnons and Neanderthals had babies with Down syndrome; even those ape-men and ape-women in the opening scene of Stanley Kubrick's *2001: A Space Odyssey*—they had kids with Down syndrome, too. For whatever reason, we've produced offspring with Down syndrome with remarkable regularity at every point in our history as hominids—even though it's a genetic anomaly that's not transmitted hereditarily (except in extremely rare instances) and has no obvious survival value. The statistical incidence of Down's in the current human population is no less staggering; there may be almost half a million people with Down's in the United States alone, or just about one on every other street corner.

But although *Homo sapiens* and all our hominid forebears have always experienced some difficulty dividing our chromosomes properly, Down syndrome was not identified and named until 1866, when British physician J. Langdon Down diagnosed it as "mongolism" (because it produced children with almond- shaped eyes reminiscent, to at least one nineteenth- century British mind, of Central Asian faces). At the time, the average life expectancy of children with Down's was under ten. And for a hundred years

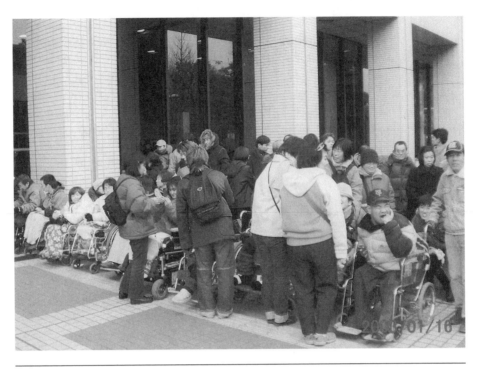

Japanese protesters with wheelchair barricade, 2004.

Source: Photo by Nagase Osamu.

thereafter—during which the discovery of antibiotics lengthened the lifespan of Down's kids to around twenty—Down syndrome was known as "mongoloid idiocy."

The 1980 edition of my college genetics textbook, *The Science of Genetics: An Introduction to Heredity,* opens its segment on Down's with the words, "An important and tragic instance of trisomy in humans involves Down's Syndrome, or mongoloid idiocy." It includes a picture of a toddler-age mongoloid idiot along with a cellular photograph of his chromosomes (called a "karyotype") and the completely erroneous information that most people with Down's have IQs in the low 40s. The presentation is objective, dispassionate, and strictly "factual," as it should be in a college textbook. But reading it again in 1991, I began to wonder: is there a connection between the official textual representation of Down syndrome in medical discourses (including college textbooks) and the social policies by which people with Down syndrome are understood and misunderstood?

You bet your life there is. Now, anyone who's paid attention to the "political correctness" wars on American campuses knows how stupid the academic left can be. We're always talking about language instead of reality, whining about "lookism" and "differently abled persons" instead of changing the world the way the real he-man left used to do. But you know, there really is a difference between calling someone a "mongoloid idiot" and calling him or her "a person with Down syndrome." There's even a difference between calling people "retarded" and calling them "delayed." These words may appear to mean the same damn thing when you look them up in Webster's, but I remember full well from my days as an American male adolescent that I never taunted my peers by calling them "delayed." Even for those of us who were shocked at the frequency with which "homo" and "nigger" were thrown around in our fancy Catholic high school, "retard" aroused no comment, no protest. In other words, a retarded person is just a retard. But *delayed* persons will get where they're going eventually, if you'll only have some patience with them. (Pp. 25–26)

In retrospect, it's beginning to look as if many of the developmental deficits attributed to Down syndrome could instead be attributed to institutionalization. Of course, the phrase "mongoloid idiocy," and its attendant policies, did not cause Down syndrome. But words and phrases are the devices by which we beings signify what homosexuality, or Down syndrome, or anything else, will mean. There surely were, and are, the most intimate possible relations between the language in which we spoke of Down's and the social practices by which we understood it—and refused to understand it. You don't have to be a poststructuralist or a postmodernist or a post-*anything* to get this; all you have to do is meet a parent of a child with Down syndrome. Not long ago, we lived next door to people whose youngest child had Down's. After James was born, they told us of going to the library to find out more about their baby's prospects and wading through page after page of outdated information, ignorant generalizations, and pictures of people with Down's in mental institutions, face down in their feeding trays. These parents demanded the library get some better material on Down syndrome and throw out the garbage. [This garbage] has had its effects *for generations.* It may look to you like it's only words, but perhaps the fragile neonates whose lives were impeded by the policies—and conditions—of institutionalization can testify in some celestial court to the power of mere language, to the intimate links between words and social policies.

Some of my friends tell me this sounds too much like "strict social constructionism"—that is, too much like the proposition that culture is everything and biology is only what we decide to make (of) it. But although James is pretty solid proof that human biology exists independent of our understanding of it, every morning when he gets up, smiling and babbling to his family, I can see for myself how much of his life depends on our social practices. On one of those mornings I turned to my mother-in-law and said, "He's always so full of mischief, he's always so glad to see us—the only thought I can't face is the idea of this little guy waking up each day in a state mental hospital." To which my mother-in-law replied, "Well, Michael, if he were waking up every day in a state mental hospital, he wouldn't *be* this little guy."

As it happens, my mother-in-law doesn't subscribe to any strict social constructionist newsletters; she was just passing along what she took to be good common sense. But every so often I wonder how common that sense really is. Every ten minutes we hear that the genetic basis of something has been "discovered," and we rush madly to the newsweeklies: disease is genetic! Homosexuality is genetic! Infidelity, addiction, adventurousness, obsession with mystery novels—all genetic! The discourses of genetics and inheritance, it would seem, bring out the hidden determinist in more

of us than will admit it. Sure, there's a baseline sense in which our genes "determine" who we are. We can't play the tune unless the score is written down somewhere in the genome. But one does not need or require a biochemical explanation for literary taste, or voguing, or faithless lovers. In these as in all things human, including Down's, the genome is but a template for a vaster and more significant range of social and historical variation. That's true even from human attributes that are clearly more "biological" than voguing and reading. Figuring out even the most rudimentary of relations between the genome and the immune system (something of great relevance to us wheezing asthmatics) involves so many trillions of variables that a decent answer will win you an all-expense-paid trip to Stockholm. Nor can you predict allergic reactions from the genes alone: because the body's immune system takes a few years to go on-line, your environmental variables (from dioxin to cat dander) are very likely going to be more important to you than most hereditary "constants" you care to name.

Yet even if you don't think that biology is destiny, and even if you don't believe evolution follows any plan, there's still something very seductive about the thought that Down syndrome wouldn't have been so prevalent in humans for so long without good reason. Indeed, there are days when, despite everything I know and profess, I catch myself believing that people with Down syndrome are here for a specific purpose—perhaps to teach us patience, or humility, or compassion, or mere joy. A great deal can go wrong with us *in utero,* but under the heading of what goes wrong, Down syndrome is among the most basic, the most fundamental, the most common, *and* the most innocuous, leavening the species with children who are somewhat slower, and usually somewhat gentler, than the rest of the human brood. It speaks to us strongly of design—if design govern in a thing so small. (Pp. 32–35)

Source: Bérubé, Michael. 1996. *Life as We Know It: A Father, a Family, and an Exceptional Child.* New York: Random House. Copyright © 1996 by Michael Bérubé. Used by permission of Pantheon Books, a division of Random House, Inc.

▣ European Union Disability Policy (1997)

The European Union's disability policy has gradually shifted from one that emphasizes disability as an individual trauma of adjustment to that of socially created barriers that inhibit disabled people's participation in society. In particular, the barriers identified here are identified as economic and attitudinal in nature. These obstacles affect the quality of life experienced by disabled people in their daily lives.

THE COUNCIL OF THE EUROPEAN UNION AND THE REPRESENTATIVES OF THE GOVERNMENTS OF THE MEMBER STATES MEETING WITHIN THE COUNCIL,

Whereas the Commission has issued a communication entitled 'Equality of opportunity for people with disabilities—A new European Community disability strategy';

Whereas people with disabilities constitute a significant proportion of the population of the Community and, as a group, they face a wide range of obstacles which prevent them from achieving equal opportunities, independence and full economic and social integration;

Whereas respect for human rights is a fundamental value of the Member States which is underlined in Article F.2 of the Treaty on European Union;

Whereas the principle of equality of opportunity for all, including people with disabilities, represents a core value shared by all Member States; whereas this implies the elimination of negative discrimination against people with disabilities and improving their quality of life; and whereas access to mainstream education and training, where appropriate, can play an important role in successful integration in economic and social life;

Whereas the Community charter on the fundamental social rights of workers, adopted at the European Council in Strasbourg on 9 December 1989 by the Heads of State or Government of 11 Member States, proclaims inter alia, in point 26:

'26. All disabled persons, whatever the origin and nature of their disability, must be entitled to additional concrete measures aimed at improving their social and professional integration.

These measures must concern, in particular, according to the capacities of the beneficiaries, vocational training, ergonomics, accessibility, mobility, means of transport and housing';

Whereas in its recommendation of 24 July 1986 on the employment of disabled people in the Community (1) the Council recommended Member States to take all appropriate measures to promote fair opportunities for disabled people in the field of employment and vocational training including initial training and employment as well as rehabilitation and resettlement;

Whereas the free movement of persons must be ensured in accordance with the existing Community legislation for the benefit of all the citizens of the European Union, including those with disabilities and those who are responsible for people with disabilities;

Whereas the overall purpose of the United Nations Standard Rules on the Equalization of Opportunities for Persons with Disabilities, adopted by the General Assembly on 20 December 1993 (2) is to ensure that all people with disabilities may exercise the same rights and obligations as others;

Whereas these Rules call for action at all levels both within States as well as through international cooperation to promote the principle of equality of opportunity for people with disabilities;

Whereas in its White Paper 'European social policy—a way forward for the Union,' adopted on 27 July 1994, the Commission indicated that it intended to prepare an appropriate instrument endorsing the principles of the United Nations Standard Rules on the Equalization of Opportunities for Persons with Disabilities;

Whereas, while responsibility in this field lies with the Member States, the European Community can make a contribution in fostering cooperation between Member States and in encouraging the exchange and development of best practice in the Community and within the policies and activities of the Community institutions and organs themselves;

Whereas the aims set out in this resolution on the equalization of opportunities for people with disabilities and the ending of negative discrimination are without prejudice to the right of each Member State to lay down its own rules and provisions for achieving the said aims, in accordance with the principle of subsidiarity and to the full extent that the resources of society permit:

I. REAFFIRM THEIR COMMITMENT TO:

1. the principles and values that underline the United Nations Standard Rules on the Equalization of Opportunities for Persons with Disabilities;

2. the ideas underlying the Council of Europe's resolution of 9 April 1992 on a coherent policy for the rehabilitation of people with disabilities;

3. the principle of equality of opportunity in the development of comprehensive policies in the field of disability, and

4. the principle of avoiding or eliminating any form of negative discrimination on the sole grounds of disability.

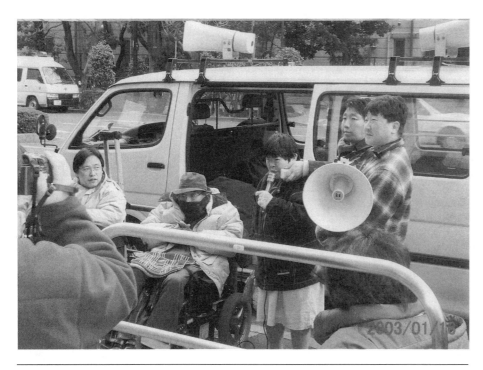

Japanese protest organizers preparing for press conference, 2004.

Source: Photo by Nagase Osamu.

II. CALL ON MEMBER STATES:

1. to consider if relevant national policies take into account, in particular, the following orientations:

- empowering people with disabilities for participation in society, including the severely disabled, while paying due attention to the needs and interests of their families and carers,
- mainstreaming the disability perspective into all relevant sectors of policy formulation,
- enabling people with disabilities to participate fully in society by removing barriers,
- nurturing public opinion to be receptive to the abilities of people with disabilities and toward strategies based on equal opportunities;

2. to promote the involvement of representatives of people with disabilities in the implementation and follow-up of relevant policies and actions in their favour.

III. INVITE THE COMMISSION:

1. to take account, where appropriate, and within the provisions of the Treaty, of the principles set out in this resolution in any relevant proposal it submits on Community legislation, programmes or initiatives;

2. to promote—in collaboration with the Member States and with non-governmental organizations of and for people with disabilities—the exchange of useful information and experience especially concerning innovative policies and good practice;

3. to submit periodic reports to the European Parliament, the Council, the Economic and Social Committee and the Committee of the Regions on the basis of information supplied by the Member States, describing the progress made and the obstacles encountered in implementing this resolution;

4. to take account of the results of the evaluation of the Helios II programme when considering whether it would be appropriate to bring forward proposals for follow up.

IV. INVITE OTHER COMMUNITY INSTITUTIONS AND ORGANS:

to contribute to the realization of the aforementioned principles in the framework of their own policies and activities.

(1) OJ No L 225, 12. 8. 1986, p. 43.

(2) United Nations General Assembly Resolution 48/46 of 20 December 1993.

Source: European Council. 1997. Resolution of the Council and of the Representatives of the Governments of the Member States meeting within the Council of 20 December 1996 on Equality of Opportunity for People with Disabilities. *Official Journal C 012* (January 13), pp. 0001–0002.

▣ Not Dead Yet

Organized in 1996 to oppose a lethal resurgence of physician-assisted suicide campaigns, Not Dead Yet began to publicly protest efforts by various factions to legalize the right to die. These efforts particularly came in the wake of some people's unwillingness to prosecute Jack Kevorkian, who devised a "suicide machine" used to end the life of those with "terminal illness." However, the group's research successfully demonstrated that such a justification both was false—Kevorkian assisted in the suicides of many individuals with nonterminal illnesses—and cultivated

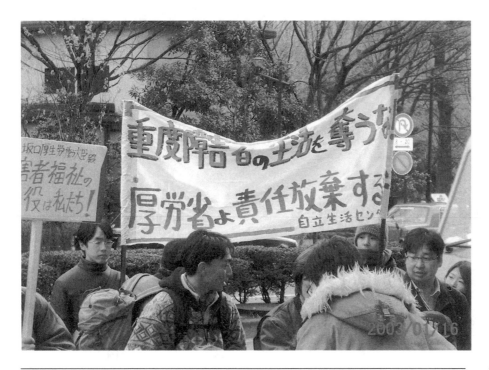

Japanese protest banner, 2004.

Source: Photo by Nagase Osamu.

a lethal atmosphere for all disabled people in the country. In recent years, the movement has also made public protests against other "pro-death" perspectives, such as Clint Eastwood's film Million Dollar Baby, *and during the court-ordered death of Terry Schiavo. For more information, contact: Not Dead Yet, 7521 Madison Street, Forest Park, IL; phone (708) 209–1500; fax: (708) 209–1735; website: www.notdeadyet.org.*

Not Dead Yet is a national grassroots organization of people with disabilities formed in response to the increasing threat of legalized physician assisted suicide and euthanasia in the United States and around the world. Not Dead Yet's mission is to advocate against legalization of physician assisted suicide, active euthanasia, and non-voluntary withholding of life-sustaining medical treatment. Not Dead Yet works to bring a disability-rights perspective to the public policy debate, and an awareness of the effects of disability discrimination in the health care system and society overall.

Formed in 1996, Not Dead Yet has worked to educate, support, coordinate and lead the disability community's effort to stop the so-called "right to die" from becoming a duty to die or a right to kill. To date, eleven other national disability groups have adopted

formal positions against assisted suicide. Twenty-six national disability organizations supported Not Dead Yet's opposition to the starvation and dehydration of Terri Schiavo based on the lack of clear and convincing evidence of her wishes.

Not Dead Yet grassroots members have undertaken specific activities in the name of the organization and in support of its mission in at least 30 states, and conducted national actions targeting Jack Kevorkian, Princeton Professor Peter Singer, the Hemlock Society, and the World Federation of Right To Die Societies. Over 500 Not Dead Yet members rallied at the U.S. Supreme Court in 1997 to oppose a constitutional right to assisted suicide. Not Dead Yet's amicus brief filed in the U.S. Supreme Court in the case of *Vacco v. Quill* was among a handful, out of over 60 such briefs, cited by the High Court in its final opinion. Not Dead Yet has also led in the filing of disability rights briefs in several other cases, including but not limited to the Conservatorship of the Person of Robert Wendland in the California Supreme Court (2000), three briefs in the Guardianship of Theresa Marie Schiavo (Florida and federal courts, 2002–2003), and *Oregon v. Ashcroft* (Ninth Cir. 2002). Not Dead Yet has also given invited testimony three times before the U.S. Congress, and its leaders have appeared on over twenty national television news and talk show broadcasts.

Reprinted by permission.

◻ Stephen Kuusisto, from "Harvest" (1997)

In "Harvest," visually impaired poet Stephen Kuusisto captures his own way of seeing as part of the pleasure of living in a visual world that is not distorted by his vision but enhanced.

My temporal task is to hear music,
drink a cup of chrysanthemum tea,
admire the white moon of the morning,
even if my eyes tell me there are two moons.

Source: Kuusisto, Stephen. 1997. "Harvest." In Fries, Kenny, ed. *Staring Back: The Disability Experience from the Inside Out.* New York: Plume Books. Reprinted by permission.

▣ Judi Chamberlin, from "Confessions of a Noncompliant Patient" (1998)

Nearly 30 years after the release of her landmark work On Our Own, *Judi Chamberlin continues to write about psychiatric survivorship and resistance to the psychiatric system. This is the closing paragraph of her 1998 article "Confessions of a Noncompliant Patient."*

Let us celebrate the spirit of noncompliance that is the self struggling to survive. Let us celebrate the unbowed head, the heart that still dreams, the voice that refuses to be silent. I wish I could show you the picture that hangs on my office wall that inspires me every day, a drawing by Tanya Temkin, a wonderful artist and psychiatric survivor activist. In a gloomy and barred room, a group of women sit slumped in defeat, dressed in rags, while on the opposite wall their shadows, upright, with raised arms and wild hair and clenched fists, dance the triumphant dance of the spirit that will not die.

Source: Chamberlin, Judi. 1998. P. 52 in "Confessions of a Noncompliant Patient." *Journal of Psychosocial Nursing and Mental Health Services* 36(4):49–52. Printed with permission from Slack, Inc.

▣ Sally Clay, "People Who" (1998)

This poem was read during the Million Mad March on May 2, 1998. Held in Washington, D.C., the march coincided with an International Day of Madness, creating an opportunity for psychiatric consumers/survivors to raise their voices and increase their visibility.

Those people lock the door before us
And stay on the other side.
They inject us with poison
And electrocute our soul.

They are those who hold the keys
And pull all the strings.

Those people take our money
And use it to build prisons.
They go home at night to suburban houses
Where we are not allowed to live.

We the people are People Who
Are cherished by none
Except our own.

Our feet move to the beat of free verse,
And our souls sing in silent places.
Warm blood flows through invisible hearts
That can't be treated.

We are not puppets, there are no strings attached.
We cut the cord and walk through open doors.

We are People Who
Leap and dare to imagine.
We spend our talent
Furnishing the place of hope.
We are people who will treat those others
By acting out, and dreaming.

Those people are People Who
Are our own.
We are people who
Also care for them.

Source: Clay, Sally. 1998. "People Who." Available at: http://home.earthlink.net/~sallyclay/z.poems/peoplewho.html. Reprinted by permission of Sally Clay.

▣ The Developmental Disabilities Assistance and Bill of Rights Act of 2000 (United States)

This act, P.L. 106–402, is the 2000 reauthorization of the original act (P.L. 95–602); it is significant in being the first introduction (in statutory terms) of the term developmental disabilities (DD). The general intent was (and largely remains) to fill in the gap on services, policy, and planning for DD populations. The national network of state DD Councils, Protection and Advocacy agencies, and University Centers for Excellence are funded under DD Act authorization.

Developmental Disability

(A) In General
The term "developmental disability" means a severe, chronic disability of an individual that—

(i) is attributable to a mental or physical impairment or combination of mental and physical impairments;

(ii) is manifested before the individual attains age 22;

(iii) is likely to continue indefinitely;

(iv) results in substantial functional limitations in 3 or more of the following areas of major life activity:

(I) Self-care.
(II) Receptive and expressive language.
(III) Learning.
(IV) Mobility.
(V) Self-direction.
(VI) Capacity for independent living.
(VII) Economic self-sufficiency; and

(v) reflects the individual's need for a combination and sequence of special, interdisciplinary, or generic services, individualized supports, or other forms of assistance that are of lifelong or extended duration and are individually planned and coordinated.

114 Stat. 1684 P.L. 106–402 (2000).

◙ Jim Ferris, "Poems with Disabilities" (2000)

The Americans with Disabilities Act signaled a change in awareness of people with disabilities in the United States. Wheelchair-accessible parking spaces and bathroom stalls became more common, and resentment toward disabled people often was expressed in absurd jokes about extreme accommodations. This poem spoofs those jokes and the attitudes that spawn them while suggesting that disabled people are deserving of prominent places in the American scene.

I'm sorry—this space is reserved
For poems with disabilities. I know
It's one of the best spaces in the book,
But the Poems with Disabilities Act
Requires us to make reasonable
Accommodations for poems that aren't
Normal. There is a nice space just
A few pages over—in fact (don't
Tell anyone) I think it's better
Than this one. I myself prefer it.
Actually I don't see any of those

Poems right now myself, but you never know
When one might show up, so we have to keep
This space open. You can't always tell
Just from looking at them, either. Sometimes
They'll look just like a regular poem
When they roll in—you're reading along
And suddenly everything
Changes, the world tilts
A little, angle of vision
Jumps, focus
Shifts. You remember
Your aunt died of cancer at just your age
And maybe yesterday's twinge means
Something after all. Your sloppy,
Fragile heart beats
A little faster
And then you know.
You just know.
And the poem is right
Where it
belongs.

Source: Ferris, Jim. 2000. "Poems with Disabilities." *Ragged Edge Online* (March/April). Available at: http://www.raggededge magazine .com/0300/b0300poem.htm. Reprinted by permission.

◙ *Parade* by Susan Nussbaum (2000)

In this dramatic satire, Susan Nussbaum takes on critical disability issues such as physician-assisted suicide and medical health care rationing. The work establishes the imperative of normative "good" health as an oppressive expectation for disabled people in late twentieth-century United States.
Two disabled women enter.

One   Glad we got here early.
Two   Mmm. Wanna get good spots.
One   Because why go to the trouble if you can't see everything.
Two   No, I agree. This is—you know, we'll be able to see the whole—
One   We won't miss a thing.
Pause while they look through their binoculars.
Two   So it's just us?
One   What? No, Jeanette couldn't come.
Two   She just couldn't make it, huh?
One   No, she wasn't—

Two Feeling well?

One She wasn't feeling—she's fine but she wasn't feeling—

Two Up to it?

One Right. I don't know. Well, she's caught in that cycle of—

Two Yeah.

One Oh, well.

Two It happens.

One Anyway, I'm glad we're here.

Two Yeah. Can I say something?

One What?

Two I don't want to sound—jumping the gun—but—and I don't want to—she has an aura of—I just don't like being with her. I like her, don't—I'm not saying I don't respect her.

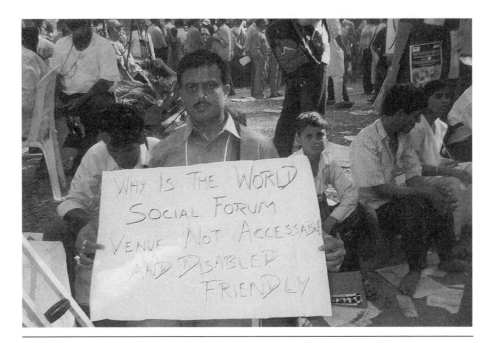

Disability protester at the 2004 World Social Forum in Mumbai, India, holding sign stating that the venue was not accessible to disabled participants.

Source: Photo by Meenu Bhambhani.

One Well, there's a difference between liking and spending time with. I like her, too, but she doesn't—I don't know . . .

Two Take care of herself.

One She doesn't take care of herself.

Two And, you know, what does that say about her? Between the two of us. It reflects back.

One I'm glad you said it, and not me. Really, thank you.

Two It can have the effect of making *us* look—like we're . . .

One No, I know. Is it wrong to be aware of the effect of how it looks to be with people who, for whatever reason, don't have a *consciousness* about what's— about priorities—the things *we* feel are important? I don't think so.

Two I'm sick of feeling guilty about it.

One Me, too! Exactly!

Beat.

Two But you look well.

One Thank you. Thanks. I am well. I feel good. What about you? How's your quality of life?

Two Very high, thanks. I've been moving up in the point range.

One Good for you. Where—do you mind if I ask—where on the scale?

Two I was a four, now I'm a five.

One You're kidding. What did you do? I mean, what'd you—?

Two I've been contributing a lot lately. Which makes me feel great and which you have to feel great in order to do! A vicious cycle. But not *vicious,* just cyclical.

One A whole point just for contributing. No, but that's great. From four to five.

Two It's a good feeling.

One Mm hmm.

Two So. What're you these days?

One Me? I'm a seven.

Two Whoa. That's—I thought I was in good shape. You're a seven?

One Yup. You know, because I don't lose credit for burdening.

Two Individual or collective?

One Oh, I was an individual burden. What about you?

Two Oh, same old. I'm a burden to several individuals and society as a whole.

One Actually, I wasn't really a burden, but my mom needed the extra credit for caretaking, so she claimed me as a burden. So, technically—

Two Officially, you were a burden.

One Uh huh.

Two Is that legal? For your mom to—?

One   What? Yeah. Well, pretty much. I mean . . .

Two   So—your mom needed the extra points . . .

One   Before she was kevorked, yeah.

Two   Huh.

One   What? It's not like we were making *money* off it. It's not like we're Point Scalpers, or anything.

Two   No, I know. I mean, it's not like you were *selling* your mom the extra credit. Which, far be it from me—I'd do the same thing, except my mom was liberated in one of the early Ethical Life Rationings. So, you know . . .

One   You must be proud.

Two   Oh, yeah. She was a great example. She was very unselfish.

One   How old was she?

Two   Sixty.

One   Well, that's the age.

Two   Yeah.

One   That's when my mom's quality of life scale started dropping. And after she broke her hip and became a burden to society herself, it just got to the point where her safeguards were really, you know, in the toilet, and finally she just said forget it and got liberated.

Two   That's show biz.

Beat.

Well, at least you got that extra point back.

One   Yeah, I'm happy about that. Let's face it, I needed the point. I'm still a collective burden.

Two   Well, who isn't? The collective burden stuff is killing me. So to speak. Ha ha.

One   I know. It's not so much the environmental category as the cosmetic. It's an automatic two points off the quality of life scale to be born this way.

Two   Sure. Plus, the extra points off as you grow out of childhood. Losing the cuteness credits.

One   Well, the kids are cuter.

Two   Yeah, they get those little wheelchairs . . .

One   Remember those telethons they used to have? With the kids?

Two   Yeah, and people would actually give money, right? They would donate all this—

One   Oh, yeah, they'd raise millions and millions of dollars and—

Two   Hundreds of millions of—

One   God, I wonder what ever happened to all that money.

Two   No one knows.

Beat.

One   And what happened to that guy? The—you know—the telethon guy?

Two   Murdered.

One   Oh, right, yeah. That real gruesome—

Two   Yeah. Anyway, it's weird, because for me, I lose a point and a half for—you know, the sight of me makes people—feel agitated—

One   So do I.

Two   Wait. You lose points in addition to the—

One   Right. Public Physical Appropriateness Ratio. Minus one point five.

Two   I'm surprised we're the same.

One   1.5's pretty standard. I mean, we probably upset people about the same amount.

Two   I guess. I get a .3 credit, though.

One   How come?

Two   For being a visual reminder to wear seat-belts. So . . .

One   Wow, that's a—lucky girl. Hey, look, that guy must be in the parade.

Two   Where? That guy?

One   Yeah, in the Eskimo outfit.

Two   Oh, right. The Eskimo float.

One   Do they still do that?

Two   What?

One   Walk out into glaciers and stuff when they're too old to be useful?

Two   I don't think there're very many of 'em left to do that. They die the regular way, I think. They just have an Eskimo thing in the parade as a, like a symbol . . .

One   Like an example . . .

Two   Yeah, like a nostalgia thing.

One   Hey, heads up. There's a doctor.

Two   Where?

One   There! There! Jesus, he's walking right toward us!

Two   Oh, shit! (*calls out*) Hello, Doctor! How's your quality of life today?

One   Beautiful day for the parade, Doctor!

Two   Fine, thank you! High quality today, Doctor! Feeling like a full ten today!

One   I feel like a twelve, Doctor!

Two   Who needs safeguards on a day like today!

One   Enjoy the parade, Doctor!

Two   Viva Voluntary Self-elimination!

They salute as Doctor passes.

One   Doctors make me nervous.

Two   Tell me about it.

One   Yeah. Hey look, there's the Global Insurance Corporation float! What—can you see what the banner says?

They take out their binoculars.

Two   "Better Dead Than Sick in Bed."

One   Oh, uh huh. Boy, I guess it's really starting now.

Two   Yeah, here goes. There's supposed to be some new stuff this year. New floats.

One   Well, new legislation. So, naturally. I—you know, I do feel kind of bad Jeanette couldn't make it.

Two   I know. Even though she drives me crazy, it's not like I don't kind of miss her.

One   Not that I think she—I mean, she's *fine*—

Two   Right. She's doing fine, she's—she's not feeling well for one *day,* it's not the end of—

One   No, it's not.

Two   Which is all it is. Right?

One   I told her she had to take *care* of herself better. Get her points up.

Two   Name of the game.

Beat.

They look through binoculars.

Two   Look, the Doctor's float is passing. I like their new uniforms, don't you?

One   Oh, absolutely, I love leather. I wonder if my doctor's up there.

Two   Mine is. He's real patriotic.

One   Didn't your doctor write that book? That real famous—what's it called?

Two   "The Depression Myth: No Excuses."

One   Right. He's really a hardliner, I guess.

Two   Let's just say I better not get a bad case of the flu.

One   Hey, remember that time we were—the three of us—you, me and Jeanette—and we were at that concert—and—god, remember that song?—about how ethical life rationing was this forced thing—

Two   And the police came and stopped the concert and Jeanette wouldn't—

One   Yeah, she refused to leave and she started shouting and stuff and—

Two   She was chanting—wait, what was it—I don't know, something really—

One   Right, right. The Supreme Court are Hit Men, that kind of—

Two   She was always a radical.

One   It's turns people off to say the Supreme Court are hit men. People don't wanna hear that.

Two   I don't wanna hear it.

One   Too extreme.

Two   Way out there.

Beat.

They look through their binoculars.

One   There's the Afterlife float. Wow. Pretty.

Two   They must spend a lot of money on that one.

One   Mmm. Well, they have it. Afterlife Industry is huge. Wow. The Afterlife must really be fantastic.

Two   You can see why people look forward to it.

One   You know, in ancient Egypt, the pharoahs would be buried with all their earthly posessions, like gold and stuff.

Two   I know. It's amazing the stuff people believe in.

One   Really.

They look through binocs.

Two   Ooh, look at that float. That's beautiful. Someone must've spent ages blowing up all those latex exam gloves.

One   Where? Oh, the Preventive Chronic Care Float. Yeah. That's new this year. I read all about it in the Liberation newsletter.

Two   Look, it's so big they had to have two floats.

One   Huh? Oh, no, the second float is for the surpluses.

Two   What?

One   You know, the surplus people.

Two   Oh, yeah. That's a new thing this year. You know, some of those people don't even look sick.

One   Oh, well, you don't have to be sick anymore. To be euthanized.

Two   What? But—

One   Well, that's the preventive part. Because they found out you can sort of predict who's gonna get sick, how much it'll cost, and you know, that kinda thing.

Two   They can predict? Boy, it's amazing what they can—

One   Uh huh. Like people from a lower income brackett, who don't have insurance—

Two   They don't take very good care of themselves—

One   Yeah, so they can predict that those people are gonna be like, Burden City.

Two   Wow.

One   And they put this float at the end of the parade, and after the parade, the deal is all the surplus people go off and get euthanized.

Two   That's why it's at the end. Sort of a *piece de resistance* thing.

One   I mean, there's all these incentives and stuff. Tax breaks for survivors. It's really a good deal for some people. Some of them, they don't have jobs, they don't have skills, so you know.

Two   Their quality of life numbers must stink. I guess, you know, the thing is, if they want to live, they'll do something about their situation. Work on their numbers, try not to burden. Like we did.

They look thru binocs.

Two   Hey, wait. Wait! Look! That's her!

One   What? Who?

Two   Jeanette! She's on that float!

One   Oh my god! What's she—? She said she couldn't come. She said she wouldn't be here. There must be a mistake!

Two   But that's her. Why would she volunteer to be liberated? She doesn't even believe in it.

One   She didn't volunteer! They—Somebody made a mistake! (*calling out*) Hey! Hey! You've got the wrong person up there! Hey!

Two   (under her breath)

Wait! Stop! Are you crazy? If she's up there it's because she's supposed to be up there. Don't make a big thing of it! You're just gonna get yourself—both of us—a lot of attention that we don't need. Just get a grip on yourself. Just calm down.

One   But—

Two   Just shut up!

They look through their binocs.

One   Well, that's it. Parade's over.

Two   Yeah.

One   I'm sorry I—I'm sorry about that outburst.

Two   Well. No harm done.

One   No.

Two   That's the main thing.

One   Right. It came as a surprise. Seeing someone you know makes you think how—it makes you aware of your own—

Two   Yeah, but we're in good shape. Our numbers are up and our safeguards are in place.

Just keep reminding yourself of that.

One   She was always a radical.

Two   That's right. I just didn't want anyone to think you and she were—Everyone is so paranoid these days.

One   We're in good shape.

Two   No, I know. We are.

One   That's right.

Two   So I guess I'll see you.

One   Yeah. Well, this was fun.

Two   It was. The floats were really—

One   They were absolutely—

Two   They were terrif.

One   So, dinner next week, okay?

Two   Sounds good.

One   Okay. Keep your numbers up!

Two   You, too.

One and Two   Viva Voluntary Self-elimination!

Blackout.

▣ From the Charter of Fundamental Rights of the European Union, (2000)

The Charter of Fundamental Rights of the European Union is the result of a unique procedure in the history of the European Union (EU). For the first time, the EU proclaimed the civil, political, economic, and social rights of European citizens and all persons living in the EU. On December 7, 2000, the presidents of the European Parliament, of the Council, and of the Commission signed and proclaimed the Charter on behalf of their institutions in Nice, France.

SOLEMN PROCLAMATION

The European Parliament, the Council and the Commission solemnly proclaim the text below as the Charter of Fundamental Rights of the European Union.

Done at Nice on the seventh day of December in the year two thousand.

PREAMBLE

The peoples of Europe, in creating an ever closer union among them, are resolved to share a peaceful future based on common values.

Conscious of its spiritual and moral heritage, the Union is founded on the indivisible, universal values of human dignity, freedom, equality and solidarity; it is based on the principles of democracy and the rule of law. It places the individual at the heart of its activities, by establishing the citizenship of the Union and by creating an area of freedom, security and justice.

The Union contributes to the preservation and to the development of these common values while respecting the diversity of the cultures and traditions of the peoples of Europe as well as the national identities of the Member States and the organisation of their public authorities at national, regional and local levels; it seeks to promote balanced and sustainable development and ensures free movement of persons, goods, services and capital, and the freedom of establishment.

To this end, it is necessary to strengthen the protection of fundamental rights in the light of changes in society, social progress and scientific and technological developments by making those rights more visible in a Charter.

This Charter reaffirms, with due regard for the powers and tasks of the Community and the Union and the principle of subsidiarity, the rights as they result, in particular, from the constitutional traditions and international obligations common to the Member States, the Treaty on European Union, the Community Treaties, the European Convention for the Protection of Human Rights and Fundamental Freedoms, the Social Charters adopted by the Community and by the Council of Europe and the case-law of the Court of Justice of the European Communities and of the European Court of Human Rights.

Enjoyment of these rights entails responsibilities and duties with regard to other persons, to the human community and to future generations.

The Union therefore recognises the rights, freedoms and principles set out hereafter.

CHAPTER III

EQUALITY

Article 20
Equality before the law
Everyone is equal before the law.

Article 21
Non-discrimination

1. Any discrimination based on any ground such as sex, race, colour, ethnic or social origin, genetic features, language, religion or belief, political or any other opinion, membership of a national minority, property, birth, disability, age or sexual orientation shall be prohibited. . . .

Article 26
Integration of persons with disabilities

The Union recognises and respects the right of persons with disabilities to benefit from measures designed to ensure their independence, social and occupational integration and participation in the life of the community.

Source: Charter of Fundamental Rights of the European Union. 2000. *Official Journal C 364* (December 18), pp. 0001–0022.

▣ Council Decision of 3 December 2001 on the European Year of People with Disabilities 2003 (2001)

The Council Decision is the document that establishes agreement among European countries to hold a year dedicated to the forwarding of the political agenda of disabled people. Full inclusion involves the development of a barrier-free Europe as an ideal of access for all individuals.

THE COUNCIL OF THE EUROPEAN UNION,

Having regard to the Treaty establishing the European Community, and in particular Article 13 thereof,

Having regard to the proposal from the Commission,

Having regard to the opinion of the European Parliament,

Having regard to the opinion of the Economic and Social Committee,

Having regard to the opinion of the Committee of the Regions,

Whereas:

(1) The promotion of a high level of employment and of social protection, and the raising of the standard of living and quality of life of the population of the Member States, are objectives of the European Community.

(2) The Community Charter of the Fundamental Social Rights of Workers recognises the need to take appropriate action for the social and economic integration of disabled people.

(3) The Resolution of the Council and the Ministers for Education, meeting within the Council, of 31 May 1990 concerning integration of children and young people with disabilities into ordinary systems of education stresses that "the Member States have agreed to intensify, where necessary, their efforts to integrate or encourage integration of pupils and students with disabilities, in all appropriate cases, into the ordinary education system."

(4) The Resolution of the Council and of the Representatives of the Governments of the Member States meeting within the Council of 20 December 1996 on equality of opportunity for people with disabilities, and the Council Resolution of 17 June 1999 on equal employment opportunities for people with disabilities, reaffirm the basic human rights of disabled people to equal access to social and economic opportunities.

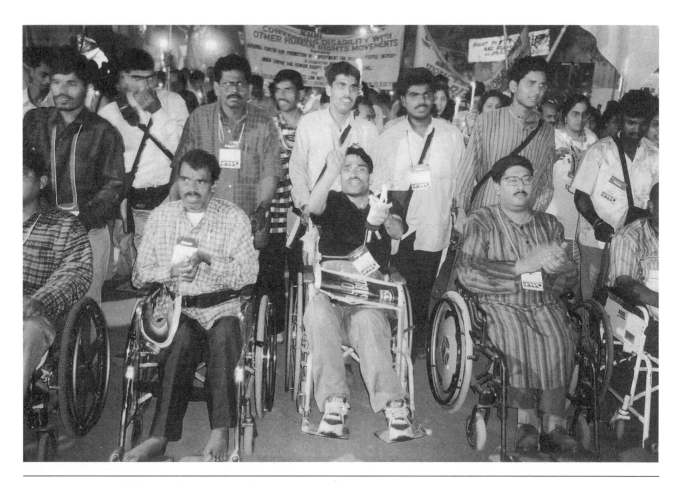

Disability protest at the World Social Forum in Mumbai, India, 2004. Participants from across India shout slogans such as "WSF Shame! Shame!" and "WSF Inaccessible, Inaccessible!"

Source: National Centre for Promotion of Employment for Disabled People, New Delhi, India.

(5) The conclusions of the Lisbon European Council of 23 and 24 March 2000 call upon Member States to take greater account of social exclusion in their employment, education and training, health and housing policies and to define priority actions for specific target groups, such as people with disabilities.

(6) The European social agenda approved by the Nice European Council meeting on 7, 8 and 9 December 2000 states that the European Union will develop, in particular during the European Year of People with Disabilities (2003), "all action intended to bring about the fuller integration of disabled people in all areas of life."

(7) The year 2003 will mark the 10th anniversary of the adoption by the UN General Assembly of the Standard Rules on the Equalisation of Opportunities for Persons with Disabilities, which have enabled considerable progress to be made in an approach to disability in accordance with human rights principles.

(8) This Decision respects fundamental rights and observes the principles recognised in particular by the Charter of Fundamental Rights of the European Union. In particular, this Decision seeks to promote application of the principles of non-discrimination and integration of people with disabilities.

(9) The European Parliament, the Economic and Social Committee and the Committee of the Regions have all urged the Community to strengthen its contribution to efforts in Member States to promote equal opportunities for people with disabilities, with a view to their integration into society.

(10) On 10 May 2000 the Commission adopted a communication entitled "Towards a barrier-free Europe for people with disabilities," in which it commits itself to developing and supporting a comprehensive and integrated strategy to tackle social, architectural and design barriers that unnecessarily restrict access for people with disabilities to social and economic

opportunities. The Parliament has unanimously adopted a similar resolution.

(11) The general framework in favour of equal treatment in employment and occupation provided for by Directive 2000/78/EC and the Community action programme to combat discrimination in order to support and supplement legislative measures at Community and Member State level set up by Decision 2000/ 750/EC aim at changing practices and attitudes by mobilising the players involved and fostering the exchange of information and good practice.

(12) Since exclusion from the labour market of people with disabilities is inextricably linked to problems of attitude and a lack of information about disability, it is necessary to increase society's understanding of the rights, needs and potential of disabled persons, and a joint effort by all the "different partners is required to develop and promote a flow of information and an exchange of good practice.

(13) Raising awareness relies primarily on effective action at Member State level which should be supplemented by concerted efforts at Community level. The European Year could act as a catalyst in raising awareness and in building momentum.

(14) Consistency and complementarity with other Community action is needed, in particular with action to combat discrimination and social exclusion, and to promote human rights, education, training and gender equality.

(15) The joint statement of 20 July 2000 provides for the budget authority to deliver an opinion on whether the new proposals with budgetary implications are compatible with the financial framework, without any reduction in existing policies.

(16) The Agreement on the European Economic Area (EEA Agreement) provides for closer cooperation in the social field between the European Community and its Member States, on the one hand, and the countries of the European Free Trade Association participating in the European Economic Area (EFTA/EEA), on the other. Provision should be made for participation, on the one hand, by the candidate countries of central and eastern Europe, in accordance with the conditions established in the Europe Agreements, in their additional protocols and in the decisions of the respective Association Councils, on the other hand, by Cyprus, Malta and Turkey, funded by additional appropriations in accordance with the procedures to be agreed with those countries.

(17) A financial reference amount within the meaning of paragraph 34 of the Interinstitutional Agreement of 6

May 1999 between the European Parliament, the Council and the Commission on budgetary discipline and improvement of the budgetary procedure is included in this Decision without thereby affecting the powers of the budgetary authority as they are defined by the Treaty.

(18) Since the objectives of the proposed action aimed at generating at European level awareness of the rights of people with disabilities, cannot be adequately achieved by the Member States on account, inter alia, of the need for multilateral partnerships, the transnational exchange of information and the Community-wide dissemination of good practice, and can therefore be better achieved at Community level, the Community may adopt measures, in accordance with the principle of subsidiarity as set out in Article 5 of the Treaty. In accordance with the principle of proportionality, as set out in that Article, this Decision does not go beyond what is necessary to achieve those objectives.

(19) The measures necessary for the implementation of this Decision should be adopted in accordance with Council Decision 1999/468/EC of 28 June 1999 laying down the procedures for the exercise of implementing powers conferred on the Commission,

HAS DECIDED AS FOLLOWS:

Article 1
Establishment of the European Year of People with Disabilities

The year 2003 shall be designated as the "European Year of People with Disabilities."

Article 2
Objectives

The objectives of the European Year of People with Disabilities shall be:

(a) to raise awareness of the rights of people with disabilities to protection against discrimination and to full and equal enjoyment of their rights;

(b) to encourage reflection on and discussion of the measures needed to promote equal opportunities for people with disabilities in Europe;

(c) to promote the exchange of experience of good practice and effective strategies devised at local, national and European level;

(d) to reinforce the cooperation between all parties concerned, namely government, the social partners, NGOs [nongovernmental organizations], the social services, the private sector, communities, voluntary sector groups, people with disabilities and their families;

(e) to improve communication regarding disability and promote a positive image of people with disabilities;

(f) to raise awareness of the heterogeneity of people with disabilities and of the various kinds of disability;

(g) to raise awareness of the multiple discrimination facing people with disabilities;

(h) to pay special attention to awareness of the right of children and young people with disabilities to equality in education, so as to encourage and support their full integration in society and to promote the development of European cooperation between those professionally involved in the education of children and young people with disabilities, in order to improve the integration of pupils and students with special needs in ordinary or specialised establishments and in national and European exchange programmes.

Article 3
Content of measures

1. The measures designed to meet the objectives set out in Article 2 may entail the development or the provision of support to:

(a) meetings and events;

(b) information and promotional campaigns throughout the Member States;

(c) cooperation with broadcasting and media organisations;

(d) surveys and studies on a Community-wide scale;

2. Details of the measures referred to in paragraph 1 are set out in the Annex.

Article 4
Implementation at Community level

The Commission shall ensure the implementation of the Community actions covered by this Decision in conformity with the Annex.

It shall conduct a regular exchange of views with representatives of people with disabilities at Community level on the design, implementation and follow-up of the European Year of People with Disabilities. To that end, the Commission shall make the relevant information available to these representatives. The Commission shall inform the Committee established under Article 6(1) of their opinion.

Article 5
Cooperation and implementation at national level

1. Each Member State shall be responsible for the coordination and implementation at national level of the measures provided for in this Decision, including the selection of projects under Part B of the Annex.

To this end, each Member State shall establish or designate a national coordinating body or an equivalent body to organise the participation of the Member State in the European Year of People with Disabilities. This body shall ensure that it is representative of a range of organisations representing people with disabilities and other relevant stakeholders.

2. The measures required to determine global grants to be allocated to the Member States to support actions at national, regional and local level shall be adopted in accordance with the procedure referred to in Article 6(2). Global grants shall be awarded only to public-law bodies or bodies which have a public-service mission guaranteed by the Member States.

3. The procedure for the use of global grants shall be subject to an agreement between the Commission and the Member State concerned.

The procedure shall detail in particular, in compliance with the Financial Regulation of 21 December 1977 applicable to the general budget of the European Communities:

(a) the measures to be implemented;

(b) the criteria for choosing beneficiaries;

(c) the conditions and rates of assistance;

(d) the arrangements for monitoring, evaluating and ensuring the financial control of the global grant.

Article 6
Committee

1. The Commission shall be assisted by a Committee, (hereinafter referred to as "the Committee").

2. Where reference is made to this paragraph, Articles 3 and 7 of Decision 1999/468/EC shall apply.

3. The Committee shall adopt its rules of procedure.

Article 7
Financial arrangements

1. Measures which are Community-wide in nature, as described in Part A of the Annex, may be subsidised up to 80 % or give rise to procurement contracts financed from the general budget of the European Communities.

2. Measures which are local, regional or national, possibly with a transnational dimension, as described in Part B of the Annex, may be co-financed from the general budget of the European Communities up to a maximum of 50 % of the total cost.

Article 8
Application and selection procedure

1. Decisions on the financing and co-financing of measures under Article 7(1) shall be adopted in accordance with the advisory procedure referred to in Article 6(2). The Commission shall ensure a balanced distribution among the different fields of activity involved.

2. Requests for financial assistance for measures under Article 7(2) shall be submitted to the Member States. On the basis of the opinion expressed by the national coordinating bodies, Member States shall select beneficiaries and allocate financial assistance to the applicants selected in accordance with Article 5(3).

Article 9
Consistency and complementarity

The Commission, in cooperation with the Member States, shall ensure consistency between the measures provided for in this Decision and other Community actions and initiatives.

The Commission shall also ensure that appropriate efforts are made to enable people with disabilities to participate equally in Community programmes and initiatives.

It shall also ensure optimal complementarity between the European Year of People with Disabilities and other existing Community, national and regional initiatives and resources, where these can contribute to fulfilling the objectives of the European Year of People with Disabilities.

Article 10

Participation by the EFTA/EEA countries, the associated countries of central and eastern Europe, Cyprus, Malta and Turkey

The European Year of People with Disabilities shall be open to participation by the following countries:

(a) EFTA/EEA countries in accordance with the conditions established in the EEA Agreement;

(b) the candidate countries of central and eastern Europe . . . in accordance with the conditions established in the Europe Agreements, in their additional protocols and in the decisions of the respective Association Councils;

(c) Cyprus, Malta and Turkey, their participation being funded by additional appropriations in accordance with procedures to be agreed with those countries.

Article 11
Budget

1. The financial reference amount for the implementation of this Decision is hereby set at EUR 12 million.

2. The annual appropriations shall be authorised by the budgetary authority within the limits of the financial perspective.

3. Actions aimed at preparing the launching of the European Year of People with Disabilities may be financed as from 1 January 2002.

Article 2
International cooperation

Within the framework of this Decision, the Commission may cooperate with relevant international organisations.

Article 13
Monitoring and evaluation

The Commission shall submit, by 31 December 2004 at the latest, a report to the European Parliament, the Council, the Economic and Social Committee and the Committee of the Regions on the implementation, results and overall assessment of the measures provided for in this Decision, including an assessment of the long-term effects of the measures. The Commission shall ensure that the report is drawn up in formats accessible to people with disabilities.

Article 14
Entry into force

This Decision shall be published in the Official Journal of the European Communities.

It shall take effect on the day of its publication.

Done at Brussels, 3 December 2001.
For the Council
The President
F. Vandenbroucke

Source: European Council. 2001. 2001/903/EC: Council Decision of 3 December 2001 on the European Year of People with Disabilities 2003. *Official Journal L 335* (December 19), pp. 0015–0020.

◎ The Disability Media Action and Awareness Project, "'Do You Mean to Say What We Hear?' A Disability Language Reference" (2000–2001)

From 2000 to 2001 a group of disabled activists, academics, artists, and community residents in Chicago compiled the following guidelines about appropriate language use in coverage of disability issues. The creation of such guidelines was intended to steer journalists toward less objectifying and demeaning portrayals of disabled people and to demonstrate the lack of objectivity in current rhetorical constructions of disability in mainstream U.S. journalism.

We include below some "street" perspectives on terms that continue to circulate around (and even impinge upon) people with disabilities. These terms have been selected as worthy of more thoughtfulness. They name affinities (and not) among a group of people with disabilities who have put some thought into the matter of representation; the mainstream media; diagnostic labels; and disability subcultures. The definitions reflect widely shared perspectives across Chicago disability groups.

Terms were compiled by the Disability Media Action and Awareness Project—a group that monitors coverage of disability communities and disability issues in the Chicago media. Our purpose? To serve as a link between Chicago media professionals and the authentic voices of disabled persons in Chicago.

Language is important because our language reflects our ideas about being human! The terms we use when referring to each other shape our values. We want to help media professionals reflect on terms that have traditionally dehumanized people with disabilities. This is not a comprehensive list and not everyone would agree. These are just the twists of language that most sock it to us in the gut—good and bad.

—The Disability Media Action and Awareness Project, University of Illinois at Chicago, Disability Studies a.k.a. Michael Ervin, Sharon Snyder, Gary Arnold, Larry Biondi, Kenneth Borst, Will Cowing, Stephen Drake, Herbert Hoffman, Ayo Maat, Gloria Nichols, Joan Porter, Harvey Rabin, and Monique Streff.

Blind People: Technically blind people recognize one another as those with 2200 or less sight with correction. Those with limited sight are usually referred to as people with low vision. But some people who are blind think this is a nit-picky distinction. They say you are either legally blind or not.

Cerebral Palsy: The most common misconception about people with cerebral palsy is that they have intellectual problems involving thinking and reasoning. Most people who bear the label C.P. have cognition that operates in similar ways to other general non disabled groups. Cerebral palsy is a misleading term when you think about it. Palsy is an archaic word meaning muscular inability to move part or all of the body. Put it all together and it implies a paralyzed brain. No one has come up with a better term so go ahead and use it. But understand its shortcomings when applied to real people.

Confined to a wheelchair: Confined means "limited, small, cramped or completely enclosed." A wheelchair is the opposite. It is liberating. Why not be accurate and say he/she is a wheelchair user or uses a wheelchair?

Courageous: Why are we insulted when someone says we are brave and courageous? Doesn't everyone want to be considered brave and courageous? Well, these words are often used to describe people with disabilities who are just living their lives. They are doing nothing spectacular, just activities everyone does. But if nothing is expected of us, when we are successful it may be viewed as extraordinary. To say we are brave and courageous just for living life implies that we would be justified in giving up and doing nothing.

Crippled: Before we get too far we should talk about out and out Hate Speech usage such as Cripple, Retard, Spastic, Freak. These are words that kept us fearful when we were growing up. Some still use crippled as "completely ruined or damaged." Of course, crippled is archaic, too, and still sounds like Victorian back bedrooms. Note: we sometimes call ourselves crippled to "be real" and nitty gritty among ourselves—or to off-set the hate tossed our way. That does not mean you should.

Deaf and dumb/mute: This was used a lot in an old Jane Wyman movie, which shows how out of date it is. Dumb implies stupid, and mute means unable to speak. Most deaf people can use their voices, though many choose not to. These terms should be consigned to the linguistic basement. Why not he/she does not speak with his/her voice?

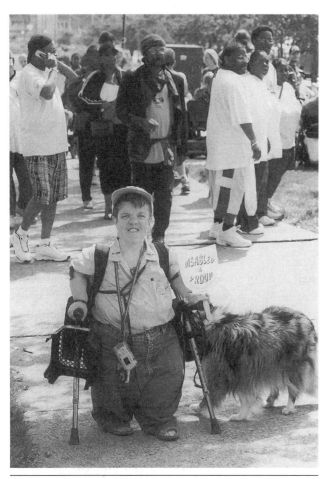

Proud Short-Statured Woman and Dog at the Chicago Disability Pride Parade, 2004.

Defects: As in "only you can prevent birth defects." Propagandizes the idea that a disabled person should be prevented instead of accepted and included. Assumes everyone's body falls short of some ideal "whole." An inaccurate and frequently abusive idea.

Guide dog: The proper term for dogs assisting blind people. Seeing-eye dog is the name of one of the guide dog training schools. Dogs that assist sighted people with disabilities are called service dogs.

Invalid: Changing the accent doesn't change the meaning of the word. It wouldn't be any less offensive to call a woman a bim-BO. No matter how you slice it, it still means In-VA-lid.

Handicapped: We don't like this one for a lot of reasons. Mainly it places the emphasis on the wrong spot by saying the disability is what handicaps us. Sounds like one is the perpetual object of charity, emblem of a telethon, or in need of pity. Barriers are what handicap. Besides, "handicapped" sounds whiney, doesn't it?

Hard of hearing: This has emerged again as a term for those who have partial hearing. And no, people who have partial sight are not hard of sight.

Mental Retardation: This sounds like a permanent unalterable predicament—that one's life and brain [are] fixed and that one will be forever stunted. Developmental delay implies that people are always catching up rather than perceiving the world in cognitively varied ways. Please say people with cognitive or developmental disabilities.

Midget: Went out of fashion with court dwarves. Seems to assume that everyone of short stature is there to entertain. Assumes that the person's size accounts for their amicable or sometimes devilish personality. Please say person of short stature.

Non disabled: Whatever.

Normal: Who's to say what is normal? Let ye who is normal cast the first stone.

Overcome: This implies that [those who don't] overcome their disability . . . are the one[s] with the problem. They are either not trying hard enough or don't have the right attitude. It's not our disabilities we have to overcome. It's the barriers that disallow our participation.

Patient: This implies that we are always ill or in need of being fixed. People with disabilities are only patients in our relations with our doctors, just like the nondisabled.

People with disabilities: This has evolved as the proper term because it puts the person first. We know it can become literarily cumbersome when used repeatedly. "Disabled people" is fine and actually preferred in some countries as a claim of pride and solidarity. "The disabled," however, makes everyone sound like an item or immovable object.

Physically Challenged, Handicapable, Differently-abled: Ridiculous terms that are used by people who seem uncomfortable with disabled people or with their own disabilities. Why bend over backward not to say disabled as if it is a bad word?

Special: The word gives an inaccurate impression that people born with disabilities get special treatment throughout life. It even perpetuates the myth that children with disabilities are spoiled. Sugar coats an experience or makes it cute. Even sounds like luck is involved!

Suffering: Bears the automatic coding that a disabled life is miserable such as in "he suffers from brain damage." Instead of saying a person suffers from, is stricken by or afflicted with (etc!) a disability, [j]ust say he/she has a disability.

Vegetable: A favorite of legal defense teams and those of pro-euthanasia persuasions. Someone who is supposed to be a burden upon family, society and country. A waste of space. No longer animal, thus no longer human. What next, mineral?

Victim: Assumes that all people with disabilities are suffering from some great tragedy. When people with disabilities are victims, it's usually for reasons that have little to do with the bodily experiences from their disability. See also "burden."

Wheelchair bound: Makes it sound as if we are tied up, being held hostage. Some people with disabilities are into bondage, but not all. No one is bound to their wheelchair. Everyone gets out of it at least once a day.

A Special Bonus for Being a Good Sport and Sticking It Out!! SLANG!

Some throw these words around with abandon while others find some of them too dangerous in any context, no matter how self-deprecating or ironic. WARNING: DO NOT ATTEMPT TO USE WITHOUT PROPER CONTEXT:

Some examples:

Blind people: Blinks, bats.

People with physical disabilities: Gimps, crips.

Nondisabled people: Uprights, verticals, walkie-talkies, bipeds.

Super duper overcoming disabled people (i.e. jocks): Supercrips.

Super duper passive and subservient disabled people: Tiny Tims.

▣ Apology on the 75th Anniversary of the *Buck v. Bell* Decision (2002)

In the most notorious sterilization case, Buck v. Bell (1927; see excerpt from the decision on pp. 390–391, this volume), the argument supporting sterilization was based on the longstanding prejudice that cognitively disabled women were more promiscuous than nondisabled women. Eugenics historians have since established that Carrie Buck (the cognitively disabled woman targeted in the case) had been raped by a relative of her foster parents. The statement, by Virginia Governor Mark R. Warner, was read by Delegate Mitch Van Yahres at a ceremony on May 2, 2002, to dedicate a highway marker commemorating the Buck v. Bell

decision. The highway marker's wording was authorized by the Virginia Board of Historic Resources.

I am sorry that I am unable to be with you on this important occasion.

In 1924, Virginia, like many states, passed a law permitting involuntary sterilization. In 1927, Carrie Buck was the first person sterilized by the Commonwealth pursuant to that law. Virginia's actions were upheld by the Supreme Court of the United States, and the government ultimately sterilized approximately 8,000 people.

Last year, the General Assembly passed a resolution expressing profound regret for the Commonwealth's role in the eugenics movement. Today, I offer the Commonwealth's sincere apology for Virginia's participation in eugenics. As I have previously noted, the eugenics movement was a shameful effort in which state government never should have been involved.

We must remember the Commonwealth's past mistakes in order to prevent them from recurring. This highway marker will serve as a constant reminder of how our government failed its citizens and how we must always strive to do better.

▣ International Commemoration Committee on Eugenic Mass Murder (2003)

On May 2, 2003, the following elegy was read in public ceremonies throughout Europe and the United States. These commemoration events sought to remind populations of the eugenics-based killings in National Socialist Germany that ultimately led to the Holocaust against Jews, Romany ("gypsy"), and gay people. The document details some of the processes and technology implemented against those with disabilities and psychiatric diagnoses in German psychiatric institutions. These practices were later exported to Nazi death camps during the implementation of the "final solution" involving mass extermination.

In Memoriam,

In 1939 at a psychiatric institution in Germany a group of patients were told to undress and take a shower. After the "shower" door was locked, one psychiatrist turned a valve, releasing poisonous gas through pipes into the "shower" room. Then the psychiatrists looked on through a glass aperture as the patients slowly asphyxiated to death in the fumes.

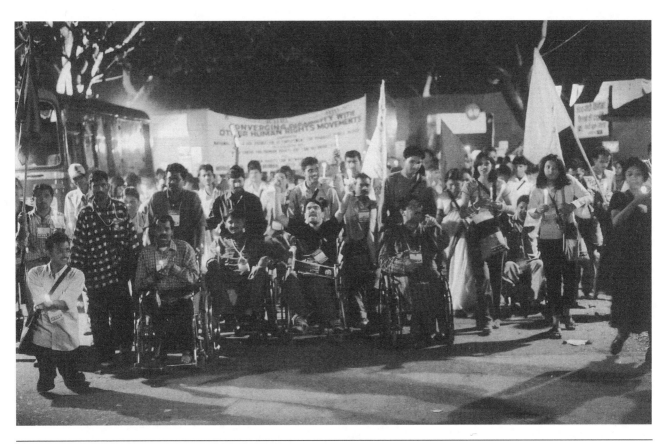

Disabled protesters at the 2004 World Social Forum in Mumbai, India, march toward the podium to press for their demands.

Source: National Centre for Promotion of Employment for Disabled People, New Delhi, India.

By 1941, before the mass murders in the concentration camps had begun, hundreds of thousands of defenseless people, men, women, children, the elderly, and infants, who had been defined by doctors as "life unworthy of living," had been gassed, drugged, shot, or deliberately starved to death. The murders continued even after 1945.

It is often incorrectly assumed that the murders were ordered by Hitler. In fact, doctors proceeded independent of government approval. In 1941 after Hitler ordered a stop to the murders, doctors committed what has since been dubbed "wild euthanasia."

These eugenic mass murders had been endorsed by the medical establishment decades before the [N]azis came to power. They were sanctioned by proponents of eugenics in other countries, including doctors in the United States and England.

History has failed to do justice to the hundreds of thousands of victims. Therefore, we, the International Commemoration Committee on Eugenic Mass Murder, set aside the date May 2 in memoriam, and demand that no person, with or without disability, ever fall victim to medical murder again.

Reprinted by permission.

◉ Disabled Students Union Meeting (2003)

The formation of the Disabled Students Union (DSU) was one of the first successful organizing efforts around disability issues in colleges and universities in the United States. Below is an excerpt from the organization's call for members at the University of Illinois at Chicago (UIC). The group's founders also went on to successfully create a National Disabled Students Union that organized disabled students and their close advocates at the national level.

January 28, 2003 11:30 a.m.–1:00 p.m.
Room 448 IIDD

ACCESS IS A CIVIL RIGHT!
About the Disabled Students Union

The purpose of this cross-disability organization is to mobilize, organize, and represent students with disabilities at UIC in order to promote empowerment and community solidarity among people with disabilities on campus. Students with disabilities at UIC are one of the most underrepresented and marginalized minority groups on campus. DSU was created (Feb. 2000) with the express intent of strengthening the political voice and power of students with disabilities on campus. DSU is a socio-political advocacy organization that seeks to build disability community, culture, pride and power.

If you are a student with a disability and you are interested in participating in the DSU to promote disability access and disability pride, then we need your input and involvement!

Los Angeles Times on Eugenics Apologies (2003)

At the outset of the twenty-first century, numerous states issued formal apologies to disabled people and their families who were negatively affected by sterilization practices. The following journalistic article discusses the larger issue of such apologies, and particularly California's longstanding lack of inquiry into the state's ambitious eugenics effort to sterilize more than 20,000 disabled people.

To make amends for a state program that sterilized 7,600 people against their will, North Carolina's governor created a panel last year to probe the history of the effort, interview survivors and consider reparations.

In Oregon, then-Gov. John Kitzhaber last year apologized in person to some of the 2,600 people sterilized there, and he created an annual Human Rights Day to commemorate the state's mistake. On the day Virginia Gov. Mark R. Warner apologized, Jesse Meadows and other victims unveiled a roadside marker.

"It felt pretty good to be there, even though it was so late," said Meadows, 80.

Some historians and advocates for the disabled had a mixed reaction to the apology issued Tuesday by Gov. Gray Davis for California's policy, the most aggressive in the nation, which sterilized an estimated 20,000 mentally disabled people and others from 1909 through the 1960s.

Davis offered his apology in a press release. No survivors or disability groups were on hand to accept it. There was no order to probe for more details of a history that, according to scholars, is still largely unexplored and not fully understood.

"It's like a preemptive apology. . . . We don't know yet who to apologize to," said Alexandra Stern, a University of Michigan historian who is writing a book about California's sterilization program.

"An apology with no attempt to find the people who deserve to receive it is meaningless," said Stephen Drake, research analyst with Not Dead Yet, a national disability rights group. "If the governor is serious about wanting to understand this shameful chapter of California history, then you need an effort to study the records of just how this was done."

"I think it's premature," said Paul Lombardo, a University of Virginia historian who revived interest in the state policy when he lectured Tuesday to a California Senate committee. The lecture, which some officials said was the first time they had heard of the sterilization policy, triggered a statement within hours from Davis and a separate apology from state Atty. Gen. Bill Lockyer.

Lombardo and Drake said the apologies were welcome as acknowledgments of past abuse. "But if they don't try to understand the history, then I don't know what it's worth," Lombardo added.

Historians have only recently begun to explore California's sterilization effort. Primarily at institutions for the mentally ill and the developmentally disabled, the state sterilized thousands of people under the premise that the "unfit" should be removed from the gene pool so their children would not burden society.

But some of the basic details still are missing. Among them: exactly how many people were sterilized.

The mentally ill and developmentally disabled were the initial focus of the policy, but some historians believe that it also targeted Mexican and Asian immigrants, criminals, juvenile delinquents and sexually active women.

Even the date that the practice ended is unclear, though it may have been as late as 1969.

"We checked that and we haven't been able to determine that," said Bertha Gorman, spokeswoman for the California Health and Human Services Agency. Because of patient confidentiality rules, historians have had little access to state records that might shed light on the state's sterilization history.

"Shouldn't we demand that the state fill in the history?" asked David Mitchell, who runs a disabilities studies program at the University of Illinois at Chicago. "That would be the foundation of a meaningful apology."

Russell Lopez, a spokesman for the governor, said he had called three state departments last week in an attempt to find survivors but was told no names could be released because of patient confidentiality rules.

"The governor just learned about this," Lopez said, "and he decided it was something he must do: apologize for what the Legislature did in the past."

In Virginia, North Carolina and Oregon, a combination of media interest and university research brought attention to past sterilization programs and led to the state apologies.

Although some details remain clouded, there is no doubt that California was once home to the largest sterilization program in the nation and to some of the most influential supporters of the practice, including the publisher of the *Los Angeles Times* in the 1930s.

At least 30 states passed laws in the first decades of the 1900s that aimed to shape society by denying the so-called unfit the ability to reproduce. Scientists already had shown how careful breeding could improve crops and livestock. Now, they were arguing that selective breeding could improve humanity and wipe out poverty, prostitution and mental illness, which were thought to have genetic roots.

The concept, known as eugenics, led to the sterilization of more than 63,000 people in the United States from about 1907 through the 1970s.

California accounted for one-third of all operations. Its sterilization law was the second in the nation, after Indiana's.

The state's enthusiasm for eugenics was so well known that it is mentioned in "The Great Gatsby." When Nazi Germany wrote its sterilization policy, it borrowed from California's law, historians say.

"Why California more than other states? That's a key question," Stern said. "I think it has to do with the need to civilize the frontier."

In better breeding practices, Californians saw a way to control the chaos of nature. And their use in human reproduction had the support of prominent citizens, including then-Stanford University President David Starr Jordan and Pasadena citrus magnate Ezra Gosney, who founded one of the most influential think tanks devoted to eugenics, the Human Betterment Foundation, in 1926.

Another cheerleader was *The Times,* whose publisher, Harry Chandler, was listed as a member of the Human Betterment Foundation in a 1938 pamphlet by the group.

"We have secured the ardent support of the *Los Angeles Times,"* Gosney wrote in a 1937 dispatch to the *Eugenical News,* a monthly periodical. "They are running an article each week in their Sunday magazine edition which, while not as good as the editor-owner of the paper would like, keeps the subject before the people and does much to encourage us in carrying on."

That Sunday column, called "Social Eugenics," ran from 1935 to 1941 and argued for strong sterilization laws, said Lombardo of the University of Virginia. The paper ran at least 120 of them, he added.

Through much of the 1930s, many sterilization advocates also cheered on the eugenics policies in Germany. "Why Hitler Says: 'Sterilize the Unfit!'" ran a headline in a 1935 issue of *The Times'* magazine. "Here, perhaps, is an aspect of the new Germany that America, with the rest of the world, can little afford to criticise."

Under California law, people with "mental disease" could be sterilized if doctors believed the condition could be passed to descendants. The superintendents of state institutions had broad authority to decide how often to use the procedure, Stern said.

"The term 'mental disease' could be interpreted broadly," she said. "People who were epileptics were lumped in there, and people with 'perverse' sexual tendencies, so you had gay men."

Some who were sterilized had landed in state institutions on grounds of theft, forgery and truancy from school. In some places, women appear to have been sterilized merely for promiscuity.

"Something like 25% of the girls who have been sterilized were sent up here solely, or primarily, for that purpose," wrote Paul Popenoe, director of the Human Betterment Foundation, during a 1926 research trip to the Sonoma State Home for the Feeble-Minded. "They are kept only a few months—long enough to operate and instill a little discipline in them; and then returned home."

Stern and Lombardo believe that hundreds of prisoners, as well as many of the women and others at the Sonoma facility, are not included in the commonly cited figure of 20,000 sterilizations in California.

They also suspect that the state's strong anti-immigrant movement of the early 1900s targeted Mexicans and other nonwhite groups with sterilization, an attempt to dilute their presence in the population. But no broad survey of the racial and ethnic profile of sterilization patients has been done.

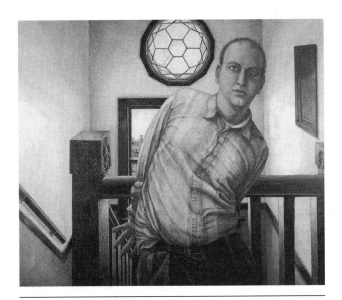

Circle Story #1: Jeff Carpenter, *by Riva Lehrer. 1997. Jeff Carpenter, a comedian, writer and teacher, works with an improvisational troupe and also performs solo work. Carpenter was injured in a random drive-by shooting several years ago, and he has written darkly sardonic pieces about its difficult aftermath.*

law allows sterilization for mentally incompetent people who cannot give informed consent. A court-appointed conservator must petition a judge for permission.

Victim Jesse Meadows said that Virginia, at least, "ought to pay people for what they did." Meadows, of Lynchburg, was sent to the Virginia Colony for Epileptics and the Feebleminded in 1940, after his mother died and his father remarried. He was sterilized there, at age 17.

"They said it was to help my health . . . and so I wouldn't have no feeble-minded children," Meadows said.

Virginia's apology and roadside marker "helped me some," Meadows said. "But it's hard to forget that somebody ruined your life like that."

Source: Zitner, Aaron. 2003, March 16. "Davis' Apology Sheds No Light on Sterilizations in California: Lack of an Inquiry into the State's Ambitious Eugenics Effort and Its 20,000 Victims Angers Some Historians and Disabled Advocates." *Los Angeles Times.* Available at: http://www.geocities.com/madelinefelkins/CAeugenics.htm. Copyright © *Los Angeles Times.* Reprinted by permission.

Joel Braslow, an associate professor of psychiatry at UCLA, says critiques of sterilization laws often misstate how the policy was practiced.

In state institutions, he says, doctors cared little about eugenics. Instead, they saw sterilization as a humane and beneficial treatment for patients, along with lobotomies and other now-discredited practices.

"In practice, we didn't sterilize the severely retarded," said Dr. William Keating, a surgeon at Sonoma State Hospital throughout the 1950s. "They had very little opportunity for sex. The people we concentrated on were people who were moderately retarded, who had a chance of going out and getting pregnant."

In an interview, Keating said he performed 500 to 600 tubal ligations and vasectomies at the institution. Individuals who could perform some sort of job outside the institution would be released, but not if they were at risk of getting pregnant or impregnating someone. In effect, sterilization was a ticket to a work furlough, or general release.

Keating recalled a young man who had an IQ he estimated to be 85. After his vasectomy, the man was released, only to return for a visit one day—in full Army uniform. He had become a first lieutenant during the Korean War.

Eugenic sterilizations tailed off through the 1950s and 1960s but remained legal until 1979. Today, state

▣ Margaret Talbot, from "The Executioner's I.Q. Test" (2003)

One of the more contentious issues in the United States at the beginning of the twenty-first century is the issue of capital punishment for people with cognitive disabilities. Given the lengthy history of IQ testing and its controversial status as a valid scientific evaluation tool, the following excerpt from a journalistic article provides an important commentary on the continuing use of such testing to determine ultimate decisions about "ability to reason" as the basis for enactments of state-sponsored murder.

Most people will never take an I.Q. test, and if they do, it probably won't have a big impact on them. Generally speaking, I.Q. tests do not carry much weight anymore. Not with vague charges of cultural bias still clinging to them. Not at a time when multiple intelligences—that happy, inclusive vision in which nearly everybody is good at something—are on the ascendancy. If you do take a Stanford-Binet or a Wechsler, and you score in the average range, well, there you'll be, with hardly a reason to mention it. If you score high, the particular number won't matter much—unless you're the sort to join Mensa, and then it will matter only to your fellow Mensa members. But if you are in the bottom 3 percent of the population that scores 70 or lower, your actual I.Q. number will mean a great deal. Scores in that range will most likely lead to a diagnosis of mental retardation, and that diagnosis will entail many things, starting with mandated special education. Since last June, across the United States, it has also entailed exemption from capital punishment. And so, for someone who has committed a capital crime, an I.Q. score can mean the difference, quite literally, between life and death. It can mean, if we want to be blunt about it, that there is such a thing as being too dumb to die, at least at the hands of the state.

Source: Talbot, Margaret. 2003, July 29. "The Executioner's I.Q. Test." *New York Times Magazine.* Available at: http://www .newamerica.net/index.cfm?sec=Documents&pg=article&DocID =1275&T2=Article

▣ Andrea Dworkin, "Through the Pain Barrier" (2005)

This is the last piece written by Andrea Dworkin, composed just a month before she died. Few knew that she had suffered from an agonizing bone disease for several years. She describes with grim humor her worst moments and why she felt she was starting to heal.

The doctor who knows me best says that osteoarthritis begins long before it cripples—in my case, possibly from homelessness, or sexual abuse, or beatings on my legs, or my weight.

John, my partner, blames *Scapegoat,* a study of Jewish identity and women's liberation that took me nine years to write; it is, he says, the book that stole my health. I blame the drug-rape that I experienced in 1999 in Paris. I returned from Paris and finished *Scapegoat* over a period of months while caring for my dying father. Shortly after he died I was in hospital, delirious from a high fever, with infection and blood clots in my legs. I was there for a month. John had been told that I was dying. I forgot that in hospitals when one is dying, nurses abrogate the rules. John was allowed in after visiting hours; nurses would pull the curtain around my bed and let him lie with me. This was my happiness. Doctors tell me that there is no medical truth to my notion that the rape caused this sickness or what happened after it. I believe I am right: it was the rape. They don't know because they have never looked.

A few months after I got out of the hospital, my knees began to change. They lost their flexibility. Slowly they stiffened. As they stiffened they became sore. They started to hurt terribly—as if injured but not visibly injured. I got a cellphone—this was before they were ubiquitous—so that if I couldn't walk any more I could call a car. I had given up on New York City subways: my knees could no longer bend enough to use them.

I went to an orthopaedic surgeon. I was diagnosed with osteoarthritis in my knees. I was treated with the anti-inflammatory Celebrex and, when that didn't work, its stronger cousin, Vioxx. Vioxx was recently taken off the market by its makers because of a risk of heart attacks or strokes; I was on it for three years. I had cortisone shots in my knees, followed by prednisone. The cortisone shots, which are painful, worked only once. Then I could walk without pain; in joy I sat on my front steps and talked with my neighbour—inconsequential chat. When I tried to stand up, my knees were rigid and excruciating. I managed to stand and swivel around; I took the remaining two steps up to my front door and used the door to drag me inside. I had had an hour-and-a-half of freedom.

My mobility lessened as the pain increased. Eventually I found myself housebound. I could walk only a few steps at a time, intimidated by the pain and the refusal of my knees to bend. John and I lived in a three-floor house. I could barely make my way up or down the steps. I'd crawl up the steps on hands and feet. I'd try to go down on my butt, step by step. The kitchen was on the first floor; the toilet on the second; my desk, books and shower on the third. My physical world became tiny and pain-racked. I stayed in my bed when I could. John brought me up food. I'd go out only to the doctors.

The orthopaedist started giving me narcotics, most of which contained acetaminophen, a common, nonprescription analgesic. My pharmacist persuaded the doctor that the liver damage caused by too much acetaminophen was more dangerous to me than stronger drugs. Through her advocacy I got a drug normally given only to cancer patients. It was a little yellow lollipop and when in pain one was supposed to lick. I licked a lot. I was told that I had to have my knees replaced. The prostheses are made out of titanium and plastic. I had both knees replaced at once, a normal practice now but unusual even a few years ago. My surgeon would later tell me that if I had had one done, I would never have returned for the second. He got that right.

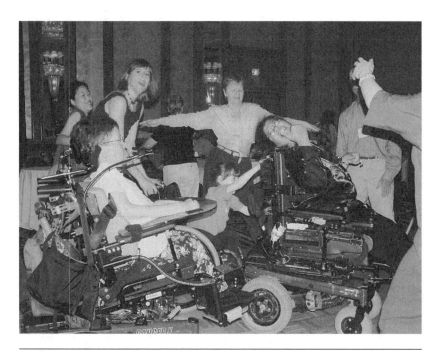

"Bodies in Commotion." Dancers at the annual Society for Disability Studies Dance, 2003.

Source: Photo by Sharon Snyder.

I still don't know what he did to me but I came to the conclusion that the operation was barbaric, involving as it did the sawing out of the arthritis, which meant sawing through bones. It was like being kneecapped, twice, or having one's knees and bones hammered and broken into bits. After the operation I was in a nightmare of narcotics and untouchable pain. There were morphine shots. I asked for them and got them often. Even morphine shots in the upper arm hurt.

I had a hallucination but it is still real as rain to me. I was in Virginia Woolf's house and I was happy. But "they" wanted me to go down the stairs. I can't, I begged, I can't. My hospital bed was at the top of the stairs and I was afraid that they were going to push me down. I saw the steep decline of the steps. I couldn't get over my visceral fear of falling or being pushed or being turned over from the bed down the flight of steps. I kept experiencing my bed as being on the edge of a precipice.

One day, I remember, a nurses' aide braided my hair and I felt cooler, cleaner. I was on the bedpan, but raising myself up to use it—knees—was so fiercely painful that I would rather lie in my piss.

Then the day came when I had to walk. There was a vinyl chair next to my hospital bed. The physical therapist's name was Carl. He was like a tree trunk, big and solid. You can do it, he said. I'll help you; we'll just go over to the chair. It was impossible, outside the realm of the imaginable. Carl let me hold on to him in a desperate, tight embrace as he carried me over to the chair. My legs dangled, my knees twisted, I sweated, I screamed. See, you could do that, he said, without a shred of irony. I had to sit there for two hours, which meant knees bent but not weight-bearing. Nurses came by and gave verbal approval: good dog, good dog. Eventually Carl carried me back to bed.

Pain is a four-letter word. There is no way to recreate it through memory. It is not like the flashback arising from traumatic events such as rape or battery. The flashback is as if it is happening now, in the present, even if it is from decades ago. Pain can be recent yet inaccessible to immediate experience. Torturers know that people can't die from pain. The consequences of pain—for instance a heart attack—yes, but not from pain itself, however intense. The horror is that no one dies from pain. This means that suffering can be immeasurable, enduring, without respite. So it would be for me for the next two years.

I was taken to an institute for physical rehabilitation. A nurses' aide took me to shower in a wheelchair. I used a walker from the cot on which I slept to the wheelchair, maybe two miserable steps. I had two responsibilities—take my pain medications (Vicodin or Percocet) and show up at the right room at the right time for the scheduled rehabilitative class. I was not allowed to go to class if I did not take the painkillers. In fact, the pain was unrelenting. I lived for the next pill.

Physical therapy is based on tiny movements, increments of change that almost defy detection; it is built on the repetition of the minuscule. Yet to the hurt person these motions or movements or minute steps are hard. The first time is daunting and the 10th is like climbing Mount Everest. I sit in a big room, my wheelchair in a big circle of wheelchairs. Big is good because it means that my turn does not come often. I stand up by holding on to a walker and take a step. Then I step back and sit down. The cycle is hideous. The steps with the walker increase to two, then three. After several weeks I am assigned a means of locomotion: crutches.

Rehabilitation also includes so-called occupational therapy: throw a ball around in a circle; put round pegs in round holes; stand up, arms on a table, and read a page of a magazine; water a plant; play checkers or cards; and the pièce de résistance, cook and serve a simple meal. I am guided in the intricacies of shopping while crippled; I learn how to use a "grabber" to latch on to things I have dropped or cannot reach; I am taught again how to put on shoes and socks and tie shoelaces.

I also have to meet the institution's psychologist once. I keep getting called back.

When I ask why, I am told that I am "interesting." Well, yes, I think, I used to be. The narcotics help me deal with the psychologist but the physical pain simply marches on. It does not lessen or change or stop.

I learn three rules in my occupational therapy classes: never hold on to anything that moves; if it rains or snows, stay inside, even if that means cancelling doctors' appointments (to those medicalised this is nearly profane); and kick the cat—if a cat curls up in front of your feet, kick it away. I learned to use my crutch to kick the cat. I will go to hell for this.

On discharge, social services are provided. My male partner is not expected to be a care-giver. I am sent an itinerant nurse, a young, poorly paid and badly trained social aide to help me with baths and to do light housework, and a freelance physical therapist who will do the drill: stand up, take steps, bend your knees, and—the killer—stand on your toes.

And on discharge a wreck like me is sent to a "pain management centre." Despite my small successes at physical rehabilitation I am in agony. I spend almost all my time in bed, a bed of nails, all through the knees. The pain management centre is run by Curly, Larry and Moe. First there is a 10-page questionnaire. Rate from 1 to 10 your pain (I modestly assert an 8; my social conscience, atavistic as it is, tells me that there are others in more pain). Rate from 1 to 10: is your mother dead; how many people in your family have died of cancer; how is your sex life; how many times a week do you have sex?

They want me to undress so they can examine me. This is absurd. I refuse. There is a table they want me to lie on that they claim lessens pain. The bottom line is that New York State regulates narcotics to such an extent that regular doctors are reluctant to write prescriptions for painkillers; and so Curly, Larry and Moe at pain management put you through whatever rigmarole and then write prescriptions, none of which,

according to state law, can be refilled. So one is in a cycle of coming back for new prescriptions and new indignities every 30 days.

Curly eventually puts me on Percocet, fentanyl patches and methadone. I am on these drugs for nearly two years. I become slightly indifferent to the awful pain. My speech slurs and my memory is impaired. It is during this time that I write my memoir Heartbreak. I want to remember some good things in my life. I work for one hour a day. The narcotics do not make me Coleridge; but I hold my own.

One day I wake up and the pain is gone from my right knee—as if God had intervened. The pain in the left one is the same. I begin to go outside on my crutches. I can walk half a block to my local Starbucks. One day I sit there, still on my meds, and I see the ballet going on outside. The sidewalk is heavy with pedestrian traffic. They are so unselfconscious, these normal walkers. They have different gaits; they move effortlessly; each dances without knowing it. I used to be one of them. I want to be again.

The anti-drama of small gesticulations continues, this time in physical therapy several blocks from where I live. My left knee is still rotten. After another year of physical therapy they give me a cane. I put away all the crutches and other signs of what I call "disability chic." I can sort of walk. The cane means victory. The pain in my left knee keeps me on my meds. Over the course of another year, that pain lessens. It's a whisper, a shadow—it goes. I give up the pills, though I go through a nasty withdrawal from methadone.

Alas, there is no happy ending. John and I move to Washington so that he can take a job as managing editor of a large-circulation magazine. We live in an apartment without steps. I am on the cane. I go into physical therapy because, unable to stand up straight, I hunch over the cane. A few days later I am at the kitchen table reading a magazine. I stand up to get something and my right knee cannot bear any weight, none. I can't use it because I can't step on it. I have no pain; I have had no warning. I get to my crutches, which are in a closet. I need both of them in order to move. My right knee remains useless. The physical therapist determines that the quadriceps above the knee has stopped working, because imperceptible pain occasions the quad muscle to give out. Then my knee buckles and I fall. It is dangerous to fall. I see the physical therapist twice a week.

The orthopaedic surgeon ("a genius with knees," says my internist) puts me in a restrictive brace that allows

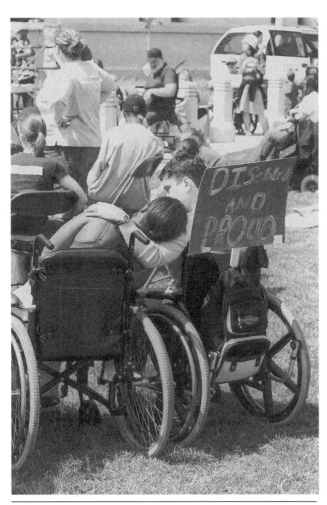

"Disabled and Proud" wheelchair lovers hug each other during the Chicago Disability Pride Parade, 2004.

my knee to bend only so far. That way, if my knee fails, I am unlikely to fall. After nearly a year of physical therapy my quad muscle is not much stronger and my knee still buckles. The surgeon sends me to a rehabilitation hospital where they make me a new brace, specifically fitted to my leg. This brace works on the opposite principle to the first one: it immobilises the knee so that no buckling is possible, thus, no fall is possible.

It takes months for artisans to make the brace. It goes from beneath my calf to the top of my thigh. It is made of a black space-age material created to go to Mars or Saturn. Nothing makes it bend or stretch or break. It is completely unforgiving. I call it Darth Vader. It is the principle of evil incarnate. The straps that attach front to back are Velcro. I am supposed to lock it when I walk and unlock it when I want to sit. The brace is worn under my pants leg so no one can see it. Each manipulation is distinct: in public locking

it makes me look as if I am masturbating, and unlocking it makes me look as if I am fondling my thigh. The brace must be very tight and positioned perfectly to work. It takes me nearly two months to learn how to put it on and use it. I lose my balance in efforts to lock it. Once I flip backward, magically landing on a chair.

Self-respect demands that I clean up the faecal mess that my cat has made. It is the immobilized knee that makes bending down to the floor fraught with peril. I start falling and know that I must not hit the floor. I fight against gravity, my fingernails clawing at the walls and my hand grasping for the door frame. I know that if I fall I probably will not be able to get up. Somehow I raise myself.

I was slow with the first brace. I had to remind myself to be patient. With Darth I make the turtle look like the hare. The landscape is one of hazard. Anything can reach up and bite me: a break in the sidewalk; leaves; sand; mud; a sudden slope up or down; a stone; some pebbles. Anything threatening balance is dangerous: first the brace itself; then wind, people running or bicycling or being too close or too many; a fast car; a step; a curb; a puddle; heavy doors; slick surfaces. Crowds are impossible and so are stairs.

I want to be able to carry a cup along with a plate to the kitchen sink in one trip. I don't want to have to make two trips. The cup slips and breaks. This happens several times. Is it a small thing? I can't bear it or accept it. I reject the extent of my disability. I find myself in a silent rage that stretches over weeks. I am utterly exhausted by my incapacity. I am worn out from walking. I am sick of physical therapy.

There are little humiliations. I keynote a conference on the Holocaust. The organiser picks me up. She is driving a truck. I try to climb up into it. She physically pushes me under my ass without permission, all the while talking to me in baby talk, put your tooshie there, keep your cute little fanny there. I turn to her and say, I am disabled, not stupid. A friend throws a party for me in Washington. I ask how many steps there are to the apartment. He doesn't know. I assume he will get back to me. John and I go to the party. There are three flights of steps. I can't get to the party being given for me. We could have given it in another venue, the friend says the next day. It cuts. I go to a bar and need to use the rest room. The men's is filthy, the bartender says; the women's is two flights up. I use the dirty one. I go to a new movie theatre that has elevators and disability bathrooms but the polished stone of the floor is so slick that my crutches cannot safely navigate it. I am walking with a friend who suddenly looks at my crutches and says, you don't want to be this way the rest of your life, do you? Her repulsion is barely masked. I feel unutterably alone.

Each disabled person has a story, often including pain, impairment, disorientation and loss of control. Each disabled person lives always on the threshold of separation, exile and involuntary otherness. Only a determined policy of public access can help to mitigate the loneliness. One needs to be able to enter buildings; have a cup of coffee; go to a restaurant, the theatre, cinema or a concert; attend school; go to lectures or readings; use public transport, bathrooms, hotel showers; go to museums and sporting events and political rallies. One needs equal opportunity in employment. One needs to be integrated into the world, not separated from it; yet one has special needs, ones that able-bodied people rarely consider. The low consciousness of the able-bodied increases alienation.

For mobility problems, one needs a new geography: kerb ramps; ramps in addition to steps; handrails; grab bars; high toilets; light doors; wheelchairs; room for wheelchairs in public bathrooms and hotel rooms; elevators; safety in floor surfaces including carpeting; entry and egress from public transport as well as acceptable seating; and a host of other considerations. Other disabilities require other remedies. In 1990 Congress passed the landmark Americans with Disabilities Act, which articulated in great detail the requirements for making the world available to disabled people. This is a civil rights law that recognises the exclusion of disabled people from the larger community as outright discrimination.

The law had its impact because disabled people found aggressive trial lawyers to sue commercial and private venues for noncompliance. The plaintiffs went after big-money damages for violating the civil rights mandated by the ADA. Eventually it became clear that compliance would be cheaper than continuing litigation. Losing money does put the fear of God into Americans.

I have to say that the ADA increases the quality of my life, Darth notwithstanding. I get through airports in a wheelchair provided by the airline; John takes me to the zoo a few blocks from where we live [and] the zoo provides a wheelchair; local coffee houses to which I gravitate have disability-standard bathrooms; there are special seats for me in cinemas and theatres and in rock venues; there are kerb ramps at pedestrian crossings and ramps or elevators in addition to steps and escalators in most public accommodations. In my neighbourhood I see many other disabled people outside all the time. We are not rare or invisible, because we are not hidden as if in shame.

And bless those nasty trial lawyers, whom George W Bush and the Republicans hate so much. Without them the ADA would be a useless pile of paper.

For myself—despite physical therapy, the breaking cups, and my immobilised knee—in the middle of the night, worn down, I listen to Yo-Yo Ma playing Bach or Loretta Lynn's Van Lear Rose; and I am, I think, healing. Surely music must be more powerful than bad luck.

Source: Dworkin, Andrea. 2005, April 23. "Through the Pain Barrier." *The Guardian*. Available at: http://books.guardian.co.uk/news/articles/0,6109,1468336,00.html. Reprinted by permission of the Guardian News Service.

CHRONOLOGY

1500 BCE ◆ Egypt: The Ebers Papyrus, a medical textbook, devotes an entire chapter to eye diseases. It also shows that deafness is well understood and that clinical knowledge has developed.

400 BCE ◆ Graeco-Anatolian Hippocratic writings coin the word *epilepsy* for a convulsive condition they view as a disease rather than a possession or punishment. Today, it is estimated that more than 80 percent of the 40 million people who currently have epilepsy throughout the world have little access or no access to contemporary treatments.

300 BCE ◆ China: *The Yellow Emperor's Internal Classic* is the first text to outline acupuncture. Ordinances on emergency relief for the disabled date to the Han Dynasty, 206 BCE–AD 220. Fiscal and administrative disability classification date at least to the Tang Dynasty, 618–907.

1250– 1350 ◆ High point of medieval medicalization during which theoretical explanations for conditions gain currency in Western Europe. Prior to this time, in the most general of terms, lay explanations held more sway, ranging from the superstitious to the spiritual to the vindictive. With the founding of the universities, medical theory, typified by the four humors, became more influential in governmental, legal, and elite social circles. Disabling conditions like epilepsy, strokes, and paralyses, as well as psychiatric conditions, increasingly fell under the social control of doctors.

1400 ◆ Turkey: Deaf people work in the Ottoman Court from the 15th to the 20th centuries. Sign language becomes a recognized means of communication among both hearing and deaf courtiers.

1593 ◆ England: The origins of disability as a social and political category emerge with the first state disability benefits being enacted by Parliament for those disabled in war.

1593 ◆ Europe and the United States: English Parliament initiates Europe's first national system of benefits for rank-and-file disabled veterans. The first veterans' homes—France's Hôtel des Invalides, Britain's Chelsea Hospital, and Frederick the Great's Invalidenhaus in Berlin—are established in 1633, 1685, and 1748, respectively. Following the American Civil War, the U.S. government responds with a system of homes, preferences in government hiring, land grants, free prosthetics, and pensions for disabled veterans (however, southern veterans were limited to usually scanty state pensions).

1601 ◆ England: The Poor Law is passed to provide family and community support for those unable to make a living for themselves.

1604 ◆ Laws on witchcraft in the colonies all evolve from a 1604 English Statute that makes "being a witch" punishable by death. During outbreaks of witch-hunting, the "different" body itself is targeted as a sign and symptom of one's confederation with demonic forces.

1697 ◆ England: The first English workhouse for people with mental and physical disabilities is established in Bristol in 1697.

1704 ◆ Bethlem Hospital in the United States has 130 residents housing the "furiously mad."

1714 ◆ Canada: The Bishop of Quebec opens the first building in Canada exclusively for the confinement of mentally disturbed individuals. It is adjacent to Quebec General Hospital.

1749 ◆ France and England: Denis Diderot pens one of the most influential treatises on the blind and education in his *Letter on the Blind* in which he argues that the blind can be educated. In 1784, Valentin Haüy opens the first school for the blind in Paris. He perfects a system of raised *letters* to enable the blind to read. In 1828, Louis Braille modifies a raised *dot* system invented by Charles Barbier, which is used today by blind persons to read and communicate. In 1847, William Moon, an Englishman, develops an embossed script based on Roman capitals that blind adults can learn to read in a few days. It is the first reading system for the blind to be widely adopted across the world, but because it is costly to print, the Braille system, which can be produced by blind individuals for themselves, overtakes Moon's system.

1755 ◆ France, the United States, and Germany: The Abbé Charles-Michel de l'Épée establishes the first state-supported school for the training of young deaf children, where he teaches sign language. The school serves as an inspiration for the establishment of other European schools and has a dramatic impact on social attitudes toward the deaf. In 1817, Thomas Gallaudet and Laurent Clerc establish the Asylum for the Deaf (now American School for the Deaf) in Hartford, Connecticut. Clerc imports the French sign system, which influences the makeup of contemporary American Sign Language (ASL). In 1778, Samuel Heinicke establishes a school in Leipzig, Germany, where the "oral method" is used.

1800 ◆ France: Victor of Aveyron, a "feral child" found in southern France, is brought to Paris. Jean Marc Gaspard Itard, a French physician, develops a systematic training program for the boy and works intensively with him for five years. Itard considered his attempt at educating Victor to be a failure because the boy did not learn to use a language. Nevertheless, Itard's disciples, including Edouard Séguin, Maria Montessori, and Alfred Binet, continue his work by establishing classes for children considered to be "mentally retarded."

1802 ◆ France: The world's first pediatric hospital, L'Hôpital des Enfants Malades, is founded.

1817 ◆ The American School for the Deaf is founded in Hartford, Connecticut. It is the first school for disabled children in the Western Hemisphere.

1817 ◆ James Parkinson, a London physician, describes what is to become known as Parkinson's disease.

1817 ◆ Thomas Gallaudet and Laurent Clerc open the American Asylum for the Education of the Deaf and Dumb in Hartford, Connecticut.

1828 ◆ Frenchman Louis Braille, blind from childhood, modifies a raised-dot system of code, one of the most important advances in blind education. It not only allows the blind to read at a much faster rate but also makes it possible for the blind to be teachers of the blind. UNESCO creates the World Braille Council in 1952.

1829 ◆ France: Louis Braille publishes an explanation of his embossed dot code.

1832 ◆ Samuel Gridley Howe is chosen to direct what is later to be called the Perkins School for the Blind in Boston. It becomes the model for schools around the nation. Laura Bridgman and Helen Keller attend Perkins. In 1837, Ohio establishes the first state-sponsored school for the blind.

1834 ◆ England: The English Poor Law Amendment stipulates five categories of those unable to work: children, the sick, the insane, defectives, and the aged and infirm. This sets the stage for the development of specialty institutions that isolate the disabled from the community.

1841 ◆ P. T. Barnum purchases Scudder's American Museum in New York City. This moment is considered to be the beginning of the "Golden Age" of freaks, which persists until the 1940s. The tension between freaks and disability rights comes to a head in 1984, when disability rights activist Barbara Baskin successfully lobbies the New York State Fair to remove Sutton's Incredible Wonders of the World Sideshow, featuring a limbless man who performs as the "Frog Boy," from the midway.

1843   Due to the influence of Dorothea Dix, an American social reformer, the Massachusetts legislature allocates funds to greatly expand the State Mental Hospital at Worcester. Dix also plays an instrumental role in the creation of 32 mental hospitals and becomes nationally known for her reform efforts. By the late 1840s, Dix focuses on developing a national plan that addresses the treatment of people with mental illness.

1846   William Thomas Green Morton discovers anesthesia and in 1867 Joseph Lister provides a model for antisepsis. These new technologies play a central role in the future of aesthetic surgery as well as surgical intervention for every type of disability that calls for it. Penicillin is discovered in 1929, cutting mortality rates in hospitals dramatically.

1848   The North Carolina School for the Deaf begins the first publication for Deaf persons with its school newspaper, *The Deaf Mute.* First published in 1907, the *Matilda Ziegler Magazine for the Blind* is an ongoing Braille publication.

1848   Samuel Gridley Howe founds the first residential institution for people with mental retardation at the Perkins Institution in Boston.

1851   In the United States there are 77 residential institutions for children, 1,151 by 1910, and 1,613 by 1933. By the 1950s and 1960s, family members and politicians throughout Western Europe, Canada, and the United States push for the deinstitutionalization of people with disabilities.

1851   The first International Sanitary Conference is held in Paris, France, with 12 countries participating. It leads to the World Health Organization, the WHO, which formally comes into existence in 1948.

1857   Edward Miner Gallaudet, youngest son of Thomas Hopkins Gallaudet, establishes the Columbian Institution for the Instruction of the Deaf, Dumb, and Blind, located in Washington D.C. Its college division, eventually known as the National Deaf-Mute College, is the world's first institution of higher education for deaf people. Abraham Lincoln signs its charter on April 8, 1864; today it is known as Gallaudet University.

1857   English philosopher Herbert Spencer is first to use the expression "survival of the fittest." The application of his idea in combination with Charles Darwin's theories in his 1859 book, *The Origin of the Species,* is called Social Darwinism. It is widely accepted and promoted in Germany in the 1920s and leads Adolf Hitler to express prejudice against the weak, sick, and disabled.

1863   Louis Agassiz, a significant American naturalist, advocates the permanence of different races and worries about the "tenacious influences of physical disability" if races were mixed.

1864   Germany: Karl Ferdinand Klein, teacher for deaf-mutes, and Heinrich Ernst Stotzner are considered the founding fathers of the *training school,* which calls for schools to be created for less-capable children with the goal of improving their lot. Training schools remain in effect today, but critics maintain that there is an over-representation of socially and economically underprivileged students in this type of setting experiencing little academic success.

1868   Sweden: The Stockholm Deaf Club is the first recorded organization of people with disabilities.

1870   England and Wales: Education for children with disabilities begins when universal elementary education is first introduced around this time. From 1895 onward, schools for "defective" children spring up. In 1899, Alfred Eichholz, an inspector of special education, draws up key recommendations, which leave their mark on the historic 1994 Education Act legislation. In 1978, the Warnock report introduces the term *special needs education,* which soon gains acceptance worldwide. With the 1994 UNESCO Salamanca Statement and Framework for Action on Special Needs Education, a major shift in organizing educational services for children with disabilities is confirmed internationally.

1876 Isaac Newton Kerlin, Edouard Séguin, and others establish the Association of Medical Officers of American Institutions for the Idiotic and Feeble-Minded Persons. Today, it is known as the American Association on Mental Retardation. Séguin, who staunchly believes in the educability of those with significant cognitive disabilities, is styled as "apostle to the idiots," by Pope Pius X, reflecting the attitude of the time.

1880 The United States National Association of the Deaf (NAD), the first organization of deaf or disabled people in the Western Hemisphere, is established. In 1964, the Registry of Interpreters for the Deaf (RID) is formed to establish a national body of professionals who are trained and certified to enable communication between deaf, signing persons and nondeaf, speaking persons.

1880 Helen Keller is born in Tuscumbia, Alabama. An illness at the age of 19 months leaves her totally deaf and blind. In 1887, Anne Sullivan, recently graduated from Perkins Institution for the Blind, joins the Keller household as Helen's teacher and remains Keller's companion for nearly 50 years. For many, Keller's story is the quintessential overcoming narrative.

1881 The Chicago City Council enacts the first American "ugly law" forbidding "any person, who is diseased, maimed, mutilated or deformed in any way, so as to be an unsightly or disgusting object, to expose himself to public view."

1882 The first major federal immigration law in the United States, the Immigration Act of 1882, prohibits entry to "lunatics," "idiots," and persons likely to become unable to take care of themselves. Most of the restrictions that apply specifically to disability are removed from U.S. law in 1990. Today, disabled immigrants are still denied an entry visa if they are deemed "likely to become a public charge."

1887 Walter Fernald serves as superintendent of the Massachusetts School for the Feeble-Minded (now known as the Fernald Center) from 1887 to 1924. Unlike most of his colleagues, Fernald moderates some of his earlier extreme views and eventually develops one of the country's largest "parole" systems for moving institutional residents back into smaller, community-based residences.

1887 The American Orthopaedic Association is founded. German and British counterparts are founded in 1901 and 1918, respectively.

1895 The chiropractic profession is founded. This type of care is used to relieve musculoskeletal pain, one of the most common causes of disability.

1899 Maria Montessori and a colleague open the Scuola Magistrale Ortofrenica in Rome, an educational institute for disabled children and a training institute for instructors. Her method relies on the concept of sensory-based instruction as a means for developing intellectual competence. Her methods allow the child the greatest possible independence in order to foster his or her own development (the child's own inner "building plan").

1904 Sir Francis Galton, half first cousin of Charles Darwin, defines the term *eugenics* (which he coined in 1883) in a paper he presents to the Sociological Society on May 16. He argues for planned breeding among the "best stock" of the human population, along with various methods to discourage or prevent breeding among the "worst stock." Galton also develops the idea for intelligence tests. The term *feeblemindedness* is defined as broadly as possible and is widely used by eugenic social reformers to conflate myriad social problems. Further naming, classification, and labeling provides eugenicists with a troubling rationale for treating people with coercion, disrespect, and profound inhumanity. Persons within the various categories of sub-normality become particularly vulnerable to state-sanctioned segregation, institutional confinement, and enforced sterilization. Eugenics is widely practiced in Europe, the United States, and Canada, culminating in the systemic murder of more than 260,000 disabled people by the Nazis between 1939 and 1945. Today, the so-called new eugenics, known as "human genetics," appeals to the needs of the individual. Critics (some of the first in Germany), however, criticize individualistic eugenic approaches and disclose the connections between human genetics, national socialist racial hygiene, and eugenics.

1905 ◆ Alfred Binet and Theodore Simon publish the first intelligence scale, known as the Binet-Simon Test.

1908 ◆ The publication of Clifford Beers's *A Mind That Found Itself* initiates the mental health hygiene movement in the United States. Speaking out against mistreatment and neglect within the system, Beers establishes the Connecticut Committee of Mental Hygiene, which expands in 1909, becoming the National Committee for Mental Hygiene and is now known as the National Mental Health Association. In 1940 there are 419,000 patients in 181 state hospitals. In 1943, the patient-doctor ratio is 277:1, and by the mid-1950s in New York state alone, there are 93,000 inpatients. The Bazelon Center for Mental Health Law, founded in 1972 by a group of committed lawyers and professionals in mental health and mental retardation, attempt to improve mental health service provision through individual and class action suits. In 1980, a group of these lawyers form the National Association of Rights Protection and Advocacy (NARPA). One-third of its board of directors must identify themselves as current or former recipients of mental health care. The association is committed to the abolishment of all forced treatment.

1908 ◆ Pastor Ernst Jakob Christoffel establishes a home in Turkey for blind and otherwise disabled and orphaned children. This grows into Christoffel-Blindenmission (CBM), an independent aid organization of Christians of various denominations united to help disabled people in third world countries. Today, it supports more than 1,000 development projects in 108 countries. In 1999, CBM, other agencies, and the World Health Organization initiate VISION 2020: The Right to Sight, a global initiative for the elimination of avoidable blindness by the year 2020.

1909 ◆ Germany: The German Organization for the Care of Cripples is created as an umbrella organization for the care of the physically disabled. The Prussian Cripples' Care Law of 1920 for the first time provides a right to medical care and scholarly and occupational education for this group.

1912 ◆ Henry H. Goddard publishes *The Kadikak Family,* supports the beliefs of the eugenics movements, and helps create a climate of hysteria in which human rights abuse of the disabled, including institutionalization and forced sterilization, increases. In 1927, the U.S. Supreme Court, in *Buck v. Bell,* rules in favor of forced sterilization of people with disabilities, further fueling eugenics movements—the number of sterilizations increases.

1914 ◆ By this date, Sigmund Freud develops his most enduring influence on the study of disability, namely, the theory of psychosomatic illness in which a psychopathological flaw is given corporeal form as a symptom, thereby establishing the notion that people succumb to disease or disability because they feel guilty about past or present repressed desires.

1918 ◆ The Smith-Sears Veterans Rehabilitation Act passes, authorizing VR services for World War I veterans. In 1916, the National Defense Act marks the beginning of the U.S. government's supportive attitude toward rehabilitation. In 1920, the Smith-Fess Act marks the beginnings of the civilian VR program. The Social Security Act of 1935 establishes state-federal VR as a permanent program that can be discontinued only by an act of Congress.

1919 ◆ Edgar "Daddy" Allen establishes what becomes known as the National Society for Crippled Children. In the spring of 1934, the organizational launches its first Easter "seals" money-making campaign. Donors place seals on envelopes containing their contributions. The seal is so well-known that it becomes part of the organization's official name. Today, Easter Seals assists more than one million children and adults with disabilities and their families annually through a nationwide network of more than 500 service sites. During the 1920s, Franklin D. Roosevelt inspires the March of Dimes.

1920 At about this time, the Shriners open hospitals for the care of crippled children. President Herbert Hoover establishes a "Children's Charter" in 1928 highlighting the need to attend to the needs of crippled children.

1921 Franklin D. Roosevelt contracts poliomyelitis. Despite damage to his legs (which makes him a wheel-chair user) and deep depression, through enormous rehabilitative effort, he eventually re-enters politics and becomes president of the United States. His triumph over personal disability becomes legendary. Critics, however, fault him for choosing to minimize his disability in what is called his "splendid deception." He establishes a center for the treatment of polio patients in Warm Springs, Georgia, called the Georgia Warm Springs Foundation (1927), which hires medical specialists from Atlanta to direct orthopedics. In 1937, President Roosevelt becomes the prime mover behind the National Foundation for Infantile Paralysis Research.

1921 Mary L. McMillan (Molly) establishes the American Women's Physical Therapeutic Association, which is known today as the American Physical Therapy Association (APTA).

1921 The American Foundation for the Blind is established.

1921 Canada: Researchers isolate the hormone insulin. In 1922, Frederick Banting, Charles Best, J. B. Collip, and J.R.R. Macleod produce and test the pancreatic extract on people with diabetes, for which they are awarded a Nobel Prize. Insulin becomes a wonderful treatment for diabetes, but not a cure.

1921 France: Three historical waves of advocacy movements can be identified beginning with the National Federation of Injured Workers (FNAT) in 1921 and other organizations that focus essentially on the protection of rights. Another factor that stimulates advocacy groups in the first wave is the wounded veterans of World Wars I and II. A second wave dates from the period after World War II. Many advocacy groups form between 1950 and 1970, such as the Union of Associations of Parents of Maladjusted Children (UNAPEI) in 1960. A third wave finds a gradual emergence of three types of associations: those that run specialized facilities (for example, Living Upright, which, in 1970, leads to the creation of the first group living facility); those interested in trade unions; and those represented by user-advocate associations. Financing comes in large part from public funds, thereby creating a government-association partnership.

1922 The founding of Rehabilitation International sets the stage for the establishment of other international organizations of and for people with disabilities that link together throughout the world. Later international organizations include, among numerous others, the World Federation of the Deaf (1951), Inclusion International (1962), the International Association for the Scientific Study of Intellectual Disability (1964), Disabled Peoples' International (1981), and the International Disability Alliance (1999).

1925 The American Speech-Language-Hearing Association, today the American Academy of Speech Correction, is established to provide high-quality services for professionals in speech-language pathology, audiology, and speech and hearing science, and to advocate for people with communication disabilities.

1928 Charles Nicolle is the first deaf person to be awarded a Nobel Prize.

1929 Seeing Eye establishes the first dog guide school in the United States.

1930 The Veterans Administration is created to administer benefits, promote vocational rehabilitation, and return disabled veterans to civil employment. There is a record of provision for disabled veterans in the United States since the Revolutionary War and the Civil War. After World War I, three agencies administer veteran's benefits.

1932 Herbert A. Everest, a mining engineer with a disability, and Harry C. Jennings collaborate to design and patent the cross-frame wheelchair, which becomes the standard for the wheelchair industry that exists today. Developed during World War I, the first powered wheelchair appears, but doesn't gain popularity for another 30 years.

1935 President Franklin D. Roosevelt signs the Social Security Act of 1935 on August 14. Beginning in 1956, SSA amendments provide disability benefits.

1935 By 1935, in the United States more than 30 states pass laws allowing for the compulsory sterilization of those deemed genetically unfit in state and federal institutions. By 1970, more than 60,000 people are sterilized under these laws.

1935 As a result of being denied participation in the Works Progress Administration (WPA), six young people with disabilities hold a sit-in at the offices of New York City's Emergency Relief Bureau, demanding jobs in non-segregated environments and explicitly rejecting charity. The League of the Physically Handicapped is born out of this activism and operates in New York from 1935 to 1938. The League identifies social problems that remain issues today.

1935 Peer support in the United States is traced to the establishment of Alcoholics Anonymous in this year. Interest in peer support increases in the 1960s and is adopted by the disabled community. Movements, such as the Center for Independent Living, and groups, such as the National Spinal Cord Injury Association, make peer support one of their major activities.

1936 The American Academy of Physical Medicine & Rehabilitation is founded, leading to the approval of the American Board of Physical Medicine & Rehabilitation by the American Medical Association in 1947.

1937 The Fair Housing Act of 1937 passes with a mandate to assist the poor, a group that includes people with disabilities, by creating public housing. However, it is not until the Rehabilitation Act of 1973 that housing law specifically deals with discrimination faced by individuals with disabilities in housing programs that receive federal funding. The 1988 amendment to the Fair Housing Act of 1968 extends protection for people with disabilities beyond those of Section 504 of the Rehabilitation Act to include private housing.

1939 The Nazi regime institutes the Aktion T4 program in Germany. Children and, later, adults with disabilities are selectively killed both in hospitals and in special centers. The program was officially terminated by Adolf Hitler in August 1941, but practitioners "informally" continued it through a phase historians have called "wild euthanasia."

1940 State activists for the blind, including Jacobus Broek, come together in Wilkes-Barre, Pennsylvania, to charter the National Federation of the Blind (NFB). In 1957, the NFB publishes the first edition of the *Braille Monitor,* which is still in print today. In 1960, dissatisfied NFB members form the American Council of the Blind (ACB).

1940 Paul Strachan establishes the American Federation of the Physically Handicapped, the nation's first cross-disability, national political organization.

1942 The American Psychiatric Association develops a position statement in favor of the euthanasia of children classified as *idiots* and *imbeciles.*

1943 The LaFollette-Barden Act, also known as the Vocational Rehabilitation Amendments, adds physical rehabilitation to federally funded vocational rehabilitation programs.

1943 The United Nations is established on October 24 by 51 countries. The global Programme on the Disability is the lead program concerning disability. Many other types of programs, activities, and instruments include the 1975 Declaration on the Rights of Disabled Persons, the 1981 International Year of

Disabled Persons, the 1982 World Programme of Action Concerning Disabled Persons, the 1983–1992 UN Decade of Disabled Persons, and the 1993 Standard Rules on the Equalization of Opportunities for Persons with Disabilities. In 1988, the first UN Disability Database (DISTAT) publishes statistics from 63 national studies covering 55 countries and the 2001 publication presents 111 national studies from 78 countries, indicating a growing interest worldwide for the collection of usable data. In 2005, a UN Ad Hoc Committee continues to consider a Convention on the Rights of Disabled Persons that is a legally binding human rights instrument. Today the UN membership totals 191 countries.

1943   Sweden: In possibly the first reference to the concept of normalization, the most significant driving force in the ongoing closure of state-run or state-funded institutions for people with a disability is made by the Committee for the Partially Able-Bodied, established by the Swedish Government. Through the advocacy of people such as Niels Erik Bank-Mikkelsen, normalization, with its profound positive effect on the lives of people who were once removed and segregated from society, remains relevant today.

1944   Richard Hoover invents long white canes known as Hoover canes that are used by many blind people.

1944   The word *genocide* first appears in a book by a Polish lawyer Raphael Lemkin titled *Axis Rule in Occupied Europe* in which he describes Nazi Germany's practices but also seeks the adoption of legal restrictions so that genocide will not occur. In 1948, the United Nations adopts a declaration and then a convention on genocide that describe both against whom genocide might be directed and acts constituting genocide. Article 6 of the Rome Statute of the International Criminal Court (ICC), established in 2002, uses language identical to that in the UN convention to define genocide. More than 90 countries are parties to the ICC, but not the United States.

1945   President Harry Truman signs into law an annual National Employ the Handicapped Week. In 1952, it becomes the Presidents' Committee on Employment of the Physically Handicapped, a permanent organization, which reports to the President and Congress.

1945   Canada: Lyndhurst Lodge, the first specialized rehabilitation center for spinal cord injury (SCI) in the world, and the Canadian Paraplegic Association, the first association in the world administered by individuals with SCI, are established.

1946   The first chapter of what will become the United Cerebral Palsy Association, Inc. is established in New York City. It is chartered in 1949, and along with the Association for Retarded Children, it becomes a major force in the parents' movement of the 1950s.

1946   The National Mental Health Foundation is founded by attendants at state mental institutions who aim to expose abusive conditions. Their work is an early step toward deinstitutionalization.

1946   The National Institutes of Mental Health (NIMH) are founded in the United States.

1946   Europe: The European Union is founded on September 17 in Paris. It consistently shows its commitment to eliminating discrimination on many fronts through joint declarations, resolutions, directives, and action programs. With regard to disability, the European Union supports actions in favor of people with disabilities, principally in the form of European Social Fund interventions. Action programs aim at facilitating the exchange of information between member states and nongovernmental organizations with a view to identifying good practices, integrating people with disabilities into society, and raising awareness of related issues. The EU Council of Ministers Recommendation on the Employment of Disabled People (1986) calls on member states to "eliminate negative discrimination by reviewing laws, regulations and administrative provisions to ensure that they are not contrary to the principle of fair opportunity for disabled people." Further steps are taken in 1996 when a communication on equality of opportunities for disabled people sets out a new European disability strategy that promotes a rights-based approach, rather than a welfare-type approach. This is strengthened in 1997 when the heads of state act to strengthen Article 13 of the European Community Charter of Fundamental Social Rights of Workers (1989), giving the European Community specific powers to take action to combat a broad spectrum of discrimination that includes disability.

1948   The National Paraplegia Foundation is established as the civilian branch of the Paralyzed Veterans of America.

1948   The World Health Organization is established. The WHO actively promotes human rights and the principle of equity in health among all people of the world, including persons with disabilities. Today it consists of 191 member states, but strives for universal membership. In 1980, the WHO publishes the International Classification of Impairments, Disabilities, and Handicaps (ICIDH) and issues a revised version in 2001, the International Classification of Functioning, Disability, and Health (ICF).

1948   The United Nations General Assembly adopts the "Universal Declaration of Human Rights," which promotes and affirms the fundamental rights to life, liberty, and security; to medical care and social services; and to the benefit from scientific progress and its uses.

1948   Sir Ludwig Guttmann organizes the first Stoke Mandeville (England) Games for the Paralysed, thus launching the Paralympic movement. The Games become international in 1952. In 1960, the first Paralympic Summer games are held in Rome and the first Paralympic Winter Games follow in 1976. The Paralympic Games are multi-disability, multi-sport competitions and have become the second-largest sporting event in the world, only after the Olympic Games.

1948   World War II bomber pilot and war hero Leonard Cheshire establishes what is to become the largest charitable supplier of services for disabled people in the United Kingdom. In the 1960s, the resistance of disabled people who live in one Leonard Cheshire home, Le Court, plays a major role in establishing the British disabled people's movement. In the late 1990s, the Leonard Cheshire organization establishes the Disabled People's Forum, which is run by disabled people and supports disabled people's involvement and empowerment.

1949   Timothy Nugent founds the National Wheelchair Basketball Association, and the first Annual Wheelchair Basketball Tournament takes place.

1949   Europe: The Council of Europe, an intergovernmental organization, is founded. Its activities cover all major issues facing European society other than defense. Human dignity, equal opportunities, independent living, and active participation in the life of the community form the heart of the Council of Europe's activities in relation to people with disabilities. The European Social Charter of 1961 and its revision in 1996 include specific wording and expand the rights of individuals with disabilities.

1950   The Social Security Amendments of 1950 provide federal-state aid to the permanently and totally disabled (APTD), which serves as a limited prototype for future Social Security assistance programs for disabled people.

1950   The National Mental Health Association is formed with the mission to continue 1908-advocate Clifford W. Beers's goals of "spreading tolerance and awareness, improving mental health services, preventing mental illness, and promoting mental health."

1950   The National Association for Retarded Children (NARC) is established by families in Minneapolis. It is the first and most powerful parent-driven human-services lobby in the nation to emerge in the 1950s.

1950 ◆ Amniocentesis is developed by a Uruguayan obstetrician. Later, advanced prenatal testing provides a battery of powerful medical tools to predict risk of disability and provide information to parents about their pregnancies.

1951 ◆ With the founding of the World Federation of the Deaf, the deaf community becomes international.

1953 ◆ Francis Crick and James Watson propose a three-dimensional structure for the DNA molecule. The paper they publish also gives clues to genetic mechanisms. Today, more than 6,000 monogenic disorders have been identified, and these affect approximately 1 in 200 live births.

1955 ◆ The polio vaccine, developed by Dr. Jonas Salk, becomes available, thus ending polio epidemics in the Western world. A new oral vaccine, developed by Dr. Albert B. Sabin, is approved for use in 1961.

1956 ◆ Social Security Disability Insurance (SSDI) becomes available through amendments to the Social Security Act of 1935 (SSA) for those aged 50–64. Other important amendments to SSA include the following: 1958: provides for dependents of disabled workers; 1960: removes age limit; 1965: Medicare and Medicaid provide benefits within the framework of the SSA (until 1977); 1967: provides benefits to widows and widowers over the age of 50; 1972: Supplemental Security Income (SSI) establishes a needs-based program for the aged, blind, and disabled; 1984: the Social Security Disability Reform Act responds to the complaints of hundreds of thousands of people whose disability benefits have been terminated; 1996: President Clinton signs the Personal Responsibility and Work Opportunity Reconciliation Act, making it more difficult for children to qualify as disabled for SSI purposes.

1959 ◆ The UN Declaration of the Rights of the Child is adopted; the UN Convention on the Rights of the Child is adopted in 1989. A central principle of both documents is access to education for all children including those with disabilities. In 1993, a related UN document, the Standard Rules for the Equalization of Opportunity, extends this to preschool children, and in 1994, UNESCO's Salamanca Statement and Framework for Action specifies the provision of special education for children with disabilities or learning difficulties. These documents constitute a universal bill of rights that can serve as a framework in the development of national policies worldwide.

1961 ◆ The American Council of the Blind is established.

1961 ◆ Europe: The European Social Charter (ESC) protects "the right of physically and mentally disabled persons to vocational training, rehabilitation and social resettlement." In 1996, it is revised, updated, and expanded to take account of social changes.

1961 ◆ Michel Foucault's work *The History of Madness in the Classical Age* becomes obligatory reading for those concerned with the archaeology of madness and its treatments. It continues to be an academic *rite de passage*.

1962 ◆ Battered child syndrome is defined. Researchers estimate that the incidence of maltreatment of children with disabilities is between 1.7 and 3.4 times greater than of children without disabilities.

1962 ◆ Russia: The Moscow Theater of Mime and Gesture is the first professional deaf theater in the world. It has been in continuous operation for more than 40 years and has staged more than 100 classic and modern plays.

1963 ◆ Congress enacts new legislation to ensure funding for a comprehensive program of research on mental retardation through the National Institute on Child Health & Human Development. In 1965, the Office of Economic Opportunity launches the Elementary and Secondary Education Act (ESEA), commonly known as Project Head Start. The goal is to prevent developmental disability by providing increased opportunities for disadvantaged children in the preschool years.

1963 ◆ The Developmentally Disabled Assistance and Bill of Rights Act (DD ACT) is authorized, with its last reauthorization in 1996. It focuses on individuals with developmental disabilities such as intellectual disability, autism, cerebral palsy, epilepsy, and hearing and visual impairments, among others.

1964 ◆ The Civil Rights Act is passed. It becomes the model for future disability rights legislation.

1964 ◆ France: L'Arche is established. By the beginning of the twentieth-first century, it includes more than 113 communities in 30 countries. "The Ark" is a distinctive style of community living, based on "core members" and "assistants," who view their commitment as sharing life *with* people with disabilities, rather than as caregivers.

1965 ◆ Newly enacted Medicare and Medicaid provide national health insurance for both elderly (over 65) and disabled persons.

1965 ◆ The Vocational Rehabilitation Amendments of 1965 are passed. They provide federal funds for the construction of rehabilitation centers and create the National Commission on Architectural Barriers to Rehabilitation of the Handicapped.

1965 ◆ The Autism Society of America is founded.

1967 ◆ Deaf actors establish the National Theatre of the Deaf (NTD). It is the world's first professional deaf theater company and the oldest continually producing touring theater company in the United States. Today, after almost 40 years, the NTD chronicles over 6,000 performances. The National Theatre Workshop for the Handicapped begins in 1977 and the Other Voices Project in 1982. These groups are among the earliest groups formally to place the disability experience at the heart of their creative endeavors.

1967 ◆ Heart transplantation is introduced. This technology is preceded by open-heart surgery developed in the 1950s and coronary bypass and internal pacemakers in the1960s. The Framingham Heart Study begins in 1948. It collects data over the next decades that help identify major risk factors contributors to heart disease.

1967 ◆ Paul Lemoine in France in 1967 and Kenneth Jones and David Smith in the United States in 1973 independently describe the condition fetal alcohol syndrome (FAS), which comprises a recognizable pattern of birth defects attributable to the adverse effects of maternal alcohol abuse during pregnancy.

1967 ◆ England: St. Christopher's Hospice in South London opens. It is the first attempt to develop a modern approach to hospice and palliative care.

1968 ◆ Congress enacts the Architectural Barriers Act. The ABA requires access to facilities designed, built, altered, or leased with federal funds.

1968 ◆ The Fair Housing Amendments to the Civil Rights Act of 1968 guarantees civil rights of people with disabilities in the residential setting. The amendments extend coverage of the fair housing laws to people with disabilities and establish accessible design and construction standards for all new multi-family housing built for first occupancy on or after March 13, 1991.

1968 ◆ Sweden: The origins of People First® go back to a meeting of parents of children with intellectual disabilities whose motto is "we speak for them." However, the people with disabilities in attendance wish to speak for themselves and start their own self-advocacy group. Similar groups quickly spread to England and Canada. The name People First is chosen at a conference held in Salem, Oregon, in 1974. People First is an international self-advocacy organization run by and for people with intellectual disabilities to work on civil and human rights issues.

1970 ◆ Landmark legal cases such as *Diana v. State Board of Education* (1970; Latino students) and *Larry P. v. Riles* (1971–1979; minority students) challenge biases inherent in standardized testing procedures used to identify students as eligible for special education. Both cases call into question the widespread use of "scientifically" objective measures to gauge intellectual ability. Today, despite reforms, a disproportionate number of students from racial, ethnic, and linguistic minorities continue to be placed in special education classes.

1970 ◆ Japan: The Disabled Persons' Fundamental Law (DPFL) becomes one of the 27 fundamental laws that stipulate basic principles in each policy area. Major revision takes place in 1993 reflecting a progress of guiding principles in disability policy that are deeply influenced by international movements such as the International Year of Disabled Persons (1981) and the UN Decade of Disabled Persons (1983–1992). Disability Studies as well as modern disability movements are born this same year, when members of Aoi Shiba, a group of people with cerebral palsy, protest publicly for the first time against sympathetic views toward the killing of disabled children by their parents. Aoi Shiba and other disability movements join in the establishment of Disabled Peoples' International in 1981. In 1986, the Rehabilitation Engineering Society of Japan (RESJA) is established. In 1992, disability movements in Japan initiate the Asian and Pacific Decade of Disabled Persons 1993 to 2002. The Japan Society for Disability Studies is established in 2003 and a unified national organization, Japan Disability Forum (JDF), is established in 2004.

1970 ◆ United Kingdom: The Chronically Sick and Disabled Persons Act (CSDPA) strengthens the provisions in the 1948 National Assistance Act (NAA). Later, the Disability Discrimination Acts of 1995 and 2005, together with the Disability Rights Commission Act of 1999, constitute the primary source of antidiscrimination legislation for disabled people.

1971 ◆ A U.S. District Court decision in *Wyatt v. Stickney* is the first important victory in the fight for deinstitutionalization.

1971 ◆ WGBH Public Television establishes the Caption Center, which provides captioned programming for deaf viewers.

1971 ◆ Gerontologist M. Powell Lawton defines *functional assessment* as any systematic attempt to objectively measure the level at which a person is functioning in a variety of domains. Over 30 years later, functional assessment, in combination with *outcomes analysis,* is considered one of the "basic sciences" of rehabilitation. In 1980, the World Health Organization proposes a series of definitions, which have a profound impact on the assessment of functional status and outcomes in rehabilitation. It is modified and revised in 1993 and 2001.

1971 ◆ The Declaration on the Rights of Mentally Retarded Persons (UN 1971), the Declaration on the Rights of Disabled Persons (UN 1975), and the World Programme of Action Concerning Disabled Persons (UN 1982) indicate the emergence of a global discourse of rights for disability.

1972 ◆ A group of people with disabilities (including Ed Roberts, John Hessler, and Hale Zukas), known as the Rolling Quads, living together in Berkeley, California, formally incorporate as the Center for Independent Living (CIL). This first CIL in the country becomes the model for Title VII of the Rehabilitation Act of 1973. In the late 1980s and early 1990s the group's advocacy efforts help pass the Americans with Disabilities Act (ADA). CILs are always controlled by disabled people. Accepted by most people as the birth of the modern independent living movement, the Berkeley concept migrates to other countries. In 1999, a global summit on independent living is held in Washington D.C. The summit brings together more than 70 countries. The Washington Declaration that comes out of the conference establishes a set of basic principles. In 1996, the Ed Roberts Campus, an international center and a service facility, is created in Berkeley, California, in memory of Edward V. Roberts, founder of the independent living concept.

1972   A young television reporter for the ABC network, Geraldo Rivera, is given a key to one of the wards at Willowbrook State School on Staten Island, New York. Established in the late 1930s as a state-of-the-art facility for the "mentally deficient," by 1972, Willowbrook becomes a warehouse for the "socially undesirable" of New York City, with a substantial minority having no disability at all. The inhumane conditions deteriorate to the extent that a visitor remarks, "In Denmark we don't let our cattle live this way." Rivera's exposé leads to a lawsuit that results in the Willowbrook Consent Decree of 1975, which creates a detailed system of monitoring and oversight of all residents living there at that time, to be met until the last of the "class clients," as they are sometimes referred to, pass on. The property has since been sold to a college.

1972   Paul Hunt's call for a consumer group to promote the views of actual and potential residents of institutional homes for the disabled in the United Kingdom results in the establishment of the Union of the Physically Impaired against Segregation (UPIAS). The group's aim is to formulate and publicize plans for alternative forms of support in the community. Hunt is regarded by many disability activists as the founder of the modern disabled people's movement.

1972   New Zealand: Three key pieces of legislation pass have long-term effects on the disabled community: the 1972 no-fault Accident Compensation Act that provides monetary compensation to victims based on level of impairment suffered; the 1975 Disabled Persons Community Welfare Act, giving assistance to disabled people, parents, and guardians, as well as voluntary associations; and the Human Rights Act of 1977, which does not include disability as a recognized grounds for discrimination. Today, disabled populations in New Zealand continue to fight to establish an identity as disabled people rather than a group needing "welfare." One task is to promote legislation that includes disability as a group against whom discrimination is outlawed.

1973   The Rehabilitation Act of 1973 lays the foundation for the disability rights movement. Its Section 504 asserts that people with disabilities have equal rights that prevent discrimination based on their disability in programs or activities that receive federal funding. This is the first major nationwide antidiscriminatory legislation designed to protect disabled Americans. These rights are further protected with the landmark Americans with Disabilities Act (ADA) of 1990.

   Section 501 of the Act requires affirmative action and nondiscrimination in employment by federal agencies of the executive branch. Section 502 creates the Access Board, which grows out of the 1965 National Commission on Architectural Barriers to Rehabilitation of the Handicapped. As a result of the commission's June 1968 report, Congress enacts the Architectural Barriers Act (ABA). Section 503 requires that to receive certain government contracts, entities must demonstrate that they are taking affirmative action to employ people with disabilities. The enduring hallmark of the act, Section 504, provides that no otherwise qualified individual with a disability shall, solely by reason of his or her disability, be excluded from the participation in, denied the benefits of, or subjected to discrimination under any program or activity receiving federal funds. However, it would take five years of lobbying and protesting before the American Coalition of Citizens with Disabilities (ACCD) wins the release of regulations that allow Section 504 to be implemented.

   The Act is in many ways the direct predecessor to the ADA. However, the primary focus is vocational training and rehabilitation, and over the next half-century, disability law and advocacy move from the medical (medical issues) and vocational (often a justification for welfare and benefits) models to a civil rights model, which seeks to remove the barriers that impede the full integration of people with disabilities into society.

1973   The term *mainstreaming* emerges within the educational jargon associated with the Education for All Handicapped Children Act (EHA), the early U.S. legislation subsequently reauthorized as the Individuals with Disabilities Act (IDEA) in 1990.

1973   Ronald Mace is the driving force behind the creation of the first accessible state building code in the United States (North Carolina, 1974) and in the drafting of national accessibility codes and standards. He coins the term *universal design* to capture and promote his expanded philosophy of "design for all ages and abilities"—curb cuts being his favorite example.

1973 ◆ Washington D.C. introduces the first handicap parking stickers. The Federal-Aid Highway Act funds curb cuts.

1974 ◆ First Lady Betty Ford and investigative reporter Rose Kushner are diagnosed with breast cancer. They help break the public silence on this topic. In 1954, Terese Lasser begins Reach to Recovery, a program of volunteers who have previously undergone radical mastectomies who provide emotional support to hospitalized women who have just had the operation. Today, one in eight women is diagnosed with breast cancer during her lifetime.

1975 ◆ The Education for All Handicapped Children Act, the first separate federal legislation authorizing special education for children and youth, passes, due, in part, to the advocacy efforts of a group of parents. In 1990, it becomes known as the Individuals with Disabilities Education Act, or IDEA.

1975 ◆ The Developmentally Disabled Assistance and Bill of Rights Act, providing federal funds for programs that provide services for people with developmental disabilities, passes.

1975 ◆ The Association of Persons with Severe Handicaps (TASH) is founded. It calls for the end of aversive behavior modification and deinstitutionalization of people with disabilities.

1975 ◆ The UN General Assembly adopts the Declaration on the Rights of Disabled Persons, which states that all persons with disabilities have the same rights as other people. This document is not legally binding and can be attributed in part to a UN Ad Hoc Committee set up in 2001 to consider a Convention on the Rights of Disabled Persons that is legally binding.

1975 ◆ United Kindom: The Union of the Physically Impaired against Segregation (UPIAS) publishes a paper that redefines the term *disability,* which becomes known as the social model of disability as it radically transforms the way disabled people see themselves and their place in society.

1976 ◆ The Higher Education Act of 1965, which establishes grants for student support services aimed at fostering an institutional climate supportive of low-income and first-generation college students, is amended to include individuals with disabilities. In March 1978, the Association on Handicapped Student Service Programs in Post-Secondary Education is founded. It later becomes the Association on Higher Education and Disability (AHEAD).

1976 ◆ Sponsored by Ralph Nader's Center for the Study of Responsive Law, the Disability Rights Center is founded in Washington D.C.

1977 ◆ Protesting the federal government's delayed enactment of the rules and regulations for the implementation of the Rehabilitation Act of 1973, disabled activists on April 1 organize protests at the federal offices of the Department of Health and Human Services in various cities across the United States. In San Francisco, protesters hold the regional offices hostage for 28 days, gaining national attention and resulting in an agreement with federal officials for the rapid establishment of the rules and regulations to implement Section 504 of the Act.

1977 ◆ Max Cleland is appointed to head the U.S. Veterans Administration. He is the first severely disabled person to hold this post.

1977 ◆ S. Z. Nagi defines *disability* as an individual's performance of tasks and activities related to achievement of social roles—a distinct concept, different from *impairment*. It is further formalized with the introduction of the World Health Organization's International Classification of Impairments, Disabilities, and Handicaps in 1980 and further refined in 2001 in its International

Classification of Functioning, Disability, and Health. Nagi's model is used as the basis for the Americans with Disabilities Act, for almost all disability social policy in the United States, and for statistics at the United Nations and in Europe.

1978 The Child Abuse Prevention and Treatment and Adoption Reform Act of 1978 and the Adoption Assistance and Child Welfare Act of 1980 promote the adoption of children with special needs, including disabilities.

1978 The Atlantis Community, the second independent living center in the country after Berkeley, is established in Denver, Colorado, in 1975. On July 5–6, 1978, twenty disabled activists from the Atlantis Community block buses with their wheelchairs and bodies and bring traffic to a standstill at a busy downtown intersection. This act of civil disobedience results in the American Disabled for Accessible Public Transit, the original name for the American Disabled for Attendant Programs Today, or ADAPT.

1978 Legislation creates the National Institute on Handicapped Research. In 1986, it is renamed the U.S. National Institute on Disability and Rehabilitation Research (NIDRR). Its mission is to contribute to the independence of persons of all ages who have disabilities. It is located in the Department of Education under the Office of Special Education and Rehabilitation Services.

1978 The World Health Organization starts to promote the concept of community-based rehabilitation (CBR) as a means of helping people with disabilities in the developing world. It emerges, in part, from the WHO primary health care campaign Health for All by the Year 2000. Around the same time, in Western countries, home-visiting programs in which a trained worker regularly visits the family to advise on ways of promoting child development become one of the success stories of modern disability services. Among the best-known programs are those based on a model originating in Portage, Wisconsin, and now used in many countries.

1978 England: The Warnock report introduces the term *special needs education*. It marks a major shift in organizing educational services for children with disabilities and results in the new conceptualization of special needs education. This change is confirmed internationally by the Salamanca Statement and Framework for Action on Special Needs Education at the UNESCO's Conference held in Salamanca in 1994. This theoretical shift is marked with the change of the term *integration* to *inclusion* or *inclusive education*.

1978 USSR: The Action Group to Defend the Rights of the Disabled is established to advocate for legal rights for Soviets with disabilities.

1979 The Disability Rights Education and Defense Fund (DREDF) establishes itself as a leading cross-disability civil rights law and policy center. It is founded by people with disabilities and parents of children with disabilities. Because its philosophy is closely aligned with other civil rights struggles, in 1981, DREDF is invited to join the executive committee of the national's largest coalition of civil rights groups, the Leadership Conference on Civil Rights. In 1987, DREDF establishes the Disability Rights Clinical Legal Education Program and begins teaching disability rights law at the University of California's Boalt Hall School of Law.

1979 The National Alliance for the Mentally Ill (NAMI) is founded. NAMI is an advocacy and education organization.

1979 Germany: The first Cripples' Group is founded as a cross-disability group with emancipatory aims. In an attempt to reinterpret disability in positive terms, the cofounders choose the term *Krüppel* over handicapped or disabled.

Chronology

Chronology

1979 ◆ Nicaragua: The Organization of the Revolutionary Disabled is set up in the wake of the Sandinista victory.

1980 ◆ The California Governor's Committee on Employment of People with Disabilities and entertainment and media industry professionals establish the Media Access Office (MAO).

1980 ◆ About the time Congress is considering passage of the ADA (1990), marketers begin to acknowledge the economic potential of the disabled community; consequently, the appearance of disabled characters in consumer goods advertising mushroom and ability-integrated advertising becomes much more commonplace. Organizations such as MAO and NOD (National Organization on Disability) provide advertising strategies and guidance.

1980 ◆ The Rehabilitation Engineering and Assistive Technology Society of North America (RESNA), an interdisciplinary association composed of individuals interested in technology and disability, is founded.

1980 ◆ The World Health Organization's International Classification of Impairments, Disabilities, and Handicaps (ICIDH), a groundbreaking, but controversial, classification system is tentatively released for trial purposes with the goal of uniform information collection worldwide. It has a negligible impact on disability statistics or data collection; however, researchers argue that it is a vast improvement over available tools. It is renamed and vastly revised in 2001.

1980 ◆ England: Graeae Theatre Group, composed of disabled actors, directors, and other theater professionals, is founded in London by Nabil Shaban and Richard Tomlinson. It takes its name from the the Graeae of Greek mythology, three gray-haired sisters who shared one eye and one tooth. Graeae's first production is *Sideshow*.

1980 ◆ Netherlands: The Liliane Foundation starts by assisting 14 children. In 2002, it helps 31,982 children spread over 80 countries. The Foundation's efforts are directed primarily toward children with disabilities living at home. Its aim is to have direct contact with the child within the home situation and to assist the personal growth and happiness of the child, thus providing "tailor-made" assistance.

1980 ◆ Taiwan: The Physically and Mentally Disabled Citizens Protection Law is promulgated. It guarantees legal rights for the disabled and creates a significant improvement in their welfare. Although most of the disabled people in Taiwan still struggle to earn their due respect, today, public awareness of this group is emerging gradually and significantly.

1980 ◆ United Kingdom and Europe: The Black Report (*Report of the Working Group on Inequalities in Health*) is published. Among other groups it targets disabled people for better conditions that lead to better health. The report does not find favor with the Conservative government, but begins to be implemented under the Labour government in 1997. With its central theme of equity, the report plays a central role in the shaping of the World Health Organization's Common Health Strategy of the European Region.

1981 ◆ The Reagan Administration begins to amend and revoke disability benefits, a policy that continues throughout his administration and leads several disabled people who are in despair over the loss of their benefits to commit suicide.

1981 ◆ Justin Dart, recognized as the founder of the Americans with Disabilities Act (ADA, 1990), is appointed to be vice-chair of the National Council on Disability. The council drafts a national policy on equal rights for disabled people; the document becomes the foundation of the ADA.

1981 ◆ The Committee on Personal Computers and the Handicapped is established in Illinois, an indicator of the disabled community's interest in information technology (IT) accessibility, but in order to stimulate the development of suitable products, activists lobby for legislative protections, which are included in the Americans with Disabilities Act of 1990. In 2000, a suit brought by the National Federation of the Blind against AOL is suspended when AOL agrees to make its software accessible by April 2001. The World Wide Web Accessibility Initiative (WAI) launches in 1997. It raises the level of awareness of disability accessibility issues within the Internet community, especially among those who design and implement web pages.

1981 ◆ The first reported cases of AIDS in the United States appear in June. Today, the World Health Organization estimates that worldwide, approximately 40 million people are living with HIV/AIDS; 22 million men, women, and children have died; and 14,000 new infections are contracted every day. Around the world, in the year 2003, the AIDS epidemic claims an estimated 3 million lives, and almost 5 million people acquire HIV, 700,000 of them children. Currently, 6 million people infected with HIV in the developing world are estimated to need access to antiretroviral therapy to survive, but only 400,000 have this access.

1981 ◆ Disabled Peoples' International (DPI) is officially founded at a meeting in Singapore. The establishment of such international organizations around this time represents the disability movement becoming a global social movement instead of a national one. DPI is directed by persons with disabilities working in human rights advocacy. It sponsors World Assemblies, which are held every four years to develop a multiyear action plan. The most recent one is held in 2002 in Sapporo, Japan, where delegates from more than 100 countries come together. A leading slogan for DPI and other disability groups, coined in the early 1990s, is "nothing about us without us."

1981 ◆ The International Year of Disabled Persons encourages governments to sponsor programs that assimilate people with disabilities into mainstream society. Despite the positive worldwide effects it has, the UN program also creates some angry activists with disabilities who protest against the charity approach officially adopted for the event. Consequently, the activists build their own infrastructure consisting of counseling and advocacy facilities as well as job creation programs.

1981 ◆ Australia: Australia's modern disability policy takes shape after the 1981 International Year of Disabled Persons. Examples: The 1980s see a shift away from institutional care; the Commonwealth Disability Service Act provides a framework for the provision of disability services; and in 1991, the federal Disability Reform Package maximizes the employment of disabled. In 1995, a legal decision represents a watershed in telecommunications policy for people with disabilities when a commission's inquiry finds the national carrier, Telstra, guilty of discrimination against people with severe hearing or speech impairments. The success of the action results in the Telecommunications Act of 1997, which includes new provisions for the deaf community.

1981 ◆ Mexico: The Program of Rehabilitation Organized by Disabled Youth of Western Mexico begins as a rural community-based rehabilitation program.

1981 ◆ Soweto: The Self Help Association of Paraplegics begins as an economic development project.

1981 ◆ United Kingdom: Disabled people set up the British Council of Disabled Persons (BCOPD), the United Kingdom's national organization of disabled people, to promote their full equality and participation in UK society.

1981 ◆ Zimbabwe: The National Council of Disabled Persons, initially registered as a welfare organization, becomes a national disability rights group.

Chronology

1982 ◆ Disability Studies originates with the formation of the Society for the Study of Chronic Illness, Impairment, and Disability. In 1986, it officially changes its name to the Society for Disability Studies (SDS). Disability Studies is a critical field of study based in human and social science.

1982 ◆ *In re Infant Doe* (commonly known as the Baby Doe case) launches the debate as to whether parents or medical authorities should choose to let a disabled infant die rather than provide the necessary medical treatment and nourishment essential to sustain life. In response to this and other cases, the U.S. Department of Health and Human Services creates a rule maintaining it unlawful for any federally funded hospital to withhold medical treatment from disabled infants. In 1984, the U.S. Congress enacts the Child Abuse Amendments, which calls for the medical treatment of newborns with disabilities unless the child would die even with medical intervention. The issue makes it to the U.S. Supreme Court in 1986 with the *Bowen v. American Hospital Association* case. The Court holds that denying treatment to disabled infants does not constitute legally protected discrimination under Section 504 of the Rehabilitation Act and that hospitals and physicians are to implement the decision of the parents. The decision results in the passage of the Child Abuse Prevention and Treatment Act Amendments of 1984. In the year 2000, a scholar argues that the Amendments, presidential commission writings, and disability advocates "have all combined to ensure that most babies who can benefit from medical interventions do receive them."

1982 ◆ Disability Awareness in Action (DAA) and other groups such as the Disabled Peoples' International (DPI) and International Disability Alliance (IDA) are the driving force behind the globalization of disability issues through the World Program of Action (1982), the United Nations Standard Rules of Equalization of Opportunities for People with Disabilities (1993), the World Summit for Social Development (1995), and the Education for All Framework for Action (2000), as well as the current campaign to secure a UN convention on the rights of disabled people.

1982 ◆ The National Council on Independent Living (NCIL) is formed in the United States. It provides an excellent example of leadership for people with disabilities by people with disabilities.

1982 ◆ Canada: The Charter of Rights and Freedoms section of the Constitution provides protection to persons with disabilities.

1982 ◆ France: Handicap International is founded in Lyon. It is active in various areas associated with all the causes of handicaps, both traumatological (land mines, road accidents) and infectious (polio, leprosy). In the 1990s it begins working on mental disability issues as a result of experience with Romanian orphanages and the war in the Balkans. In 1992, Handicap International creates its first two mine clearance programs and in 1997 it is the joint winner of the Nobel Peace Prize for its leading role in the fight against landmines.

1983 ◆ Rights-based approaches to disability rapidly gain currency in many developing countries since the UN Decade of Disabled Persons, 1983–1992. UNESCAP's Biwako Millennium Framework for Action towards an Inclusive, Barrier-Free and Rights-Based Society for People with Disabilities in Asia and the Pacific sets the priorities for the extended Decade of Disabled Persons, 2003–2012.

1983 ◆ Access and accessibility are concepts discussed throughout the World Programme of Action Concerning Disabled Persons passed by the UN General Assembly. The General Assembly in 1993 passes the Standard Rules on the Equalization of Opportunities for Persons with Disabilities.

1983 ◆ England: The first Covent Garden Day of Disabled Artists is held in London.

1983 ◆ Thailand: DPI-Thailand is established.

1984 ◆ The Access Board issues the "Minimum Guidelines and Requirements for Accessible Design," which today serves as the basis for enforceable design standards. The 1990 Americans with

Disabilities Act (ADA) expands the board's mandate to include developing the accessibility guidelines for facilities and transit vehicles. The Rehabilitation Act Amendments of 1998 give the Access Board additional responsibility for developing accessibility standards for electronic and information technology. In 2001, Section 508 of federal law establishes design standards for federal websites, making them accessible to individuals with disabilities.

1985   The U.S. Department of Health and Human Services issues the first comprehensive national minority health study, which shows racial disparity in health and concludes that the difference in mortality is not acceptable. In 1998, studies indicate that racial disparity has not improved as much as hoped; consequently, President Bill Clinton launches an initiative that sets a national goal of eliminating disparities in six key areas by the year 2010. Some of these areas include diseases and conditions considered to be disabling as well as life threatening.

1986   The Air Carrier Access Act (ACAA) passes. It requires the U.S. Department of Transportation to develop new regulations that ensure that disabled people are treated without discrimination in a way consistent with the safe carriage of all passengers. The relevant regulations, Air Carrier Access rules, are published in March 1990.

1986   The National Council on the Handicapped publishes its report *Toward Independence.* It recommends that "Congress should enact a comprehensive law requiring equal opportunity for individuals with disabilities" and suggests that the law be called "the Americans with Disabilities Act." In its 1988 follow-up report, *On the Threshold of Independence,* the council takes the somewhat unusual step of publishing its own draft of the ADA bill.

1986   The Equal Opportunities for Disabled Americans Act allows recipients of federal disability benefits to retain them even after they obtain work, thus removing a disincentive that keeps disabled people unemployed.

1986   Australia: The Disability Services Act provides that a person with disability has the right to achieve his or her individual capacity for physical, social, emotional, and intellectual development. In 1992, the Disability Discrimination Act supports nondiscrimination in education and training. It also makes it unlawful to discriminate in relation to access to premises, including public transportation.

1986   Canada: The Employment Equity Act mandates the institution of positive policies and practices to ensure that persons in designated groups, including persons with disabilities, achieve at least proportionate employment opportunities.

1986   England: The first issue of the magazine *Disability Arts in London* (DAIL) is produced in London.

1986   Southern Africa: The Southern Africa Federation of the Disabled is formed as a federation of nongovernmental organizations of disabled persons.

1988   The Technology Act (Technology-Related Assistance for Individuals with Disabilities Act of 1988 and its 1994 amendments), and, in 1998, the Assistive Technology Act (AT) provide financial assistance to states to support programs of technology-related assistance for individuals with disabilities of all ages. The1988 act defines *assistive technology* (AT). The Americans with Disabilities Act of 1990 prohibits discrimination against people with disabilities in employment, public institutions, commercial facilities, transportation, and telecommunications, which includes accessibility to all entrances, bathrooms, program areas, and parking spaces as well as interpreters for the deaf and Braille and large-print materials for the blind. The Telecommunications Act of 1996 requires the telecommunication industry to make equipment that will support transmission of information in forms accessible to people with disabilities including broadband and television program captioning. By 2000, approximately 10 percent of the U.S. population uses AT devices and/or modifications to their home, work, or school that allow them to participate in major life activities.

1988 ◆ Congress introduces a series of amendments to the Civil Rights Act of 1968, including a prohibition of housing discrimination against people with disabilities. These amendments are known as the Fair Housing Act Amendments of 1988.

1988 ◆ China: Deng Pufang, a wheelchair user and son of the late Chinese leader Deng Xiaoping, is the driving force behind a series of laws and programs initiated to improve life for the disabled. In 1984, he sets up the China Welfare Fund for Disabled Persons and, in 1988, the China Disabled Persons' Federation, which endeavors to improve public images of disabled people. Today, there are 60 million disabled people in China.

1989 ◆ The European Network on Independent Living (ENIL) is set up. It focuses on personal assistance as a key component of independent living.

1990 ◆ ADAPT, the American Disabled for Attendant Programs Today, originally called the American Disabled for Accessible Public Transit, continues to gain public awareness through tactics of civil disobedience until regulations are finally issued with the passage of the Americans with Disabilities Act (ADA).

The ADA passes, after ADAPT uses tactics of civil disobedience, in the tradition of other civil rights movements, in one of the largest disability rights protests to date (600 demonstrators), the "Wheels of Justice March," during which dozens of protesters throw themselves out of their wheelchairs and begin crawling up the 83 marble steps to the Capitol to deliver a scroll of the Declaration of Independence. The following day 150 ADAPT protesters lock wheelchairs together in the Capitol rotunda and engage in a sit-in until police carry them away one by one.

George H.W. Bush signs the ADA on July 26. It provides employment protections for qualifying persons with disability. It is the most prominent and comprehensive law prohibiting discrimination on the basis of disability in the United States, expanding the mandate of Section 504 of the Rehabilitation Act of 1973 to eliminate discrimination by prohibiting discrimination in employment, housing, public accommodations, education, and public services.

In June 2000, the National Council on Disability issues a report, *Promises to Keep: A decade of Federal Enforcement of the Americans with Disabilities Act,* which includes 104 specific recommendations for improvements to the ADA enforcement effort. On December 1, 2004, the council issues a final summary report, *Righting the ADA,* in order to address "a series of negative court decisions [that] is returning [Americans with disabilities] to 'second-class citizen' status that the Americans with Disabilities Act was supposed to remedy forever."

1990 ◆ The ADA requires public entities and businesses to provide effective communication to individuals with disabilities. Title IV of the ADA mandates that nationwide telecommunication systems be accessible to persons with speech or hearing disabilities. The Federal Communications Commission (FCC) requires relay services to be in place by July 26, 1993. The Telecommunications Act of 1996 adds provisions to the Communications Act of 1934 that requires manufactures and providers of telecommunications equipment and services to ensure accessibility to persons with disabilities. In 2000, President Bill Clinton establishes regulations governing the accessibility to people with disabilities of the electronic and information technology used within the federal government.

1990 ◆ The Individuals with Disabilities Education Act (IDEA) is enacted. It guarantees the right to free and appropriate education for children and youth with disabilities and focuses on higher expectations, mainstreaming students where possible, and an increased federal rule in ensuring equal educational opportunity for all students. IDEA requires schools to provide a free and appropriate public education to eligible children with disabilities. It also requires schools to develop an individualized education plan (IEP) for each child and placement in the least restrictive environment (LRE) for their education. IDEA is amended in 1997 and reauthorized again in 2004 as the Individuals with Disabilities Education Improvement Act.

1990 ◆ Legislation establishes the National Center for Medical Rehabilitation Research (NCMRR), whose mission is to foster development of scientific knowledge needed to enhance the health, productivity, independence, and quality of life of persons with disabilities. It has primary responsibility for the U.S. Government's medical rehabilitation research that is supported by the National Institutes of Health (NIH).

1990 ◆ The World Declaration on Education for All (EFA) is adopted in Jomtien, Thailand, by more than 1,500 persons representing the international community. Article 23 of the UN Convention on the Rights of the Child states that disabled children have the right to a "full and decent life" and that member nations provide free education and training to disabled children whenever possible in order to provide the "fullest possible social integration and individual development." UNESCO is the lead UN organization for special needs education.

1990 ◆ Korea: The disability movement celebrates the passage of the Employment Promotion Act for People with Disabilities. The government imposes control over the disabled population in the 1960s and 1970s by forwarding institutionalization under the banner of "protection," promoting sterilization, and violating the rights of disabled people in general. The 1981 International Year of Disabled Persons influences the government, and new laws, such as the Welfare Law for Mentally and Physically Handicapped, are enacted, and the human rights of disabled people becomes the dominant rhetoric of the disability movement.

1990 ◆ United Kingdom: The National Disability Arts Forum is launched at the UK-OK Conference at Beaumont College in Lancashire, UK.

1991 ◆ The Resolution on Personal Assistance Services is passed at the International Personal Assistance Symposium. Personal assistance services are the most critical services for individuals. Critical aspects of these services are that they must be available up to 24 hours a day, 7 days a week, to people of all ages, and with access to governmental payments. In the United States alone, personal assistance services affect the lives of more than 9.6 million citizens with disabilities.

1991 ◆ Australia: The federal Disability Reform Package is introduced; the Disability Discrimination Act, which covers issues of discrimination in education, is enacted in 1992; and the Commonwealth Disability Strategy, designed to provide equal access to government services for people with disabilities, is first introduced in 1994 and then revised in 2000. During the 1990s similar discrimination legislation emerges in other countries, such as New Zealand's Human Rights Act, the U.K.'s Disability Discrimination Act, Israel's Disabled Persons Act, Canada's Human Rights Act, and India's Disabled Person's Act.

1991 ◆ China: The most important laws and initiatives reside in the 1991 Law on Protection of Disabled Persons and a series of National Work Programs for Disabled Persons (1988, 1991, 1996, 2001), which integrate disability into the government's Five-Year Plans. China participates heavily in the United Nations Decade of Disabled Persons, 1983–1992, and initiates the Asia Pacific Decade of the Disabled Persons, 1993–2002. China continues to collaborate with UN projects involving the disabled and will host the 2007 International Special Olympics in Shanghai.

1991 ◆ Serbia and Montenegro: From the 1960s to the 1980s, post–World War II Yugoslavia is lauded for being a socially advanced nonaligned nation, but the contemporary wars that decimate Yugoslavia begin in 1991, and today there are more than one million disabled citizens, refugees, and casualties due to the wars. Disabled people in Serbia and Montenegro (formally named the Federal Republic of Yugoslavia—FRY) are left with shattered pieces of the spent past with little hope for the near future. Although the FRY constitution prescribes special protection of disabled persons in accordance with legal provisions and Serbia is party to numerous UN documents and acts, a disabled expert in 2004 admits that discrimination against persons with disability in Serbia and Montenegro is a long-term problem that people without disability tend to ignore. Two of the most effective advocacy groups making in-roads today are the Association of Students with Disabilities and the Center for Independent Living in Belgrade.

1992   The UN Economic and Social Commission of Asia and the Pacific (ESCAP) proclaims a 10-year program known as the Asian and Pacific Decade of Disabled Persons 1993–2002 with goals of full participation and equality for persons with disabilities.

1993   The United Nations publishes the Standard Rules on the Equalization of Opportunities for Persons with Disabilities, which becomes the international legal standards for disability programs, laws, and policies. Although not legally enforceable this instrument sets an inclusive and antidiscriminatory standard that is used when national policies are developed. It marks a clear shift from the rehabilitation and prevention paradigm to the human rights perspective on disability.

1993   Slovak Republic: The Czech and Slovak Republics separate into two independent countries. They both join the European Union in 2004. In Slovakia, a large number of highly innovative and resourceful grassroots nongovernmental organizations emerge to address the human rights, quality-of-life, and independent living priorities of citizens with disabilities. They pursue this mission, however, with extremely limited resources and with varying degrees of support from a multiparty parliament.

1993   Sweden: The Independent Living Institute (ILI) is founded.

1994   Two networks, one for elderly persons and the other for persons with disabilities, join together to form the U.S. National Coalition on Aging and Disability. In following years, policy makers and advocates begin to see the benefits of merging some services.

1994   Germany: The disability rights movement is successful in using for its own aims the reform of the German constitution, which is made necessary by the reunification process. An amendment to the constitution forbids discrimination on the grounds of disability. Other such laws as the Rehabilitation of Participation Law (2001) and the Federal Equal Rights Law (2002) are formulated with the active contribution of disability rights activists, and in 2003, the official German program of the European Year of People with Disabilities is organized by a prominent activist.

1994   Sweden: The Swedish Disability Act (LSS) comes into force. It expands the 1985 Special Services Act. The LSS is also more ambitious than its predecessor, calling for "good living conditions" rather than just an "acceptable standard of living."

1995   The National Council on Disability, a federal agency, makes recommendations to the president and Congress on disability issues. Among other issues, it calls for the end to the use of aversives (techniques of behavior control such as restraints, isolation, and electric shocks) because they are abusive, dehumanizing, and psychologically and physically dangerous. Other organizations follow, such as the Autism National Committee in 1999, TASH in 2004, and the International Association for the Right to Effective Treatment in 2003.

1995   The Commission for Case Management Certification (CCMC) incorporates. Case management is a process of care planning and coordination of the services and resources used by people with disabilities and their families.

1995   Europe: The Association for the Advancement of Assistive Technology in Europe (AAATE) is founded as an interdisciplinary association devoted to increasing awareness, promoting research and development, and facilitating the exchange of information. AAATE is composed of more than 250 members from 19 countries. It interacts with sister organizations in North America, Japan, and Australia to advance assistive technology worldwide. The Tokushima Agreement, signed in 2000 by AAATE, the Rehabilitation Engineering and Assistive Technology Society of North America

(RESNA), the Rehabilitation Engineering Society of Japan (RESJA), and the Australian Rehabilitation and Assistive Technology Association (ARATA), promotes exchange of information and collaboration.

1995 United Kingdom: The campaign for antidiscrimination legislation begins in earnest with the emergence of the disability movement in the late 1970s. The Disability Discrimination Act of 1995 (DDA) together with the Disability Rights Commission Act of 1999 constitute the primary source of antidiscrimination legislation for disabled people in the United Kingdom. The Disability Discrimination Act 2005 extends the protection.

1996 There are 1.4 million fewer disabled older persons in the United States than would have been expected if the health status of older people had not improved since the early 1980s.

1996 Advocates for mental health parity such as the National Alliance for the Mentally Ill (NAMI; 1979) believe that mental illnesses are real illnesses and that health insurance and health plan coverage for treatment should be equal with coverage of treatment for all other illnesses. Due in part to advocacy, the Mental Health Parity Act becomes law in 1996. In 1999, mental illness ranks first in causing disabilities among many industrialized nations, including the United States, which experiences a loss of productivity in this year of $63 billion. In the United States, 5 to 7 percent of adults suffer from serious mental disorders and 5 to 9 percent of children suffer from serious emotional disturbances that severely disrupt their social, academic, and emotional functioning.

1996 Costa Rica: Approval of a law called Equal Opportunities for People with Disabilities is a turning point for the population with disabilities, which is among the most excluded sectors of society. The law is inspired in part by the United Nations Standard Rules on the Equalization of Opportunities for Disabled People (1993). Disability experience in Costa Rica is definitely transformed as a result of the mandates of this generic law, as people with disabilities and their families start to use this legal instrument as a strategy to empower themselves.

1996 Europe: Created in 1996, the European Disability Forum (EDF) is today the largest independent, trans-European organization that exists to represent disabled people in dialogue with the European Union (EU) and other European authorities. Its mission is to promote equal opportunities for disabled people and to ensure disabled citizens full access to fundamental and human rights through its active involvement in policy development and implementation in the EU. The EDF has national councils in 17 European countries and has 127 member organizations. The European Year of People with Disabilities 2003 is one of the EDF's most important campaigns.

1996 India: The Persons with Disabilities (Equal Opportunities, Protection of Rights and Full Participation) Act, 1995, becomes law. It is the first legislation for equal opportunities for disabled people. Prior to this, disabled persons receive services but not legal protection. Improvements in conditions begin in 1981 with the International Year of Disabled Persons. India is a signatory to the UN resolution of 1976 establishing it and is thereby committed to improving the lot of the disabled. The Lunacy Act of 1912 is repealed and the National Mental Health Act is passed in 1987. Nonetheless, with approximately 70 million disabled people residing in India (in a population of over a billion), the government does not include the domain of disability in the 2001 census, which reflects the attitudinal barriers in acknowledging the disabled identity.

1997 Government expenditures on behalf of persons with disabilities may total as much as $217.3 billion (taking into account the costs that would be expected among persons with disabilities in the absence of the disability), the equivalent of 2.6 percent of the gross domestic product in the United States for 1997.

1997 The landmark 1997 UNESCO Universal Declaration on the Human Genome and Human Rights frames the actual application of the new scientific developments raised by genetics. As a policy statement, it provides the first signs that genetics will be applied in ways that maintain human rights. In 2003, the Council of Europe and the council's Steering Committee in Bioethics issue policy statements in a working document titled Application of Genetics for Health Purposes. In the case of gene therapy, in 1994, the Group of Advisors on the Ethical Implications of Biotechnology of the European Commission voices concern regarding equity, maintaining that all genetic services that are available for the entire population should be equally available for persons of disability. Today, UNESCO's Human Genome Organization's Ethics Committee, the World Health Organization, the Council of Europe, and consumer organizations such as Inclusion International, Rehabilitation International, and Disabled Peoples' International play major roles in translating genetic innovations into health service and public health fields, helping develop policies that focus on the general recognition, respect, and protection of the rights to which all people, whether disabled or nondisabled, are entitled. Concerns related to the possible undermining of human rights are expressed in 2003 when Disabled People's International demands a prohibition on compulsory genetic testing.

1997 Colombia: The General Act for People with Disabilities, also known as the Disability Act: Law for Opportunity, passes. The 2003–2006 National Plan of Attention to Persons with Disabilities estimates that 18 percent of the general population has some type of disability. Despite the existence of at least 37 disability-related legal policies (2001), the government provides limited spending on programs that protect the rights of people with disabilities, and the lack of enforcement of rights remains a major concern. Today's awareness efforts include marathons with the participation of the general population to raise money for educational programs for children with special needs, Special Olympics, new organizations such as the Colombian Association for the Development of People with Disabilities, and media awareness campaigns.

1998 President Bill Clinton issues an executive order ensuring that the federal government assumes the role of a model employer of adults with disabilities.

1998 President Clinton signs into law the Rehabilitation Act of 1973 Amendments. Section 508 requires that electronic and information technology (EIT), such as federal websites, telecommunications, software, and information kiosks, must be usable by persons with disabilities.

1998 Ireland: The Irish Employment Equality Act entitles all individuals, including disabled persons, equal treatment in training and employment opportunities. The Education Act of 1998 requires schools to provide education to students that is appropriate to their abilities and needs. The Education for Persons with Disabilities Bill passes in 2003. A Disability Bill published in 2001 fails to underpin a rights-based approach and is withdrawn amid a storm of protest in 2002; a redrafting of a new Disability Bill is suffering from continuing delays. Traditionally, Irish voluntary organizations play a reactionary role in the development of services for people with disabilities and a key role as pressure groups trying to keep disability issues on the political agenda.

1999 The National Center on Physical Activity and Disability (NCPAD) is established as an information and resource center that offers people with disabilities, caregivers, and professionals the latest information on fitness, recreation, and sports programs for people with disabilities.

1999 Established by a panel of experts brought together to evaluate the UN Standard Rules on the Equalization of Opportunities for Persons with Disability, the International Disability Alliance (IDA) encourages cross-disability collaboration and supports the participation of international disability organizations in the elaboration of a proposed UN convention on disability.

1999 England: The first disability film festival, Lifting the Lid, is held at the Lux Cinema in London.

2000 ◆ The National Telability Media Center collects documentation of 3,000+ newsletters, 200 magazines, 50 newspapers, 40 radio programs, and 40 television programs dedicated to disability in the United States alone. *The Ragged Edge, Mainstream* (Internet-based), and *Mouth* are examples of disability rights-focused publications.

2000 ◆ *Healthy People 2000,* the second edition of the Surgeon General's report on health promotion and disease prevention (the first edition published in 1979), includes some reference to the health and well-being of people with disabilities, but few data are available. In the mid-1990s, the U.S. Department of Health and Human Services begins a dialogue with the Centers for Disease Control and Prevention to include people with disabilities in the third edition, *Healthy People 2010.* The resulting report includes more than 100 objectives that include "people with disabilities" as a subpopulation for data gathering.

2000 ◆ The World Bank, increasingly concerned with how to include disabled persons in the economies and societies of developing nations, establishes an online clearinghouse to make documents concerning the disabled readily available to member nations and the general public and holds its first course on disability issues in 2004 in Guatemala.

2000 ◆ Africa: The African Decade of Persons with Disabilities, 2000–2009, is adopted by the Declaration of the Organization of African Unity. The African Network of Women with Disabilities (2001) and the community-based rehabilitation organization CBR Africa Network (CAN) are examples of the many activities that result from the African Decade.

2000 ◆ Brazil is one of the few countries to include an entire section on disability in its 2000 census. Results show that 14.5 percent of the population, roughly 24 million people, report having some form of disability, the poorest region, the northeast, reporting the highest percentage and the richest, in the south, the lowest. People with disabilities in the first half of the twentieth century have no voice or representation. In 1932, the first Pestalozzi Society, a community-based school for children with intellectual disabilities, is founded. By the end of the twentieth century, there are 146 Pestalozzi Societies and more than 1,700 chapters of the Association of Parents and Friends of the Exceptional. The first center for independent living is established in 1988 (CVI-RIO). In 1992 and 1995, CVI-RIO organizes two international conferences on disability issues called DefRio, out of which comes "Goals of the ILM," a document that delineates the basis for the independent living movement in Brazil; however, financial support is not provided by the government, creating a struggle for sustainability. Brazil has progressive policies toward disability. The constitution includes sections on the rights of people with disabilities, and laws have been passed with regard to accessibility, education, and employment.

2000 ◆ Europe: A European Community directive requires all member states to have introduced antidiscrimination laws in the fields of employment and training by the end of 2006. It seeks to establish a general framework for equal treatment in employment and occupation and to render unlawful discrimination based on, among other categories, disability. The European Union Charter of Fundamental Rights sets out in a single text, for the first time in the EU's history, the whole range of civil, political, economic, and social rights of European citizens. Disability is included in the general nondiscrimination clause (Article 21), but Article 26 specifically states that the Union recognizes and respects the rights of persons with disabilities to benefit from measures designed to ensure their independence, social and occupational integration, and participation in the life of the community.

2000 ◆ The Human Genome Project (HGP), an international effort to specify the 3 billion pairs of genes that make up the DNA sequence of the entire human genome, produces its first draft in June 2000. Formally begun in October 1990, it is completed in 2003.

2001 ◆ President Clinton declares in Executive Order No. 13217 the commitment of the United States to community-based alternatives for individuals with disabilities. This ensures that the *Olmstead v. L.C.* decision (1999), which mandates the right for persons with disability to live in the least-restrictive setting with reasonable accommodations, is implemented in a timely manner. The executive order directs federal agencies to work together to tear down the barriers to community living.

2001 ◆ In the United States, census data indicate that only 48 percent of citizens 25 to 64 years old with severe disabilities have health insurance compared with 80 percent of individuals with nonservere disabilities and 82 percent of nondisabled Americans. Women with disabilities in general are more likely to live in poverty than men. Minorities with disabilities are more likely to live in poverty than nonminorities with disabilities. In 2003, in the United States, about 28 percent of children with disabilities live in poor families compared with 16 percent of all children.

2001 ◆ A UN Ad Hoc Committee begins discussions for a legally binding convention under the draft title Comprehensive and Integral Convention on the Protection and Promotion of the Rights and Dignity of Persons with Disabilities. Its fifth session is held in early 2005.

2001 ◆ A new World Health Organization classification of people with disabilities, the International Classification of Functioning, Disability, and Health (ICF), replaces the old International Classification of Impairments, Disabilities, and Handicaps (ICIDH). The ICF definition shifts the focus from disability as an innate deficit ("medical model") to disability as constructed through the interaction between the individual and the environment ("social model"). This shift encourages a focus on the kinds and levels of interventions appropriate to the needs of individuals.

2001 ◆ UNESCO launches pilot education projects for disabled children in Cameroon, the Dominican Republic, Egypt, Ghana, India, Madagascar, Mauritius, Nicaragua, Paraguay, South Africa, Vietnam, and Yemen. The global initiative Education for All 2000 has as its primary millennium development goal universal education by the year 2015.

2002 ◆ The U.S. Supreme Court rules that executing persons with mental retardation is unconstitutional.

2002 ◆ Disabled Peoples' International's 2002 Sapporo Platform, developed by 3,000 delegates from more than 90 countries, urges members to take every opportunity to seek publicity and awareness in order to change negative images of disabled people.

2002 ◆ Canada: The Canadian International Development Bank announces the approval of the Canada-Russia Disability Program, a four-year $4 million project, focusing on education, disability studies, social work practice, social policy, and information dissemination.

2003 ◆ A national survey that updates the Disability Supplement to the 10-year-old National Health Interview Survey highlights barriers to care among the uninsured. The uninsured are four times as likely to postpone care and three times as likely to go without needed supplies.

2003 ◆ The National Association of Social Workers (NASW) issues a policy statement that discusses their core values with respect to working with people with disabilities, including self-determination, social justice, and dignity and worth of the person. The statement emphasizes that social workers are responsible to take action with people who have disabilities in advocating for their rights to fully participate in society.

2003 ◆ The Disability Awareness in Action (DAA) database contains a total of 1,910 reports of known abuse affecting nearly 2.5 million disabled people. In the area of education alone, it documents

118 cases affecting 768,205 people in 67 countries. Responding to this documentation and other reports, the United Nations Commission on Human Rights creates the Global Rights campaign to address human rights abuses. Disability rights organizations use this information to insist on a UN convention on the rights of disabled people that would be legally binding on nation-states.

2003 The International Association for the Study of Pain has more than 6,700 members, representing more than 100 countries and 60 disciplinary fields. Chronic pain is one of the leading causes of recurrent and permanent disability in the developed world today, yet less than 1 percent of the U.S. National Institutes of Health's budget supports research into mechanisms and management of pain. The U.S. Congress declares 2000–2010 the Decade of Pain Control and Research.

2004 The *Journal of Gene Medicine* (January) reports that 636 gene therapy clinical trials are completed or ongoing, involving 3,496 patients. The first gene therapy clinical trials begin in the early 1990s.

Today Seventy to eighty percent—approximately 400 million—of the world's disabled people (600 million, or 10 percent of the world's population) live in the developing world, and of the world's poorest of the poor, 20 to 25 percent are disabled. In most countries, 1 out of 10 persons has a disability. Many international efforts are under way to address poverty and disability, such as those of the Action on Disability Development and the Chronic Poverty Research Centre.

Today E-health is the use of emerging interactive telecommunications technologies such as the Internet, interactive TV, kiosks, personal digital assistants, CD-ROMs, and DVD-ROMs to facilitate health improvement and health care services, including those with disabilities. E-health relies on environments that use a variety of technologies that can compensate for the lack of sensory ability. Telerehabilitation is an example of services delivered information technology and telecommunication networks.

Today Celebrating difference is the mantra and visible manifestation of disability culture in all regions of the world.

SEARCHING FOR AND EVALUATING WEBSITES

Anne Armstrong

The Internet, or Web, provides a vast number of channels through which researchers can find information on virtually any subject. The expansiveness of the Web can be daunting to new researchers. On the other hand, researchers often assume that they have mastered the Web in its entirety when indeed they have merely scratched the surface in terms of the numbers of resources they have consulted and searches they have performed.

Because the field of disability studies is continually evolving and inherently multidisciplinary, Web searchers can draw on previously conducted research from disciplines within the humanities, social sciences, and health sciences. This guide aims to expose beginning researchers to a mixture of general and subject-specialized Web-based search tools, as well as strategies for performing sophisticated Web searches and criteria for evaluating websites. In addition to its broad subject coverage, the field of disability studies differs from most fields in that many researchers may themselves have disabilities affecting their ability to perform research on the Web. For this reason, this description concludes with an overview of accessibility issues on the Web and suggestions for further reading.

OVERVIEW OF WEB-BASED RESEARCH TOOLS

When approaching Web searching, researchers should be aware of the multitude of search tools available to them, in addition to the varying purposes of these tools. Many users approach Web searching with the assumption that "everything is in Google," but this is a limiting misconception. No single search engine contains everything on the Web. Furthermore, all search engines function differently and rank results differently. Therefore, sampling various search tools increases the comprehensiveness of results on any topic. This discussion outlines multiple types of search tools available on the Web and offers potential starting points for Internet research on issues related to disability studies, whether from a health sciences, social sciences, or humanities perspective.

The Web-based search tools outlined in this chapter include general search engines, subject-specialized search engines, directories, indexes, catalogs, and Listservs. It is important to note that different types of search tools cover different parts of the Web. The Web is composed of layers. The top layer is detectible by general search engines, while a deeper layer termed "the invisible Web" can be penetrated only by specialized search engines, indexes, and catalogs. Readers should be aware that because the Web is in a constant state of flux, currently available resources may become obsolete over time, and newer, more sophisticated search tools will undoubtedly evolve.

General Search Engines

Most people who have searched the Web are familiar with sites such as Google, HotBot, or Lycos, which allow them to enter a string of keywords into a search box to retrieve a list of relevant websites (see Table 1). These sites, referred to as search engines, search the Web by means of a program called a *spider* (also

Table 1   Selected General Search Engines

Name	URL
AltaVista	www.altavista.com
Excite	www.excite.com
GO	www.go.com
Google	www.google.com
HotBot	www.hotbot.com
Lycos	www.lycos.com
Yahoo!	www.yahoo.com

called a *robot* or *crawler*). Since search engines tend to index millions of websites, they are most useful for entering specific search terms rather than broad concepts such as disability studies.

While Web searchers tend to pick a favorite search engine and return to it repeatedly, it is important to note that different search engines produce varying results, and that a truly comprehensive Web searcher should compare the results of multiple search engines. The variation between search engines can be attributed to differences between the spiders fueling the search engines as well as differences in the level of indexing and the order in which results are ranked. While some search engines index the full text of documents, others may index only the first page, or merely the *meta-tags*, which are lines of code containing keywords. Web searchers should be aware that developers of websites may intentionally increase their usage of certain words or meta-tags to increase the prominence of their website among search results. This practice has been referred to as *spamdexing* and is most prevalent among the developers of commercial websites advertising products and services. Due to the constant fluctuation of the Web, no search engine is entirely up-to-date; results produced by identical searches can vary greatly from one day to the next, even when one is using the same search engine.

Subject-Specialized Search Engines

Subject-specialized search engines (also referred to as subject portals) developed by educational institutions, associations, government agencies, and corporate entities narrow the broad scope of the Web, providing a focused channel by which researchers can search for information when they have determined the discipline from which their topic stems. Examples of such search engines are listed in Table 2. While subject-specialized search engines index considerably fewer websites and documents than general search engines, the information contained within them has been preselected, ideally by experts within a given field. Many subject-specialized search engines expose searchers to parts of the "invisible Web" not indexed by general search engines. Subject-specialized search engines can ease the research process by whittling down the Web to a more manageable size. However, researchers who use them should take the time to view the criteria for selection of

Table 2   Examples of Subject-Specialized Search Engines

Name	URL	Subject Coverage
Center for International Rehabilitation Research Information and Exchange (CIRRIE)	http://cirrie.buffalo.edu	Rehabilitation research
FamilyDoctor.org	http://familydoctor.org	Health sciences
FirstGov	www.firstgov.gov	Government
Google's Uncle Sam	www.google.com/unclesam	Government
Health*Web*	www.healthweb.org	Health sciences
Mayo Clinic	www.mayoclinic.com	Health sciences
MedlinePlus	http://medlineplus.gov	Health sciences
National Center for the Dissemination of Disability Research (NCDDR)	www.ncddr.org	Disability studies
Social Science Information Gateway (SOSIG)	www.sosig.ac.uk	Social sciences
Thomas	http://thomas.loc.gov/	Legislative information
Voice of the Shuttle	http://vos.ucsb.edu	Humanities
*Web*MD	www.webmd.com	Health Sciences

Web Research

information contained within them. This information is usually posted within online "help" or "about" pages on the home page.

Table 3 contains search tools that have been developed distinctly for the purpose of locating specialized search engines by subject.

Directories

Directories are hierarchically arranged subject guides composed of websites chosen by or recommended to editors of the directory (Table 4). Usually, directories follow a template in which major subject categories such as health, sciences, social sciences, or humanities are posted on the top-level page. Each of these links leads to lists of narrower subcategories. The links on the second level lead to narrower subcategories, and so on. A sample hierarchy from the directory created by Google (available at http://directory.google.com) lists the following subject breakdown: Society → Disabled → Disability studies.

Directories provide Web searchers with the ability to browse recommended resources in various subject areas without having to enter specific search terms. Other useful attributes of directories are that they often contain summaries and evaluations of websites.

Article Indexes

Article indexes allow researchers to search by topic for published articles in magazines and scholarly journals. Researchers could certainly locate journal and magazine articles using a freely available search engine such as Google, but they would merely be skimming the surface of what has been published. While the Web provides access to *more* content, it does not provide comprehensive access to research published in journal articles. Article indexes are for the expressed purpose of finding journal articles. With a few exceptions (such as PubMed, an article index of health sciences journals developed and maintained by the National Library of Medicine), article indexes are not freely available on the Web. Libraries purchase subscriptions to multiple article indexes covering a wide spectrum of disciplines. The indexes available through a given library are often dictated by the curriculum of the college or university that the library serves. Thus, large research institutions offer a greater number of specialized article indexes than smaller institutions and public libraries. Due to licensing agreements between article

Table 3 Resources for Finding Subject-Specialized Search Engines

Name	URL
CompletePlanet	www.completeplanet.com
Direct Search	www.freepint.com/gary/direct.htm
InfoMine	www.infomine.com
Invisible Web Directory	www.invisible-web.net
Librarians' Index to the Internet	www.lii.org
Search Engine Colossus	www.searchenginecolossus.com

Table 4 Selected Directories

Name	URL
eBlast	www.eblast.com
Google Directory[a]	http://directory.google.com
Internet Public Library	www.ipl.org
LookSmart	www.looksmart.com
Yahoo! Directory[a]	www.yahoo.com

a. These sites contain both directories and general search engines.

index providers and libraries, off-site access to indexes is usually limited to faculty and students of a college or university. However, there are many libraries that allow members of the public to use their article indexes from within the library. A local public library would be a good starting place for those not connected with academic or commercial organizations.

Since article indexes are proprietary products developed by companies for sale to libraries, they tend to offer specialized search features that are not always available on freely available search engines. These features include subject headings, thesauri, abstracts (summaries of articles), and frequently the full text of articles. Researchers should familiarize themselves with online tutorials, "help" screens, and "about" pages to increase the effectiveness of their searching.

Freely available article indexes relevant to disability studies include the following:

- PubMed: A product of the National Library of Medicine, which includes more than 14 million citations for biomedical articles dating back to the 1950s. URL: http://www.ncbi.nlm.nih.gov/entrez

- CIRRIE: Center for International Rehabilitation Research Information and Exchange, a database containing more than 24,000 citations of international research published from 1990 to the present. URL: http://cirrie.buffalo.edu

Catalogs

While researchers can search indexes to find articles on specific topics, they can search online catalogs to find books. Some catalogs list the books available at individual libraries, while others contain the holdings of multiple libraries and institutions. The individual catalogs of public libraries and universities are usually freely available on the Web. The most comprehensive catalog is called WorldCat, developed by an organization called OCLC (Online Computer Library Center). WorldCat lists books available at public and academic libraries throughout the world. Like most article indexes, WorldCat is not freely available on the Web and must be accessed through a library.

Listservs

Listservs are mailing lists on the Internet that facilitate online discussions on various subjects. They allow researchers within a given field to communicate about scholarly issues via email. People customarily sign up for Listservs by sending an e-mail to the Listserv address stating that they wish to subscribe. Several Listservs related to disability studies are listed in Table 5. In addition, Web searchers can perform a search on a database called tile.net to search for Listservs by topic.

SEARCH STRATEGIES

Since search capabilities vary from site to site, Web searchers should use online "help" screens and tutorials to learn search tips and strategies for improving their search results. Some search techniques common to several Web-based search tools are summarized below.

Quotation Marks

When entering a search, users should enter phrases in quotation marks to stipulate that they would like the results to contain a specific word combination and order. For instance, multiword concepts such as "disability studies," "adaptive technology," and "section 508" should be entered within quotation marks. Proper

Table 5   Disability Studies Listservs

Name	URL
ADA-LAW	http://listserv.nodak.edu/archives/ada-law.html
Disability-Research Discussion List	http://www.leeds.ac.uk/disability-studies/discuss.htm
Disability Studies at Yahoo.com	http://www.groups.yahoo.com/group/disabilitystudies
Disabled Student Services in Higher Education (DSSHE-L)	http://listserv.acsu.buffalo.edu/archives/dsshe-l.html
Women's International Linkage on Disability (D-WILD)	http://groups.yahoo.com/group/d-wild

names can also be entered within quotation marks.

Truncation

Truncation symbols allow Web searchers to simultaneously search for multiple endings of a given word. For instance, assuming that the asterisk is the designated truncation symbol in a search engine, entering the word "impair*" would produce results including all forms of the word after the root, including "impair," "impaired," "impairment" and "impairments." In addition to adding truncation symbols to the end of words, users may also insert internal truncation symbols if there are potential variations for the spelling of the middle of a word. For instance, entering the word "colo*r" would simultaneously search for the words "color" and "colour." "Help" screens or "search tips" usually list the designated truncation symbol for a given database.

Boolean Logic

Developed by the English mathematician George Boole, Boolean logic is a mathematical framework that Web searchers can apply to broaden or refine their searches. There are three words, or *operators*, that Web searchers can use to combine their keywords to perform more complex searches: AND, OR, and NOT. The three Boolean operators are summarized below, along with potential applications. It is important to read the online "help" section of a database before performing a Boolean search, as Boolean searching does not work in all databases.

Using the Boolean Operator "AND"

Combining words with "AND" narrows a search, as the database retrieves only items that contain *all* the words entered. The second search example below will produce fewer results than the first, since there are three keywords that must appear within the content of each result.

"disability studies" AND theory
"disability studies" AND theory AND history

Using the Boolean Operator "OR"

Entering the term "OR" between keywords stipulates that any, but not all, of the words entered must appear within the search results. Using "OR" is a way of searching for synonyms or related terms when there are multiple words for the same concept. The example below shows how you could broaden your search if you wanted to search for multiple adaptive technology applications in a search engine. The second search example will potentially produce more results than the first, since there is an additional keyword that the results could include.

JAWS OR "Ruby OpenBook"
JAWS OR "Ruby OpenBook" or "window eyes"

Using the Boolean Operator "NOT"

Entering the Boolean operator "NOT" after a word stipulates that the word should not appear within the results. Using "NOT" in a search can be particularly useful if a word is frequently used in multiple contexts and you wish to eliminate results dealing with a particular topic. In the example below, the second search will ideally eliminate items relating to the state of New Mexico, given that the researcher is looking for information on legislation related to disabilities in the country of Mexico. The use of NOT can be too limiting. The second search would eliminate results that discussed both Mexico and New Mexico.

Disabilities AND legislation AND Mexico
Disabilities AND legislation AND Mexico NOT "new mexico"

Nesting

Nesting allows Web searchers to simultaneously search for multiple search terms relating to the same topic.

The grouping of synonymous terms within parenthesis is referred to as nesting, as multiple terms relating to the same idea are clustered together as a single concept. When using nesting, the words within the parenthesis are connected by the Boolean operator "OR."

To find information about software for people who are visually impaired, search results are increased by using nesting to group multiple words for each facet of the topic:

(software or "adaptive technology") AND ("visually impaired" or blind)

Plus and Minus Signs

Most general search engines allow users to enter plus or minus signs before a particular word. Entering a plus sign before a word (e.g., +ADA) stipulates that the word must appear within the search results. A minus sign before a word (e.g.,–mobility) stipulates that the word should not appear within the results. Since some search engines also use plus and minus signs as substitutes for Boolean operators, it is important to view online "help" or "search tips."

Search Limits

Most search engines allow users to limit their results by date, language, or document type. Limiting capabilities vary from site to site and are customarily outlined in online "help" screens. In general, article indexes have more sophisticated limiting capabilities than search engines that are freely available on the Web.

EVALUATING WEBSITES

A researcher weighing the quality of a journal article faces a lesser challenge than a researcher considering a website as a potential resource. The publishing industry applies labels to periodicals of varying type: Scholarly journals, popular magazines, trade publications, and newspapers comprise the major categories. Articles submitted to scholarly journals undergo a peer review process by experts in a given field. If in doubt as to the suitability of journal for scholarly purposes, a researcher can consult a directory of periodicals such as *Ulrich's Periodicals Directory,* which indicates whether or not a journal is peer reviewed.

The fact that the Web has no comparable methods of control complicates the task of determining whether a website is appropriate for research purposes. While websites produced by certain types of agencies and organizations certainly undergo a form of *internal* review, the Web is a free forum; people can post anything they want, and no one has the right to force to take it down if it fails to meet certain standards of quality or accuracy. To complicate the matter, inaccurate or inexpert information can hide like a wolf in the sheep's clothing of sophisticated graphics, layout, and design. The Web has no peer review process to ensure quality. While none of the evaluation criteria outlined below can provide the final word as to the suitability of a website for scholarly use, a researcher who searches the Web with multiple evaluation criteria in mind expedites the process of finding quality information.

Authorship

When determining the credibility of a website, researchers should use multiple techniques to determine the credentials of the author as well as the character of the organization hosting, or sponsoring, the site. If individuals are listed as authors, researchers should take steps to determine their credentials and reputation in the field by performing a search in a general search engine to find biographical information or other documents written about the author. This will also produce references to the author on the sites of other authors within a field. Researchers can also consult a number of biographical sources available at libraries, such as *Who's Who in the America* or sources tailored to particular fields of study, such as *Who's Who in Science and Engineering.*

Website addresses, or URLs (Uniform Resource Locators) can also provide hints as to author affiliations and potential bias. Personal websites are often hosted on commercial ISP (Internet Service Provider) Web servers such as aol.com, or geocites.com. URLs of personal websites often contain first or last names, as well as percent (%) or tilde (~) signs. While personal websites may contain authoritative information, researchers should question why the same content does not appear on a site sponsored by an educational or research organization.. Was the site created as a pastime or to serve as a forum for airing personal views? Or does the site reflect serious scholarship backed up by other credentials and research published in scholarly publications?

Every website URL ends with a *domain name*, usually a series of three letters preceded by a period. The domain name denotes the type of institution that hosts the website and can often provide clues as to the purpose or potential bias of a site. Common domain names include the following:

Educational sites: .edu
Government sites: .gov, .mil, or country codes
   (e.g., .uk = United Kingdom, .au = Australia,
   .do = Dominican Republic)
Nonprofit organization sites: .org
Commercial sites: .com

Most URLs contain multiple levels separated by slashes (e.g., http://www.nod.org/stats/). To learn more about the sponsor or publisher of a particular site, you can remove levels of the URL one by one to see where the site is hosted and determine the character of the sponsoring entity. For instance, if a site is hosted on the site of an association, viewing the mission statement on the home page of the association can provide clues as to the bias or purpose of the content. When judging the credentials of the publishing entity, researchers should look for contact information and institutional logos. In general, sites devoid of identifying information or contact numbers and addresses should raise suspicion.

Audience

When evaluating a site, researchers should determine whether the content succeeds in addressing the stated audience through tone and presentation. Sites for adults should not have a childlike appearance or tone. Likewise, sites may be deliberately overrun by technical language or jargon to confuse or mislead a particular audience. High-quality sites clearly define their intended purpose.

Currency

Medical research findings or population statistics may become obsolete at a faster rate than research in the humanities. Web researchers should check sites for copyright dates and the date of the last update. Broken links are a sign of neglect, as they may indicate that URLs have changed or become obsolete since the last update of the site. To verify the currency of information on a site, researchers should check for several sites covering the same subject matter.

Accuracy

Determining accuracy involves further research to ensure that the claims or findings on a site are substantiated by other sources. If a site presents original research, the methods of the research and instruments used should be clearly explained, as well as potential limitations of the research. If authors make claims or conclusions, they should cite their sources, and these sources should be tracked down to ensure their existence and authenticity. Websites should contain a list of works cited or footnotes on par with any print book or article. Since websites sometimes include fabricated resources, and erroneous or incomplete citations, sources should be verified using library tools such as indexes and catalogs. Lists of works cited with multiple errors reflect irresponsible research. If a website contains links, the links should be checked. Researchers should be wary of websites populated by broken links or links to defunct websites.

Quality

In general, sites that are poorly organized or sloppy should be approached with caution. Shoddy design may point to further weaknesses. Poor grammar and spelling errors are also red flags.

Bias

While bias is not always a negative attribute, Web searchers should be cognizant of bias as the search for information. The bias of a website can be partially discerned by the domain name (as discussed above under "Authorship"). Commercial websites may be motivated by the goal to market a product or service. Nonprofit organizations may promote a political agenda. While bias may be clearly stated in mission statements and "about" pages, many websites deliberately shroud their bias. Thorough research involves consulting additional sources to determine the history and activities of a particular organization. If a site contains links to other sites, those links should be checked to discern the character and activities of the other organizations listed. If a site is sponsored by other organizations, researchers should consider the relationship between the sponsors and the creators of the site.

Special Considerations for
Evaluating Health Information on the Web

The American Medical Association (AMA) has published "Guidelines for Medical and Health Information Sites on the Internet" outlining evaluation criteria for websites publishing health information, whether for consumers or health professionals. While these guidelines are technically enforced only on sites sponsored by the AMA or affiliated organizations, they could be applied to all sites containing health information. Many of these guidelines mirror the previously outlined criteria for evaluating all websites,

but there are certain factors that are heavily emphasized in the AMA guidelines, including the importance of peer review by experts in the field, the importance of clearly identifying sources of funding, an explanation of the relationship between individual researchers and the institutions sponsoring the research, the importance of clearly stating the purpose and intended audience of a site, and the need to address the stated audience in a consistent and effective tone. Seven criteria for assessing the quality of health information on the Internet have been developed by the Health Summit Working Group (Health Information Technology Institute 1999).

Information on health-related websites should be verified by checking sources such as journal articles, books, and other websites. These measures are needed as health information on the Web frequently includes unsubstantiated claims.

OVERVIEW OF ACCESSIBILITY ISSUES ON THE WEB

Disability studies research is unique in that many scholars in the field have disabilities that may impact their ability to effectively search the Web. While in many ways the Web "evens the playing field" by making a vast number of resources available electronically, inaccessible design frequently places barriers on Web searchers with disabilities.

Principles of Web accessibility have been developed by the World Wide Web Consortium's (W3C) Web Accessibility Initiative (WAI). The WAI establishes guidelines for creating accessible websites, browsers, and authoring tools to increase the ease of use of the Web for users with disabilities. Multiple scenarios outlining potential challenges to Web searchers with disabilities are summarized in a W3C working draft titled "How People with Disabilities Use the Web" (2001). Among other scenarios, the document emphasizes that many Web searchers with cognitive or visual disabilities use OCR (optical character recognition) software, which reads Web page text and transmits the information to a speech synthesizer and/or refreshable Braille display. Many users with visual disabilities use text-based Internet browsers instead of standard graphical browsers. The successful use of these tools requires that images on websites be accompanied by descriptive text and *ALT tags*. ALT tags are textual labels that appear on the computer screen when a mouse moves over an image. Since visually impaired

Web searchers often enlarge Web-based text using screen magnification programs, Web designers must create pages with nonfixed font sizes that can be altered as necessary. These are only a few of the issues facing Web searchers with disabilities. Other population groups with disabilities discussed in the guidelines include individuals with cognitive disabilities, hearing impairment, and mobility-related disabilities. Readers should consult the WAI website for the complete guidelines (http://www.w3.org/WAI/).

To support the goals of WAI, an online tool called Bobby™ helps website developers test the accessibility of their sites and adhere to accessibility guidelines. By entering a URL into the Bobby website, a Web developer can generate a report outlining which features of the site need to be adjusted to make it "Bobby compliant" and adhere to both W3C accessibility guidelines and guidelines established by the U.S. government's Section 508, a 1998 amendment to the Rehabilitation Act requiring that all federal agencies make their electronic and information technology accessible to people with disabilities. Complete information about these guidelines can be found on the Section 508 website (www.section508.gov).

CONCLUSION

While "one-stop shopping" in Google may be tempting, there is no single search engine leading to everything on the Web. Comprehensive and effective research in disability studies involves consulting multiple search tools, including but not limited to general search engines, subject-specialized search engines, directories, and indexes. In addition to using multiple search tools, Web searchers should experiment with multiple search strategies to maximize the effectiveness of their searching. As there are no standards of quality on the Web, researchers should apply multiple evaluation criteria to every website, verifying that research findings posted on sites are supported by other sources. Web accessibility is a crucial component to disability studies, as the Web has the potential to deliver equal content to all users but frequently presents barriers to people with disabilities by failing to adhere to standards of accessible design. Researchers can develop an awareness of accessibility issues on the Web by familiarizing themselves with the standards outlined by W3C's Web Accessibility Initiative and Section 508.

Further Readings

Ackermann, Ernest C. and Karen Hartman. 2000. *The Information Specialist's Guide to Searching & Researching on the Internet & the World Wide Web*. Chicago: Fitzroy Dearborn.

Blasiotti, Ellen Liberti, Iwao Kobayashi, and John Westbrook. 2001. "Disability Studies and Electronic Networking." Pp. 327–347 in *Handbook of Disability Studies*, edited by Gary L. Albrecht, Katherine D. Seelman, and Michael Bury. Thousand Oaks, CA: Sage.

Bradley, Phil. 2002. *Internet Power Searching: The Advanced Manual*. New York: Neal-Schuman.

Conner-Sax, Kiersten and Ed Krol. 1999. *The Whole Internet: The Next Generation—A Completely New Edition of the First and Best User's Guide to the Internet*. Beijing and Cambridge, MA: O'Reilly.

Davoren, J. B. 1998. "Searching the Internet." Pp. 129–144 in *Evidence Based Medicine: A Framework for Clinical Practice*, edited by D. J. Friedland. Stamford, CT: Appleton & Lange.

Harris, Robert H. 2000. *A Guidebook to the Web*. Guilford, CT: Dushkin/McGraw-Hill.

Health Information Technology Institute. 1999. "Criteria for Assessing the Quality of Health Information on the Internet— Policy Paper." Mitretek Systems. Retrieved June 22, 2004 (http://hitiweb.mitretek.org/docs/policy.html).

Johnstone, David. 2001. *An Introduction to Disability Studies*. London: David Fulton.

World Wide Web Consortium (W3C), Education and Outreach Working Group. 2001. "How People with Disabilities Use the Web: W3C Working Draft, 4 January 2001." Retrieved June 29, 2004 (http://www.w3.org/WAI/EO/Drafts/PWD-Use-Web/Overview.html).

Websites

American Medical Association, "Guidelines for Medical and Health Information on the Internet," http://www.ama-assn .org/ama/pub/category/ print/1905.html

Olin & Uris Libraries, Cornell University Library, "Evaluating Web Sites: Criteria and Tools," http://www.library.cornell.edu/ olinuris/ref/research/webeval.html

Schnall, Janet G., HealthLinks, University of Washington, "Navigating the Web: Using Search Tools and Evaluating Resources," http://healthlinks.washington.edu/howto/navigating

Section 508, http://www.508.gov

Sheridan Libraries of the Johns Hopkins University, "Evaluating Information Found on the Internet," http://www.library.jhu .edu/elp/useit/evaluate/

UC Berkeley Library, "Finding Information on the Internet: A Tutorial," http://www.lib.berkeley.edu/TeachingLib/Guides/ Internet/FindInfo.html

University of Illinois at Chicago, Library the Health Sciences Peoria, "Finding Information on the Internet: Evaluating Web Sites," http://www.uic .edu/depts/lib/lhsp/resources/evaluate.shtml

Web Research